Manual of FORENSIC EMERGENCY MEDICINE

A Guide for Clinicians

Edited by

RALPH J. RIVIELLO, MD, MS, FACEP, FAAEM

Jefferson Medical College of Thomas Jefferson University

JONES AND BARTLETT PUBLISHERS

Sudbury, Massachusetts

BOSTON TORONTO LONDON SINGAPORE

World Headquarters
Jones and Bartlett Publishers
40 Tall Pine Drive
Sudbury, MA 01776
978-443-5000
info@jbpub.com
www.jbpub.com

Jones and Bartlett Publishers
Canada
6339 Ormindale Way
Mississauga, Ontario L5V 1J2
Canada

Jones and Bartlett Publishers
International
Barb House, Barb Mews
London W6 7PA
United Kingdom

Jones and Bartlett's books and products are available through most bookstores and online booksellers. To contact Jones and Bartlett Publishers directly, call 800-832-0034, fax 978-443-8000, or visit our website www.jbpub.com.

Substantial discounts on bulk quantities of Jones and Bartlett's publications are available to corporations, professional associations, and other qualified organizations. For details and specific discount information, contact the special sales department at Jones and Bartlett via the above contact information or send an email to specialsales@jbpub.com.

The authors, editor, and publisher have made every effort to provide accurate information. However, they are not responsible for errors, omissions, or for any outcomes related to the use of the contents of this book and take no responsibility for the use of the products and procedures described. Treatments and side effects described in this book may not be applicable to all people; likewise, some people may require a dose or experience a side effect that is not described herein. Drugs and medical devices are discussed that may have limited availability controlled by the Food and Drug Administration (FDA) for use only in a research study or clinical trial. Research, clinical practice, and government regulations often change the accepted standard in this field. When consideration is being given to use of any drug in the clinical setting, the healthcare provider or reader is responsible for determining FDA status of the drug, reading the package insert, and reviewing prescribing information for the most up-to-date recommendations on dose, precautions, and contraindications, and determining the appropriate usage for the product. This is especially important in the case of drugs that are new or seldom used.

Production Credits
Senior Editor: Nancy Duffy
Custom Projects Editor: Kathy Richardson
Editorial Assistant: Sara Cameron
Production Director: Amy Rose
Associate Production Editor: Melissa Elmore
Marketing Manager: Ilana Goddess
V.P., Manufacturing and Inventory Control: Therese Connell
Composition and Text Design: Shawn Girsberger
Illustrator: Louis Andre Ochoa
Cover and Title Page Design: Kristin E. Parker
Cover and Title Page Image: © Pitris/Dreamstime.com
Printing and Binding: Replika Press
Cover Printing: Replika Press

Library of Congress Cataloging-in-Publication Data
Riviello, Ralph.
Manual of forensic emergency medicine : a guide for clinicians / Ralph Riviello.
p. ; cm.
Includes bibliographical references.
ISBN-13: 978-0-7637-4462-5
ISBN-10: 0-7637-4462-X
1. Medical jurisprudence—Handbooks, manuals, etc. 2. Emergency medicine—Handbooks, manuals, etc. I. Title.
[DNLM: 1. Emergency Medicine—methods. 2. Forensic Medicine—methods. 3. Violence. W 700 R625m 2009]
RA1053.R62 2009
614'.1—dc22

2008038389

6048
Printed in India
13 12 11 10 09 10 9 8 7 6 5 4 3 2 1

TO MY FAMILY,
especially my parents, Ralph and Gilda,
for all their love and support over the years.

TO FORMER, CURRENT, AND FUTURE RESIDENTS:
Thanks for all you have taught me.
I am amazed by your abilities
and am glad I was able to play a role in your education.
Continue your hard work and dedication to your patients.

TO MY PATIENTS,
especially those who were victims of violence/injury,
for whom this book is written.
Throughout my career, it is you who have taught me the most.
It is my privilege to write this book for you
so that you and countless others will have
expert forensic care in an emergency department when you need it.

Contents

Preface vii

List of Contributors ix

1 **Forensic Emergency Medicine** 1
Ralph Riviello, MD, MS, FACEP, FAAEM

2 **Forensic Nursing in the Emergency Department** 4
Kathleen Brown, RN, PhD

3 **Suicide** 10
Pierre Detiege, MD, and Matthew Brooks, MD

4 **Evidence Collection and Preservation in the ED** 22
Shannon L. Maier, MS, BSN, RN, and Jennifer Barger, MS, BSN, RN

5 **DNA** 29
Mahshid Abir, MD

6 **Forensic Toxicology** 36
Paul Francis Kolecki, MD, FACEP

7 **Forensic Photography** 44
William M. Green, MD, and Elliot Schulman, MD, MPH

8 **Forensic Bite Mark Evidence** 54
Scott W. Brown, MD, and Allyson A. Kreshak, MD

9 **Forensic Documentation** 59
Ralph Riviello, MD, MS, FACEP, FAAEM

10 **Blunt Force Trauma** 65
Paul Ko, MD, and Christine Dang, MD

11 **Sharp Force Injury** 77
Marianne Hamel, MD, PhD, FCAP

12 **Firearms** 83
Ralph Riviello, MD, MS, FACEP, FAAEM

13 **Gunshot/Shotgun Injuries** 89
Ronald F. Sing, DO, FACS, and J. Michael Sullivan, MD

14 **Mechanisms of Injury Related to Motor Vehicle Crashes** 98
Edward T. Dickinson, MD, FACEP

15 **Sexual Assault** 107
William M. Green, MD

16 **Interpersonal Violence** 122
Janelle Martin, MD

17 **Male Interpersonal Violence Overview** 128
Mark Zwanger, MD

18 **Physical Child Maltreatment** 133
Raquel Mora, MD

19 **Pediatric Sexual Abuse: Evaluation in the Emergency Department** 156
Amita Sudhir, MD, Sarah Anderson, PhD, RN, CEN, SANE-A, and William J. Brady, MD, FACEP, FAAEM

20 **Elder Abuse and Neglect** 165
Matthew R. Bartholomew, MD, FAAEM, Jean Cheek, RN, FNE, and Jennifer Hoyt, MD

21 **Sudden Infant Death Syndrome (SIDS)** 171
Jennifer Sellakumar Tom, MD, Ron V. Hall Jr, MD, and Neil Gandhi, MD

22 **Youth and Gang Violence: Identification and Prevention Strategies** 186
S. Ivan Riley Jr, MD, and Jayne Batts, MD, FACEP
Special Thanks to Mitchell J. Goldman, DO

23 **Suspect Evaluation and Evidence Collection** 204
Bohdan (Dan) M. Minczak, MS, MD, PhD, FACEP, FAAEM

24 **Forensics for EMS** 210
James P. McCans, MS, NREMT-P

25 **In-Custody Death** 214
Kenneth G. Lavelle, MD, NREMT-P, and Theodore Corbin, MD, MPP

APPENDIX I Adult Forms 219

APPENDIX II Pediatric Forms 263

Glossary 287

Photo and Illustration Credits 293

Index 295

Preface

Clinical forensic medicine is a rapidly growing field and interest in Emergency Medicine. Emergency departments are among the first medical settings to care for victims surviving crime and violence. In addition to stabilization and evaluation techniques, emergency department personnel need to consider the forensic needs of their patients. The *Manual of Forensic Emergency Medicine: A Guide for Clinicians* provides emergency personnel the tools necessary to meet this patient need. This book offers information in caring for almost any victim of violence, crime, or injury.

This book provides the reader with clear, easy-to-understand explanations of forensically important topics for the emergency medicine practitioner. It is organized by specific topic (e.g., Forensic Toxicology, Evidence Collection, and Forensic Photography) or by specific injury type (e.g., Sharp Force Injury, Blunt Force Trauma, and Sexual Assault). Several of the chapters are enhanced with illustrations and photographs. Several photographs are reproduced in color in the insert section. The Appendix sections contain sample forms for documentation and are followed by a forensically relevant glossary. Several of the forms are from the State of California Governor's Office of Emergency Services and can be accessed through the California Clinical Forensic Medical Training Center at their Web site, www.ccfmtc.org. In addition, other sexual assault forms, policies, sample consent forms, and job descriptions can be obtained through the Sexual Assault Forensic Examiner Technical Assistance Forms Library section of the IAFN, available at www.safeta.org.

A unique feature of the book is the chapter on Gang Violence. Other informative chapters include Forensic Photography, Forensic Documentation, and Forensic Toxicology. In addition, there is a chapter dedicated to the timely topic of In-Custody Death and another chapter on forensics in the Pre-hospital/EMS setting.

In addition to the authors who contributed to the book, I would like to thank Dr. Steven Selbst; Dr. Chris Haines; Johan Duflou, MMed; Isadore Mihalakis, MD; and Vincent Tranchida, MD, who contributed photographs to the book. Thanks to Chief James Tiano and Lt. John Hrywnak of the Philadelphia Police Department for their assistance with the weapon photographs. I would also like to personally thank the Editorial and Production staff at Jones and Bartlett Publishers, especially Kathy Richardson and Melissa Elmore for all of their help, guidance, and ability to keep me mostly on time. Finally I would like to thank my Chairman, Theodore Christopher, MD, who allowed me the time and resources to get this book completed.

I am proud to present this book to emergency medicine practitioners and personnel. My hope is that it will be a useful tool in the provision of quality forensic emergency care. After all, our patients deserve and demand nothing less.

Ralph Riviello, MD, MS, FACEP, FAAEM

List of Contributors

EDITOR

Ralph Riviello, MD, MS, FACEP, FAAEM
Associate Professor and Director of Clinical Research
Department of Emergency Medicine
Jefferson Medical College of Thomas Jefferson University

Medical Director, Sexual Assault Treatment Center
Thomas Jefferson University Hospital

Philadelphia, Pennsylvania

CONTRIBUTOR LIST

Mahshid Abir, MD
Thomas Jefferson University
Philadelphia, Pennsylvania

Sarah Anderson, PhD, RN, CEN, SANE-A
UVA Emergency Department Clinician IV
School of Nursing Research, Assistant Professor
University of Virginia
Charlottesville, Virginia

Jennifer Barger, MS, BSN, RN
Forensic Nurse Specialist and Assistant Nurse Manager
Emergency Department
Hospital of the University of Pennsylvania
Philadelphia, Pennsylvania

Matthew R. Bartholomew, MD, FAAEM
Assistant Professor of Emergency Medicine
Medical Director of Clinical Forensics and Forensic Nurse Examiners
Virginia Commonwealth University Medical Center/ Medical College of Virginia Hospital
Richmond, Virginia

Jayne Batts, MD, FACEP
Director of Clinical Forensic Medicine Program
Department of Emergency Medicine
Carolinas Medical Center
Charlotte, North Carolina

William J. Brady, MD, FACEP, FAAEM
Professor of Emergency Medicine and Medicine
Vice Chair, Department of Emergency Medicine
University of Virginia School of Medicine
Charlottesville, Virginia

Matthew Brooks, MD
Thomas Jefferson University
Philadelphia, Pennsylvania

Kathleen Brown, RN, PhD
Practice Assistant Professor, University of Pennsylvania School of Nursing
Philadelphia, Pennsylvania

Scott W. Brown, MD
Department of Emergency Medicine
Thomas Jefferson University
Philadelphia, Pennsylvania

Jean Cheek, RN, FNE
Department of Emergency Medicine
Virginia Commonwealth University Medical Center
Richmond, Virginia

Theodore Corbin, MD, MPP
Assistant Professor of Emergency Medicine
Drexel University College of Medicine
Philadelphia, Pennsylvania

Christine Dang, MD
Thomas Jefferson University
Philadelphia, Pennsylvania

Pierre Detiege, MD
Clinical Assistant Professor
Department of Medicine, Section of Emergency Medicine
Louisiana State University Health Sciences Center (LSUHSC)
New Orleans, Louisiana

Edward T. Dickinson, MD, FACEP
Associate Professor
Department of Emergency Medicine
University of Pennsylvania
Philadelphia, Pennsylvania

Neil Gandhi, MD
Thomas Jefferson University
Philadelphia, Pennsylvania

William M. Green, MD
UC Davis Medical Center
CA Clinical Forensic Medical Training Center
Sacramento, California

Ron V. Hall Jr, MD
Instructor Department of Emergency Medicine
Thomas Jefferson University
Philadelphia, Pennsylvania

Marianne Hamel, MD, PhD, FCAP
Office of the Chief Medical Examiner of the City of New York
New York, New York

Jennifer Hoyt, MD
Department of Emergency Medicine
Virginia Commonwealth University Medical Center
Richmond, Virginia

Paul Ko, MD
Assistant Professor of Emergency Medicine
Department of Emergency Medicine
SUNY Upstate Medical University
Syracuse, New York

Paul Francis Kolecki, MD, FACEP
Associate Professor, Department of Emergency Medicine
Thomas Jefferson University
Philadelphia, Pennsylvania

Allyson A. Kreshak, MD
Medical Toxicology Fellow
Division of Medical Toxicology
University of California San Diego Medical Center
San Diego, California

Kenneth G. Lavelle, MD, NREMT-P
Attending Physician, Department of Emergency Medicine
Albert Einstein Healthcare Network
Philadelphia, PA

Shannon L. Maier, MS, BSN, RN
Clinical Assistant Professor Department of Pathology, Microbiology, Immunology & Forensic Medicine
Philadelphia College of Osteopathic Medicine
Philadelphia, Pennsylvania

Janelle Martin, MD
Thomas Jefferson University
Department of Emergency Medicine
Philadelphia, Pennsylvania

James P. McCans, MS, NREMT-P
Philadelphia College of Osteopathic Medicine
Instructor, Forensic Medicine Program
Philadelphia, Pennsylvania

Bohdan (Dan) M. Minczak, MS, MD, PhD, FACEP, FAAEM
Assistant Professor
Academic Director EMS Education
Department of Emergency Medicine
Thomas Jefferson University Hospital
Philadelphia, Pennsylvania

Raquel Mora, MD
Assistant Professor of Emergency Medicine and Pediatrics
St. Christopher's Hospital for Children
Philadelphia, Pennsylvania

S. Ivan Riley Jr, MD
Department of Emergency Medicine
Carolinas Medical Center
Charlotte, North Carolina

Elliot Schulman, MD, MPH
Santa Barbara County Public Health Department
Santa Barbara, California

Jennifer Sellakumar Tom, MD
Clinical Assistant Professor, Department of Emergency Medicine
Thomas Jefferson University
Philadelphia, Pennsylvania

Ronald F. Sing, DO, FACS
F. H. Sammy Ross Jr. Trauma Center
Carolinas Medical Center
Charlotte, North Carolina

Amita Sudhir, MD
Department of Emergency Medicine
School of Medicine
University of Virginia
Charlottesville, Virginia

J. Michael Sullivan, MD
Department Director
Mecklenburg County Medical Examiner's Office
Mecklenburg County, North Carolina

Mark Zwanger, MD
Associate Professor, Department of Emergency Medicine
Thomas Jefferson University
Philadelphia, Pennsylvania

1 | Forensic Emergency Medicine

Ralph Riviello, MD, MS, FACEP, FAAEM

INTRODUCTION

Clinical forensic medicine is the application of forensic medical knowledge and techniques to living patients. This specialty has been practiced in Europe, Great Britain, and other countries for centuries. In some settings, practitioners of clinical forensic medicine are referred to as police surgeons, forensic medical officers, or forensic medical examiners. Clinical forensic medicine has only recently been recognized in the United States. The discipline has had modest beginnings in the United States but is starting to become increasingly recognized and needed.

In the United States, the coroner or medical examiner is responsible for the investigation of suspicious or unnatural deaths; however, these officials typically do little for surviving victims. Many crime victims survive their insult but do not have their forensic needs met by the health system. In addition, a large number of patients receive some form of medical care prior to expiring from their injuries. Improper actions taken by emergency department (ED) personnel can hamper investigation by the medical examiner and law enforcement. Common clinical forensic mistakes made by inadequately trained emergency physicians include destroying, throwing away, or losing pertinent evidence; writing illegible records; creating partial documentation or incomplete medical records; delaying forensic examination; missing subtle injuries because of lack of pattern recognition; and making "educated guesses" about projectile mechanism.

In 1973, Root and Scott first addressed the issues in the United State concerning the practice of forensic medicine on the living.[1] These forensic pathologists felt that if forensic issues were not addressed in the living, justice would suffer. It took several years before the medical community reacted. So, the question is, what medical specialty is best suited to answer the forensic needs of the living patient? Emergency medicine (and trauma surgery) is the obvious answer.

EMERGENCY MEDICINE AND FORENSICS

The unique nature of emergency medicine (EM) makes it the perfect specialty to incorporate forensic medicine into practice. Emergency specialists are available 24 hours a day and in almost all cases are the first physicians who care for crime victims who seek medical treatment.

In 1983, Smialek was the first to write on forensic medicine in the US emergency department. He found that evidence of crimes was disappearing from the ED. The evidence was not being lost on purpose but rather through lack of knowledge by the staff.[2] That same year, an article appeared in the *American Journal of Nursing* emphasizing the importance of evidence recognition and preservation in the ED.[3] These two articles mark the starting point for US clinical forensic medicine.

Emergency nursing was quicker to respond to the call for improved forensic care in emergency departments. Through their efforts, forensic nursing was born. (See Chapter 2 for a discussion of forensic nursing.)

Dr. Carmona, former US Surgeon General and a trauma surgeon, published his review of 100 charts at his Level 1 trauma center.[4] He found that 70% of the cases contained improper, poor, or inadequate documentation. Also, in 38% of cases, evidence was improperly secured, improperly documented, or inadvertently discarded. Harry McNamara, a New York medical examiner, realized that evidence was being discarded or destroyed, wounds were repaired or surgically altered without adequate documentation of their appearance, and forensic opinions were being given without any factual basis.[5]

The need was obvious. Training was needed for physicians and nurses in forensic matters.

In 1990, Dr. William Smock from the University of Louisville School of Medicine initiated the first formal clinical forensic medicine consultation service in the United States. In his program, a forensic physician (either a forensic pathologist or forensically trained emergency physician) was available to respond to the ED or inpatient unit on a 24-hour basis.[5] The program has grown and now includes six forensic pathologists, two clinical forensic emergency physicians, one forensic pediatrician, one forensic odontologist, one forensic pathology fellow, and full-time clinical forensic nurses. Clinical forensic evaluations are performed at the request of local, state, and federal law enforcement as well as adult/child protective services.[5]

In 1991, Dr. Smock established the first formal clinical forensic medicine training program for emergency physicians. The program was a cooperative effort between the University of Louisville Department of Emergency Medicine and the Kentucky Medical Examiner's Office. It was designed to introduce forensic topics and techniques into the EM residency program and created a 1-year fellowship in clinical forensic medicine. The fellowship was for emergency medicine residency graduates and provided advanced forensic training comparable to forensic pathology fellowships with focus on the unmet needs of survivors of violent crimes and trauma.[6] A second fellowship was established at the University of Maryland. However, these fellowships are no longer offered.[7]

Recently, other options have emerged for physicians interested in forensic training. Several colleges in the United States have begun offering advanced degree programs in forensic medicine. These programs are of varying lengths and offer a wide variety of training opportunities and modalities. They are designed to be multidisciplinary in their approach and often involve practical experiences for students. In Philadelphia, two such programs are offered: a Master's in Forensic Science (MFS) at Drexel University College of Medicine and a Master's in Forensic Medicine at the Philadelphia College of Osteopathic Medicine.

In 2004, the Joint Commission on Accreditation of Healthcare Organizations (JCAHO) addressed clinical forensic medicine in its accreditation manual for hospitals. It stated that evidentiary materials must be identified, retained, and safeguarded as part of the screening and assessment processes.[8]

RESOURCES

Forensic nurses have been very successful in organizing themselves and advancing their goals and objectives. Forensic nursing training programs have become widely accepted, and these nurses are working in hospitals all over the United States. The International Association of Forensic Nursing (IAFN) was established in 1991. It publishes a journal (*Journal of Forensic Nursing*) and hosts an annual scientific assembly. The IAFN does allow associate membership status to physicians, forensic scientists, law enforcement, prehospital providers, and students. The Web site is www.iafn.org.

Emergency medicine has not been as successful. The American College of Emergency Physicians (ACEP) has a policy statement regarding the care of the sexual assault victim and in 1999 published the handbook *Evaluation and Management of the Sexually Assaulted or Sexually Abused Patient.* There are no other formal policy statements or guidelines regarding forensic medicine, although American College of Emergency Physicians has supported the use of sexual assault nurses in the ED.[9]

Some training opportunities for emergency physicians exist. In the past, lectures on sexual assault care and management, child abuse, child sexual assault, and general forensic medicine principles were hosted at ACEP scientific assemblies. From 1994 through 1999, the University of Louisville Department of Emergency Medicine and the Kentucky Chapter of ACEP sponsored an annual clinical forensic medicine conference. The conference attracted a wide variety of participants including nurses, physicians, law enforcement officers, and prosecuting attorneys.[5] Other courses throughout the United States have offered various lectures on child abuse, sexual assault, interpersonal violence, and other forensically related topics.

In 2006, Dr. William Green, Dr. Michael Weaver, and Dr. Smock started a strong movement to create a Forensic Medicine section of ACEP. They developed subsections focusing on the major areas of adult and adolescent sexual assault, child abuse and sexual assault, and research/education. The section held its first official meeting in October 2007 at the ACEP Scientific Assembly. The section's objectives can be found on the ACEP Web page.

Most recently, an article by Wiler and Bailey appeared in the *Annals of Emergency Medicine* discussing the need to include clinical forensic medical training in emergency medicine residency programs.[7] The article reviews the importance of forensic medicine to emergency medicine and reviews the history of the specialty in the United States. The article outlines potential training, including "evidence collection and preservation, awareness and use of SANE and Sexual Assault Response Team programs, case preparation and trial testimony, interviewing techniques, forensic photography, ballistics and firearms analysis, courtroom and expert testimony, examination of the assaulted adolescent, sexual assault, or pediatric victim, and the forensic evaluation of penetrating trauma."[7]

TABLE 1-1 **Forensic Emergency Medicine Curriculum Topics**

Forensic evaluation of gunshot wounds
Forensic photography
Pediatric sexual assault/abuse
Pediatric physical abuse/assault
Courtroom presentation and expert testimony
Forensic evaluation of blunt trauma and domestic violence
Firearms and ballistics
Forensic odontology and bite marks
Adult sexual assault
Evidence collection and chain of custody in the ED
Determination of driver versus passenger
Forensic anatomy and injury mechanisms
Forensic toxicology and pharmacology
Crime scene investigation
Forensic serology and DNA
Motor vehicle accident reconstruction
Investigation of pedestrian collisions
Introduction to clinical forensic medicine

Source: Smock WS. Genesis and development. In Lynch VA, ed. *Forensic Nursing*. St. Louis: Elsevier Mosby; 2006:13–18.

CONCLUSION

Unfortunately, US medicine has fallen behind many other countries in the development of forensic medicine as a specialty. Although some progress has been made, we have a long way to go. Clearly, emergency physicians are well poised to further the cause. Future goals need to include the development of standardized protocols for patient care, a curriculum for residency programs, and research programs focusing on clinical forensic medicine. Efforts should be made to expand fellowship training opportunities.

ADDITIONAL RESOURCES

ACEP Forensic Medicine Section: Committee information and objective located at www.acep.org. Under the membership, use the sections of membership tab.

REFERENCES

1. Root I, Scott W. The clinician and forensic medicine. *Calif Med.* 1973;119:68–76.
2. Smialek JE. Forensic medicine in the emergency department. *Emerg Med Clin North Am.* 1983;1(3):1685.
3. Mittleman RE, Goldberg HS, Waksman DM. Preserving evidence in the emergency department. *Am J Nurs.* 1983;83:1654.
4. Carmona R, Prince K. Trauma and forensic medicine. *J Trauma.* 1989;29(9):1222.
5. Smock WS. Genesis and development. In Lynch VA, ed. *Forensic Nursing.* St. Louis: Elsevier Mosby; 2006:13–18.
6. Smock WS, Nichols GR, Fuller PM. Development and implementation of the first clinical forensic medicine training program. *J Forensic Sci.* 1993;38(4):835–839.
7. Wiler JL, Bailey H. The need for emergency medicine resident training in forensic medicine. *Ann Emerg Med.* 2007;50:733–738.
8. Joint Commission on Accreditation of Healthcare Organizations (JCAHO). *Accreditation Manual for Hospitals, Core Standards, and Guidelines.* Oak Park, Ill: Joint Commission; 2004.
9. American College of Emergency Physicians. Management of the patient with the complaint of sexual assault. ACEP Policy Statement 400130. October 2002. Available at: http://www.acep.org . Accessed September 13, 2007.

2 | Forensic Nursing in the Emergency Department

Kathleen Brown, RN, PhD

INTRODUCTION

The word *forensic* means pertaining to legal processes. Forensic nursing is the application of nursing principles and practice to matters that are legal in nature. Nurses work with patients, people they encounter in a healthcare setting; therefore, forensic nurses work with patients whose situation may include a legal component.

According to the International Association of Forensic Nurses:

> Forensic Nursing is the application of nursing science to public or legal proceedings; the application of the forensic aspects of health care combined with the bio-psycho-social education of the registered nurse in the scientific investigation and treatment of trauma and/or death of victims and perpetrators of abuse, violence, criminal activity and traumatic accidents.
>
> The forensic nurse provides direct services to individual clients, consultation services to nursing, medical and law related agencies, and expert court testimony in areas dealing with trauma and/or questioned death investigative processes, adequacy of services delivery, and specialized diagnoses of specific conditions as related to nursing.[1]

Nurses working in an emergency department (ED) encounter many patients whose situation includes a legal component. Nurses are well educated to deal with the health-related component of care for all patients who enter an emergency department. With additional education, nurses can add new skills to their background and experience that will assist in creating a foundation for a law enforcement investigation. Nurses who obtain these additional skills are forensic nurses. This chapter will discuss the role of the forensic nurse in the emergency department and opportunities available to them. It will also discuss the process of becoming a forensic nurse and resources available to the forensic nurse.

THE TEAM ENVIRONMENT

When providing care for patients, nurses in an emergency department work within a team. This team consists of medical personnel, laboratory personnel, social work, and pastoral care. The team may include members other than those listed, but the overall goal of the team is to provide the best health care possible on an episodic basis in the emergency department.

Forensic nurses in an emergency department work within the healthcare team, but also work within a forensic team. This forensic team is composed of law enforcement, crime laboratory personnel, victim advocates, and prosecutors.

Victims of crime, accident victims, and perpetrators of crime are frequently patients in an emergency department. The role of forensic nursing within an emergency department developed to help ensure that the legal aspects of these patients' cases are appropriately addressed in the emergency department healthcare setting.

HISTORY OF FORENSIC NURSING

Once considered a problem exclusively for the criminal justice system, violence is now regarded as a public health issue.[2] The efforts of the healthcare community to stem the tide of violence in the United States gained momentum in 1985, with the Surgeon General's Workshop on Violence and Public Health. In his opening remarks, US Surgeon General C. Everett Koop, MD, encouraged the 150 attendees to develop recommendations that could become the "stimuli of change and progress everywhere." He championed a multidisciplinary approach that could be embraced by professionals in medicine, nursing, psychology, and social services. "Our focus will be squarely on how the health professions might provide better care for victims of violence and also how they might contribute to the prevention of violence," he said.[3]

At the same time, nursing was enjoying new strength as a provider of healthcare services to victims. Doors opened for nurses to collaborate with other providers, initiate courses and programs of research on victimology and traumatology, influence legislation and healthcare policy, provide expert testimony in criminal and civil court cases, and ultimately, create a new specialty.[2]

Forensic nursing has its roots in the 18th century, when midwives testified in court on matters such as virginity, pregnancy, and rape.[4] (By contrast, the discipline of forensic medicine began early in the 16th century and focused on pathology and cause of death.)[4] The current model of forensic nursing evolved from the role of the police medical officer found in the United Kingdom and other countries.[5]

The skills of the forensic nurse—observation, documentation, and preservation of evidence—are critical in determining the legal outcome of violent crimes.[6]

EDUCATION OF FORENSIC NURSES

According to the *American Journal of Nursing*, there are four primary routes for obtaining training in forensic nursing:[2]

1. Continuing education courses supplement nursing degree programs and are used for professional education and to fulfill renewal criteria for state licensure.
2. Certification programs have specific content, entrance requirements, and often a written examination. Clinical internships may be required.
3. A minor or concentration in forensics is available in some university undergraduate and graduate nursing programs.
4. Formal graduate study builds on the foundation of the baccalaureate.

In 1997, the American Nurses Association (ANA) published *The Scope and Standards of Forensic Nursing Practice*, which calls for the synthesis of education and experience for forensic nursing proficiency. ANA recommends that in addition to attending core graduate nursing courses, graduate students carry out a clinical internship and complete the forensic nursing curriculum required for the degree.[2]

INTERNATIONAL ASSOCIATION OF FORENSIC NURSES

The International Association of Forensic Nurses (IAFN) is an international membership organization made up of forensic nurses working around the world and other professionals who support and complement the work of forensic nursing.[1]

The mission of the IAFN is to provide leadership in forensic nursing practice by developing, promoting, and disseminating information internationally about forensic nursing science.

IAFN organizational goals are as follows:

1. To incorporate primary prevention strategies into its members' work at every level in an attempt to create a world without violence.
2. To establish and improve standards of evidence-based forensic nursing practice.
3. To promote and encourage the exchange of ideas and transmission of developing knowledge among its members and related disciplines.
4. To establish standards of ethical conduct for forensic nurses.
5. To create and facilitate educational opportunities for forensic nurses and related disciplines.[1]

ROLES OF THE FORENSIC NURSE IN AN EMERGENCY DEPARTMENT

The roles forensic nurses can play in the emergency department are many. A brief description of each is given in the following subsections.

Sexual Assault Nurse Examiner

Sexual assault nurse examiners or sexual assault forensic examiners provide health care to victims/survivors of sexual assault. The examiner carefully observes the victim for any injuries, provides or recommends treatment for injuries, and administers medication to prevent sexually transmitted infections and pregnancy. In addition, the sexual assault examiner collects any biological and trace evidence from the victim's body, documents all injuries in writing and with photography, and carefully records a history of the event based on victim recall.

Forensic Psychiatric Nurse

Psychiatric patients in an emergency department require specialized care. Stabilization of the patient and prevention of the patient from harming him- or herself or others is of paramount importance. The forensic psychiatric nurse assists with maintaining safety and carefully documents the behavior of the patient in anticipation of legal processes.

Forensic Nurse Examiner

In many emergency departments, a forensic nurse is on staff at all times. The role of the forensic nurse is to anticipate legal aspects of patient care and ensure that the healthcare responsibility for those needs are met. The nurse may provide the necessary forensic care herself or himself, or another forensic nurse with specialized skills may be called to the ED as needed.

Forensic Nurse Investigator

A forensic nurse investigator is salaried by a law enforcement team. These nurses work closely with members of the law enforcement community and may be called to an emergency department for consultation on evidence collection and documentation.

Forensic Correctional Nurse

Nurses who work with suspects and offenders are called correctional nurses. Most of these nurses work in jails and prisons providing health care for inmates. These nurses may accompany suspects or convicted offenders to the emergency department for treatment.

Emergency department patients who are suspected of committing a crime may be transferred to a jail from the ED. These suspects are screened for health-related concerns by a correctional nurse upon arrival at the jail. In such cases, good communication between the ED nurse and the correctional nurse is helpful to the patient.

Legal Nurse Consultant

Nurses who work with attorneys on legal cases that include a healthcare aspect are legal nurse consultants. The role includes interpreting healthcare records and giving opinions on standards of care. Emergency department nurses join legal teams in cases where emergency department background and experience are of assistance to legal experts.

Nurse Attorney

Nurse attorneys have completed law school. Nurses with law degrees often practice in areas of the law that include a healthcare component.

FORENSIC PATIENT AND FORENSIC CASE MANAGEMENT

The basic forensic skills added to the provision of health care in the ED are observation, photography, evidence collection, and forensic documentation.

Adding these basic skills to the case management of the following patients in the ED greatly enhances law enforcement investigations.

Victims of Violent Crime

When a victim of violence presents to the ED, medical and trauma nursing care is the first priority. The survival and health of the victim is the primary focus of the ED personnel's response. Forensic work can be done simultaneously with medical and trauma nursing, or it can be done after the patient is stabilized.

The following are forensic skills appropriate for patients who have been victimized by a violent act or acts:

1. **Collect the victim's clothing.** Clothing worn by the victim should be saved and placed into paper bags if possible. (Plastic bags encourage mold that influences the analysis of DNA.) If the victim's clothing is dry, place each item of clothing in a separate paper bag to prevent cross contamination from one piece of clothing to another. Give the clothing to law enforcement personnel present in the ED. If clothing is wet from blood or some other liquid, it should be placed in a biohazard bag and given to law enforcement in the ED.

   Law enforcement will take the clothing to the police crime laboratory where it is analyzed. The crime laboratory will examine the clothing for any evidence that may have transferred from the offender to the victim such as gun shot residue, DNA, or tears from a knife.

   It is frequently necessary for emergency department personnel to cut through clothing to facilitate removal prior to administering care. If this must be done, they can avoid cutting through bullet holes and stab wounds in the clothing to be helpful to the law enforcement investigation. Placing the clothing after it is removed from the victim into paper bags for law enforcement to collect is the next step.

2. **If time and safety permit, take a few photographs of the crime victim.** If nurses can take a picture of the victim and the injuries he or she received, this is helpful for recall in a legal setting. Pictures can be taken with a camera loaned to the nurse by law enforcement or with a camera housed in the ED. A chain of custody must be followed with photographs. Law enforcement will assist the nurse in following an appropriate chain of custody.
3. **Document injuries.** Clear documentation of any injuries sustained by the victim assists the investigation.

If a forensic nurse is available to the emergency department when a victim of violent crime arrives, the forensic nurse should assist with the care of the victim. She or he will collect evidence including clothing, take photographs following a chain of custody, and document forensic findings.

The investigative process for victims of violent crime includes law enforcement investigation of the crime scene, the weapon, and the suspect. Investigative information related to the victim can be greatly enhanced by nurses in an ED setting.

Victims of Sexual Assault

Victims of sexual assault benefit greatly from the services provided by a sexual assault forensic examiner. Every emergency department should have access to a sexual assault forensic examiner. In most ED settings, a sexual assault forensic examiner is available to victims of sexual assault on an on-call basis. When the patient is medically stable, a sexual assault forensic examiner can collect evidence, photograph, and document.

If a sexual assault forensic examiner is not available to the emergency department, law enforcement may be able to suggest to the emergency department nurse how to collect evidence, take photographs, and document the situation.

Victims of Domestic Violence

Forensic nurses are a resource for victims of domestic violence. Victims of domestic violence who come to an emergency department are often physically injured. These victims require documentation of their injuries, photographs of their injuries, and a forensic interview. Forensic nurses can assist victims of domestic violence with issues related to reporting of the crime. Victims of domestic violence utilize the forensic nurse's documentation for legal matters such as restraining orders, divorce, and supervised child visitation.

If a forensic nurse is not available to the emergency department, the ED nurse should document and photograph any injury found on the victim whether or not the injury required medical intervention. The documentation and photographs can be utilized by the victim in a court of law at a later date.

Substance Abuse

Crime is often related to alcohol and substance abuse. Alcohol and drugs impair judgment and can contribute to automobile accidents, workplace injuries, assaults, and other crimes. A forensic nurse can be of assistance in cases in which substance abuse is considered as part of an investigation.

Blood alcohol levels and drug screenings are obtained in an emergency department setting for clinical reasons. Forensic nurses obtain a forensic toxicology screening in addition to the clinical screening. This forensic sample is analyzed in a forensic laboratory and is used for legal, not clinical, purposes.

Victims of Assault

Emergency departments frequently care for victims of assault. Simple and aggravated assaults are very common crimes. Injuries from assault should be carefully documented and photographed by a forensic nurse. Many injuries related to assault heal quickly. Accurate documentation of all injuries, including those that do not require medical intervention, assist in the investigation of simple and aggravated assault.

Patients Involved in Automobile or Pedestrian Accidents

When an accident occurs, health and safety are the first priorities. Patients who are injured are treated as soon as possible. After the accident, police reports are filed that include drawings and photographs of the accident scene. Insurance companies and law enforcement investigate the accident. Clear documentation of all injuries of the people involved in the accident, including injuries that require medical intervention and injuries that do not require medical intervention, can be of assistance in the investigative process.

Forensic nurses clearly document any and all injuries including by using photographs and can interview patients about the incident.

Worker's Compensation Cases

Accidents can and do occur in the workplace. Keeping employees safe is a serious responsibility placed upon employers. If an accident occurs in the workplace, an investigation will ensue. Questions will be asked related to responsibility of both the employer and the employee.

Good observations as well as clear and concise documentation of injury can be of assistance in this investigative process. Forensic nurses carefully document any and all injuries. Forensic nurses also make referrals to specialists who may enhance the investigation.

Victims of Elder Abuse and Neglect

Abuse and neglect of elders are currently recognized as all-too-common crimes. The growing number of elders in the United States increases the possibility of abuse and neglect of this vulnerable portion of the population.

Elder physical abuse is a difficult crime to prosecute. One of the important reasons for this is the normal physical changes that accompany aging. Changes in skin related to aging, common diseases of the elderly, fragility of vessels, and increased susceptibility to head injury are just a few of the physical changes that occur with age. These changes make it difficult for prosecutors to positively correlate an injury with abuse.

Neglect of an elder can be difficult to prove as well. Is the elderly person refusing food, or is he or she not being fed? Is the elderly person refusing medication or treatment, or is it being withheld? These are important questions that require definitive answers.

In cases of elder abuse and neglect, a fact pattern must be established that demonstrates intent and can show cause and effect of abuse or neglect. Forensic nurses can assist with evidence collection and documentation of injury and signs of neglect. Experts in geriatrics who may render an opinion on the cause and effect can analyze photographs taken by the forensic nurse.

The forensic nurse can begin a mental status examination in the emergency department that can be useful for competency examinations to be performed at another time. The forensic nurse will make appropriate referrals to social work, geriatrics, and psychiatry. A complete forensic evaluation in addition to a complete medical evaluation contributes to the future safety of the elder.

Victims of Child Abuse and Neglect

Children are a vulnerable portion of our population. Children cannot care for themselves and therefore require protection and care by adults. Physical abuse of children is responsible for the death and injury of children at a rate much higher than any other medical malady.

Emergency department personnel are charged with determining when injuries to a child are the result of an accident or the result of physical abuse. In some cases, a pattern of the same child returning to the ED with injuries cues the ED nurse to possible abuse. At other times, the appearance of the injury or the history given by the caregiver cues the nurse to possible child abuse.

If the ED nurse suspects that the injury or injuries were intentional, a forensic nurse should be called in for consultation. The forensic nurse will conduct an interview with the child if at all possible, and he or she will examine the child's injuries. The forensic nurse will document and photograph the injuries and make appropriate referrals to pediatric medical specialists and pediatric social workers.

Neglect of a child can be observed by the ED nurse through signs such as malnutrition, lack of medical care, poor hygiene, and symptoms of exposure. If an ED nurse suspects child neglect, referral to a forensic nurse will assist social work and law enforcement in the investigative process.

Victims of Institutional Abuse or Neglect

Abuse of people can occur in a home setting as well as in nursing homes and care facilities. Assault and sexual abuse can and do occur in various institutional settings such as detention facilities, prisons, and psychiatric facilities.

When a crime occurs in institutional settings, a forensic nurse is required. The forensic nurse will contact the appropriate authorities that have jurisdiction over the issue. Institutions are held to different standards than individuals are. Contacting the appropriate authorities that will conduct an investigation is important for the current patient and is also important for the other individuals residing in the institution.

Death in the ED

If at all possible, a forensic nurse should be called in to assist in cases in which a patient expires in the ED. If a patient expires in the ED, an investigation follows. The office of the medical examiner will determine whether the cause of death was natural, accidental, homicide, suicide, or undetermined. ED nurses can assist the medical examiner in making this determination by saving the clothing from the patient and releasing it to law enforcement.

The ED nurse can also follow several procedures to assist the investigation. Not cutting through bullet marks and cut marks in the person's clothing is helpful, as is documenting in the patient's record any injury created by or during the treatment of the patient.

If the patient is the victim of a gunshot wound, the ED nurse should not try to determine the exit wound versus entrance wound; the medical examiner will determine this during autopsy. If the patient is a victim of a stabbing, the ED nurse should not attempt to determine the type of knife that made the cut; if at all possible, stabbing wounds should not be extended for therapeutic purposes because extending the wound alters the ability of the medical examiner to determine the type of weapon used. Nurses should also be very careful about probing any wounds made by a knife because a knife can break off in a wound and the nurse can be cut by a piece of the blade. If a weapon or bullet is retrieved in the ED, the nurse should give it to law enforcement, and law enforcement will assist the ED nurse in securing the chain of custody for the bullet or weapon.

Sudden Infant Death

It is difficult to determine sudden infant death versus other causes of infant death. Preservation of evidence is helpful to the medical examiner. A forensic nurse can assist the medical examiner in determining cause and manner of death by preserving any evidence of suffocation, battering, or any other form of violence that may have been inflicted upon the child. A forensic nurse should be called in to assist in all cases in which a child expires in the ED.

VICARIOUS TRAUMA IN THE ED

The invention of the term *vicarious traumatization* is attributed to McCann and Pearlman (1990)[7] who observed that working with trauma victims can cause severe and lasting psychological effects in healthcare personnel. Vicarious traumatization can lead to changes in self and changes in professional identity. A wide range of symptoms and psychological reactions has been suggested to result from vicarious traumatization, including post-traumatic stress disorder.

Working in an emergency department subjects nurses to vicarious traumatization. Nurses are observers of many different forms of trauma that people experience. Forensic psychiatric nurses may be of assistance to ED nurses who are experiencing vicarious trauma.

RESOURCES

This section contains lists of resources related to forensic nursing.

Web Sites Related to Forensic Nursing

International Association of Forensic Nursing: www.iafn.org
International Association of Chiefs of Police: www.iacp.org
National Alliance to End Sexual Violence: www.naesv.org
National Center for Injury Prevention and Control: www.cdc.gov/ncipc.dvp.dvp.htm
National Center for Prosecution of Child Abuse: www.ndaa-apri.org/apri/programs/ncpca/ncpca_home
National Sexual Violence Resource Center: www.nsvrc.org
Office on Violence Against Women: www.usdoj.gov/ovw
National Center for the Prosecution of Violence Against Women: www.ndaa-apri.org/apri/index.html
Tribal Law and Policy Institute: http://www.tribal-institute.org/lists/tlpi.htm

Government Agency Web Sites

Bureau of Justice Statistics: www.ojp.usdoj.gov/bjs
FBI Uniform Crime Reports: www.fbi.gov/ucr/ucr.htm
Office for Victims of Crime: www.ojp.usdoj.gov/ovc
US Department of Defense, Sexual Assault Prevention and Response: www.sapr.mil

Professional Organizations

American Academy of Forensic Science: www.aafs.oprg
American Academy of Psychiatry and the Law: www.aapl.org
American Board of Forensic Psychology: www.abfp.com
American Board of Medicolegal Death Investigators: www.slu.edu/organizations/abmdi/
American College of Forensic Examiners: www.acfei.com/programs.php
American College of Obstetricians and Gynecologists: www.acog.org

IAFN Home Office

1517 Ritchie Highway, Suite 208
Arnold, MD 21012-2461
Phone: 410-626-7805
Fax: 410-626-7804

CONCLUSION

Forensic nurses can play an important role in the evaluation, management, and treatment of many kinds of patients in the emergency department, particularly, those who are victims of crime, abuse, and/ or neglect. The forensic nurse is an invaluable resource between the victim, the healthcare system, law enforcement, and the criminal justice system. Hospital emergency departments across the country should consider developing a program for their patients. Several resources are available to help.

REFERENCES

1. International Association of Forensic Nurses. About IAFN. 2008. Available at: http://www.iafn.org/displaycommon.cfm?an=3. Retrieved July 23, 2008.
2. Burgess AW, Berger AD, Boersma RR. Forensic nursing. *Am J Nurs.* 2004, March;104(3): 58–64.
3. US Public Health Service. *Surgeon General's workshop on violence and public health report.* 1986. Available at: http://profiles.nlm.nih.gov/NN/B/C/F/X/_/nnbcfx.pdf. Retrieved July 23, 2008.
4. Lynch VA. Forensic nursing. In: Burgess AW, ed. *Advanced Practice in Psychiatric Mental Health Nursing.* Stamford, Conn: Appleton-Lange; 1998.
5. Lynch VA. Clinical forensic nursing: a new perspective in the management of crime victims from trauma to trial. *Crit Care Nurs Clin North Am.* 1995;7(3):489–507.
6. Malestic SL. Fight violence with forensic evidence. *RN.* 1995;58(1):30–32.
7. McCann L, Pearlman LA. Vicarious traumatization: a framework for understanding psychological effects of working with victims. J Traumatic Stress. 1990;3:131-149.

SUGGESTED READING

Sullivan LW. Forum on youth violence in minority communities. The prevention of violence—a top HHS priority. *Public Health Rep.* 1991;106(3):268–269.

American Association of Colleges of Nursing. Violence as a public health problem. 2002. Available at: http://www.aacn.nche.edu/Publications/positions/violence.htm. Retrieved July 23, 2008.

Shepherd J. Violence as a public health problem. Combined approach is needed. *BMJ.* 2003;326(7380):104.

Littel K, US Department of Justice. Sexual Assault Nurse Examiner (SANE) programs: improving the community response to sexual assault victims. 2001. Available at: http://www.ojp.usdoj.gov/ovc/publications/bulletins/sane_4_2001/welcome.html. Retrieved July 23, 2008.

American Nurses Association. *Scope and Standards of Forensic Nursing Practice.* Washington, DC: American Nurses Publishing; 1997.

Burgess AW, Frederich A. Sexual violence and trauma. Policy implications for nursing. *Nurs Health Pol Rev.* 2002;1(1):17–36.

3 | Suicide

Pierre Detiege, MD, and Matthew Brooks, MD

INTRODUCTION

Few things in society are more difficult to discuss than suicide. Part of the problem is the mixed messages on the issue. By definition, suicide is a "death arising from an act inflicted upon oneself with the intent to kill oneself."[1] This behavior seems contrary to what we are taught is the basic human instinct for self-preservation. However, suicide has been documented throughout the centuries and in many different societies: Ancient warriors threw themselves on their spear to avoid capture, *seppuku* (ritual suicide) was practiced by Japanese samurai to maintain honor, and broken-hearted lovers ingested poison because of unrequited love throughout history. Many famous figures have committed suicide: Ernest Hemingway, Vincent Van Gogh, Virginia Woolf, to name a few. Fame and the relationship between suicide and popularity further confuse the subject. Why, some ask, would someone rich and famous commit suicide? Why does a person's art or music suddenly become popular after he or she commits suicide?

Another difficulty with this subject stems from the wide range of emotions provoked by a suicide. The anger, guilt, or grief of family members, the frustration felt by healthcare providers, and the confusion and search for reasons by the community are just the initial emotions. One estimate is that a suicide affects six other people intimately,[2] and those effects are carried on with those people forever. Other barriers to discussing suicide involve historic factors including legal and moral statutes prohibiting suicide. At one time in Britain, the government could seize the property and possessions of someone who committed suicide.[3] Religions often do not allow someone who dies from suicide to be buried in church cemeteries, and they teach followers that a loved one's soul could suffer damnation after a suicide.

Today the medical community and much of society view suicide as the outcome of mental illness, a failure of prevention, intervention, and treatment. However, some argue that suicide is a dignified choice in certain situations. It can be viewed as the ultimate act of self-determination and free will. All these factors combine to make this one of society's greatest taboos. How do we approach this complex issue from a forensic standpoint? What information do we have about suicide, and what additional information can we gather? How does research and the information gathered help in a situation that by definition is fatal?

RISK FACTORS

Volumes of data and studies relate the risk factors for suicide. What does research tell us are risk factors for suicide? A mental health disorder or a substance abuse disorder is present in 90% of suicide deaths. Family history of suicide, prior suicide attempt, physical or sexual abuse, and stressful life events are all factors. Another important factor is access to a firearm in the home.[4] In the United States, firearms are the leading method used in suicide. Additionally, many studies examine the relationship of alcohol and suicidality. Alcohol use increases impulsivity and aggressive behavior, and both are major factors in suicide. Studies have shown high rates (33–69%) of suicide victims with positive blood alcohol levels. Alcohol abuse leads to chemical changes in the brain, most notably low serotonin levels, which also have been shown to be present in people with depression, prior suicide attempts, and in suicide completers. Finally, alcohol abuse is known to affect interpersonal relationships, is related to abuse situations, and leads to life stressors such as job and financial woes.[5]

EPIDEMIOLOGY

In 2005, suicide was the 11th leading cause of death in the United States. That year more than 32,600 people died because of intentional self-harm. Almost 90 people per day committed suicide. By comparison, homicide ranked as the 15th leading cause of death, with a death rate of 6.1 per 100,000 people. This was almost half the suicide rate of 11.0 per 100,000 people.[2]

Suicide affects all demographics (see Table 3-1). Males commit suicide much more frequently than females do (3.7 to 1) and use firearms more frequently. However, studies show that there are three female attempted suicides for every male attempt. Divided by race, the suicide rate by white males is at least double that of almost every other group. However, this problem touches every race. Suicide is rare in children younger than 14 years, but is a factor in every age group, even elderly people older than 85 years.

In the United States, the majority of suicides (52%) involve firearms, a method which far outdistances the second leading method of hanging/suffocation (23%). Poisoning is the third leading method (18%). Gender differences in methodology shed light on the gender demographics mentioned earlier. Whereas the majority of male suicides are by firearms, females are more likely to use poisoning as their preferred method. This difference in preference affects survival, and the lower survival rate in males relates to the overall higher suicide rate among men. Less lethal methodology among females leads to increased survival and might translate into repeat attempts and higher attempt rates by women.[4] See Table 3-2.

TABLE 3-1 **Suicide Demographics in the United States, 2005**

	Rate (per 100,000 population)
Nation	11.0
Male	17.7
White male	19.7
Black male	8.7
Female	4.5
White female	5.0
Black female	1.8
White	12.3
Black	5.1
Hispanic	5.1
Native American	12.4
Asian/Pacific Islanders	5.2
Elderly (65+ years)	14.7
Young (15–24 years)	10.0

Source: American Association of Suicidology, http://www.suicidology.org.

TABLE 3-2 **Suicide Causes by Gender**

Suicide by:	Males (%)	Females (%)
Firearms	57	32
Suffocation	23	20
Poisoning	13	38

Source: Centers for Disease Control and Prevention, National Center for Injury Prevention and Control. WISQARS, http://www.cdc.gov/ncipc/wisqars.

The suicide rate has fallen somewhat in recent years. In 1998, suicide ranked as the eighth leading cause of death in the United States but has since been surpassed by Alzheimer's disease, nephritis, and sepsis.[6] However, when we look at the suicide rate by year since the 1950s, the decreased trend is less dramatic (see Figure 3-1). What does that say regarding education, prevention programs, and treatments? Are we just saving more people with better medical and traumatic resuscitation? Is this all we can find with current data collection?

CLASSIFICATION

How is a death classified as a suicide? In most areas, classification is done by the coroner or the medical examiner. These terms are often used interchangeably by the public but in fact are very different positions. A *coroner* is usually an appointed or elected official, placed in office to be the administrator of the area's death investigation system. A *medical examiner* (ME) is typically a forensic pathologist with medical training in pathology and additional training

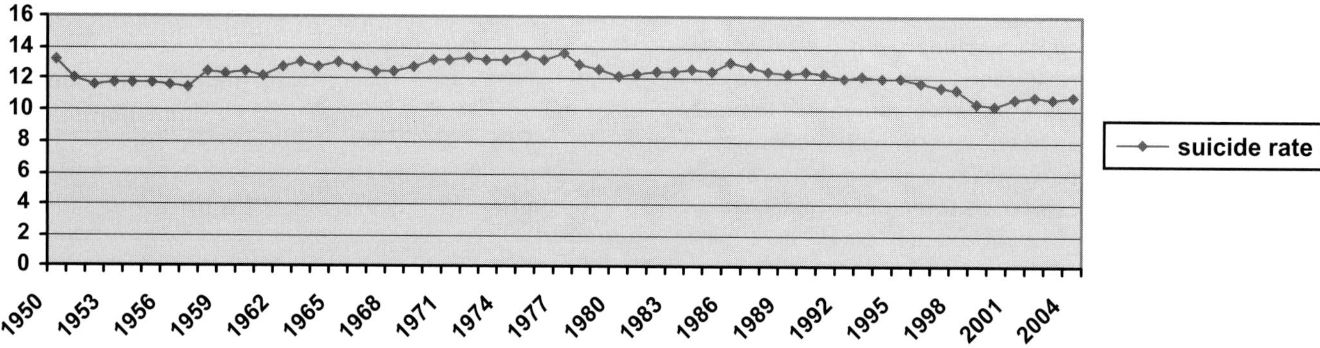

FIGURE 3-1 **US suicide rate per 100,000 population 1953–2004.**[7]

in forensic sciences. Forensics is the connection between the medical and legal aspects regarding injury and death[8]—it is the window into what happened and how. In large cities, a coroner may have multiple medical examiners as well as other investigators, such as toxicologists, working in his or her office. MEs use their scientific training to decipher what happened that lead to a death. Small jurisdictions may have only a coroner who outsources the autopsy to a pathologist and forensic studies to outside labs. For the most part, though, the types of death investigation systems that the coroner or the medical examiner use overlap, and it is important to realize there are both administrative and forensic portions to death investigations.[9]

Many other people and factors play roles in a suicide death investigation. The initial suspicion of suicide may be based on family, emergency medical system (EMS)/first responder, or even emergency department staff (physician or nurse) feelings. Occasionally, the victim leaves evidence to the fact, such as a suicide note or makes a call prior to the attempt. When hard evidence is not present, information must be found to help distinguish between natural, accidental, homicide, and suicide deaths, but this information can be hard to obtain. Although an autopsy can be performed, sometimes despite the forensic investigation there is no firm proof of the person's intention. Sometimes family may interfere with an autopsy; they may exert pressure against or withhold evidence to prevent the determination of suicide for moral or insurance reasons. The limited resources of the ME's office and a heavy workload investigating homicides for legal proceedings can also hinder a thorough investigation. Finally, some cases just may not provoke suspicion of suicide or may involve other confounding medical issues that lead to a classification as natural death. All this leads to a question to which we do not know the answer: How many suicides are we missing?

TYPES OF SUICIDE

Suicide can be accomplished by various manners. Several of the more common manners are reviewed here with emphasis on the forensic implications for the ED personnel.

Firearm Suicide

In the United States, among both genders firearm-related suicide is the most common method, accounting for 55% of all yearly suicides.[10,11] Although the majority of firearm suicides are men, women account for 20% to 30% of suicides committed in this manner. Compared to other methods of suicide, firearm-related suicide is usually more impulsive, more closely related to alcohol consumption, and more lethal than other forms. It is also closely linked with a household that contains a firearm. In contrast to other forms of suicide, those who committed firearm-related suicide were less likely than other suicides to have a previous suicide attempt in their history.[12] This makes firearm suicide somewhat distinct from the "typical" suicide victims.

When examining a suspected case of firearm suicide, careful examination of the wound is important. Contact wounds leave different wound patterns than either close shot wounds or distance shots. Therefore, the wound should correlate with the postulated manner of death. Also, if a death is to be ruled a suicide, the wound should correlate with the victim's ability to inflict such a wound. In other words, is the distance indicated by the wound pattern reasonable considering the victim's arm length? Sometimes additional instruments are present to aid the victim's reach, such as a stick to help depress the trigger of a long gun. To duplicate the observed wound pattern, it is often prudent to test shoot the weapon at varying distances to determine the most likely distance the victim's body was from the gun barrel.[13]

When a gun is fired, in addition to the bullet, several other materials are expelled from the barrel: a 1400°F jet of flame 1 to 2 inches in length, a cloud of gas, burning and unburned grains of gunpowder, carbon from the burnt gunpowder, and vaporized metal from the bullet. When these materials are considered in relation to the distance of the gun from the target, they create distinct patterns at varying distances that are loosely categorized as contact, near contact, intermediate, and distant. Most suicide wounds fall into the first two categories: contact and near contact.[11,14,15]

In all contact wounds, the entrance wound is usually circular and about the size of the gun muzzle. Contact wounds have slightly different patterns depending on whether the gun had hard or loose contact with the skin. A hard contact wound occurs when the gun is pushed into the skin hard enough to create a seal ensuring that all the material that exits the gun is forced beneath the skin. In these cases, the skin is seared by the flame that exits the gun and soot is impregnated into the wound area. If a hard contact wound occurs in the abdomen or the chest, the escaping gas causes the area to bulge against the muzzle of the gun and produces an imprint on the skin. If the contact wound is on the head, the victim may have a stellate (star-like) pattern because when this area of the skin balloons out, it can tear. The type and severity of the wound is usually related to the size and caliber of the weapon, with shotguns or rifles having the ability to create large tears in the skin. The caliber of the weapon also affects the amount of back splatter of tissue onto the gun. Larger caliber weapons tend to create more back splatter.[11,16]

Slightly different than hard contact injury is the loose contact wound. In this wound, there is usually a small gap between the gun muzzle and the skin during firing, and a ring of soot is deposited at the entrance wound. A near contact wound, which typically occurs at a range of less than 10 mm, has a larger area of soot around the wound than the hard contact wound. The wound has seared and blackened edges. These wounds never have a muzzle mark because the muzzle does not contact the skin at any point.[11,16]

Because most studies show that only approximately 80% of suicide wounds are contact or near contact, it is also possible to see intermediate distance wounds on the skin. With handguns, intermediate pattern occurs starting at 10 mm and continues to approximately 2 m depending on the type of powder in the gun. What characterizes intermediate shots is the presence of *powder tattooing* around the wound. Powder tattooing occurs when the powder grains that exit the gun produce punctuate abrasions on the skin. Unlike soot marks, these cannot be washed off. At a distance of up to 1 m, there can still be burning of the skin. As the distance from muzzle to skin increases, soot marks diminish and powder tattooing increases. The diameter of powder tattooing also increases as the distance from the gun barrel does.[11,16] Intermediate wound patterns vary for smooth bore weapons (no lands or grooves) such as a shotgun. At distances between 20 cm and 1 m, the spread of shotgun pellets causes the wound to be irregular. This has been referred to as "rat-holed" wounds. The wound is round with scalloped edges.[16]

A distant gunshot wound is very unlikely in a suicide and should instead raise suspicion that a homicide has taken place. These wounds have no powder tattooing and produce a round wound with punched-out margins. The edges of the wound also have an abrasion ring caused by the bullet scraping the skin and compressing the edges as it enters the body.[11] In smooth bore weapons such as shotguns fired at a distance of 2 to 3 m, satellite pellets begin to appear around the central wound. Roughly, the spread of the shot in centimeters equals 2 to 3 times the range in meters. For example, a wound 20 cm across was made by a gun fired at approximately 10 m and cannot be a suicide.[16]

The location of the gun at the time of death can also help a physician determine whether the death is a suicide. In the case of handgun use, the gun is found in the hands of the deceased person 25% of the time, and when the gun is a long gun, it is found in the victim's hand approximately 20% of the time. In addition, the gun is much more likely to be found in the victim's hand if the victim was sitting or lying down at the time of the incident as opposed to standing up. When not in the victim's hand, most firearms are either on or touching the body, or they are within 30 cm of the body. In one study, only 7% of suicide firearms were more than 30 cm from the body of the deceased. If the gun is not present at the scene, it almost instantly rules out suicide unless someone has removed the firearm.[17]

Oftentimes, the most concerning issue in a firearm suicide is whether or not this was, in fact, a homicide. We can use several characteristics to help differentiate between suicide and homicide, although no one characteristic is absolute. Instead, we must view the entire circumstance, and then make a decision based on all information.

The age distribution of homicide victims is usually younger when compared to suicides. The mean age, in one study,[14] of homicide victims was 34 years versus 51 years in the suicide category. Homicide victims also have a lower frequency of high blood alcohol than suicide victims do. Suicide victims commonly fire only one shot as opposed to homicide victims, who usually sustain multiple wounds; however, from 1–7% of suicide victims fire more than one time because immediate incapacitation occurs only when essential centers of the central nervous system (CNS) are injured. Therefore, the only way that a suicide could be ruled out by the number of shots is if it is determined that these CNS centers were wounded by the first shot.[14] Extreme care should always be taken when ruling a wound as instantly fatal because even individuals who have suffered destruction of the heart or severe brain damage as a result of the shot may still be capable of repeated firings.[16]

Suicide victims have preferred shot sites, which have been validated in many studies. The most common sites for a suicide victim are shots in the forehead, the temple, the mouth, and the left chest, although some suicide victims occasionally have shots in atypical places as well. Discharges to the temple are usually on the same side as the dominant hand, although approximately 5% of right-handed people shoot themselves in the left temple. Also, people almost never shoot themselves in the eye, the abdomen, or in spots difficult to reach such as the back.[11,14,16] In homicides, the main target is the head, but as a result of the fact that the victim and the perpetrator often are moving at the time of the shooting, the wounds in homicides tend to be more evenly distributed across the body.[14] Clothing is less often damaged in suicide likely because of the preference of suicide victims to choose sites that are unclothed rather than to expose the part of the body prior to shooting.

An important test to perform on any suspected suicide victim is to check for the presence of gunshot residue. This is soot, gunpowder, primer components, and vaporized metal that has been discharged from the gun. This residue may be present on the skin or clothing of the person who fired the gun. Tests can be performed to identify whether the residue is present and if the distribution and quantity are consistent with firing the weapon. Note that if the test is negative, it does not automatically indicate a homicide because the test is positive only in about half the cases in which the individual is known to have fired the gun.[11]

Another tool that can aid in differentiation is the previously mentioned back splatter onto the gun. Usually, if a gun is fired at a person in close proximity, evidence of blood is on the weapon. The distribution of this blood often gives clues as to whether there was a suicide. When analyzing handguns, it was found that 53% of revolvers and 57% of pistols used in suicides had evidence of blood in the gun barrel. This suggests that the gun was very close to the target. It has been shown that a handgun must be approximately 7.6 mm from the target to have blood inside the barrel. In suicides, blood is detected outside the barrel on 74% of revolvers and 76% of pistols. Therefore, a positive test for blood inside the barrel, as opposed to simply blood on the outside of the gun, suggests a very close proximity injury, which is overwhelmingly more prevalent in suicide cases. Of long guns tested, 58% had blood inside the barrel and 81% had blood on the barrel. These figures must be interpreted more carefully though: Because most long guns tend to have a higher caliber and shot velocity, the gun could be several feet away from the victim and still get blood on it. But blood inside the muzzle end does require that the target be within centimeters of the gun.

A final tool that helps determine the difference between a homicide and a suicide is the path of the bullet. At the time of death, suicide victims are typically in a stable and comfortable position, allowing them to point the gun in a predetermined way. In contrast, the dynamic situation of homicide creates multiple different paths that the bullet may take. Gunshots to the right temple tend to show a front to back or upward bullet path in suicides. Therefore, a downward shot or a back-to-front shot should raise suspicion despite its typical shot site location. When they place the gun in their mouth, suicide victims have shown a clear preference for an upward trajectory. Downward trajectory does occur but is a rarity. Also, gunshots to the left chest tend to show a preference for moving in a right-to-left path when the suicide shoots. Finally, in the rare instances when a suicide chose to shoot in the back of the head or neck, they tended to fire with an upward-directed trajectory.[14]

Suicide by Cop

When discussing firearm-related suicides, special cases must be considered. One such case is suicide by cop, also referred to as "police-assisted suicide." This is defined as an incident in which an individual engages in life-threatening criminal behavior to provoke the use of lethal force from law enforcement personnel. Police-assisted suicide is different from "victim-precipitated homicide," which refers to people who initiate or contribute to the events of their death and which is a much broader term and does not necessarily indicate the person had suicidal intent.[18–20] Although data determining the percentage of police shootings that are suicide by cop are fairly sparse, one study of the Los Angeles Police Department (LAPD) indicated that 10.5% of the shooting deaths over a 10-year span were in fact suicide by cop.[20]

There is much speculation as to why a person will choose this particular form of suicide, and many reasons have been suggested. Ultimately, most people who have chosen this form of suicide are found to have multiple reasons in mind, such as to avoid the consequences of criminal acts, to avoid the exclusion clause in life insurance, to circumvent the spiritual problem that suicide is wrong, to exact revenge and possibly commit homicide as well, and to draw attention to important personal issues.[19] In one studied instance, 10% of the police-assisted suicides were facing jail terms of 25 years to life imprisonment for their participation in multiple crimes.[20]

After review of the known cases of suicide by cop, several patterns start to emerge both about the victims and the indicators of intended suicide. In the cases studied, most of the victims were male Caucasians. One study showed a mean age of 32 years.[19,20] As with other forms of suicide, a substantial portion of the victims had diagnosed psychological disorders, alcohol and drug abuse problems, and a previous suicide history at the time of their death. In one study, 40% of the victims were intoxicated with alcohol at the time of their death and 47% had previous suicide attempts. In addition, 40% had documented psychiatric disorders and 60% had evidence of psychiatric disorders.[19,20]

When the incidents are reviewed, several commonalities are present. The first is that all incidents were, not surprisingly, perceived as life-threatening by the police officer or the hostages and all victims resisted arrest and threatened homicide during the incident. All victims possessed a weapon or an object they passed off as a weapon, as in some instances the weapon was a replica gun or was an unloaded gun. During the incident, 60% of the victims used their weapon with intent to harm and approximately 66% took hostages.[20]

The presence of several verbal and behavior clues can help determine if an incident is in fact a suicide by cop. Examples of the verbal cues include the victim demanding that the police officer kill him or her, wanting to go out "in a blaze of glory," saying a verbal will, offering to surrender to the person in charge, indicating that "jail is not an option," and making biblical references especially to the Book of Revelation or passages about resurrection. Behavioral clues include the victim being demonstrative with the weapon by showing it or waving it at officers, clearing a path for the officer to fire a weapon, attaching the weapon to the body, performing a countdown to kill the hostages, refusing to negotiate, calling the police to report the crime, failing to make escape demands, and performing self-mutilation with police present. Finally, certain types of police calls have an increased likelihood of being or becoming suicide by cop. Examples include suicidal citizen, barricaded suspect, hostage situation, "three strikes" criminals facing apprehension, and police pursuit of wanted criminal.[20]

Suicide by cop is a rapidly evolving form of suicide with trends showing an increase in its prevalence. Most instances occur within 30 minutes of police arrival, giving minimal time for effective intervention. In addition, the shooting officer often experiences profound psychological effects, causing many to second-guess their response in such incidents.[18]

Russian Roulette

Another special case when considering firearm-related suicides is their relationship to Russian roulette. Russian roulette is defined as "a game of high risk in which each player in turn, using a revolver containing one bullet, spins the cylinder of the revolver, points the muzzle at the head, and pulls the trigger."[21] Russian roulette-type suicide is a form of high risk taking behavior in which the person shoots himself or herself, making it appear in some ways as a suicide; however, the person participating is not necessarily suicidal.

Several reasons for why people tend to play Russian roulette have been postulated. To adolescents the game may represent an extension of their need to engage in risk. It is also viewed as an extreme form of the ordeal or rite of passage of a boy into manhood. Also, high risk for some people is a form of addiction, and the risk of death gives them an otherwise unattainable high. It has also been suggested that recklessness may have an antidepressant effect on young males and that it is engaged in as a form of self-treatment.[22]

When compared to typical firearm-related suicide, in Russian roulette cases several patterns emerge about the person and the situation. Russian roulette players are predominantly men. Even when the greater tendency of men to use guns for suicide is factored in, women are still less likely to engage in the game. Russian roulette players are also predominantly younger than their other suicide counterparts. One study found the mean age for Russian roulette victims was 27 years compared to 50 years for firearm suicides.[22] This may be linked to young people being more prone to risk taking behavior.

Russian roulette, in most instances, is a group activity. One study showed that all Russian roulette victims died in the presence of others. Russian roulette victims were also significantly less likely than other suicides to die in the morning, to die in their beds, or to leave suicide notes. They were, however, much more likely to have alcohol and drugs in their body at the time of death and to have a history of drug or alcohol abuse. Russian roulette victims often exhibit varying degrees of the amount of risk taking and the person's desire to die. It was noted that among the game's players 57.8% had fired more than once, 26.3% had played the game before, and 15.7% loaded more than one bullet into the gun.[22]

This game may also be an emerging problem among adolescents, who are some of the most likely candidates to engage in risky behavior. This form of risk taking behavior is rarely asked about by physicians when interviewing adolescents. When adolescents at inpatient psychiatric hospitals and juvenile detention centers were asked, an alarming 20% of individuals stated that they had participated in the game at least once. Many had to be asked directly about it because few openly volunteered the information.[23] For this reason, a physician should consider specifically questioning adolescents about such risk taking practices.

Asphyxia Suicides

The term *asphyxia* is often used to convey a broad range of conditions that are characterized by inadequate oxygenation of the tissue. In most cases, this implies a force applied to the neck such as in hanging or manual strangulation. Contrary to what is commonly believed, inadequate oxygenation need not entail a cutoff of oxygen supply to the lungs, but instead may be the result of impaired circulation of blood to the brain. The different types of asphyxia can be broadly divided into two types: suffocation or strangulation. The most common type among suicide victims is strangulation and therefore is discussed most extensively in this section. Suicide by asphyxia accounts for 22.6% of all suicides in the United States, making it the second most common behind firearms.[10,12,15]

Suffocation results from either a reduced amount of oxygen in the air in the lungs or a mechanical obstruction that prevents the delivery of oxygen. The first type is usually accidental, although there are occasional cases of suicide. Examples of this type of suffocation is when a person is trapped in a farm silo that has accumulated carbon dioxide and when a person intentionally locks himself or herself in an abandoned refrigerator. There are no classic signs to differentiate accidents from intentional suicide, so to distinguish accident from suicide you must rely on psychological data about the victim and typical suicide risk factors such as suicidal ideation, previous attempts, or presence of a note.[15]

The second type of suffocation described as mechanical obstruction may also be termed *smothering*. Smothering may also be homicidal, suicidal, or accidental, although most are homicides. Examples of each, respectively, include a gag placed over the mouth and nose, a plastic bag placed over one's head, or an infant who becomes trapped under pillows and blankets. Another example of accident is when a person abuses inhalants placed in a plastic bag. As described earlier, the evidence of whether a case is a suicide, homicide, or accident is often related to the situation and history because there are very rarely pathological findings present to differentiate the three. When examining the gag on a victim, care must be taken to establish whether or not it was an obstructing device capable of suffocating the individual. In cases of homicidal smothering, occasionally evidence of trauma is present. Bruises and abrasions on the cheeks and chin as well as hemorrhages and bite marks on the lips and oral mucosa all indicate a struggle during smothering more suggestive of homicide. However, in suffocations there is often postmortem blanching around the mouth and nose, and this should not be mistaken for evidence of a struggle. In the special cases of solvent inhalation from a plastic bag, the person should be tested for presence of the inhalant to establish whether he or she had been abusing the drug.[13,15]

The second broad category of asphyxia is strangulation, which refers to a device being placed around the neck to occlude the blood vessels in the neck and cause cerebral hypoxia. Strangulation is further divided into hangings, ligature strangulation, and manual strangulation. Although most think the cause of death is related to airway obstruction, the majority of strangulation deaths occur as a result of compression of the victim's carotid arteries and jugular veins. Two-thirds to three-quarters of the cerebral blood flow comes from the carotid arteries and the rest comes from the vertebral arteries. It takes approximately 11 pounds of pressure applied to the neck to cut off blood supply from the carotids. Because only 4.4 pounds of pressure are needed to compress the jugular vein, almost all cases of carotid compression also include jugular compression. In these cases, the blood supply continues from the vertebral arteries, but no drainage can occur. The faces of these victims often appear blue as a result of vascular congestion. In addition, because of the raised venous pressure in the face and neck, these victims usually have petechiae on their face, eyelids, and conjunctiva. If the vertebral arteries are also occluded during strangulation, there is no blood flow to the head, but the secondary vertebral venous system still provides some drainage. These victims often have extremely pale faces and often show no petechiae.[13,15]

In hangings, the pressure for the strangulation comes from the weight of the body itself. Hangings are almost uniformly suicidal. Mostly males attempt this form of suicide, and the preferred place is at home.[24] This form of suicide can be accomplished in any position, even standing, because the weight of the head alone is enough to occlude the carotids. However, the most common position for hanging suicides tends to be sitting or half-kneeling position with the noose suspended from a low point such as a door handle. Because the direction of force in hanging is downward, the noose usually leaves an inverted V shape on the skin with the apex indicating where the knot was placed. The furrow is most often above the larynx of the individual. Furrows are usually variable depending on the noose material, with ropes often leaving prominent weave patterns. Hanging victims often appear very pale because of complete occlusion of the vessels. As a result of the upward pressure from the noose, the jaw is pushed upward, causing the tongue to protrude and dry out. When these individuals are completely suspended, there is pooling of blood in the forearms and lower extremities. It is very uncommon for these types of hanging victims to have fractures or cervical spine injuries, which are patterns more often associated with judicial hangings involving a long drop on the rope.

Most hangings are suicides because homicidal hanging is difficult to accomplish in an awake and resisting person. For a homicidal hanging to be accomplished, the victim would have to be drunk or drugged or unconscious from other means. Evidence of additional injuries, which might indicate an incapacitating blow or physical restraint of the individual, should be carefully sought if homicide is suspected.[15]

For suicidal hangings, a special note should also be made about hangings that occur in prison. Many times, hanging is the suicide method of choice for people who have been incarcerated. When accomplished, most victims use a belt because this is the most convenient object. Most prison suicide hangings occur within a day or so of incarceration.[24]

Ligature strangulation occurs when an object is wrapped around the neck to compress the vessels and the compression force is applied by something other than the victim's own body weight. Although most cases of ligature strangulation are homicide in nature, there have been instances of suicide. It is possible for an individual to wrap an instrument around his or her neck multiple times before losing consciousness from the pressure. As opposed to hanging suicides, the marks in ligature strangulation are usually horizontal in nature and are at or below the larynx level. In a homicide, if the person was capable of resisting, the person often has scratch marks around the ligature as the person tries to pull it off. In these cases, the person tends to have a congested face pattern with scattered petechiae on the face.[13,15]

Some forensic factors can aid in differentiating a ligature strangulation homicide from a suicide. Obviously, if the ligature is not present at the scene, homicide must be suspected unless a family member or the police have removed the device. A suicide victim is unable to remove the ligature because it must be wrapped around the neck tight enough to cause continued pressure after loss of consciousness. Often with homicides, the situation is obvious from the scene itself because signs of a struggle exist, or the ligature is missing, or there is the presence of defensive wounds on the victim.[13,15]

When you compare the ligature marks and injury patterns of homicides and suicides, there are differences between the two. In most homicides, the ligature marks show evidence of real mechanical skin injury, including abrasion and hemorrhages. In most suicides, evidence of skin injury is rare and if it is present, it is often mild, consisting of lines of petechiae only.[25]

Additional damage to the neck and its internal structures is usually the hallmark of a homicide. Although there are cases of severe injury in suicide, it occurs rarely. This is easily explained by the nature of the incident: Homicides tend to be much more violent events, and as a result a greater amount of force is applied to the individual's neck. In less than 20% of all homicides, but in more than 50% of all suicides, there was no evidence of internal injury to the neck. In suicides, the most common injury is to the sternocleidomastoid muscle. It is also extremely rare for suicide cases to have fractures of either the hyoid bone or laryngeal cartilage. When these fractures do occur in suicides, the damage is usually limited to one broken upper thyroid horn. This is not always helpful. This injury does not definitively exclude suicide because these fractures occur in approximately 12.5% of cases. In addition to this, only 20% of homicides have no injuries other than those of the strangulation, which is the case in 80% of the suicides. There is usually additional evidence of abuse and blunt force trauma in most homicide cases.[15]

When comparing the noose knots in homicide and suicide, the use of only one ligature occurs in the vast majority of both types of cases. Because it is possible for a person to wrap material around his or her own neck several times, the number of ligatures and the presence of repeated knotting is not necessarily indicative of homicide. When suicide victims tie the knots, the knots are most often present in the frontal or lateral neck regions, but there have been cases in which the person tied the knots at the back of the neck.[25]

The final type of strangulation is manual strangulation. This is virtually always a homicide. When a victim is asphyxiating, loss of consciousness occurs before death. After a victim loses consciousness, if asphyxiation continues, in the case of manual strangulation by continued pressure on the ligature, death will occur. Because a suicide victim would release his or her grip on the ligature upon a loss of consciousness, suicide is not possible in this manner. Like ligature strangulations, these victims appear congested with the presence of petechiae on the face. These victims also have abrasions and fingernail marks caused by both the perpetrator and their own hands during the struggle. There is also the presence of semicircular finger marks on the neck from the applied pressure and underlying neck trauma such as muscle hemorrhage and cartilage fractures.[15]

As stated earlier, asphyxiation cases often have little in the way of definitive forensic evidence. Rather, each case must be evaluated from all sides before reasonable conclusions can be reached. It is often the situation and the mental state of the person that provide more clues than the forensics.

Autoerotic Asphyxiation

When you consider suicide related to asphyxia, the special case of autoerotic asphyxiation must be addressed. Autoerotic asphyxiation is the practice of using some injurious instrument, such as a rope around the neck or a plastic bag over the head, during sexual stimulation to cause cerebral hypoxia and bring about a profound sexual euphoria. The intent of the victim is not to commit suicide; however, miscalculation by the individual or failure of the device to release results in unconsciousness and death. The circumstances in which one finds the body often makes this an easy incident to confuse as either homicide or suicide.[26,27]

Autoerotic asphyxiation is not a new phenomenon and has been described by anthropologists and in literature for centuries. However, its prevalence has been overlooked until rather recently. In the United States, it is estimated that approximately 1000 deaths every year can be attributed to this form of sexual practice. Usually, the practice is kept secret from others, and oftentimes the person is not discovered until they have died as a result of the practice.[26,28]

The predominant practitioners of this in North America are white males between the ages of 15 and 25 years. Although women have been shown to engage in this practice, the ratio of males to females is greater than 50:1. It occurs among people of all socioeconomic backgrounds, and the men are often happily married with several children. Evidence shows that the practice has been increasing over the past 25 years. This may be in part attributed to the fact that the practice is more well known, leading some to try it out of curiosity.[28]

Men engage in autoerotic asphyxiation in different ways based on age and experience. Because the behavior is repetitive, it tends to become more complex in older individuals. Preadolescent boys are often found fully clothed and the noose is simple in nature. For teenagers, the genitals are usually exposed and the victim is often found with pornographic materials. Older men often have more complex mechanisms for asphyxia and demonstrate a tendency for transvestitism and masochism.[28]

When you encounter a typical scene of autoerotic asphyxiation, several clues can help you to indicate it was a suicide rather than a homicide. People who practice autoerotic asphyxiation are usually found in secluded locations because secrecy is very important to the practice. A typical scenario is a door barred from the inside. Most cases involve incomplete hanging of the individual, although cases of inhalant use, suffocation, and chest compression have been documented.[28] The hanging construction usually includes a release or escape mechanism or some way for the individual to control the amount of asphyxia. One example case showed a male with a noose around his neck that was wrapped over a rod in the closet and then tied to the victim's left wrist so that he could control the pressure exerted. Also of important note, there is usually evidence that the act was repetitive. In the same case, the victim's closet rod had evidence of old abrasions showing that it had been used multiple times for the hanging practice.[26] Another major commonality is that the hanging device is usually padded so as to reduce the evidence of furrow marks on the user's neck.[26–28]

Male participants are often found wearing women's clothing, with pornographic materials, and in various permutations of masochism. Males may be found with foreign bodies in their rectums, electrodes attached to their genitals for stimulation, or sitting in front of a mirror. Mirrors have also been implicated in suicides, however—and you should be careful not to jump to conclusions.[27,28] Also, evidence of masturbation and seminal fluid exists in these cases. This should be interpreted with care because the ejection of seminal fluid can occur in any form of death secondary to rigor mortis.[26]

Women who engage in this type of behavior differ in several respects from their male counterparts. In most cases, women will rarely use unusual attire, pornography, or masochism. Most women are typically found with a simple ligature around their neck. The only clues to differentiate these cases from homicide tend to be the barred room, evidence of repetitive nature, padded ligature device, and some escape device.[28]

Because many of the findings described are not uniformly present in all cases of autoerotic asphyxiation, differentiating it from a suicide can sometimes be difficult on forensic grounds. Often further psychological information is needed to aid in the diagnosis. The differentiation from a homicide is often determined from the evidence of a struggle. If there are fingernail marks indicating the person had been trying to tear the instrument off, homicide should instead be suspected.[28]

Death by Stabbing or Piercing Object

Suicide by stabbing is a rarely used and very dramatic-appearing scene among causes of death. Often, when presented with this scenario, it is not always immediately clear whether the death was suicide or homicide. If there is a question of this, several clues can lead the physician to a conclusion.

When completed suicides are examined, this method is an uncommon choice among both sexes. Stabbing death accounts for only 1.8–2% of suicide mortality. Men predominantly use this method; however, the number of females who use this method increases if you also include attempted suicides without true self-destructive intent. Younger females often use cutting as a "cry for help" because the degree of cutting can be directed and made to different grades, giving the person more control over the amount of injury.[9,29]

When a person decides to use this method, the instrument chosen is often one of convenience. The type of killing strike can be broadly divided into *suicidal stabs* and *suicidal incisions*. A stab wound occurs when the weapon is driven into the body. When a suicide victim decides to use a stabbing motion, most often the site of choice is the left chest with the intent of stabbing through the heart. The head, the neck, and the abdomen are rarely choices for a stab site. A suicidal incision is when the blade is dragged across the skin. When suicide victims choose this method, they use an easily accessible area and clearly prefer the wrist or the antecubital fossa. Right-handed individuals are more likely to cut the left side and vice versa. Some people will cut both sides.[10]

To differentiate between homicide and suicide in questionable cases, several factors must be examined and considered. A thorough investigation involves the victim, the victim's mental state, the location, and the types of wounds inflicted. When considering these factors together, you can often reconstruct the incident.

When stabbing victims are compared, several factors can help differentiate suicide from homicide. In most studies, the percentage of men in the suicide group is greater. There is also an age difference between the two groups, with the suicide group composed of older people (in their 40s and 50s). The younger population instead tend to be victims of homicide. However, stabbing deaths routinely occur across a broad range of ages. Although previous suicide attempt, alcohol, and drug use have been cited as risk factors for repeat attempts, many suicide by stabbing victims have no risk factors. So, although all three of these risk factors were present for some suicide victims, their absence does not preclude the determination of suicide. A suicide note is, of course, highly predictive of a suicide, but they are left by a minority of victims.[29–31]

Both victims of suicide and homicide tend to be found at home, and in the overwhelming number of stabbing cases the instrument was a knife, usually a kitchen knife. This is usually a result of the convenience of obtaining such an instrument.[31]

The wound pattern often demonstrates the nature of the victim's death. Many suicides have fewer wounds than homicide victims do, with the suicide victim usually having one fatal wound or bilateral arm involvement. The larger number of homicide wounds is related to the patient sustaining multiple defensive wounds prior to the mortal wound. The presence of multiple cuts and stabs to a patient's arms and hands indicates that the victim was attempting to shield himself or herself from a perpetrator at the time of the incident and is highly suggestive of homicide. These wounds may be either stab or incised wounds and most often occur in the upper extremity. It is rare to see lower extremity defensive wounds, although it does occur. The presence of slashes in addition to stab wounds is also high suggestive of homicide.[11]

The neck, the wrists, the heart area, and the epigastrium are the most frequent areas chosen for suicide stabs whereas the shoulders, lower extremities, and buttocks are among the most rarely targeted areas. Prior to the final mortal blow in suicide, some victims show hesitation marks, which are shallow cuts directly adjacent to the final cut and highly indicative of suicide. Hesitation marks most often occur when a person cuts the wrists or neck, and they are usually multiple and parallel to the deeper mortal cut. The number of cuts varies from person to person. It is important to note that hesitation marks may also be present in incised neck wounds in a homicide; in this case, they are caused by the victim's struggling or attempting to pull away from the assailant.[11]

When examining the cut throat of suicide versus homicide victims, the direction of the cuts gives clues to the incident. In right-handed victims, the cuts are often the deepest on the left side, and then tail off. They often pass obliquely through the larynx of the individual. In homicides, the orientation varies depending on whether the strike occurred from the front or from behind. When the incision occurs from behind, the wound usually begins at the ear opposite the hand holding the knife, continues across the neck in a horizontal fashion, and ends on the opposite side usually at a point lower than the initial cut. The deepest portion of the cut in this case is at the larynx. If cut from the front, the wound is often short and angled. Many times, multiple irregular wounds that tend to skid away from the main cut are caused by movement of the victim.[11]

In questionable cases, the orientation of the wounds also demonstrates the type of incident. For a suicide victim, it is much easier to hold a knife in a horizontal fashion and attempt to maneuver between the ribs while trying to stab in the chest. These people tend to hold the knife in the right hand or with both hands to access the heart. They also attempt to stab upward from the subcostal region. Suicide victims usually have only one fatal strike to the heart because this type of blow makes it unlikely that they could continue the act. In contrast, the homicide victim often has wounds in a vertical pattern because this is the normal orientation of the blade when gripped by another person. Homicide victims also tend to have multiple fatal strikes; however, there are known cases of suicide in which the person had multiple fatal strikes to the body.[29–31]

Surprisingly enough, damage to the clothing is also highly predictive of whether a case is homicide or suicide. Many suicide victims expose the area that they are preparing to stab, so they sustain no damage to their clothing. By contrast, most homicide victims have cuts through their clothing. Also, if the cut was made in the clothing, the relationship of the clothes to the wound should be examined. In cases where a struggle occurred, the clothing may have been moved while fighting the assailant, resulting in anatomic wound location not corresponding to cuts in the clothing. Although the absence of damage to the surrounding clothing is not 100% predictive, it is suggestive of suicide.[29–31]

To truly differentiate, the factors must all be taken together, along with what is known by witnesses and the police, to construct a complete picture of what happened. Exceptions to all the stated differences between suicides and homicides have been noted in all studies of the subject.

Drowning Suicides

Suicide by immersion in water poses many challenges when trying to determine the manner of death. No specific test can confirm that the method of death was drowning. As a diagnosis, it is one of exclusion. The diagnosis of drowning is made only after autopsy and toxicology testing have not determined the cause. Also, there is often no perceivable difference between an accidental, suicidal, or homicidal drowning.[32]

This method of suicide has a high variability from area to area. For obvious reasons, it is much higher in coastal areas and areas bordering large bodies of water. Although the method is used by both sexes, there is a preponderance of white males older than 40 years. Drugs and alcohol are sometimes involved, but in many cases the person had a negative toxicology at the time of death.[11]

When trying to differentiate a suicide from a homicide from an accident, only a few physical clues can help. In suicides, many times this is not the victim's first attempt and the body may have evidence of previous attempts such as scars on the wrists. Also, a suicide does not have further injuries indicating the struggle that would have taken place in a homicide. However, if the person had been incapacitated entering the water, there also would be no evidence of a struggle. Although it is far from universal, suicide victims will often remove their coats, hats, and glasses prior to entering the water.[33]

When considering any drowning death, the physician should always take into account the psychiatric history of the patient. Prior suicide attempts and the presence of a note point toward suicide. The physician should also inquire as to whether the patient knew how to swim.[32]

Many times when a body is found with weights tied to it, the immediate conclusion is homicide. This is not always true because there have been several documented cases of suicide in which the person used weights to hold himself or herself down. If weights are tied to the body, you must consider whether the person would have been able to carry and attach them without any assistance.[32]

Drug Abuse Suicides

In drug-related fatalities, the state of mind of the victim is paramount in discovering whether the case is a suicide or accidental in nature. A large overdose of prescription medications, other than controlled substances, usually raises suspicions of suicide and not an accidental death. Often, the victim may have abused illegal drugs or controlled substances prior to the event, making it very difficult to determine in these scenarios. To determine whether the death was related to drug misuse or abuse or whether the death was the intention, it is often necessary to try to reconstruct the person's state of mind just prior to death. Because of the often ambiguous nature of drug-related deaths, many times these cases are labeled as "could not be determined." For example, in studies of drug-related deaths in 2003, 75% of cases in Maryland and more than 90% of cases in Utah were classified in this manner. As with all suicides, presence of a note or previous suicide attempts can aid in clarifying the matter.

Single-Vehicle Accidents

Car accidents are not generally thought of as a means of suicide. However, we do recognize a car as a weapon in cases of homicide. People can be convicted of vehicular manslaughter or even murder for actions while driving. So, because a vehicle can be viewed as a weapon, and one with a high degree of lethality, the information necessary to determine if an automobile crash is actually a suicide is the driver's intent. Proof of intent is rarely present, unless suicide committers leave a note (which happens in less than 25% of cases) or call someone to explain their actions.[34]

Situations that raise suspicion of suicide are accidents that contain no evidence that the driver attempted to avoid the accident or brake, accidents that occur after the individual received bad news, when victims have legal or financial issues, and when the victim was known to have a psychiatric history and recent deterioration. A few studies have looked at the drivers of single-car, single-occupant fatal accidents and characterize the victims as young, male, unmarried, with prior traffic violations and shown to have been driving at excessive speeds. These risk taking behaviors do lead to more accidents, but risk taking behavior may also be an expression of self-destructive behavior. Individuals may choose this manner because a car is easily accessible and offers an opportunity to risk death spontaneously and without consciously viewing it as suicide.[34] It is also a way to hide a suicide so that the stigma, moral, legal, and insurance issues are avoided. One study found that 2.7% of single-car fatal accidents were actually suicide.[35] Even when suicide is a high suspicion, though, the case will be listed as "accidental" or "unable to be determined" unless proof of intent is found.[34]

SUICIDE AND THE EMERGENCY DEPARTMENT

What happens when a possible suicide presents to the emergency department? As medical providers, we may feel angry or frustrated with the person for the damage they have inflicted upon themselves. We may have personal beliefs or opinions that we have to keep from expressing or may feel like our efforts to save someone who "wants to die" are in vain. Most medical providers' exposure to suicide is during their short time on the psychiatry ward during medical training. At that time, as it is in much of the literature, suicide is viewed from the standpoint of prevention. But what happens when it is an active event occurring in front of your eyes? How do you treat the patient? What happens if your medical care fails and the suicide is successful? How do you address concerns that a death may have been a suicide?

In medicine, we believe that to the best of our abilities we should treat anyone brought to us for care. This can occasionally put us in awkward positions: treating the gunshot victim and the shooter, treating a convicted criminal, an enemy soldier or terrorist, or treating someone who does not want to live. This last situation presents itself during a suicide attempt. We may be required to expend significant resources to save the life of a person that just inflicted the injury on himself or herself. We must not be cynical or judgmental in these cases. Our most important job after an attempted suicide is to perform a medical or traumatic resuscitation as we would in any other case. Modern advances in EMS systems, advanced cardiac life support (ACLS), and trauma care may be the direct cause of the decrease in the overall suicide rate.

If the medical care fails and the patient expires, the physician should report the case to the local Death Investigation System (coroner or ME). Most jurisdictions require official notification of any unexpected or suspicious death. Next, the physician should focus on the forensic investigation to follow. The physician is not required to conduct the investigation but should take several simple steps (discussed in the following paragraph) to aid the accuracy of the findings. Many physicians feel intimidated by the legal process. Others feel it is not part of their job; they think their duty is to treat a patient, but once the patient expires, the job ends. Some feel that protecting forensic evidence will take an excess of their time during and after patient care. However, we must remember that as members of the medical community we also have a responsibility to address medical issues that can affect our local population. An unexpected death such as a suicide has effects beyond just the victim: Family and close contacts of a suicide might develop the need for counseling; justice and community safety can be at stake if the case turns out to be homicide rather than suicide; and correct epidemiologic data aid prevention programs.

The biggest aid to the death investigation is a well-documented chart. Ideally, every chart is documented completely, but when a suspicious death is involved, we should take extra care to be thorough. Comprehensive documentation should have three components: narrative, diagrammatic, and photographic.[36] The narrative should be detailed and objective. An important piece is history and information from other sources including family, friends, police, and emergency medical services (EMS). Collecting and documenting their input and the identity of the source while the case is fresh can be very valuable. Notes on the victim's recent behavior and demeanor can give insight to possible mind-set and intent just prior to the event. However, documentation should avoid legal conclusions. It is acceptable to express clinical opinions if they are based on and consistent with the facts and findings.

To supplement the narrative documentation, diagrams can add details that may be difficult or lengthy to describe. Many charts have human body outlines that allow for easy documentation of location and type of wound, especially when the wounds are numerous. Also, the irregular shapes of wounds can be shown. Diagrams, however, should only supplement written documentation, not stand alone because they may cause confusion without a corresponding narrative.[8]

Photographic documentation is gaining use in emergency departments possibly because of the ease of use of digital photography. Reasons to use photography include for documenting evidence or injuries that will be affected by medical treatment, for documenting lesser features of an injury, or as a reference and memory aid.[36] Photographs, if properly obtained, can be a powerful tool in a death investigation or any other legal proceeding. The photo should be an accurate portrayal of the subject matter. A complete lesson in forensic photography is beyond the scope of this chapter, but the following few simple points should be remembered. Forensic photos should have a picture area mostly filled by the injury. Photos should be in focus and show details of the injury. The background should be plain and not include any people, medical instruments, or bloody gauze or material. A small ruler or some other easily recognizable reference of size, such as a coin, in the same plane as the wound should be included. The photograph must be taken at 90° from the subject so as to not distort the scale. Finally, to document an injury or wound completely, a photograph record should show the location on the body, the size, and the details of the wound. This usually requires three photos: a distant "staging" photo, a medium-range photo, and a close-up with scale to show details. Similar to diagrams, photographic documentation is a supplement to the narrative description and the two should correspond. Finally, in suicide cases, after the death of a patient, consent is not required and taking photographs for the purpose of investigating the death or education is accepted practice.[35]

Evidence preservation is also important to the death investigation. When the medical team understands a few forensic principles, simple steps can be taken to help the investigation that will not interfere with patient care. For clothing, remember these guidelines:

- Avoid cutting through holes created by gunshots or knife wounds.[8] A natural tendency is to start cutting clothing at the hole, but the size, shape, and edges of the hole will be ruined for the forensic examination.
- Pack pieces of clothing separately to avoid cross-contamination of blood or ballistic residue.
- Avoid placing clothing in plastic bags. If moist or bloody clothing is placed in plastic bags and closed, the moisture leads to mold development that destroys the evidence. Clothing should be placed in paper bags, closed, and tagged with the patient name for later collection by the police or ME.[8]

Following are other guidelines:

- Place paper bags over the hands of self-inflicted gunshot wound (GSW) victims to protect the area for a gunshot residue test later.[36]
- Avoid washing areas of the body unless medically necessary because blood patterns and weapon residue may be washed off.
- If objects such as bullets are removed from the victim, handle them only with gloved hands or gauze-covered instruments. Metal to metal contact can destroy the microscopic markings on bullets that identify the gun from which they were fired.
- Avoid rubbing bullets to clean them, and do not place bullets in airtight containers. Place bullets in a paper envelope or cardboard box, document the location from which the projectile was removed, and seal the container until handed over to the police.[8]
- The chain of evidence is important in legal cases, and evidence should be kept in one person's possession until signed over to and accepted by the police.[36] Medical departments should have a written protocol for who (physician, charge nurse, security) is responsible for evidence when it is collected.

CONCLUSION

Suicide is a tragic situation for those left behind. Investigation of a death should always be sensitive to the grief of those close to the deceased and should never become an inquisition of the survivors or a trial of the victim's every past deed. As a leading cause of death in the United States, suicide is a part of society, a major public health problem, and therefore a legitimate focus of study.[2] The first step in suicide prevention is to understand the size of the problem. To study suicide, we must first be able to separate suicide deaths from accidents and homicides. Forensic death investigation is an important part of the scientific approach to the medical process. The study of injury patterns and death may not help the victim, but it adds to the overall knowledge base and ultimately may prevent future illness and death.

REFERENCES

1. Rosenberg ML, Davidson LE, Smith JC, Berman AL, Buzbee H, Gantner G, Gay GA, Moore-Lewis B, Mills DH, Murray D, O'Carroll PW, Jobes D. Operational criteria for the determination of suicide. *J Forensic Sci.* 1998;33(6):1445–1456.
2. Kung HS, Hoyert DL, Xu J, Murphy SL. Deaths: final data for 2005. National Vital Statistics Reports, 2008; 56(10). Available at: http://www.cdc.gov/nchs/data/nvsr/nvsr56/nvsr56_10.pdf. Retrieved February 12, 2008.
3. Minois G. *History of Suicide: Voluntary Death in Western Culture.* Baltimore, Md: Johns Hopkins University Press; 1999.
4. National Institute of Mental Health. *Suicide in the US: Statistics and Prevention.* NIH Publication No. 06-4594. Available at: http://www.nimh.nih.gov/publicat/harmsway.cfm. Retrieved July 24, 2008.
5. Sher L. Alcohol consumption and suicide. *Q J Med.* 2006;99:57–61.
6. McKeown RE, Cuffe SP, Schulz RM. US suicide rates by age group, 1970–2002: an examination of recent trends. *Am J Public Health.* 2006;96(10):1744–1751.
7. Centers for Disease Control and Prevention, National Center for Health Statistics. National Vital Statistics System, mortality data. Available at: http://www.cdc.gov/nchs/deaths.htm. Retrieved July 24, 2008.
8. Ryan MT, Houry DE. Clinical forensic medicine. *Ann Emerg Med.* September 2000;36(3):271–273.
9. Randall B. *Death Investigation: The Basics.* Tucson, Ariz: Galen Press; 1997.
10. Ajdacic-Gross V, Killias M, Hepp U, Gadola E, Bopp M, Lauber C, Schnyder U, Gutzwiller F, Rossler W. Changing times: a longitudinal analysis of international firearm suicide data. *Am J Public Health.* October 2006;96(10):1752–1755.
11. Knight B. *Simpson's Forensic Medicine.* 11th ed. Hodder Arnold Publishing, London, England; 1997.
12. Spitz W, ed. *Spitz and Fischer's Medicolegal Investigation of Death.* 4th ed. Springfield, Ill: Charles C Thomas; 2006:607–611.
13. Karger B, Billeb E, Koops E, Brinkmann B. Autopsy features relevant for discrimination between suicidal and homicidal gunshot injuries. *Int J Legal Med.* October 2002;116(5):273–278.
14. Karlsson T. Multivariate analysis: a new tool in forensic medicine. Differentiation between firearm related homicide and suicide. *Forensic Sci Int.* April 1999;101(2):131–140.
15. DiMaio V, et al. *Handbook of Forensic Pathology.* New York, NY: Taylor and Francis; 2007:107–152.
16. Garavaglia JC. Weapon location following suicidal gunshot wounds. *Am J Forensic Med Pathol.* March 1999;20(1):1–5.
17. Stone IC. Characteristics of firearm and gunshot wounds as markers of suicide. *Am J Forensic Med Pathol.* December 1992;13(4):275–280.
18. Mohandie K, Meloy JR. Clinical and forensic indicators of suicide by cop. *J Forensic Sci.* 2000;45:384–389.
19. Hutson HR, Anglin D, Yarbrough J, et al. Suicide by cop. *Ann Emerg Med.* 1998;32:665–669.
20. Wilson EF, Davis JH, Bloom JD, et al. Homicide or suicide: the killing of suicidal persons by law enforcement officers. *J Forensic Sci.* 1998;43:46–52.
21. *Random House Unabridged Dictionary.* New York, NY: Random House Reference; 2006.
22. Fishbain DA, Fletcher JR, Aldrich TE, et al. Relationship between Russian roulette deaths and risk-taking behavior: a controlled study. *Am J Psychiatry.* 1987;144:563–567.
23. Denny KM. Russian roulette: a case of questions not asked? *J Am Acad Child Adolesc Psychiatry.* 1995;34:1682–1683.
24. Guarner J, et al. Suicide by hanging: a review of 56 cases. *Am J Forensic Med Pathol.* 1987;8(1):23–26.
25. Maxeiner H, et al. Homicidal and suicidal ligature strangulation: a comparison of post-mortem findings. *Forensic Sci Int.* 2003;137(1):60–66.
26. Garza-Leal JA, Landron FJ. Autoerotic asphyxial death initially misinterpreted as suicide and a review of the literature. *J Forensic Sci.* November 1991;36(6):1753–1759.
27. Tournel G, Hubert N, Rouge C, Hedouin V, Gosset D. Complete autoerotic asphyxiation: suicide or accident? *Am J Forensic Med Pathol.* June 2001;22(2):180–183.
28. Gosink PD, Jumbelic MI. Autoerotic asphyxiation in a female. *Am J Forensic Med Pathol.* June 2000;21(2):114–118.
29. Scolan V, et al. Homicide-suicide by stabbing study over 10 years in the Tolouse region. *Am J Forensic Med Pathol.* March 2004;25:33–36.
30. Byard R, et al. Clinicopathologic feature of fatal self-inflicted incised and stab wounds: a 20 year study. *Am J Forensic Med Pathol.* March 2002;23:15–18.
31. Karlsson T, Isaksson B, Ormstad K. Patterns of sharp force fatalities: a comprehensive forensic medical study. J Forensic Sci. March 1988;33:448–461.
32. Wirthwein DP, Barnard JJ, PRahlow JA. Suicide drowning: a 20-year review. *J Forensic Sci.* January 2002;47:131–136.
33. Byard R, et al. Characteristics of suicidal drownings: a 20-year study. *Am J Forensic Med Pathol.* June 2001;22(2):134–138.
34. Peck DL. Accident or suicide? single-vehicle accidents and the intent hypothesis. *Adolescence.* Summer 1995.
35. Schmidt CW Jr, Shaffer JW, Zlotowitz HI, Fisher RS. Suicide by vehicular crash. *Am J Psychiatry.* 1977;134:175–178.
36. Olshaker JS, Jackson MC, Smock WS. *Forensic Emergency Medicine.* Philadelphia, Pa: Lippincott Williams & Wilkins; 2007.

4 | Evidence Collection and Preservation in the ED

Shannon L. Maier, MS, BSN, RN, and Jennifer Barger, MS, BSN, RN

Physical evidence cannot be intimidated. It does not forget. It sits there and waits to be detected, preserved, evaluated, and explained.

—Herbert Leon MacDonell, *The Evidence Never Lies*

INTRODUCTION

This chapter is intended to be a guideline for all hospital personnel and is not intended to meet specific requirements of various jurisdictions or to override existing hospital policy. When developing emergency department (ED) forensic policies, it is helpful to involve all the key players, including the police department, crime lab, and district attorney. Internally, representatives from the ED, trauma service, security department, and risk management/legal office should be involved. Policy should focus on defining what evidence is pertinent in specific cases and include the best method to preserve, package, and collect that evidence.

All emergency department personnel should have some type of formal forensic education and training. This can be provided during initial orientation to the ED. Yearly mandatory educational sessions of the staff are crucial to ensure competency. It is the authors' position that all emergency departments should have at least one forensically trained nurse.

Healthcare professionals are increasingly faced with victims of violence, and the need for proper forensic evidence collection and preservation is critical. The process of forensic evidence collection and preservation is just another aspect of the healthcare professional's responsibility to advocate for patients. But remember, your patient may be the perpetrator and not the victim.

THE VICTIM OF VIOLENCE

Recognizing that an ED patient is a victim of violence is often the first hurdle. The multiple variants of a violent crime cannot be detailed in precise terms, but the following list includes examples of cases for which evidence can and should be collected:

- Sexual assault
- Abuse
- Suspicious deaths or traumas
- Motor vehicle versus pedestrian
- Interpersonal violence
- Drug involvement
- Attempted suicide or homicides
- Death or injury of unknown causation

The guidance of policy, procedure, and standards put forth by the healthcare institution and the logical determination of the healthcare provider can help these victims be recognized.

Mandatory reporting of abuse, such as abuse of a child, elderly person, or person with disabilities, is covered by the law and is not a breach of patient confidentiality. Other reporting of violent crimes varies state by state, and in the situation of interpersonal violence, you must be careful and dutiful of the privacy of the victim.[1]

TOOLS FOR PROCESSING THE PATIENT

It is important to know that your patient and all of his or her belongings now constitute a crime scene. It can benefit the emergency department as a whole to have the evidence collection materials in one easily accessible area—a bag, large plastic tote, or wheeled cart all may be used. Table 4-1 lists suggested items to keep in the department evidence collection kit.

Medical evaluation and intervention and forensic evidence collection can be done in conjunction with one another. It is imperative to understand that medical intervention takes precedence over evidence collection. It is highly recommended that a designated forensic nurse take primary responsibility for evidence collection, thus maintaining the chain of custody.

PROCESSING THE PATIENT AS A CRIME SCENE

When conducting an examination of the patient, make a thorough inspection. *Forensic evaluation* refers to the detection, collection, and preservation of evidence. Pattern injury recognition, interpretation of injuries, documentation of testimonial and injuries (including photography), reporting requirements, and regulations are all vital components of a forensic evaluation. Optimally, at least two emergency department personnel should be involved during the initial patient evaluation. One should be conducting the medical evaluation and the other conducting the forensic evaluation. Once the forensic evaluation begins, it is crucial that the health professional doing the forensic evaluation stays with the evidence collected to maintain chain of custody. Example case studies are discussed later in the chapter.

Take note of the patient's general appearance. During the examination, be sure to note the patient's demeanor and

TABLE 4-1 **Suggested Items for Forensic Evidence Kit**

Item	Explanation
Brown bags (various sizes)	Maintain forensic integrity of separated items Smaller bags used for preservation of gunshot residue (GSR) on hands
Evidence tape	Seal and maintain integrity of items collected
Sterile cotton-tip applicators	Sample body fluids and unknown materials
Distilled water	Premoisten swabs or gauze; seal envelopes
Coin envelopes	Store trace evidence and/or missiles
Specimen containers	For storage of smaller evidence
Sterile gauze	For padding of missile in specimen container Premoistened for body fluid retrieval
Sticky notes	Collect trace evidence with sticky side folded inward, and then package in coin envelope
Camera	Photodocument injury
Gray scale ruler	Assists photographing dimensional injuries Serves as reminder to photograph all injuries parallel to film plane
Powderless gloves	Must be changed frequently to avoid cross-contamination
Alternate light source/Wood's lamp	Assist with visualization of biological evidence
Lint roller	For trace evidence pickup, helpful for glass pieces
Silk tape	For trace evidence pickup
Plastic tweezers	Pick up trace evidence
Rubber-tipped forceps	Maintain individual missile markings

statements that are made, using quotations whenever possible. The patient should be completely undressed and all body surfaces inspected. When removing the patient's clothing, immediately separate each piece into brown paper bags. Using plastic bags to store clothing is not recommended because the plastic can trap moisture that can cause mildew and biological breakdown.[2] If clothing is wet, package the items with a sterile drape between folds. Realistically, wet clothing should be air-dried before packaging. In a "controlled chaotic" environment such as the emergency department, this is often extremely difficult to do, if done at all. In this case, it is appropriate to package the items in separate brown bags, and then place them in a red biohazard bag. Notify law enforcement to process the items immediately to avoid degradation of biological evidence.

Try to keep the clothing in its original state; avoid folding, shaking, and manipulating it. Trace evidence does not need to be removed unless there is a fear it will be lost. Once clothing is collected in bags, seal each bag with evidence tape; label, initial, date, and write the time on the label. Mark the contents of each bag either on the bag itself, in the chart, or even better, on an evidence collection form (Figure 4-1). Weapons, money, and drug paraphernalia must be immediately secured by either law enforcement or hospital security. If such a policy is not in place, one needs to be drafted and put into practice.

Victims of violent crimes in the emergency department should receive the same diligence of evidence collection up to the point of expiration. Once pronounced dead, evidence collection can be halted. What has been collected should be accounted for, packaged, labeled, sealed, dated, and timed. If possible, the hands of victims involved in firearm-related cases should be placed in brown paper bags secured around the wrists with rubber bands. This preserves not only trace evidence but also possible gunshot residue (GSR) that indicates whether the person has recently fired a weapon.[3]

CHAIN OF CUSTODY

Chain of custody (Figure 4-2) is a record that identifies each person that comes in contact with evidence. It is a paper trail that maintains the integrity of the evidence by documenting patient name, medical record number, and the date and time the evidence was transferred to another party. The department should work with local law enforcement officials and risk management personnel in developing a chain of custody policy and standard form that can be used in all cases.

A number of individuals have the potential to handle evidence, so if at all possible, it is best to designate one person to collect the specimens and label them. Anyone else who handles the final collection of evidence must be documented appropriately on an accompanying evidence collection form (Figure 4-1). The chain of custody form maintains that one individual has been overseeing the evidence and ensuring that it has not been tampered with or disrupted in any way. If law enforcement is unavailable for immediate retrieval, it is recommended that evidence be stored in a locked cabinet, drawer, refrigerator, or closet with limited key access. Ideally, a forensic nurse or hospital security officer should be the custodian of the key and signatures should be required each time the key changes hands. Failure to maintain an appropriate chain of custody can allow the evidence to become null and void in a court of law.

CONCLUSION

"Recommendations have been made by the Joint Commission on Accreditation of Healthcare Organizations (JCAHO) regarding the management of forensic cases within health care institutions providing patient care."[4] Patient advocacy through diligent documentation and care is the primary goal of healthcare professionals. Often the law and health care coexist for one reason or another. Now more than ever, it is important to embrace forensics and incorporate it into the practice of all emergency departments. Through forensics and proper evidence collection and preservation, we can give victims the voice that they may not have otherwise.

CASE STUDY 1

A woman is the victim of a hit-and-run accident as she crossed a busy intersection. The EMS providers have cut her clothing off, and it is laying underneath the patient. The trauma team is present upon patient arrival in the ED.

What forensic information would be crucial to collect on this patient?

Documentation

You should record the patient's general condition and demeanor upon arrival. Also record any statements about the incident that the victim makes.

Clothing

In this particular case, the evidence obtained from clothing can range from paint chips, glass, hair, fibers, and other trace elements. Paint chip evidence may indicate a specific model or type of vehicle. The Paint Data Query (PDQ) is a database that provides information on paint composition, color, paint layer sequence, and source of paint.[5] A less used method, since the advent of the PDQ and streamlining of auto paints, is a catalog encompassing the paint chip, vehicle identification number (VIN), paint layer sequence, and information about the car itself.[5]

Collection of glass may help determine the part of the vehicle that impacted the patient. Glass is manufactured in different ways, for example, when different elements are mixed together during the manufacturing process and in the way the glass is annealed or cooled. Examples are laminated glass that is used in the front and back windshields, tempered glass that is used in the side windows and that cubes when broken, and the vehicle headlamps that have extra borosilicate added to make them more heat resistant.[5]

[PATIENT LABEL]

Evidence Collection Form

CLOTHING

- ❑ Jacket ______
- ❑ Shirt ______
- ❑ Undershirt ______
- ❑ Bra ______
- ❑ Pants ______
- ❑ Underwear ______
- ❑ Socks ______
- ❑ Nightgown/Pajamas ______
- ❑ Other: ______
- ❑ Other: ______

MISCELLANEOUS EVIDENCE

- ❑ None ______
- ❑ Bullet(s) ______
- ❑ Glass ______
- ❑ Paint ______
- ❑ Firearm(s) ______
- ❑ Arson Evidence ______
- ❑ Other: ______
- ❑ Other: ______

PHOTOGRAPHS

Taken: ❑ Yes No ❑ ______

Type: ❑ Digital Camera ❑ Polaroid ❑ Film

Number of Photographs: ______

Photographer(s): ______

PERSON COMPLETING FORM:

Print ______

Signature ______

Date ______

Time ______

FIGURE 4-1 **Sample evidence collection form.**

[PATIENT LABEL]

Chain of Custody

All items listed are labeled and sealed.

Name: ______________________________

To: ______________________________ Title/Badge # ____________

Date: ____________ Time: ____________

Signature: ____________________ / ____________________

Name: ______________________________

To: ______________________________ Title/Badge # ____________

Date: ____________ Time: ____________

Signature: ____________________ / ____________________

Name: ______________________________

To: ______________________________ Title/Badge # ____________

Date: ____________ Time: ____________

Signature: ____________________ / ____________________

FIGURE 4-2 **Sample chain of custody form.**

You should collect the clothing from under the patient, placing a clean sheet under her instead. Place each article of clothing in a pile to be packaged. It is much more helpful to have brown paper bags, preferably seamless, open and ready for the clothing items to be dropped in separately. Seal each bag with evidence tape and label, date, and initial them.

Trace Evidence

Trace evidence can be found on or around the woman's body. Many medical professionals use the adhesive edge of silk tape to pick up glass shards and pieces that may interfere with medical intervention, especially around the head. A lint roller can also be used. Used silk tape should be folded on itself and placed in a coin envelope (use distilled or sterile water to seal envelope) or a specimen container. The sheet the patient is lying on can contain forensic evidence as well and should be collected in a brown bag. Again, it should be labeled and sealed with evidence tape.

Photographs

You can photograph patterned injuries while the patient is being grossly examined. Patterned injury could include a car emblem imprint, or if the patient was run over, you could potentially photograph tire imprints. Patient consent should be obtained prior to taking photographs. If photographic capabilities do not exist in the ED, notify the investigators so that they might be able to obtain photographs themselves.

Chain of Custody

Establishing a chain of custody should be done in conjunction with the initial documentation and as evidence collection proceeds. If law enforcement is not able to take custody of the evidence, lock the evidence in a secure, designated location per hospital policy.

CASE STUDY 2

Patient arrives in the ED via paramedics after sustaining multiple gunshot wounds. He arrives intubated with IV fluids running. His shirt has been removed, but he remains in his pants and shoes. The only history available is that someone called 9-1-1 to report hearing gunshots and the police found him lying in the street. Mechanism of injury is multiple gunshot wounds.

What forensic information would be crucial to collect on this patient?

Documentation

Record the patient's general condition and demeanor upon arrival. Also record any statements about the incident that the victim makes.

Remember: Do not document wounds as "entrance" or "exit" wounds regardless of what any staff member reports. Such wound designation is made only if the patient goes to the operating room and the surgeon documents the wound path or if the patient dies and the medical examiner determines the wound path at the time of autopsy. It is, however, very important to document the approximate size, number, and location of wounds on the body diagram. Gunshot wounds should be documented by shape and length, and presence or absence of an abrasion ring, stippling, or powder residue.

Clothing

Clothing is just as important and revealing as the wound documentation of the body. When a gun discharges, soot, powder, and hot gases are released that, when in close enough contact with a victim, can impart powerful evidence. Clothing may stop powder and soot that would wind up within or around an unclothed wound. Clothing also alters the appearance of a wound in the skin.[3] When removing clothing, do not cut through holes or deformities in the clothing; rather, cut along the seams or as far as possible from sites of possible evidence.[1]

When packaging clothing, take care to handle it as little as possible when placing each item into separate brown bags. Manipulation of the clothing, such as folding or rolling, should be done minimally so that the soot evidence can be preserved. If there are items that are fluid soaked and that cannot be air-dried, it is appropriate to package them in brown bags, and then in biohazard plastic bags. Care must be taken to immediately prioritize this evidence to law enforcement for delivery to the crime lab. Date, time, and initial each evidence bag and seal it with evidence tape.

Trace Evidence

Place brown paper bags over the patient's hands and fasten them with tape around his wrists after injury to the hands is ruled out. This preserves any gunshot residue present if the patient has recently fired a gun. Develop a protocol with your local law enforcement agency regarding this practice.

Photographs

Photo documentation can yield a concrete picture of the wound and the presence or absence of soot deposition in or around the wound. Photos help to preserve the initial integrity of the wound in case of interruption by surgical procedures and interventions.

Missiles

Collection of missiles or fragments will need special attention with respect to preservation and safety. You can collect missiles with gloved hands, but keep in mind that they may be sharp. It is the authors' suggestion to not use gloved fingers if at all possible. Instead, use plastic, padded, or rubber-tipped forceps, which maintain bullet markings that are characteristic to the gun that fired the bullet.[6]

Tissue, hair, fiber, or other trace evidence may be found on the missile. Take care to preserve this evidence by not washing or rinsing the missile, and package each item as retrieved. Place missiles in an envelope or a padded (gauze) specimen container. Document where the missile was found or retrieved, and secure each package with evidence tape. Missiles or fragments might be recovered in the operating room or might remain in the victim. A firearm may be recovered. A forensic protocol should be established with hospital security to collect the firearm as soon as it is found if law enforcement is not present.

Chain of Custody

Establishing the chain of custody should be done in conjunction with the initial documentation and as evidence collection proceeds. If law enforcement is not able to take custody of the evidence, lock it in a secure, designated location per hospital policy.

REFERENCES

1. Fisher BAJ. *Techniques of Crime Scene Investigation.* 6th ed. Boca Raton, Fla: CRC Press; 2000.
2. Assid PA. Evidence collection and documentation: are you prepared to be a medical detective (forensics in the ED)? *Top Emergency Med.* 2005;27(1):15–26.
3. Di Maio VJM. *Gunshot Wounds: Practical Aspects of Firearms, Ballistics, and Forensic Techniques.* 2nd ed. Boca Raton, Fla: CRC Press; 1999.
4. Benak LD. Forensics and the critical role of the ER nurse. *On the Edge.* 2001;7(3):1, 20-22.
5. Caddy B, ed. *Forensic Examination of Glass and Paint Analysis and Interpretation.* New York, NY: Taylor and Francis; 2001.
6. Lynch VA. Clinical forensic nursing: a new perspective in the management of crime victims from trauma to trial. *Crit Care Nurs Clin North Am.* 1995;7(3):489–507.

SUGGESTED READING

Aiken MA, Speck PM. Forensic considerations for the emergency department. *Tennessee Nurse.* 1996;59(3):19–21.

Emergency Nurses Association. *Orientation to Emergency Nursing: Concepts, Competencies, and Critical Thinking,* Des Plaines, Ill: Emergency Nurses Association; 2000:1–34.

Ledray LE, Netzel L. DNA evidence collection. *J Emerg Nurs.* 1997;23(2):156–158.

Lynch VA. *Forensic Nursing.* St. Louis, Mo: Mosby; 2006.

Russell MA, Noguchi TT. Gunshot wounds and ballistics: forensic concerns. *Top Emerg Med.* 1999;21(3):1–10.

Saferstein R. *Criminalistics: An Introduction to Forensic Science.* 9th ed. Upper Saddle River, NJ: Prentice Hall; 2003.

O'Brien CA. Forensic patients, nursing and the law. *Chart, J Illinois Nurs.* 2006;103(2):21. Available at: http://www.illinoisnurse.com.

Santucci KA, Hsaiao AL. Advances in clinical forensic medicine. *Curr Opin Pediatr.* 2003;15(3):304–308.

5 DNA

Mahshid Abir, MD

INTRODUCTION

Forensic science plays an essential role in the justice system by providing critical, scientific information to the courts. DNA technology is a powerful forensic tool that aids in convicting criminals and freeing the innocent. By 2004, 110 innocent prisoners were exonerated secondary to the use of DNA evidence.[1] Otherwise known as DNA fingerprinting, this technology provides a unique profile that can aid in the identification of individuals much in the same way as fingerprints can.[2] The importance of this technology to the field of law enforcement and criminology is demonstrated by the allocation of $1 billion by the Bush administration in 2004 toward a 5-year plan for the Department of Justice to improve DNA collection, analysis, and use in courts.[3]

Utilization of DNA evidence is now a very important aspect of forensics not only in the United States but in other industrialized nations such as the United Kingdom.[4] The realization of the power of DNA technology in crime detection has placed a significant demand on this field. A recent Attorney General report approximated a backlog of more than half a million criminal cases awaiting DNA analysis, including homicide and rape cases.[5] Cost and long processing and analysis times have been cited as causes for this backlog,[6] especially in sexual assault cases.[7–9]

SOURCES OF DNA EVIDENCE

Forensic laboratories can successfully retrieve DNA from a number of sources (see Table 5-1).[10] Studies have shown that the rate of recovery of DNA suitable for running against DNA databases similar to the Combined DNA Index System (CODIS) is highest for semen, followed by blood.[4] The importance of timely DNA collection for the ultimate successful use of this evidence in arresting offenders has been demonstrated in different studies.[11]

TABLE 5-1 **Common Sources of DNA Evidence**

Type	Possible Sources
Blood	Pools Drops Splashes Smears Taken as a reference sample by lab personnel
Saliva	Cigarette butts Skin of victim Chewing gum Eating utensils Inanimate objects
Hair	Hair roots and scalp cells around root (nuclear DNA) Hair shaft (mitochondrial DNA only) Trace evidence on victim Comb
Semen—may be liquid or dried	Vaginal, anal, or oral swabs Underwear/clothing Condom Bed linens Skin of victim Other inanimate objects
Cellular—not from any of the above DNA sources	Inanimate objects Clothing Toothbrush

HANDLING OF DNA EVIDENCE

Biological evidence needs proper collection, documentation, packaging, and preservation to meet the legal and scientific requirements for admissibility in court. Of importance are the type and amount of evidence, and the method of collection and preservation to minimize degradation. The adequate handling of biological evidence is especially critical in violent crime cases, including homicide, assault, sexual assault, child abuse, and hit-and-run accidents to preserve permissibility of the evidence.[12]

Collection

Most times, forensic examiners in the emergency department are called upon to collect DNA from sexual assault victims. However, other patients who were victims of violence or the perpetrators themselves, may present to the ED for care. The forensic examiner may be called upon to collect DNA evidence from these patients as well. The process and techniques are the same as for sexual assault victims.

The interview of a sexual assault victim should focus on the timing of the event and whether the patient showered after the incident or had other sexual contact within the preceding 72 hours (may require collection of evidence for cross-reference). Investigating a claim of sexual assault begins with the sexual assault nurse examiner (SANE) or clinician collecting evidence using an evidence collection kit. Collection of sexual assault evidence is different from evidence collection for other crimes in that medical personnel (not law enforcement) collect the evidence. Medical staff, in general, are not as familiar with evidence collection and maintenance of chain of custody when compared with law enforcement. However, trained SANEs have been found to complete more precise and comprehensive evidence kits than non-SANE trained clinicians.[13] The collection of bodily fluid, semen in particular, is very important for successful prosecution[14] where finding semen in the vagina or other orifice is taken by courts as proof of penetration.

Standardized collection protocols exist in each jurisdiction that help guide the practices of law enforcement, forensic scientists, and hospital staff. Also, sexual assault kits must be used according to the accompanying instructions. Typical specimens collected include genital, oral, anal stains and swabs; clothing of victim or suspect; foreign head or pubic hair; fibers; known hair and fiber samples; blood and saliva samples for reference from victim and suspect; and fingernail scrapings and clippings. Each swab needs to be placed in a designated cardboard box or envelope as dictated by the particular rape kit used.

Blood and other stains on the victim's skin should be collected gently to minimize collection of skin cells. Pubic combings are used to collect any foreign hair or fibers. Collection of fingernail clippings or scrapings may be indicated if you suspect that tissue from the assailant is present underneath the victim's fingernails. Minimal force should be used in collecting this evidence to decrease retrieval of the patient's skin and blood. Seminal specimen directly deposited on the patient's garment may penetrate down to underclothing. Such drainage stains must be recognized and labeled appropriately.[15]

The patient's clothing should be collected, and any tears, cuts, stains, and smears should be documented. Of note, biological evidence may be transferred by direct deposit from an individual to an object, the crime scene, or another person, or by secondary transfer via an intermediary without direct contact.

Buccal swabs are commonly collected for a comparison of a suspect's DNA with collected DNA evidence. The DNA obtained from buccal swabs is equivalent to that obtained from blood. Buccal swabs have the advantage of being less invasive to collect and less hazardous to those who collect the samples.[15]

Statutory sexual assault cases may go unreported for weeks or months. Therefore, sexual assault kits are not collected. In such cases, the products of conception may serve as proof of crime. Samples include maternal and fetal blood or aborted tissue. Because consent is not a defense, the products of conception are proof of crime. Preservatives such as formalin degrade DNA and should not be used to preserve products of conception or abortion.[16]

Documentation

Documentation of all collected evidence is of paramount importance and may determine admissibility of this evidence in court. Any injuries, markings, or stains on the patient's body should be noted and described in detail. Ideally, diagrams, sketches, and/or photographs should be used for precise documentation of the location of any findings.

Storage

The critical step after collection and documentation of evidence is appropriate storage until the specimen is transferred to the forensic lab. Every article of clothing should be packaged separately because packaging articles of clothing together can compromise evidence. Wet clothing should be air-dried prior to storing in paper packaging as opposed to plastic or other airtight containers that can retain moisture and promote bacterial growth. A cool, dry environment such as a refrigerator is the best place to keep biological evidence. Collected evidence should be submitted to a forensic lab in a timely manner.[15,16]

SEROLOGICAL SCREENING

At the turn of the 20th century, ABO blood-typing was discovered,[17] which lead to serological testing of evidence, including blood, saliva, bone, and other tissue to identify individuals involved in crimes.[18] With scientific advancement, red blood cell (RBC) antigen systems, isoenzyme markers, RBC protein variants, serum protein markers, and human leukocyte antigens (HLAs) have been used in the field of forensics.[19–21]

Variation has been detected in a number of ways, including antigen-antibody reactions such as ABO blood group system and secretor status, Rh blood typing system, HLA histocompatibility antigens, or by electrophoretic separation of isoenzymes and proteins such as PGM, ADA, or GC variants.[22–24] The use of these techniques is now limited to identifying the type of evidence (blood, saliva, semen, etc.), which then undergoes confirmatory testing to recheck for the presence of the material, and then the material is subjected to DNA testing for individualization.

Serologic screening tests, which include the reaction of the heme component of hemoglobin with chemicals such as o-toluidine, phenolphthalein (Kastle-Meyer), liminol, and tetramethylbenzidine, are very sensitive, but false-positive tests have been reported. Tests such as the Takayama microcrystal test can confirm that blood is present but do not tell if it is human blood. Immunologic, one-step methods can be used to determine whether a sample is human blood.[16]

The presence of amylase may be a clue in the detection of saliva. To detect semen, the presence of acid phosphatase can be tested for. Acid phosphatase (AP) is found throughout the body, including in saliva and vaginal secretions, but it exists in highest concentrations in secretions from the prostate gland. If a sample tests positive for AP, direct visualization of sperm with a microscope can be attempted. If the patient douched or bathed after the incident or if the rapist has had a vasectomy or has low sperm count, sperm may not be visualized. If a sample tests positive for AP and prostate-specific Ag P30, it will be retained for DNA analysis.[15]

Many different laser- and ultrasound-operated portable devices are being investigated as screening tools for detecting bloodstains, saliva, and seminal fluid. An argon ion laser light or mini crime scene scope can help the serologist locate suspected semen and saliva stains to be tested. Products such as Polilight, which is an alternative light source that uses different wavelengths of light to detect stains of different bodily fluids, are being investigated.[25] Such products may eventually replace chemical testing for these substances such as AP for semen detection and luminol for blood detection.[26–29]

DNA ANALYSIS

DNA analysis is reliable if national guidelines and standards[30] are adhered to. Genetic variability is detected through techniques such as polymerase chain reaction, DNA sequencing, and restriction fragment length polymorphism (RFPL). Every year private and public labs in the United States process more than 40,000 cases of DNA analysis,[31] the majority of which are paternity testing and for criminal investigations. In criminal cases, the quality of DNA retrieved from the site of a crime is highly scrutinized and in many cases determines admissibility of evidence. Methods of DNA collection, storage, preservation, and the reliability of DNA typing techniques and statistical methods used to calculate DNA profile frequencies can potentially present challenges to DNA admissibility. National and international committees address the use of DNA in criminal cases.[32]

With the exception of mitochondrial DNA, biological samples need to contain nucleated cells to have DNA for analysis. For example, hair roots contain nucleated cells, whereas hair shaft DNA can only be typed by mitochondrial DNA analysis. Tears, sweat, and serum do not contain nucleated cells and are therefore not amenable to standard DNA analysis. DNA has been isolated from fecal matter and gastric fluid but not in sufficient quantities. DNA quantity, sample degradation as a result of environmental exposure or bacterial contamination, and sample purity (contamination with dirt, grease, fabric dye, etc.) can all affect the ability to type DNA.[16]

Inherent characteristics of DNA such as sequence variability and variation in numbers of tandem repeats are exploited by forensics.[33] Variable number tandem repeats (VNTRs) are stretches of genomic DNA that are highly polymorphic, containing repeater units that vary in size and number between individuals.[34] VNTRs are enveloped with restriction enzyme recognition sites. Samples are treated with restriction endonuclease, and DNA fragments of 500–22,000 base pairs are obtained by gel electrophoresis.[16] Restriction fragment length polymorphism (RFLP) is the oldest DNA typing method used for criminal and paternity cases.

Polymerase Chain Reaction

Polymerase chain reaction (PCR) is a technique that has revolutionized DNA technology by copying a fragment of DNA and amplifying it 1 to 10 million times (see Figure 5-1).[35] Compared with RFLP, PCR requires significantly less sample (1–10 ng as opposed to 300–500 ng), and much less time to produce a large amount of DNA. There is less concern with

STEP 1: DNA segment to be duplicated by PCR:

*-G-G-C-T-C-A-A-G-C-T-***C-C-A-G-**

-C-C-G-A-*G-T-T-C-G-A-G-G-T-C-*

STEP 2: Short sequences of DNA on each side must be identified. These short sequences must be available in a pure form, known as a primer.

STEP 3: Heat the strands of DNA to 94°C to separate the DNA strands.

-G-G-C-T-C-A-A-G-C-T-C-C-A-G-

-C-C-G-A-G-T-T-C-G-A-G-G-T-C-

STEP 4: Add the primers to the separated strands and allow them to hybridize with the strands.

-G-G-C-T-C-A-A-G-C-T-C-C-A-G-

C-C-G-A

C-C-A-G

-C-C-G-A-G-T-T-C-G-A-G-G-T-C-

STEP 5: Add DNA polymerase and a mixture of free nucleotides to the separated strands and heat to 72°C. The polymerase enzyme will rebuild the double-stranded DNA molecule.

G-G-C-T-C-A-A-G-C-T-C-C-A-G-

-C-C-G-A-G-T-T-C-G-A-G-G-T-C-

G-G-C-T-C-A-A-G-C-T-C-C-A-G-

-C-C-G-A-G-T-T-C-G-A-G-G-T-C-

FIGURE 5-1 **Polymerase chain reaction.**

degradation of DNA with PCR because it amplifies a product many times. In comparison, RFLP needs high-molecular-weight DNA (relatively undegraded) because the DNA fragments analyzed by RFLP are much larger.[16]

The first PCR tests routinely used for forensics purposes were DQA1, polymarker (PM), and D1S80. DQA1 and PM alleles have sequence variations that are detected by a colorimetric assay, where the DNA profile is determined by the pattern of blue dots that develop. D1S80 typing, otherwise known as amplified fragment length polymorphism (AMP-FLP), detects length variation in DNA. Like RFLP, D1S80 alleles contain different numbers of repeats. DQA1, PM, and D1S80 are very sensitive and pick up very small amounts of DNA, yet RFLP is significantly more discriminatory.[16] Real-time PCR is now the method of choice in quantifying human DNA in forensics laboratories, replacing slot blot techniques previously used.[36,37] PCR is also used in quantifying male DNA from a sample of mixed human DNA.[38]

Short Tandem Repeats

Short tandem repeat (STR) technology uses a combination of PCR and RFLP. This is a pivotal technology in forensics and DNA evidence collection that has replaced conventional PCR. STRs have variations in the number of repeated units, and this characteristic makes the technology very discriminatory and sensitive. Multiple STRs can be run in a single reaction, so the wasting of samples is not a concern. Commercial kits are available for the amplification of core STR loci from small DNA samples.[39]

It has been a decade since 13 genetic markers that compromise the basis of the FBI Laboratory's Combined DNA Index System (CODIS) were chosen. These genetic markers are STRs that are also used in other DNA databases such as the US National DNA Database (NDNAD) and other such databases.[40–42] Criminal DNA databases in the United States and United Kingdom contain a cumulative 5 million DNA profiles that contain these STRs.[43,44] Using a predesignated set of STRs in DNA databases helps the exchange of information between organizations both domestically and internationally. The Human Genome Project has helped elucidate many other STR loci. Other loci are being developed that may become part of the core loci in the future.[39] The current 13 CODIS STRs are listed in Table 5-2 along with their probabilities of identity. The probability of biological evidence having a particular combination of STR types is determined by the product of their frequency of occurrence in a population. So, the combination of the first four STRs in the table produces a frequency of occurrence of about 1 in 47,000.

Short tandem repeat technology has the potential to provide information on ethnicity of offenders by comparing allele frequencies between the collected DNA and those found in different population data sets. Such technology may help narrow the number of suspects and aid in the correct identification of criminals. However, questions are raised regarding whether the data on existing allelic frequencies for different ethnic groups are truly representative of the individuals belonging to each ethnic group. The high mutation rate in STRs poses a challenge for its use to identify identical stretches of DNA that can be solely attributed to descent. Single nucleotide polymorphisms may prove to be more useful for the identification of suspect ethnicity.[39]

TABLE 5-2 **The 13 CODIS STRs and Their Probability of Identities**

STR	African-American	US Caucasian
D3s1358	0.094	0.075
VWA	0.063	0.062
FGA	0.033	0.036
TH01	0.109	0.081
TPOX	0.090	0.195
CSF1PO	0.081	0.112
D5S818	0.112	0.158
D13S317	0.136	0.085
D7S820	0.088	0.065
D8S1179	0.082	0.067
D21S11	0.034	0.039
D18S51	0.029	0.028
D16S539	0.070	0.089

Source: The Future of Forensic DNA Testing: Predictions of the Research and Development Working Group. Washington, DC: National Institutes of Justice, Department of Justice, 2000, p. 41.

Mitochondrial DNA

Mitochondrial DNA (MtDNA) is extranuclear, circular DNA with multiple copies per cell. MtDNA can be amplified by PCR, and then sequenced. It is especially good for analysis of old skeletal remains and hair shafts that contain only MtDNA[45] and in cases where there is inadequate nuclear DNA. MtDNA has the potential of surviving in skeletal remains for millennia, and because it is inherited maternally without recombination, one maternal reference sample (i.e., blood or buccal mucosa) may be adequate for analysis.[46] MtDNA is a great supplement for other sources of evidence.[47] Because it is from maternal origin, all individuals from the same maternal lineage will be indistinguishable by MtDNA analysis. However, reference samples are available from family members sharing the same mother, grandmother, great-grandmother, and so on. MtDNA will not have the discrimination power of STR analysis of nuclear DNA, so it should be reserved for samples for which nuclear DNA typing is simply not possible.

DNA Data Banks

The Federal Bureau of Investigation developed the Combined DNA Index System (CODIS), a national data bank, to assist law enforcement laboratories in comparing forensic evidence with DNA profiles nationwide. It is used in conjunction with states that maintain DNA profiles of known convicted offenders. The major benefit of CODIS is the creation of a collaborative effort between local, state, and federal law enforcement agencies.

For crimes in which no suspect has been identified, a comparison of unknown DNA to felon DNA data banks can be made.[31] All states can use data from CODIS. CODIS combines forensic DNA technology with computer software applications to solve violent crimes. Access to CODIS allows local, state, and federal law enforcement crime labs to exchange and compare DNA profiles.[16]

Within CODIS there are several indexes. The Convicted Offender Index contains DNA profiles from individuals convicted of felony sex crimes and other crimes based on state legislation. The Forensic Index contains DNA profiles lawfully obtained from individuals during the course of a criminal investigation. The Population File contains DNA types and allele frequency information from anonymous people representing major population groups in the United States; this database is used to estimate statistical frequencies of DNA profiles. The Unidentified Persons Index contains DNA from individuals whose identities are not known; the source of DNA for this index includes human remains, unidentified body parts, and persons who do not or cannot disclose their identity to the police. The Relatives of Missing Persons Index contains DNA profiles from missing persons and their close relatives. And finally, the Victims Index contains DNA records of victims from whom DNA may have been carried away by perpetrators; this index is used to search DNA profiles found on, but foreign to, a suspect.

The information in CODIS is limited but sufficient enough to enable profile searching. The majority of information in CODIS is created and maintained by state and local crime laboratories. CODIS can store and search both restriction fragment length polymorphism (RLFP) and polymerase chain reaction (PCR) DNA profiles. The identification record in CODIS contains a laboratory identifier, a specimen identifier, DNA characteristics, and information to classify and review the integrity of the DNA record. It does not contain criminal history information, case-related information, or social security numbers.

If a possible match is made in CODIS, the identified laboratories of the match contact each other to verify the match. After a match is confirmed, the laboratories may exchange additional information including case details. If the match is made against the Convicted Offender Index, the identity and location of the convicted offender are provided.

CHALLENGES OF DNA TECHNOLOGY

Reliability of DNA technology has been challenged by trial lawyers and others from the time of its inception. DNA typing methods, algorithms used to assess for DNA matching between two samples, and concern about differences in allele frequency among different populations were early focuses of the challengers. Despite widespread acceptance and usage of DNA technology by the court system, individual cases may still be challenged from the perspective of adequacy of analysis techniques used in the laboratory.[48]

CONCLUSION

Current research is directed at reducing the number of steps and time needed to process DNA collected with rape kits. Collection of adequate evidence relies on the separation of the suspect's DNA from the victim's. Historically, the separation of male and female DNA has involved a multistep process that can require incubation overnight.[49] Microdevice cell separation techniques have been and continue to be developed that condense this multistep process, resulting in a smaller DNA sample requirement, less processing time, and less handling of the DNA sample.[50–55] Further development of such methods will undoubtedly contribute to enhanced cell recovery from cotton swabs and allow utilization of low-copy number samples.[49] Application of Y-chromosome STRs in sexual assault cases has been very useful in distinguishing mixes of male and female DNA, an area where autosomal STR testing has met with difficulty.[56] Commercially available Y-STR kits amplify all core Y-STR loci in a single assay, producing male-specific amplification even if intermixed with 1000-fold excess female DNA.[39]

REFERENCES

1. Hackenschmidt A. Advancing justice for sexual assault survivors and innocent inmates, or threat to privacy? A controversial DNA technology proposal. *J Emerg Nurs.* 2004;30:575–577.
2. Jeffreys AJ, Wilson V, Thein SL. Individual specific "fingerprints" of human DNA. *Nature.* 1985;316:76–79.
3. National Institute of Justice. Home page. Available at: http://www.ojp.usdoj.gov. Retrieved July 23, 2008.
4. Bond JW. Value of DNA evidence in detecting crime. *J Forensic Sci.* 2007;52:128–136.
5. Lovrich NP, Gaffney MJ, Pratt TC, Johnson CL, Lane SA, Asplen CH, et al. *Attorney General's Report on the DNA Evidence Backlog.* Pullman, Wash: Division of Government Studies and Services; April 2, 2004.
6. Aspleen CH, Gaffney MJ, Hurst LH, Johnson CL, Lovrich NP, Pratt TC, et al. *National Forensic DNA Study Report.* Washington, DC: National Institute of Justice; 2003.
7. Comey CT, Koons BW, Presley KW, Smerick JB, Sobieralski CA, Stanley DM, et al. DNA extraction strategies for amplified fragment length polymorphism analysis. *J Forensic Sci.* 1994;39:1254–1269.
8. Gill P, Jeffreys AJ, Werrett DJ. Forensic application of DNA "fingerprints." *Nature.* 1985;318:577–579.
9. Iwasaki M, Kubo S, Ogata M, Nakasono I. A demonstration of spermatozoa on vaginal swabs after complete destruction of the vaginal cell deposits. *J Forensic Sci.* 1989;34:659–664.
10. Association of Chief Police Officers (England and Wales). *The DNA Good Practice Manual.* London: ACPO; 2005:5.
11. Tilley N, Ford A. Forensic science and criminal investigation. *Crime Detection and Prevention.* Paper 73. London: Home Office; 1996.
12. Lee HC, Palmbach TM, Miller MT. *Henry Lee's Crime Scene Handbook.* Boston, Mass: Academic Press; 2001.
13. Sievers V, Murphy S, Miller JJ. Sexual assault evidence collection more accurate when completed by sexual nurse examiners: Colorado's experience. *J Emerg Nurs.* 2003;29:511–514.
14. De Forest PR, Gaensslen RE, Lee HC. *Forensic Science: An Introduction to Criminalistics.* New York, NY: McGraw-Hill; 1983.
15. Bowman R, Labbe TJ, Mullings KA. Serology and DNA evidence. In: *Forensic Emergency Medicine.* Philadelphia, Pa: Lippincott Williams & Wilkins; 2007.
16. Lee HC, Ladd C. Biological evidence in criminal investigations. In: *Forensic Nursing.* St. Louis, Mo: Elsevier Mosby; 2006.
17. Landsteiner K. Zur Kenntnis der antifermentaiven lystischen and agglutinierenden Wirkungen des Blutserums und der Lymphe. *Sent. Bact.* 1900;27:357–362.
18. Gaensslen RE. *Sourcebook in Forensic Serology, Immunology, and Biochemistry.* Washington, DC: US Government Printing Office; 1983.
19. Lee HC. (1982). Identification and grouping of bloodstains. In: R. Saferstein, ed. *Forensic Science Review.* Englewood Cliffs, NJ: Prentice Hall; 1982:267–337.
20. Lee HC, Gaensslen RE, Pagliaro EM, et al. *Physical Evidence in Criminal Investigation.* Westbrook, Conn: Narcotic Enforcement Officers Association; 1991.
21. Lee HC, ed. *Physical Evidence.* Enfield, Conn: Magnani and McCormic; 1995.
22. Gaensslen RE, Desio PJ, Lee HC. Genetic marker systems for the individualization of blood and body fluids in forensic serology. In: G. Davies, ed. *Forensic Science.* Washington, DC: American Chemical Society; 1986.
23. Gaensslen RE, Lee HC. *Procedures and Evaluation of Antisera for the Typing of Antigens in Bloodstains: Blood Group Antigens ABH, RH, MNSs, Kell, Dufy, Kidd, Serum Group Antigens GmlKm.* Washington DC: National Institute of Justice, US Government Printing Office; 1984.
24. Lee HC, Gaensslen RE, eds. *Advances in Forensic Science.* Foster City, Calif: Biomedical; 1985.
25. Vandenberg N, et al. The use of Polilight in the detection of seminal fluid, saliva, and bloodstains, and comparison with conventional chemical-based screening tests. *J Forensic Sci.* 2006;51:361–370.
26. Stoilovic M. Detection of semen and bloodstains using the Polilight as a light source. *Forensic Sci Int.* 1991;51:289–296.
27. Kobus HJ, Silenieks E, Scharnberg J. Improving the effectiveness of fluorescence for the detection of seminal stains on fabrics. *J Forensic Sci.* 2002;47:819–823.
28. Lloyd JBF. Forensic significance of fluorescent brighteners: their qualitative TLC characterization in small quantities of fiber and detergents. *J Forensic Sci Society.* 1977;17:145–152.
29. Bray T, Stenlake N, Armitage S. Fluorescein vs luminol and leuco crystal violet (LCV) as an alternative for bloodstain detection. *Proc 17th Int Symposium Forensic Sci.* March 28–April 2, 2004. Wellington, NZ: ANZFSS; 2004:118.
30. DNA Advisory Board Standards. *Quality Assurance Standards for DNA Testing Laboratories.* Washington, DC: US Department of Justice, Federal Bureau of Investigation; 1998.

31. *CODIS Statistics.* Washington, DC: US Department of Justice, Federal Bureau of Investigation; 2003.
32. US Congress, Office of Technology Assessment. *Genetic Witness: Forensic Uses of DNA Tests.* OTA-BA-438. Washington, DC: US Government Printing Office; 1990.
33. Wyman AR, White R. A highly polymorphic locus in human DNA. *Proc Natl Acad Sci USA.* 1980;77:6754–6758.
34. Weising K, Nymbom H, Wolff K, Mayer W. *DNA Fingerprinting in Plants and Fungi.* Boca Raton, Fla: CRL Press; 1995.
35. Saiki RK, Scharf S, Faloona F, et al. Enzymatic amplification of beta-globin genomic sequences and restriction analysis for diagnosis of sickle cell anemia. *Science.* 1985;230:1350–1354.
36. Nicklas JA, Buel E. Use of real-time *Alu* PCR for quantitation of human DNA in forensic samples. *J Forensic Sci.* 2003;48:936–944.
37. Nicklas JA, Buel E. An alu-based, eclipse real-time PCR method for the quantitation of human DNA in forensic samples. *J Forensic Sci.* 2005;50:1081–1090.
38. Nicklas JA, Buel E. Simultaneous determination of total human and male DNA using a duplex real-time PCR assay. *J Forensic Sci.* 2006;51:1005–1015.
39. Butler JM. Genetics and genomics of core short tandem repeat loci used in human identity testing. *J Forensic Sci.* 2006;51:254–262.
40. Butler JM. *Forensic DNA Typing: Biology, Technology, and Genetics of STR Markers.* 2nd ed. New York, NY: Elsevier; 2005.
41. Gill P. Role of short tandem repeat DNA in forensic casework in the UK—past, present, and future perspectives. *Biotechniques.* 2002;32:366–372.
42. Jobling MA, Gill P. Encoded evidence: DNA in forensic analysis. *Nat Rev Genet.* 2005;5:739–751.
43. Federal Bureau of Investigation. CODIS. Available at: http://www.fbi.gov/hq/lab/html/codis1.htm. Retrieved July 25, 2008.
44. Forensic Science Service. Home page. Available at: http://www.forensic.gov.uk. Retrieved July 25, 2008.
45. Budowle B, Allard MW, Wilson MR, Chakraborty R. Forensics and mitochondrial DNA: applications, debates, and foundations. *Ann Rev of Genom Hum Genet.* 2003;4:119–141.
46. Holland MM, Fisher DL, Roby RK, Ruderman J, Bryson C, Weedn VW. Mitochondrial DNA sequence analysis of human remains. *Crime Lab Digest.* 1995;22:109–115.
47. Nelson K, Melton T. Forensic mitochondrial DNA analysis of 116 casework skeletal samples. *J Forensic Sci.* 2007;52:557–561.
48. Reilly P. Legal and public policy issues in DNA forensics. *Nat Rev Genet.* 2001;2:313–317.
49. Voorhees JC, Ferrance JP, Landers JP. Enhanced elution of sperm from cotton swabs via enzymatic digestion for rape kit analysis. *J Forensic Sci.* 2006;51:574–579.
50. Horsman K, Barker SLR, Ferrance JP, Forrest KA, Koen KA, Landers JP. Separation of sperm and epithelial cells on microfabricated devices: potential application to forensic analysis of sexual assault evidence. *Anal Chem.* 2005;77:742–749.
51. Lagally ET, Medintz I, Mathies RA. Single-molecule DNA amplification and analysis in an integrated microfluidic device. *Anal Chem.* 2001;73:565–570.
52. Khandurina J, McKnight TE, Jacobson SC, Waters LC, Foote RS, Ramsey JM. Integrated system for rapid PCR-based DNA analysis in microfluidic devices. *Anal Chem.* 2000;72:2995–3000.
53. Giordano BC, Ferrance J, Landers JP. Toward an integrated electrophoretic microdevice for clinical diagnostics. In: Heller MJ and Guttman A, eds. *Integrated Microfabricated Biodevices.* New York, NY: Marcel Dekker; 2002:1–34.
54. Reyes DR, Iossifidis D, Auroux PA, Manz A. Micro total analysis systems. 1. Introduction, theory, and technology. *Anal Chem.* 2002;74:2623–2636.
55. Auroux PA, Iossifidis D, Reyes DR, Manz A. Micro total analysis systems. 2. Analytical standard operations and applications. *Anal Chem.* 2002;74:2637–2652.
56. Mulero JJ, Chang CW, Calandro LM, Green RL, Li Y, Johnson CL, Hennessy LK. Development and validation of the AmpFlSTR Yfilter PCR amplification kit: a male specific, single amplification 17 Y-STR multiplex system. *J Forensic Sci.* 2006;51:64–75.

6 | Forensic Toxicology

Paul Francis Kolecki, MD, FACEP

INTRODUCTION

Forensic toxicology, one of the three branches of toxicology, focuses on the medicolegal (and the nonmedical) aspects of the harmful effects of chemical and poisons.[1,2] Clinical toxicology is another branch of toxicology that focuses mainly on the harmful effects of chemical and poisons and patient care. Environmental toxicology is the third branch. Toxicologic analyses are used in clinical and forensic medicine (and environmental toxicology) to facilitate medical care, diagnosis, and treatment.[1] Toxicology analysis is also used for mandatory or voluntary testing in the workplace and to determine the cause of death.

Pathologists collect most of the samples used for forensic toxicology (postmortem analysis). However, clinicians and medical personnel also play an essential role in forensic toxicology because they often are the first people to examine, diagnosis, and collect samples from patients who may be the subject of legal investigation. The proper collection, storage, and testing of forensic specimens is important because improperly collected specimens can yield improper or misleading results. Accurate interviews and histories are also important because the patient's or victim's history of drug use is needed for proper interpretation of laboratory results.

There are three major subdisciplines of forensic toxicology: human performance, postmortem, and forensic drug testing. *Human performance* refers to mental or physical effects of drugs that may impair judgment or coordination. *Postmortem* refers to toxicologic analysis in circumstances of death to determine the cause of death. *Forensic drug testing* is used most often in the workplace, the military, and in the emergency department.

This chapter reviews the typical forensic investigation, sample handling (for both living and postmortem cases), the common laboratory analysis techniques used in forensic toxicology, and the important aspects concerning the interpretation of these results. In addition, the trends in drug use along with the basic pharmacology, clinical features, and laboratory testing of the drugs are reviewed. Finally, a brief review is made of drug-facilitated sexual assault and in utero and newborn drug exposure.

TOXICOLOGY INVESTIGATION

The toxicologic investigation is typically performed to explain whether a drug was involved or the cause of a patient's morbidity or mortality. The investigation is also important in revealing which specific drug was involved, how much was taken, and when it was taken. Ordinarily, toxicologic samples are collected at the time of the incident, such as a motor vehicle accident, sexual assault, or suicide attempt. The duration and effects of drugs depend on the dose administered, individual metabolism, frequency of use, and the presence of other drugs or chemicals. The toxicologic investigation can be difficult because the previously mentioned features (dose, metabolism, frequency, presence of other substances) are often unknown at the time of the incident.[1] Therapeutic and toxic concentrations of drugs are often useful in the investigation but must be interpreted with caution because of the variations of clinical effects among individuals. Thus, the toxicologic interpretation is usually based not only upon the toxicology results but also upon observations by clinicians and or trained law enforcement personnel at the scene.

Toxicologic samples are typically collected as part of a complete autopsy.[3] Lethal concentrations of drugs are often useful in the investigation but also must be interpreted with caution because of the variations of clinical effects among individuals. Many autopsies are performed with the consent of the family. In the case of an unexplained manner of death, a forensic pathologist may perform a medical-legal autopsy. If the family does not consent for a complete medical-legal autopsy, the pathologist may only obtain toxicologic fluid samples. Postmortem toxicologic samples can be obtained minutes to years after the event.[3]

Specimen Handling for Living Cases

Forensic toxicologic specimens used for analysis are frequently collected in the emergency department.[1] Occupational-related toxicologic investigations may collect samples at the workplace, the emergency department, or a private laboratory. Appropriate selection, collection, preservation, and storage of biological evidence are essential during a toxicological investigation.[1] Specimens should be collected as quickly as possible because delays can affect the interpretation of the results and establishing causation. Two such scenarios in which delays in specimen collection can affect outcome are patients arrested for driving while intoxicated (DWI) and alleged drug-facilitated sexual assault.

The selection and collection of biologic samples are often predetermined by the circumstances of the case. Blood and urine are the most common specimens obtained because of the ease of collection and availability of testing in a timely manner in the hospital setting. The analysis of other body parts and fluids (hair, sweat, saliva, and breast milk) is often difficult and thus infrequently used in the hospital setting.

Glass containers are routinely used for blood specimen collection and storage. Commercial gray-top Vacutainer or Venoject blood tubes that contain sodium fluoride and potassium oxide should be used for the collection of toxicologic specimens.[1] Urine collection (typically in plastic containers) ideally should be observed by trained personnel to reduce the likelihood of dilution or substitution. Frequently, the donor will dip the urine collection cup into the toilet or another source of water, thus diluting the specimen and potentially altering the laboratory analysis. Urine substitution also frequently occurs, thus emphasizing the importance of observation during collection. Adulteration is also popular among illicit drug users because successful adulteration produces a false-negative urine drug screen. Common household products and commercially available urine adulterant kits typically are used to adulterate urine.[4–7](See Table 6-1.)

In cases of DWI and alleged sexual assault, toxicologic specimens are considered evidence. Thus, the integrity of the specimens should be maintained at all times by first witnessing the collection of the specimen (blood and, more important, urine), and then tracking the handling and storage of the specimen from the time of collection to final disposition. A chain of custody (COC) form often is used to document the date, time, and purpose of collection. In addition, the COC form documents the location of the specimen and the name of the person handling the specimen. A COC form is used not only in hospital laboratory analysis but also in cases

TABLE 6-1 **Substances Used for Adultering Urine Drug Screens**

Acetic acid (vinegar)	Nitrite (Klear, Whizzies, Purafyzit, Krystal, Klean)*
Ammonia	Papain
Bleach	Peroxidase and peroxide (Stealth)*
Drano (Sodium hydroxide)	Pyridinium chlorochromate (PCC) (Urine Luck, LL-148, Sweet Pea's Spoiler)*
Eye drops	Soap
Glutaraldehyde (Clean-X, Instant Clean, Urine Aid)*	Table salt
Niacin	Toilet bowl cleaner

* Commercially available urine "adulterant" kit

where specimens are transported to private, commercial laboratories. Specimen handling and disposition of evidence are often scrutinized by the courts, especially in cases of DWI and alleged sexual assault. Thus, specimens must be stored in secure locations with limited access where they are not vulnerable to adulteration.[1,8]

Postmortem Specimen Handling

During postmortem examination, body fluids, tissues, and organs may provide insight into drug intoxication, which is highly relevant during a death investigation. Blood samples typically are collected from the femoral or subclavian vein. Postmortem drug concentrations are often difficult to analyze because drugs may be redistributed from fat and muscle stores into the blood following death. Collection of hair and nails may provide historical information on long-term exposure to toxic drugs or substances. Vitreous humor, urine, gastric fluid samples, and solid organ samples are also used in postmortem examination.[1,3]

TOXICOLOGIC ANALYSIS

Toxicologic analysis typically is directed at the identification of drugs or poisons followed by the quantification of the results. There are numerous toxicology laboratory tests, including spot tests, spectrochemical tests, immunoassays, on-site drug tests, and gas chromatography–mass spectrometry (GC-MS). Most hospital laboratories perform a rapid screening test such as an immunoassay, which precedes a more rigorous and labor-intensive analysis using gas chromatography–mass spectrometry.[1,9]

Spot Tests

Spot tests are simple tests that involve the reaction of a drug with a chemical to produce a colored product. Although very popular in the past, spot tests are rarely used today because of limited sensitivity, variability in interpretation of test results, and the development of more sophisticated laboratory testing methods.

Spectrochemical Tests

Spectrochemical tests are very similar to spot tests except that they rely on a chemical reaction to produce a light-absorbing substance.[9] Co-oximetry is an example of a spectrochemical test that is used frequently in hospital laboratories. In simple terms, colorimetric measures the different hemoglobin states (oxygenated hemoglobin, deoxygenated hemoglobin, carboxyhemoglobin, and methemoglobin) existing in a blood sample. Co-oximetry is used typically when evaluating patients with suspected carbon monoxide poisoning (burn or smoke inhalation victims) or methemoglobinemia (cyanotic patients exposed to oxidant stress).

Immunoassays

Immunoassays are highly selective antibody-based tests that provide toxicologic results in minutes to hours. Most immunoassays rely upon competitive binding between anti-drug antibodies and either labeled or unlabeled drug.[1,9] In an enzyme immunoassay, drug in a donor urine sample competes with enzyme-labeled drug for binding sites on an antibody molecule. If there is no drug in the urine, the enzyme-labeled drug binds to the antibody. However, if the urine sample contains a quantity of drug, the enzyme-labeled drug will not bind as readily. The more drugs in the sample, the less enzyme-labeled drug will bind, and vice versa. The amount of enzymes that are bound can be determined colorimetrically, and the intensity of the color is related to the concentration of drug in the sample. In general, these assays are automated, require small sample volumes, and are not technically demanding. A wide variety of immunoassay techniques are commercially available, many of which rely on the use of enzymes, radioisotopes, or fluorescent-labeled species for detection purposes.[1,9] Most hospital laboratories and workplace drug screening programs use immunoassays for testing urine for drugs of abuse, and typically the results are available within 1 hour. (See Table 6-2.)

The degree of specificity does not limit the usefulness of the test because some immunoassays are designed to be nonspecific to cross-react with several drugs within a drug class.[1,9] The immunoassay for opiates is such an example. The immunoassay for opiates uses antibodies that bind with substances structurally similar to morphine, thus also detecting codeine, hydrocodone, and hydromorphone. However, this immunoassay does not detect the synthetic opiates (fentanyl, meperidine, methadone, propoxyphene, tramadol). This immunoassay also can detect the low concentrations of morphine found in poppy seeds, thus producing a positive urine drug screen for opiates.

Lack of specificity can also be a drawback of the immunoassays because structurally similar molecules may also bind to the antibody to varying degrees.[1,9] An example of such is the test for amphetamines. The test for amphetamines detects the base structure and thus might produce a positive "amphetamine" result for many structures with that structure (ephedrine, methamphetamine, pseudoephedrine, and phenylpropanolamine). This lack of specificity may also produce false-positive results. Dextromethoraphan, a cough-suppressant drug, classically produces a false-positive result for the presence of phencyclidine because of a similar base structure. Because of the limitations of immunoassays, these results alone are not forensically defensible. The immunoassay screens are excellent tests to indicate which drugs or classes of drugs are present, but a more rigorous and specific test must be performed to unequivocally confirm the presence of a particular drug for forensic purposes.

TABLE 6-2 **Drugs of Abuse Detected in Typical Urine Drug Screens**

Amphetamines	Marijuana
Barbiturates	Opiates
Benzodiazepines	Phencyclidine
Cocaine	

The effectiveness of an immunoassay depends on the cut-off concentration below which the sample is deemed negative. The cut-off concentrations established by most testing facilities are set at the lowest concentration of drug that can be reliably confirmed using other tests (GC-MS).[1] These low cut-off points are necessary to identify very low concentrations of drug that could be present after a single dose.

On-Site Drug Tests

On-site drug tests, also known as point-of-care tests, rely on conventional immunoassay-based principles and rapid qualitative drug screen results. When blood or urine is added to one of these devices, capillary action allows any drug in the sample to migrate through the test medium. The progression of the antibody-antigen reaction can be easily seen; a positive reaction typically produces a concentrated blue or purple color in the test result window.[1] These on-site tests are popular in private sector toxicology screening. In addition, some emergency departments use on-site testing. However, on-site testing results are not widely used in forensic toxicology because these devices have elevated cut-off concentrations, and thus, higher concentrations (higher than the typical laboratory immunoassay) of a drug need to be present to produce a positive result. In addition, many on-site testing kits detect only a small selection of drugs.[1]

Confirmatory Toxicologic Analysis (GC-MS)

Because of the cross-reactivity and lack of specificity of immunoassays, most positive immunoassay drug screen results are confirmed using a more rigorous technique.[1,9] GC-MS is the most widely used confirmatory laboratory device in forensic toxicology because it specifically identifies and quantifies the drug or drugs present in the specimen. Another major advantage of GC-MS over immunoassays is that GC-MS detects the presence of multiple drugs in a single analysis.[9] Prior to analysis by GC-MS, the drugs must be extracted from the biological matrix. The most common extraction techniques are liquid-liquid extraction (LLE) and solid-phase extraction (SPE). When using LLE, drugs are extracted from biological fluids or tissues using solvents that are subsequently evaporated, concentrated, and analyzed. SPE uses similar principles as those of LLE.[1,9]

A major disadvantage of GC-MS is that it is not available at most hospital laboratories. Thus, positive immunoassay samples necessitating GC-MS analysis are usually sent out to advanced toxicology laboratories or major medical centers. Because of this transfer process, the timing of the results is typically delayed by hours to days. In addition, the chain of custody (COC) principles may also delay test results sent to outside facilities. This delay in receiving the results is more problematic for the clinical aspect of toxicology as compared to the forensic aspect.

INTERPRETATION OF TOXICOLOGIC ANALYSIS

The interpretation of toxicology results can be difficult at times because patients may have positive laboratory results with minimal or no signs of intoxication. Reasons for such a scenario include drug tolerance or the prolonged presence of the drug's metabolite. In fact, numerous drugs can be detected in the urine days to weeks after initial exposure to the drug and long after the clinical effects have resolved. (See Table 6-3.) Thus, positive toxicology results along with an asymptomatic patient typically indicate only past use of the drug and not current intoxication.

The reverse scenario can also occur, where a patient has negative toxicology results and clinical signs and symptoms consistent with drug intoxication. Reasons for this scenario include the inability of immunoassays to detect the presence of drugs below the cut-off concentration. In addition, some drugs have low cross-reactivity with the immunoassay, thus producing a false-negative result.[1,9]

Urine adulteration prior to laboratory analysis can also produce a false-negative result. Adulteration of urine occurs in places where urine drug screens are frequently performed, including emergency departments, jails, substance abuse treatment centers, schools, and the workplace. The reasons behind urine adulteration are obvious and pertain to the potential consequences associated with a positive urine drug screen. Potential consequences for these users include citations, incarceration, fines, suspensions, expulsion, or termination of employment.[6]

Prior to a drug screen, a urine sample can be tampered with by either ingesting a chemical prior to urinating, adding a chemical to the urine sample, or substituting the urine sample with some other substance-free sample. Many adulterants are household products that are added to the collected urine sample prior to laboratory analysis. Table 6-1 lists some easily available commercial urine adulterant kits that involve the addition of a chemical to the urine sample, thus producing the false-negative result. Adulterants are used mainly to mask the detection of marijuana, amphetamines, opioids, cocaine, and/or benzodiazepines in the urine.

Many of the adulterants can be detected by visual inspection of the urine along with routine integrity tests, focusing on creatinine, pH, temperature, and specific gravity.[7] Spot tests and urine dipsticks are commercially available to detect the presence of urine adulterants.[7] Careful observation

TABLE 6-3 **Common Drugs of Abuse and the Detection Time in Urine**

Common Drugs of Abuse	Detection Time in Urine
Cocaine	1–3 days 1 week (prolonged use)
Ecstasy	1–2 days
Gamma-hydroxybutarate (GHB)	12 hours
Heroin	1–4 days
Marijuana	1–3 days Several weeks (prolonged use)
Methamphetamine	1–3 days
Phencyclidine (PCP)	4–7 days Several weeks (prolonged use)

during the collection of the sample is probably the most useful method to detect and prevent urine adulteration or substitution. Other recommendations to potentially prevent urine adulteration include turning off all sources of running water where the sample is to be collected, adding a bluing agent to toilet water, not allowing personal items into the collection area, and having the donor wash his or her hands prior to urinating.[6]

TRENDS IN DRUG USE AND ABUSE

Illicit drugs are used and abused mainly to obtain a high or euphoria. In 2004, the Drug Abuse Warning Network (DAWN) reported approximately 2 million emergency department (ED) drug-related visits.[10] Of these 2 million visits, DAWN estimated that 1.3 million (65%) were associated with drug misuse or abuse.[10] DAWN further estimated that of the 1.3 million ED visits associated with drug misuse or abuse:

- 30% involved illicit drugs only[10]
- 25% involved pharmaceuticals only[10]
- 15% involved illicit drugs and alcohol
- 14% involved illicit drugs with pharmaceuticals and alcohol[10]
- 8% involved illicit drugs with pharmaceuticals[10]

In 2004, DAWN also reported approximately 940,000 drug-related ED visits involving a major substance of abuse.[10] These major substances included the following:

- Cocaine
- Marijuana
- Heroin
- Methamphetamine and ecstasy
- Phencyclidine
- Gamma-hydroxybutyrate (GHB)

Trends in Drug Use and Crime

Unfortunately, the use of illicit drugs is strongly associated with violent and/or criminal acts. In 2004, the Bureau of Justice Statistics (BJS) reported that there were 5.2 million violent victimizations of residents age 12 or older. Victims of violence were asked to describe whether they perceived the offender to have been drinking alcohol or using drugs prior to the violent act. Approximately 30% (approximately 1.6 million) of the victims of violence reported that the offender was using drugs or alcohol.[11]

In 2006, the BJS reported that 32% of state prisoners and 26% of federal prisoners confessed that they had committed their current offense while under the influence of drugs.[12] In 2003, the BJS reported that 41% of violent crimes against college students were committed by an offender perceived to be using drugs.[13] In addition, the BJS also reported that 40% of all rape/sexual assaults and about 25% of all robberies against a college student were committed by an offender perceived to be using drugs.[13] In 2001, the BJS reported that 35% of workplace victims of violence believed the offender was drinking alcohol or using drugs at the time of the incident.[14] Approximately 29% of convicted jailed inmates reported that they had used illegal drugs at the time of the offense. Marijuana and cocaine were the most common drugs convicted inmates said they had used.[15]

Trends in Drug and Alcohol Use and Driving Accidents

Alcohol use and intoxication are also strongly associated with motor vehicle accidents. According to the Fatality Analysis Reporting System (2006) of the National Highway and Transportation Safety Administration, approximately 41% (17,602) of the 42,642 fatal traffic crashes in 2006 were alcohol related. The blood alcohol concentration was measured at 80 mg/dL or higher in 15,121 of these alcohol-related fatalities. The total number of alcohol-related fatal traffic crashes in 2004 has declined from the estimated 2003 total (17,105).[16] The exact number of yearly traffic fatalities involving drugs other than alcohol is not known.

BACKGROUND, PHARMACOLOGY, CLINICAL FEATURES, AND LABORATORY DETECTION OF THE COMMON DRUGS OF USE, MISUSE, AND ABUSE

Emergency department personnel and forensic examiners often deal with patients who are under the influence of drugs and/or alcohol. Knowledge of the pharmacology and clinical features of the common intoxicants is important. Equally important is the ability to detect the intoxicant in patients and interpret what that means.

Alcohol

Alcohol, a sedative-hypnotic-like substance, is one of the oldest substances used by humankind for social purpose. Presently, alcohol continues to be one of the most commonly abused substances. Alcohol levels are usually determined by using serum samples and typically are measured in milligrams per deciliter (mg/dL). The legal driving limit in most states is either 80 mg/dL or 100 mg/dL. Laboratory testing for the presence of alcohol is performed using mainly serum or plasma samples. Breath analyzers for alcohol and saliva alcohol analyzers are also available. These measurements are not as precise as laboratory assays and may produce false-positive results with other organic substances. Because of these limitations, positive breath analyzer results should be confirmed using serum laboratory analysis.[9]

Alcohol has numerous toxic effects on the human body. The acute, lethal complication of acute intoxication is respiratory depression. Other clinical features of alcohol toxicity include impaired sensory function, impaired muscle coordination, reduced memory and concentration, faulty judgment, and increased perceptions of own activities with decreased performance. Marked mental impairment (impaired ability to drive a car, for instance) occurs at serum alcohol concentrations of 5–100 mg/dL. Acute alcohol-related mortality typically occurs with levels greater than 400 mg/dL.

Alcohol is rapidly absorbed following ingestion, although absorption may be delayed with a full stomach. Alcohol is metabolized mainly in the liver. Chronic alcohol abusers (alcoholics) typically eliminate alcohol from their serum at a rate of 25–30 mg/dL/hour. Nonalcoholics typically eliminate alcohol from their serum at a rate of 20 mg/dL/hour.

Cocaine

Cocaine is a stimulant-like drug derived from the plant *Erythroxylon coca*. The water-soluble salt form of cocaine can be snorted or injected intravenously. The free-base form of cocaine is exceptionally popular because this drug can be smoked. Intravenous and inhalational use of cocaine produces clinical effects within seconds, whereas intranasal use produces symptoms within 5 minutes. The symptoms of cocaine use last for approximately 20–30 minutes regardless of route of administration.

The main clinical features of cocaine toxicity are euphoria and hallucinations. Numerous potentially harmful clinical features are associated with cocaine use, including agitation, seizures, coma, myocardial infarction, ventricular arrhythmias, hyperthermia, severe hypertension, aortic dissection, and intestinal ischemia. Urine drug screens detect benzoylecgonine, the main metabolite of cocaine. This metabolite is present in the urine after 5 minutes following the IV use of cocaine. In addition, benzoylecgonine may be present up to 36 hours following a one-time use of cocaine.[9] With long-term use, urine metabolites of benzoylecgonine may be present for up to 3 weeks after discontinuation of cocaine use. Cocaine exhibits very low immunoassay cross-reactivity; thus, false-positive results are exceptionally rare.[9] Because the immunoassay detects the metabolite of cocaine, positive cocaine results do not necessarily indicate current intoxication but rather may only indicate past use.

Marijuana

Marijuana abuse became popular in the United States in the early 20th century. Marijuana, a plant-derived hallucinogen, is abused mainly via the inhalational and oral routes. Inhalation of marijuana produces symptoms within several minutes, whereas oral ingestion takes slightly longer (approximately 30 minutes). The symptoms of marijuana use typically last 2–6 hours.

The main clinical features of marijuana toxicity are euphoria and hallucinations. Other clinical features include drowsiness, paranoia, panic, increased appetite, mood fluctuations, and psychotic episodes. The main pharmacologically active substance produced following marijuana use is tetrahydrocannibinol (THC). Immunoassays detect the inactive metabolite of THC (tetrahydrocannabinoic acid).[9] Approximately 40% of THC and the metabolites of THC are excreted in the urine. Urine drug screens (UDS) typically are positive for up to 5 days following marijuana use. Because the metabolites of marijuana are stored in lipids and muscle tissue, chronic use may produce a positive UDS for up to 21 days. False-positive results are exceptionally rare. Because the immunoassay detects the metabolite of marijuana, a positive result does not necessarily indicate current intoxication but rather may only indicate past use. Metabolites of marijuana can also be detected in serum samples, hair analysis, and saliva samples.

Heroin

Heroin is an opiate-like drug derived from naturally occurring alkaloids. Heroin use is exceptionally popular both by the inhalational and intravenous routes. Both routes produce clinical effects within minutes. The main clinical features of heroin use include euphoria and hallucination. Other clinical features include miosis, decreased gastrointestinal motility, depressed level of consciousness, and depressed respiratory rate. Anoxia secondary to respiratory depression is a potentially deadly feature of many heroin overdoses.

Heroin is metabolized mainly in the liver. The metabolites are then excreted in the urine. Urine screens for heroin metabolites are typically positive for 36–48 hours following the use of this drug.

Ecstasy and Methamphetamine

Ecstasy and methamphetamine are synthetic amphetamines that are easily produced in clandestine laboratories. Methamphetamine and ecstasy are probably the two most popular amphetamine derivatives abused today. Methamphetamine typically is abused either intravenously or by the inhalational route. Ecstasy typically is ingested. Both produce rapid onset of clinical features. The duration of clinical features associated with methamphetamine use typically is 10–20 hours, whereas the clinical features of ecstasy last approximately 4–8 hours.

Both methamphetamine and ecstasy produce euphoria and hallucinations. Methamphetamine, and to a lesser extent ecstasy, can produce the same harmful clinical effects as seen with cocaine. Ecstasy may produce bruxism, and many ecstasy users typically suck on lollipops and pacifiers. Potentially life-threatening complications of ecstasy toxicity are severe hyponatremia and cerebral edema.[17,18]

Both methamphetamine and ecstasy are metabolized in the liver, producing amphetamine metabolites that are excreted in the urine. These amphetamine metabolites are typically detected in the standard UDS. False-positive amphetamine results are common and problematic because numerous over-the-counter cough and cold medicines are structurally similar to amphetamines.

Phencyclidine

Phencyclidine (PCP), a dissociative anesthetic, is easily synthesized in clandestine laboratories. PCP can be taken orally, intravenously, or by the inhalational route. The intravenous and inhalational routes provide rapid onset of action (2–5 minutes). Ingestion of PCP causes toxicity in approximately 30–60 minutes.

PCP is metabolized mainly by the liver, and the resultant metabolites are excreted by the kidneys. PCP and the resultant metabolites remain in the urine for an average of 2 weeks but may persist for up to 1 month.

PCP first became popular in the 1960s and 1970s and continues to be commonly abused. PCP has many street names, including hog and angel dust. Marijuana cigarettes are often adulterated with PCP and treated with embalming fluid. PCP-laced marijuana cigarettes also have many street names, including dip and wet.

PCP abuse can cause serious clinical features. Classic signs and symptoms of PCP toxicity include hallucinations, delusions, agitation, and violent, bizarre behavior. Patients also typically suffer tachycardia, hypertension, and diaphoresis. Nystagmus, a blank stare, and coma may also occur.

Acute PCP toxicity typically lasts 4–6 hours. Large overdoses of PCP may last 24–48 hours or longer for the chronic user. However, the relationship between dosage of PCP, clinical features, and serum levels is not predictable or reliable.

Gamma-Hydroxybutyrate

Gamma-hydroxybutyrate (GHB) is a sedative-hypnotic-like drug. In the 1980s, GHB was easily obtained at health food stores, gyms, and mail-order outlets. This drug was very popular because it was purported to act as a fat burner and a growth hormone promoter. The Food and Drug Administration (FDA) prohibited the sale and manufacture of GHB in 1990. Since then, GHB use and abuse has continued as a result of its ease of synthesis. GHB is commonly used and abused today at dance music scenes and night clubs.

GHB typically is available in pure powder form that is then either ingested or mixed with water. When mixed with water or another liquid, GHB is tasteless, odorless, and colorless. GHB is rapidly absorbed following ingestion and causes clinical effects within 5–15 minutes. GHB is eliminated by pulmonary expiration. GHB is often sold on the streets in small plastic containers that resemble hotel shampoo bottles. There are many street names for GHB, including scoop, liquid ecstasy, liquid X, and easy lay.

There are several classic clinical features of GHB intoxication. Initially, the user may suffer a brief period of agitation and seizure-like movements. Overdoses of GHB typically produce euphoria followed by a profound depressed level of consciousness, respiratory depression, and possible coma. Bradycardia may also occur. The clinical features typically only last approximately 3–6 hours. Amnesia is common following awakening from GHB toxicity. GHB has been used in numerous occasions as a date-rape drug. Even though GHB is not detected on the typical urine drug screen, GHB can be detected in urine and serum samples using GC-MS.[19]

Benzodiazepines

Benzodiazepines are sedative-hypnotic drugs that are commonly abused. The clinical features of intoxication are very similar to that of ethanol, except for the odor on the breath typically produced by ethanol-intoxicated patients. Testing for benzodiazepines frequently produces false-negative results, especially with clonazepam or lorazepam. The main reason for these false-negative results is that some benzodiazepines (clonazepam and lorazepam) are excreted in the urine almost entirely as glucuronide metabolites and not the parent compound. These glucuronides have little to no cross-reactivity with the immunoassay antibody and thus produce a false-negative result.[9]

Barbiturates

Barbiturates are sedative-hypnotic drugs with clinical features of intoxication very similar to that of ethanol and benzodiazepines. Phenobarbital, a long-acting barbiturate, can be detected both qualitatively in the urine and quantitatively in the serum.

DRUG-FACILITATED SEXUAL ASSAULT

The majority of sexual assaults in the United States are reported to be acquaintance rapes, also known as "date rapes." Drug-facilitated sexual assault occurs when a chemical is used to assist or procure nonconsensual sexual contact, typically by making the victim somnolent, lethargic, or comatose. Under these circumstances, the victim is unable to resist or consent to sexual contact. Alcohol and marijuana are two of the most common drugs implicated in drug-facilitated sexual assault cases. Two sedative-hypnotic-like drugs, GHB and flunitrazepam (Rohypnol), have received particular attention from the media as agents used for date rape. However, recent studies report that GHB and flunitrazepam account for very few cases of drug-facilitated sexual assault.[1]

GHB and flunitrazepam both possess ideal features of a date rape drug because they come as a powder that, when mixed into a drink, becomes odorless, colorless, and tasteless. The victim typically is lethargic and/or comatose for approximately 3–6 hours and awakens suddenly with no memory of the event. Both rarely cause complete respiratory arrest, so the victim typically does not sustain permanent pulmonary or anoxic injury. US formulations of flunitrazepam can potentially be identified because they turn blue or hazy blue in clear, colorless beverages. Illicit sources, however, remain colorless.

Rapid urine and blood specimen collection of drug-facilitated sexual assault cases is imperative because delays can affect the prosecutorial and toxicologic outcomes. Immediate action must be taken to preserve the COC. The victim should be urged not to urinate until the specimen can be properly collected. In addition, 20 mL of blood should be preserved with sodium fluoride and potassium oxalate (gray-top tube), especially if the drug was ingested within the last 24 hours.[1] Rapid blood collection can potentially corroborate involvement of the drug in the sexual assault. Positive urine toxicology is only indicative of prior exposure to the drug. Collected samples should be dated, timed, and refrigerated immediately.

Important historical information surrounding the sexual assault also needs careful documentation. Documentation of the events leading up to the sexual assault are best left for the legal authorities because discrepancies between the medical and legal records can interfere with the prosecution of the alleged perpetrator. Prosecution of drug-facilitated sexual assault and interpretation of toxicologic findings can also be complicated in cases of multiple drug use by the victim. An example of such is the presence of alcohol in victims of drug-facilitated sexual assault.

IN UTERO AND NEWBORN DRUG EXPOSURE

Illicit substances are frequently used and abused by a woman during her pregnancy.[20] High rates of fetal distress, growth retardation, and abnormal neurodevelopment have been reported in babies when the pregnant mother commonly abuses drugs. In utero drug exposure can lead to significant medical complications in the child during multiple stages of his or her life.[20] Drug use in nursing mothers is also a concern because many drugs are transported by passive diffusion across the mammary epithelium into the breast milk. Acute toxicity and withdrawal effects are possible when drugs are passed to baby from mother via the breast milk.

Prenatal or neonatal drug exposure can be determined using immunoassays or GC-MS.[1,20] Interpretation of these results is often difficult because the drug dose, route of abuse, and time of administration is often unknown.

CONCLUSION

Unfortunately, drug and alcohol abuse is a serious problem. Drugs and alcohol often contribute to crime and violence. Emergency department personnel need to be aware of how common intoxicants will affect their patients and use that data to assist in their care. A better understanding of the urine drug screen will allow clinicians to determine whether a particular drug is playing a role in the patient's presentation.

REFERENCES

1. Kerrigan S, Goldberger BA. Forensic toxicology. In: Lynch VA, Duval JB, eds. *Forensic Nursing.* St Louis, Mo: Elsevier Mosby; 2006:123–139.
2. Langman LJ, Kapur BM. Toxicology: then and now. *Clin Biochem.* 2006;39(5):498–510.
3. Rao RB, Flomenbaum M. Postmortem toxicology. In: Goldfrank LR, Flomenbaum NE, Lewin NA, et al, eds. *Goldfrank's Toxicologic Emergencies.* 7th ed. New York, NY: McGraw-Hill; 2002:1781–1788.
4. Burrows DL, Andrea N, Rice PJ, et al. Papain: a novel urine adulterant. *J Anal Toxicol.* 2005;29(5):275–395.
5. Mittal MK, Florin T, Perrone J, et al. Toxicity from the use of niacin to beat urine drug screening. *Ann Emerg Med.* 2007;50(5)587–590.
6. Jaffee WB, Trucco E, Levy SL, Weiss RD. Is this urine really negative? A systematic review of tampering methods in urine drug screening and testing. *J Sub Abuse Treat.* 2007;33(1):33–42.
7. Dasgupta A. The effects of adulterants and selected ingested compounds on drugs-of-abuse testing in urine. *Am J Clin Path.* 2007;128(3):491–503.
8. LeStrange W, Porter K. Risk management and legal principles. In: Goldfrank LR, Flomenbaum NE, Lewin NA, et al, eds. *Goldfrank's Toxicologic Emergencies.* 7th ed. New York, NY: McGraw-Hill; 2002:1768–1780.
9. Rainey PM. Laboratory principles and techniques for evaluation of the poisoned or overdosed patient. In: Goldfrank LR, Flomenbaum NE, Lewin NA, et al, eds. *Goldfrank's Toxicologic Emergencies.* 7th ed. New York, NY: McGraw-Hill; 2002:69–93.
10. Drug Abuse Warning Network (DAWN). Home page. Available at: http://dawninfo.samhsa.gov/. Retrieved July 25, 2008.
11. Bureau of Justice Statistics. *Criminal Victimization in the United States, 2004 Statistical Tables.* NCJ 213257. June 2006:Table 32. Available at: http://www.ojp.usdoj.gov/bjs/pub/pdf/cvus04.pdf. Retrieved July 25, 2008.
12. Mumola CJ, Karberg JC. *Drug Use and Dependence, State and Federal Prisoners, 2004.* Bureau of Justice Statistics. NCJ 213530. October 2006. Available at: http://www.ojp.usdoj.gov/bjs/pub/pdf/dudsfp04.pdf. Retrieved July 25, 2008.
13. Hart TC. *Violent Victimization of College Students, 1995–2000.* Bureau of Justice Statistics. NCJ 196143. December 2003. Available at: http://www.securityoncampus.org/schools/research/vvcs00.pdf. Retrieved July 25, 2008.
14. Duhart DT. *Violence in the Workplace, 1993–99.* Bureau of Justice Statistics. NCJ 190076. December 2001. Available at: http://www.ojp.usdoj.gov/bjs/pub/pdf/vw99.pdf. retrieved July 25, 2008.
15. Karberg JC, James DJ. *Substance Dependence, Abuse, and Treatment of Jail Inmates, 2002.* Bureau of Justice Statistics. NCJ 209588. July 2005. Available at: http://www.ojp.gov/bjs/pub/pdf/sdatji02.pdf. Retrieved July 25, 2008.
16. Fatality Analysis Reporting System. National Highway Traffic Safety Administration (NHSTA). Home page. Available at: http://www-fars.nhtsa.dot.gov/. Retrieved July 25, 2008.
17. Gahlinger PM. Club drugs: MDMA, gamma-hydroxybutyrate (GHB), Rohypnol, and ketamine. *Am Fam Physician.* 2004;69(11):2619–2627.
18. Hall AP, Henry JA. Acute toxic effects of "Ecstasy" (MDMA) and related compounds: overview of pathophysiology and clinical management. *BJA.* 2006;96(6):678–685.
19. Mason PE, Kerns WP II. Gamma hydroxybutyric acid (GHB) intoxication. *Acad Emerg Med.* 2002;9(7):730–739.
20. Huestis MA, Choo RE. Drug abuse's smallest victims: in utero drug exposure. *For Sci Int.* 2002;128(1–2):20–30.

7 | Forensic Photography

William M. Green, MD, and Elliot Schulman, MD, MPH

INTRODUCTION

Forensic medicine is the discipline that addresses the interface between medicine and the law. Clinical forensic medicine deals with the evaluation and management of living victims. The most common venue for these encounters is the emergency department (ED). The victimized individual who presents to the ED has two sets of needs. First is patient care concerns involving medical and emotional issues. The second category is the forensic needs of the criminal justice system. The fundamental forensic objective is to provide an independent reconstruction of the events in question that is accurate, scientifically sound, and evidence-based. Ideally, the rigor and precision of the reconstruction provided by the clinical forensic medical evaluation and analysis are robust enough to stand independently from the testimony of witnesses, perpetrator, or victim. The best example of this forensic ideal is the use of DNA to conclusively establish the identity of the source of biological evidence.

Unfortunately, most clinical forensic medical evaluations don't allow this level of certainty. Typically, the clinical forensic examiner obtains the history of events from the victim, and then performs a detailed physical examination that includes documentation of physical findings and collection of potential evidence. The final assessment is usually a determination regarding the degree of consistency among the history, physical findings, and analyzed evidence. Obviously, the documentation of physical findings (e.g., injuries) and discovered evidence (trace and biological) is critical in the forensic process. Forensic photography is a fundamental component of documentation along with a diagrammatic depiction and a written description of every visible finding. Forensic photography may also be employed to document the absence of visible findings.

A forensic photo "stops the clock" to reveal injury or other findings as they originally appeared before any treatment, manipulation, healing, or removal. Forensic imaging must provide a fair and accurate rendering of the original finding to allow independent review by all parties involved in the investigation and prosecution. High-quality images may provide the basis for exact measurements, comparison to published literature, or the standard for a subsequent examination. Additionally, forensic photos are invaluable for training forensic professionals and in peer review and continuous quality improvement.

FORENSIC PHOTOGRAPHY HISTORY

The first documented forensic use of photography occurred one month after the initial photographic process was patented in 1839. The plaintiff in a divorce case hired Louis Daguerre to photograph her husband and his mistress in front of the Paris Opera House. The French court accepted the photograph (Daguerreotype) as evidence and awarded the plaintiff a divorce. Unfortunately, the photograph was lost to artillery fire during the Franco-Prussian War of 1870. Again in Paris, in 1841, Detective Rogue established the first primitive mugshot database of repeat offenders using Daguerreotype arrest photographs. This investigative tool became known as a Rogue's Gallery. In the United States, in 1859, the Supreme Court ruled in favor of a runaway slave seeking his freedom, in part because of the evidence of injuries from repetitive beatings documented by a photograph.

Crime scene photography soon became more common, with documentation of homicides, arson, autopsies, evidence (fingerprints, bloodstains, impressions), and traffic collisions. The medical use of photography in violence assessment was variable, but minimal, prior to 1980. In the early 1980s initial reports appeared regarding the use of colposcopy for child sexual assault exams and the photographic recording of findings. The American Medical Association published guidelines recommending that all visible lesions be photographed, for both consultative and medicolegal reasons. It became well understood that when injuries have healed, photographs in the medical record could provide the most accurate visual proof of injuries. Photography has thus become the standard of care, and best practice, for documenting the physical effects of domestic violence, elder abuse, child maltreatment, and sexual assault.

FORENSIC PHOTOGRAPHY IN THE EMERGENCY DEPARTMENT

Forensic photography is a huge discipline involving a myriad of imaging techniques to document anatomic details, physical evidence, human interactions/activities, and crime scenes of all types. The focus for this chapter is the photographic documentation of the body (and potentially the clothing) of the living victim who presents to the emergency department after an alleged crime. The most common application is the documentation of injuries after violent interpersonal contact in which the crime scene is the victim's body.

Most clinical forensic examiners are not photographic experts. Many novice or first-time forensic photographers may be intimidated or deterred by the overwhelming array of technical issues involved in creating high-quality images. Because photographic documentation is such a critical tool for clinical forensic medicine, it is essential for every examiner to have at least modest competency in forensic imaging. The objective of this chapter is to present the basic principles and techniques necessary to facilitate the production of good quality, useful forensic images.

In the forensic world, digital photography has almost completely replaced film-based formats. This chapter focuses on digital imaging. Further, the emphasis is on user-friendly, moderately priced, entry-level digital equipment and systems.

DIGITAL IMAGING

The digital format offers a number of advantages over film-based slides and prints. The ability to instantly review digital images provides immediate feedback on both the composition and the technical quality of the image. This review may be on the camera's LCD screen or downloaded for viewing on a computer screen. If the image is not optimum, it can be reshot until it is. Because there are no film or processing costs, digital is much cheaper and should naturally stimulate the examiner to take as many images as necessary to adequately document the findings.

The electronic nature of digital photos greatly simplifies and expedites image organization, filing, storage, and transport. By using image enhancement, the examiner can adjust photos to optimal quality so that the images depict a fair and accurate view of the original scene. Multiple presentation options are readily available in the digital format. Images can be e-mailed to investigators, experts, or attorneys. They may be embedded in PowerPoint presentations or directly projected onto a screen. High-quality prints can be generated if hard copy is required. Storage of digital images is much more compact than the corresponding number of slides or prints would be. Legal chain of custody may be simpler with digital format than it is with film.

It is helpful to understand the key differences between a digital camera and a film camera. This is especially true for those examiners with some familiarity with film who are new to digital. Both types of cameras use a lens, aperture, and shutter to capture a certain amount of reflected light from the subject and bring it into the camera body. Instead of stimulating a chemical reaction on film, the digital camera focuses the light on an electronic image sensor made up of thousands of light-sensitive picture elements called *pixels*. With the aid of the in-camera computer (image processor), each pixel converts brightness and color into a discreet numeric code. These digital data are then stored on the camera's removable memory card. The greater the number of pixels, the smoother the gradation of tone and the finer the detail in the final image. The total number of pixels also influences the maximum size print of acceptable quality that can be generated. For most forensic applications, 6 megapixels (6 million pixels) is the minimum.

The number of pixels per image is a selection variable on most digital cameras. This may be described as image size (expressed in pixel dimensions) or as resolution. For forensic applications, always choose the maximum number of pixels or the highest resolution.

Imaging data on the memory card may be stored in different file formats. The three most common are TIFF (Tagged Image File Format), RAW (uncompressed), and JPEG (Joint Photographic Experts Group). The choice of format affects image quality, download speed, and storage space. TIFF and RAW are termed *lossless* because their images can be stored and reconstituted without a loss of digital code. The downside is that TIFF and RAW create large file sizes per image and transfer slowly. The most commonly used format is JPEG, which is *lossy*. JPEG images can be compressed (to a variable degree), which saves storage space (more images per memory card) and speeds transfer time. The price for these conveniences with JPEG is that when the image is reconstituted, some digital code is lost, which may slightly degrade or alter the image. The most practical compromise is to use JPEG format with the least amount of compression (JPEG Fine). The loss of digital code is minimal, is not clinically significant, and is unlikely to be detectable to the human eye.

Photographic film is selected based on its sensitivity (speed or ISO rating) and color balance (temperature) to match the light source (daylight, incandescent, fluorescent, etc.). Digital format uses the electronic versions of these variables. The sensitivity of the image sensor is controlled by adjusting the ISO value. The lower the ISO number, the more light is required; the higher the value, the less light is needed for the exposure. Lower values produce more detail but require longer exposures; higher values allow faster shutter speeds but may produce images that are "grainy" or that contain artifacts (digital noise). A good compromise is to select an ISO of 100.

Color balance is adjusted on a digital camera using the white balance (WB) control. The correct WB setting is needed to accurately reproduce the original colors of the subject and to keep white as a true neutral. If a single, predictable light source is always used (e.g., fluorescent lights in the exam room), that specific setting can be selected. The best overall choice is to select "auto WB" and let the camera calculate the best value. Some experimentation with WB settings followed by careful critique of the images is prudent.

A very important feature of digital cameras not shared by film cameras is the LCD screen. This is the functional equivalent of having a small computer monitor screen on the back of the camera. It allows the examiner to see and evaluate the image during composition and immediately after capture. The LCD also provides access to information about current settings and allows interaction with the various camera programs and controls.

PHOTOGRAPHY BASICS

It is useful for the forensic examiner to understand the rudiments of photographic theory. A detailed knowledge of the physics involved or knowing all the "bells and whistles" (that even entry-level cameras contain) is unnecessary. Basic knowledge is helpful for two reasons. First, some commonly encountered photographic challenges in forensic documentation (e.g., body cavities, curved surfaces, very small findings, etc.) require minor adjustment in camera settings or technique for satisfactory images. Second, every forensic examiner must carefully critique their own images and identify errors (both technical and compositional). Understanding the basics facilitates both error recognition and corrective action. As discussed previously, digital imaging offers the opportunity for immediate feedback, analysis, and a second chance to capture the optimum image.

The camera lens is actually several pieces of polished glass that gather and focus light reflected off the subject onto the electronic image sensor. The focal length of the lens controls the size of the image reaching the sensor. The smaller the focal length number, the wider the view and smaller the subjects appear (wide angle). The larger the focal length number, the narrower the view and the larger the subjects appear (telephoto). If the lens creates an image as seen by the unaided eye, it is said to be a normal lens. Most digital cameras in use today offer the best of all with a zoom lens that has an adjustable focal length so that the forensic examiner can control the size of the image.

An important point about digital cameras is the difference between *optical* zoom and *digital* zoom. For forensic work, only optical zoom should be used because it is a function of movement of the glass lens elements and affords reasonable quality throughout the zoom range. Digital zoom starts at the upper end of optical zoom range (telephoto) and magnifies the image further electronically, which gives a lower quality end product. Digital zoom should be disabled or turned off for forensic applications. Another important lens capability in forensic documentation is the ability to magnify small findings. These close-up shots are possible with a macro lens or macro setting. Most digital cameras have this feature.

Another basic photographic concept relates to controlling the amount of light that reaches the sensor. This is *exposure* and is primarily controlled by two reciprocating variables: aperture (or f-stop) and shutter speed. The aperture is determined by adjusting a circular opening, or diaphragm, inside the lens and is measured by the f-stop number. The smaller the number, the larger the opening (and the larger amount of light that passes through the lens). The larger the f-stop, the smaller the opening, and the less light enters. (See Figure 7-1.) The shutter is like a curtain in the lens that is opened for a specific amount of time (shutter speed), and this controls the amount of light that enters the lens and strikes the sensor. The reciprocal relationship is illustrated by the fact that a low f-stop (large opening) plus a brief shutter speed may allow exactly the same total amount of light to strike the sensor as a high f-stop (small opening) plus a long shutter speed. (See Figure 7-2.)

Even though the same exposure can be achieved by infinite pairings of aperture and shutter speed, two important practical considerations influence the choice for a given photographic situation. The choice of shutter speed has a bearing on how sharp the image is when the camera is handheld (i.e., not on a tripod). It is nearly impossible to hold a camera

FIGURE 7-1 **The iris on the left is stopping more light than the iris on the right; consequently, it has a higher f-stop value. Adapted from *Complete Digital Photography* 3rd Edition by Long. 2004. Reprinted with permission of Delmar Learning, a division of Thomson Learning: www.thomsonrights.com.**

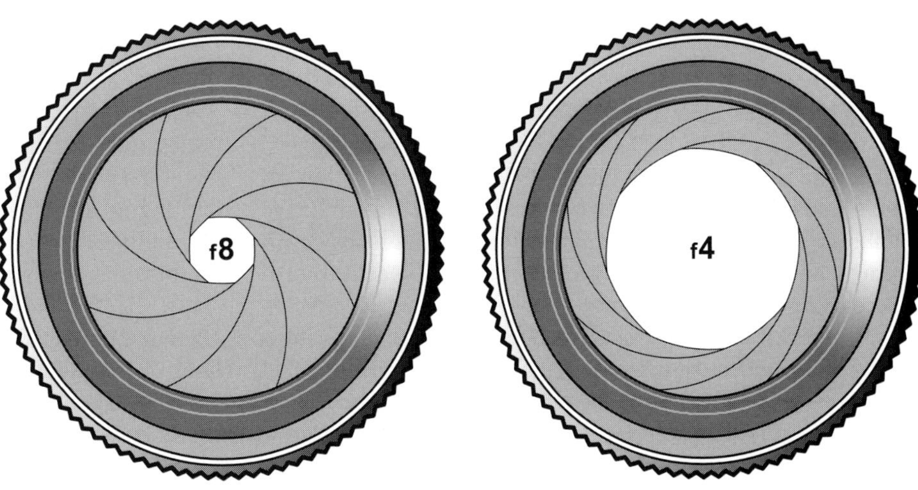

Equivalent Exposures

Shutter Speed (in seconds)

15th 30th 60th 125th 250th

Aperture (f-stop)

f8 f11 f16 f22 f32

Shutter Speed (in seconds)

15th 30th 60th 125th 250th

Aperture (f-stop)

f8 f11 f16 f22 f32

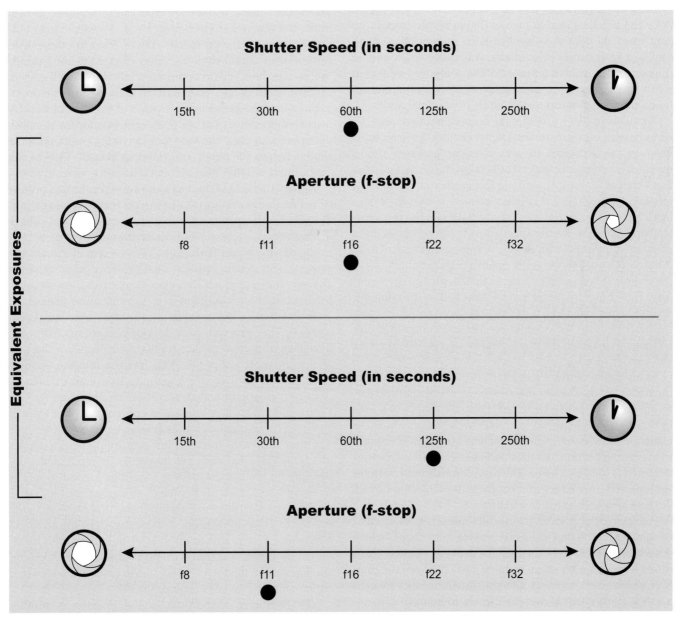

FIGURE 7-2 **Because of the reciprocal nature of exposed parameters, if you change one parameter in one direction, you can move the other parameter in the opposite direction and still yield the same overall exposure. Adapted from *Complete Digital Photography* 3rd Edition by Long. 2004. Reprinted with permission of Delmar Learning, a division of Thomson Learning: www.thomsonrights.com.**

completely motionless. The longer the shutter is open (slow shutter speed), the greater the risk of camera motion that could result in a blurred image. Practically speaking, a shutter speed faster than 1/60 s (depicted as "60" on the camera) should be used to prevent blurring. New technology has affected this issue. Some digital cameras now include an image stabilization or vibration reduction feature that helps counteract camera shake and allows slower shutter speeds to produce sharp, handheld images.

The other exposure variable, aperture, influences how much of an entire scene is in sharp focus. This factor is called *depth of field* and controls the nearest and farthest distance from the camera between which objects in the scene appear in focus. The lower the f-stop number (larger opening), the narrower the depth of field. The higher the f-stop number (smaller opening), the broader the depth of field. (See Figure 7-3.) The practical significance of this principle comes into play when the forensic objective is to sharply photograph a subject with curves or contours. A broader depth of field (higher f-stop) will render more of the contoured subject in sharp focus. Obviously, photography requires a number of trade-offs and compromises to obtain the optimal result.

Again, technology provides the forensic photographer assistance with exposure issues. Digital cameras have multiple exposure mode choices. In "automatic" or "program" mode, the camera's computer selects the best aperture/shutter speed combination for most situations. This mode suffices for most forensic applications. In "aperture priority" mode, the examiner chooses the aperture and the camera sets the appropriate corresponding shutter speed. This is a good choice for a situation requiring the maximum or minimum depth of field. "Shutter priority" mode is the opposite: The examiner picks the shutter speed and the camera calculates the proper aperture. This choice might be helpful if the victim is having difficulty staying still and a faster shutter speed could decrease the blurring from subject motion. The last common choice is "manual" in which the photographer selects both aperture and shutter speed.

Many digital cameras also offer a choice of the area within the scene that the camera analyzes to calculate exposure (metering mode). The two basic selections are spot (a tiny area in the center of the scene) or center-weighted in which the camera considers the entire frame but assigns more weight to the central portion. For most forensic applications, center-weighted is the best choice. The main forensic indication for spot metering is a circumstance where the subject is a small, discrete area such as inside a body cavity.

Achieving sharp focus is critically important in forensic imaging. Most digital cameras provide auto focus, which quickly and accurately focuses the lens. A manual focus mode is available on many cameras, which allows the photographer focus control in difficult situations. Spot focus is a useful feature that allows the camera to automatically focus on a tiny area in the scene. If available, this may be very helpful forensically in situations where the subject of interest is in a different plane than other close-by features in the scene. Using spot metering in conjunction with spot focus increases the likelihood of creating a high-quality image in difficult circumstances.

Good lighting is critical for successful photography. The issues of white balance and temperature control have already been discussed. For most forensic applications, ambient lighting in the ED suffices if the camera is properly set up. The built-in (on camera) flash can supplement room lighting but may give harsh or "hard" results with shadows and sharp edges. Close-ups with the built-in flash may wash out color and details. Cavity photography may require a separate light source, separate flash unit (off camera), or a ring light (or ring flash). It is essential to experiment with macro and cavity imaging.

EQUIPMENT AND SETUP

The digital camera market has experienced explosive growth in the last few years, which presents an overwhelming number of choices to the prospective buyer. There are three main categories of digital cameras. Entry-level units are typically "point-and-shoot" cameras that are about the size of a deck of cards or slightly larger. They perform all the basic photographic functions and generally have some of the control features discussed previously but are really designed for the nonphotographer who does not want to do anything except push the shutter button for family and travel snapshots. They are an "any camera is better than nothing" choice for forensic work.

At the other end of the spectrum are sophisticated professional single-lens reflex (SLR) cameras that have nearly infinite technical capabilities and adjustments. SLRs also have many potential accessories (interchangeable lenses, a multitude of off-camera flash units, filters, etc.). These are the cameras and systems professional evidence photographers choose. They are expensive, complicated, and for the nonprofessional, have a long and steep learning curve to mastery.

In the middle are compact or advanced amateur digital cameras. They generally provide good compromises for cost, flexibility, and good quality results. Compacts are the best choice for most nonprofessional forensic imaging applications. Some may have the capability to use an off-camera flash or a ring light source for better macro imaging. (See Figure 7-4.) Whatever camera is chosen, read the manual and keep the manual with the camera.

Other essential forensic imaging equipment includes plenty of extra batteries (rechargeable or replaceable, depending on the camera). There should be a good supply of memory cards, each with enough storage space (at least 1 gigabyte) to document an "average" case that presents to the ED for forensic evaluation. A 1-gigabyte (1-GB) card will hold about 130 images at the JPEG Fine setting with maximum image size. A tripod is useful at times when maximum sharpness is mandatory. A scale and/or color bar is standard equipment for forensic imaging. See Table 7-1.

The computer support for digital imaging is another system decision with many variables and personal preferences. A card reader facilitates downloading images from the memory card to the computer hard drive (faster than direct connection from camera to computer). Many image

Shutter Speed (in seconds)

Handheld shake

1 Stop

15th 30th 60th 125th 250th

Slower Less Motion Stopping More Motion Stopping Faster

More Light Less Light

Aperture (f-stop)

1 Stop

f8 f11 f16 f22 f32

Larger Less Depth of Field More Depth of Field Smaller

More Light Less Light

ISO (Sensor Sensitivity)

1 Stop

50 100 200 400 800

Slower Less Sensitive Less Noise More Noise Faster More Sensitive

FIGURE 7-3 **Shutter speed, aperture, and ISO are the three exposure parameters over which you have control. Each one provides a different way of controlling the amount of light that strikes the focal plane. Each adjustment, in turn, affects your image in different ways. Adapted from *Complete Digital Photography* 3rd Edition by Long. 2004. Reprinted with permission of Delmar Learning, a division of Thomson Learning: www.thomsonrights.com.**

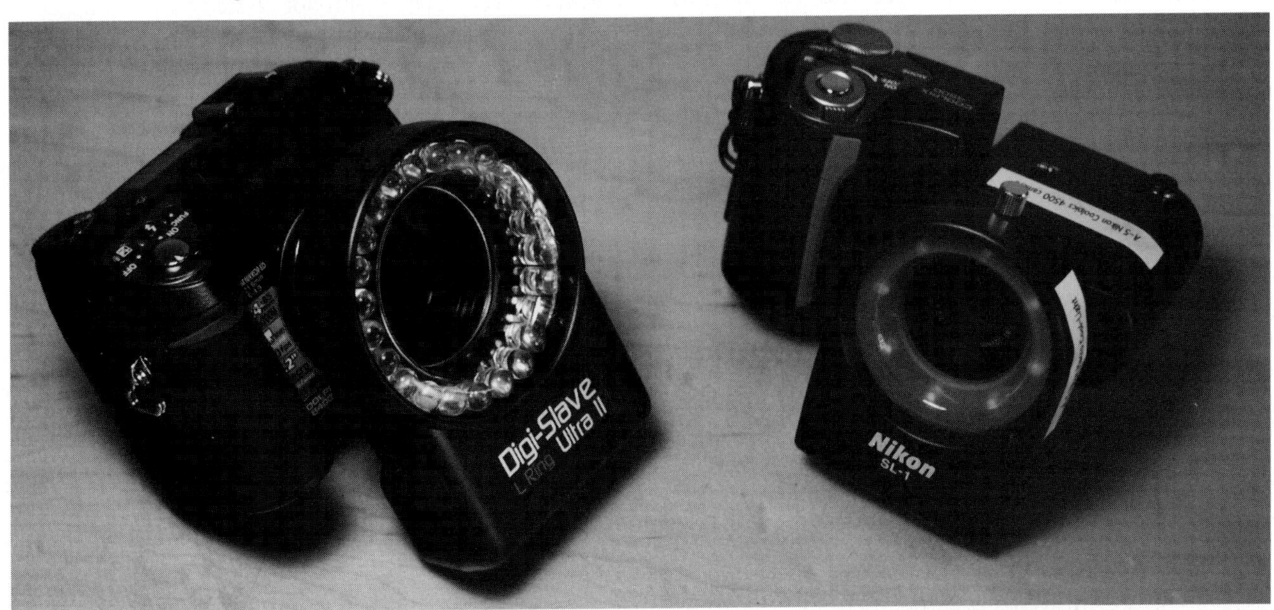

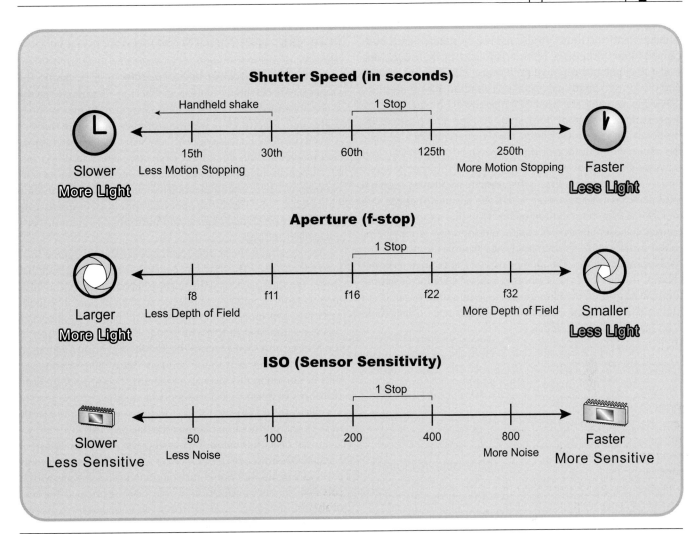

FIGURE 7-4 **Two examples of compact digital cameras equipped with LED (light emitting diode) light sources for better macro (close-up) images.**

management software programs are available, and both cameras and computers often are sold with their own version. Caseload and personal preference will drive the choice. The computer should have as much random access memory (RAM) as possible (at least 512 megabytes) to speed image processing. Amount of hard drive storage is dependent on caseload; again, more is better. The computer must also have the capacity to duplicate original images (CD or DVD) and transmit them electronically over a secure Internet connection. A backup system for all images may require an external hard drive, an off-site server, or off-site storage of duplicates on CD or DVD. Information technology (IT) support for the computer-based aspects of digital photography is very helpful for initial setup, maintenance, and troubleshooting.

Keeping in mind the perspective of a compact digital camera in the hands of a photographically nonprofessional forensic examiner, the camera can be configured to facilitate high-quality imaging with minimal experience. (See Table 7-2.) Just follow these steps:

1. First, set the time and date (consult the camera manual).
2. Set the file format to JPEG with the least compression ("Fine" image quality) and the resolution to the largest size image.
3. Set the ISO sensitivity to 100 (some cameras offer "auto" ISO, which is also a good choice).
4. Set the metering mode to center-weighted.
5. Set the focus mode to auto (if available, know how to adjust to spot focus).
6. Set the exposure mode to auto or programmed (P). Know how to change to macro mode for close-ups.
7. Set the white balance (WB) to auto.
8. Set the flash to auto (if a separate light source is to be used, set the on-camera flash to off).
9. Set the digital zoom to off.

When the camera battery is charged and the camera is configured, start taking pictures—lots of pictures. Download the images, critique them, retake the shots that need improvement, and then critique again.

TABLE 7-1 **Useful Features, Adjustments, or Accessories for Digital Forensic Imaging**

Image stabilization or vibration reduction
Aperture priority
Shutter priority
Spot metering
Spot focus
Macro (close-up) capability
Accessory ring light or ring flash
Tripod
Extra batteries
Extra memory cards
Scale or color bar
Memory card reader
Image management software

FORENSIC TECHNIQUES AND COMPOSITION

The goal of forensic imaging is to *fairly and accurately* document findings as realistically as possible and to depict the subject as it originally appeared. "Do not disturb the crime scene" is a forensic maxim. Any finding should first be photographed exactly as it was found. Every time anything is moved, removed, cleaned, or in any way manipulated, separate images should document each step. Every finding must be shown in adequate detail but also in context to its surroundings. There should be multiple images of every finding. (See Figure 7-5.) This means photographing all findings from varying perspectives (angles) and multiple distances or variable zoom settings.

As a general forensic rule, each finding should appear in at least four images. The first is an overview or orienting shot that shows the finding from a distance sufficient to show the finding's size and orientation in relation to obvious anatomic landmarks (two or more). More than one finding may be shown in this view. The next shot is a midrange shot, which is closer to the finding and reveals more detail and preferably includes at least one obvious anatomic landmark. More than one finding may be shown in this view also. The next two images are both close-ups (macro) that document the detailed appearance of a single finding. One of these close-ups must include a scale next to and in the same plane as the finding. This scale allows accurate measurement of the finding. The American Board of Forensic Odontology (ABFO) No. 2 Angled Rule is commonly used as a scale, but some jurisdictions prefer a scale with a color bar for standardization of colors in the images. The second close-up image without the scale is necessary to reveal any findings (or lack of findings) that were under the scale.

Framing of the scene should generally place the subject or finding of interest in the center. This is helpful for those who will review the image and maximizes the accuracy of the camera's autofocus and exposure functions. The background (parts of the scene not related to the finding or its anatomic orientation) must be as plain or neutral as possible. Background clutter is distracting and should be avoided or minimized. It may be necessary to reposition the subject or use uniformly colored drapes to mask unwanted background items (blue or green surgical towels or operative drapes work well and are usually readily available in the ED).

TABLE 7-2 **Suggested Settings for Digital Forensic Imaging**

Format	JPEG
Quality	Fine
Resolution	Maximum
ISO	100 or Auto
White balance	Auto
Metering mode	Center-Weighted
Digital zoom	Off
Exposure mode	Auto or Program (P)
On-camera flash	Auto
Focus mode	Auto

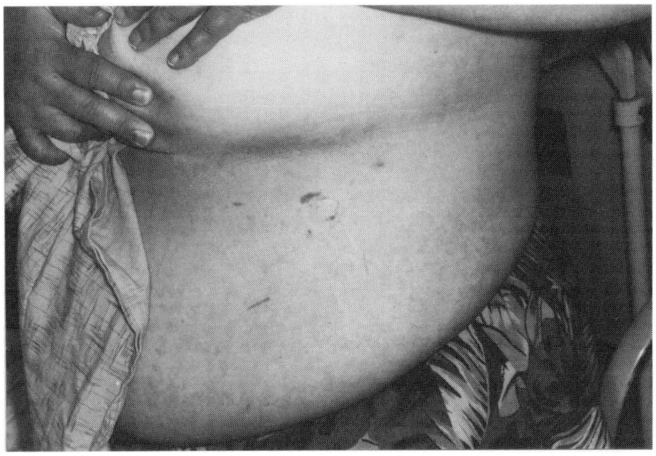

(a)

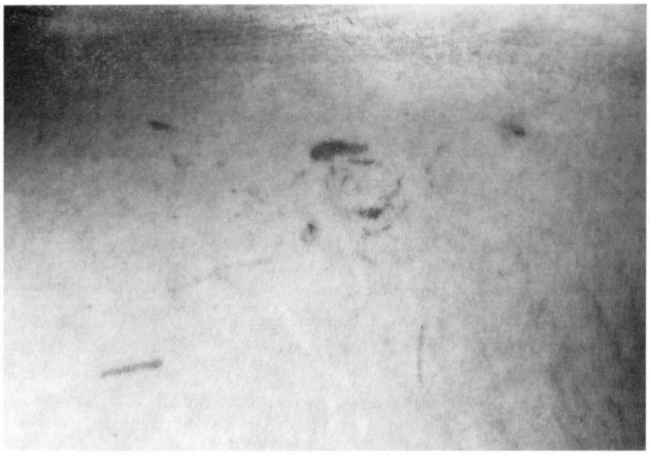

(b)

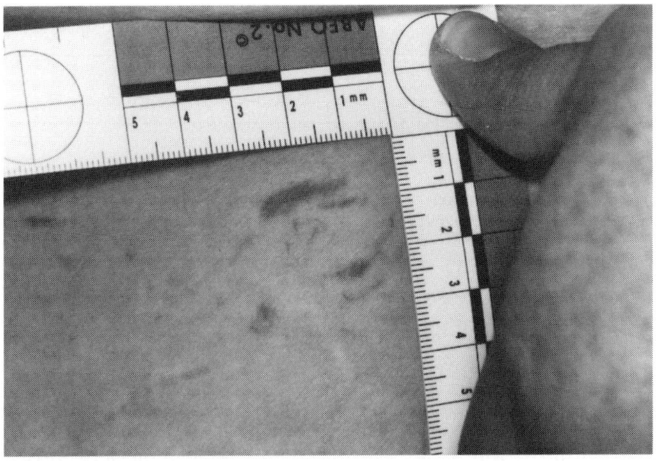

(c)

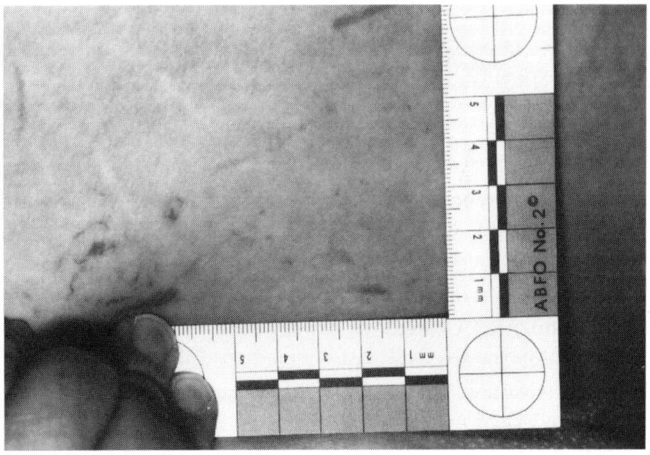

(d)

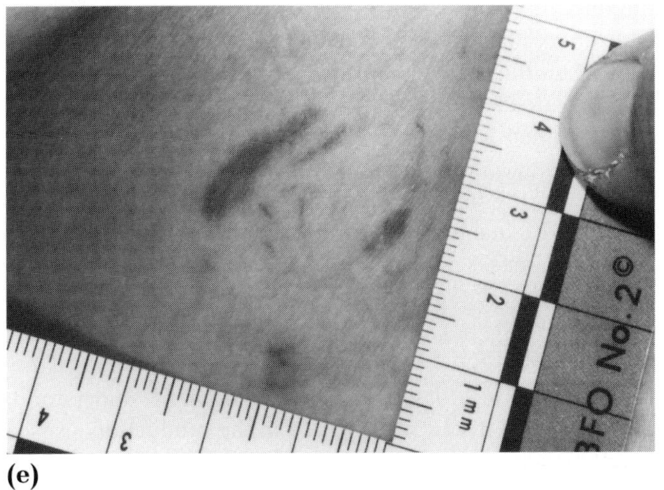

(e)

FIGURE 7-5 **45-year-old female who was sexually assaulted 40 hours prior to forensic examination. Injuries included multiple burns from a hot cigarette lighter pressed into the left upper quadrant of her abdomen several times. (a) Orienting view showing burns between left breast and waistband of skirt. (b) Midrange view showing more details. (c) and (d) Closer views showing scales for dimension. Note different positions of the scale reveal all findings. (e) Close-up view with scale showing best detail. See Color Plate 1 for 7-5 (c) and (e).**

COMMON ERRORS

Errors may be compositional or technical. (See Table 7-3.) The most common compositional error is not taking enough images to document the findings adequately. When in doubt, take more images. Related to this problem is failure to adhere to the "four images per finding" principle either by taking only a distance shot without significant detail, or the converse, taking only a close-up (or series of close-ups!) that leaves the reviewer uncertain as to which finding is which. Not including at least one scale image for each finding precludes the possibility of measurement. The plane of the sensor must be parallel to the plane of the finding. If it is not, perspective distortion will result in which part of the image is in focus and part blurred, or part of the subject will appear inappropriately larger than another part. A related problem occurs if the plane of the scale, the plane of the finding, and

TABLE 7-3 **Common Errors and Solutions**

Compositional Error	Solution
Too few images	Take more images
Lack of detail	Four Images per Finding Rule
Uncertain position, orientation, or size	Four Images per Finding Rule
Background distraction	Reposition subject or use drapes
Technical Error	
Distorted perspective	Plane of image sensor and subject must be parallel
Distorted scale	Plane of image sensor and scale must be parallel
Blurred image	Image stabilization/vibration reduction Faster shutter speed Use tripod
Inadequate depth of field	Higher f-stop (smaller aperture)
Distorted color	Adjust white balance Image enhancement
Wrong exposure	Spot metering Manual metering

the plane of the image sensor are not all parallel. An advantage of the ABFO No. 2 rule are the circles. If the sensor plane is not parallel to the rule, the circles will appear as ellipses.

Technical errors include poor focus (blurred), over- or underexposure (washed out or very dark), or distorted color. The remedy for these is usually camera adjustments. A tripod can eliminate blurring because of camera motion.

As discussed earlier, it is critical to review all images for accuracy and completeness before the patient is no longer available for corrective imaging. It may be possible to uncover gross errors using the camera's LCD, but downloading images and reviewing them on a computer screen gives the examiner much more detail for the critique.

WORKFLOW

Workflow is the organized process that includes all the steps for image management from capture to storage. The handling of forensic images must be controlled by strict protocols developed in conjunction with the clinical forensic examiner, law enforcement, and prosecution. There are many possibilities and variations in workflow that depend on volume of caseload, community resources, and personal preferences. Whatever system is created, it must be a consensus of involved parties and faithfully adhered to by all. Flow diagrams and checklists are often helpful to maintain and ensure consistency, quality, and predictability of both the images and the system.

A typical workflow begins with having all equipment present, ready for use (monitored and checked regularly), and backups (e.g., memory cards, batteries, CDs, etc.) available. A fresh (blank after reformatting) memory card should be used for each case. All images for the case should go into a new file in the camera with sequential numbers and embedded Exchangeable Image File Format (EXIF) data about each image. Proper patient consent should always be obtained, and then images are captured. Specific protocols for technique and camera settings optimize quality and consistency.

After all images are captured, the memory card is removed, placed in a card reader, and downloaded onto the computer. Many image management programs are available. All the images from the case should go into a separate file. Images can then be reviewed by the forensic examiner on the computer monitor screen and analyzed for technical quality and composition. Assuming the patient is still present, problem images can be reshot, downloaded into the same case file, and critiqued again.

Primary images on the memory card become original images when they are downloaded. All original images should be duplicated and stored separately (CD, DVD, external hard drive, server) for security and backup. If image enhancements are needed, the original images are duplicated into a file of working images. Any enhanced images are added to both the original image file and to the backup image file. All preserved images must be secure, retrievable, and unequivocally linked to the specific case/patient.

LEGAL ISSUES

A number of legal issues must be recognized, understood, and addressed by anyone involved in the production, use, or maintenance of photographs for forensic purposes. These issues may include consent, identification, relevance, authentication, admissibility, and the development of standard operating procedures (SOPs). Although consent for crime scene recording is generally not necessary, photographing a patient in the ED requires specific and separate consent from the general consent for examination and treatment.

Because these photographs may become evidence in the criminal justice system, they must be identified as to person, time, and place and any other appropriate notation as required for the chain of custody requirements of the local jurisdiction. Relevance is a judicial process; the examiner must be able to testify that the photographs accurately and fairly portray the findings noted during the exam and are related, by history and mechanism of injury, to the action being adjudicated.

The examiner must be able, in order to have the photographs admitted as evidence, to declare under oath that the photograph being used is the original or a duplicate that fairly and accurately reproduces the original. It is essential that a written standard operating procedure (SOP) be developed and followed meticulously to preserve the chain of custody and admissibility. The SOP should address issues that include image preservation, security, information regarding their creation (settings, date, time, etc.), enhancement procedures, and custody (release and availability procedures).

CONCLUSION

Photodocumentation of injuries is an invaluable tool. It can recreate the "crime scene" (the patient) for use at criminal trial. Although not technically difficult, one should be familiar with basic photographic techniques and principles to provide the best photographs possible. Emergency departments should have equipment available and provide staff with training to use this resource.

8 | Forensic Bite Mark Evidence

Scott W. Brown, MD, and Allyson A. Kreshak, MD

INTRODUCTION

Teeth serve a variety of functions beyond their role in digestion. Presented here is a description of their use as weapons of aggression or defense. *Bite marks*, defined as a tooth-imposed physical change in a medium, have been found on victims and perpetrators after violent crimes such as homicide, sexual assault, and child abuse.[1–4] Human bites may compose up to 20% of all bites evaluated by inner-city physicians[5] with an incidence of 10.7 human bites per 100,000 people in one large urban setting.[3] When bitemarks are inflicted as part of a criminal behavior, both genders are affected; however, females are more frequently bitten. A bimodal age distribution also exists in which children up to 10 years of age and adults 21–50 years of age are at the most risk.[4]

Bite marks are of forensic value, and their evidence has been used to help identify perpetrators.[4,6] Given the prevalence of bite wounds among the general population and their potential forensic importance, emergency physicians and other acute care providers should be knowledgeable about identifying and collecting evidence from these wounds when present. This chapter focuses on the identification and collection of human bite evidence in the acute care setting.

IDENTIFICATION

Human bite marks typically appear as a circular or oval pattern made up of two U-shaped arches with a gap between them (Figure 8-1). The space between is created by the posterior portion of the mouth or throat. The area within the pattern may be ecchymotic as a result of the teeth's rupture of small vessels or from negative pressure created by sucking or tongue thrusting. Typically, bite marks are made by the anterior six teeth, occasionally including the molars, but partial bite marks (only a few teeth marks showing) and double bite marks (a bite within a bite) may confuse the appearance of the mark.[6–11]

Surrounding and including the tooth marks may be abrasions, striations, lacerations, contusions, or avulsions. Animal bites, by contrast, tend to puncture and tear and may be more severe.[11–13] Adult human bites are characterized by an intercanine distance of 25 to 40 mm. Bites inflicted by children typically have an intercanine distance less than 30 mm.[11,12] If a bite occurs through clothing, it may appear less distinct and the fabric may imprint on the skin overlying the mark. Additionally, individual teeth marks and impressions will become less discrete as time from infliction passes.[6,7]

Each type of tooth produces a specific pattern of impressions, known as class characteristics. Lower incisors form rectangular marks; canines produce triangular marks; premolars leave wounds described as single or dual triangles or diamonds; and molars rarely leave marks.[6,7] Additionally, each person has a unique bite, which results from the accumulation of dental changes throughout the lifetime. These individual-specific dental patterns are essential to the linking of bite mark to biter.[7] Distinct teeth marks, however, are not always seen. Because of the mobility of the lower jaw, the biting process is dynamic and skin slippage across the upper teeth can occur, leaving a vague impression pattern.[6]

Two atypical bites are described by the behavior involved with their infliction. The *fight bite* results from a punch to the mouth of another person thereby causing a laceration over the metacarpophalangial (MCP) joint of the hand. Though this type of bite does not demonstrate the typical characteristics of a bite mark, the medical practitioner should maintain a high index of suspicion for this mechanism when evaluating any laceration over the MCP joints.[4,5,14] The other atypical bite is a *love bite.* Love bites range from small nibbles performed prior to orgasm to traumatic avulsions caused by uncontrolled spasm during orgasmic climax.[15] Although these two bites differ in their properties and origin, they should be treated as true bites with regard to evidence collection.

LOCATION ON THE BODY

Multiple studies have attempted to describe the incidence of bites to various parts of the body. The extremities and breasts seem to be most frequently involved, with bite incidences ranging from 13–76% and 10.4–31.3%, respectively.[16–20] Freeman and colleagues tried to better define these ranges by studying 259 bite mark cases involving a total of 778 bites. Their results suggest that the extremities, specifically arms, were the most often bitten (incidence of 22.7%) for both sexes combined. Among women, the back and breasts were the second most common bite sites. In men, the legs and face were the next most commonly bitten. The authors also reported that frequency of anatomic bite location varies with type of crime. Bites inflicted during homicides commonly involve the arms, legs, and breasts; bites inflicted during sexual assault similarly involve the arms and breasts, but frequently include the face. In child abuse cases, a wide variety of sites were involved, including the arms, legs, back, buttocks, face, and shoulders.[4,21]

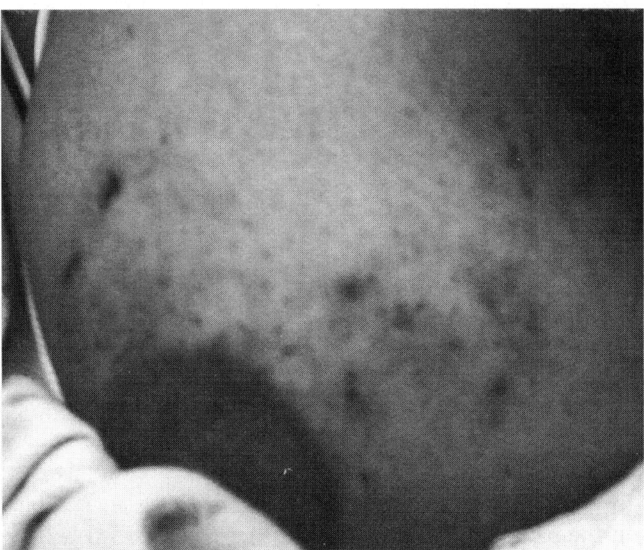

FIGURE 8-1 **Bite marks to a breast. See Color Plate 2.**

DIFFERENTIAL DIAGNOSIS

Multiple dermatologic conditions may be considered in the differential diagnosis of bite wounds. Drug reactions often have multiple lesions but may also present as a single, erythematous, well-demarcated lesion. Subacute cutaneous lupus erythema presents as scaly erythematous papules that coalesce to form larger annular lesions that may mimic bite marks. Pityriasis rosea initially manifests as a herald patch that is oval and easily confused with a bite mark. There is often a central area of salmon-pink that clears from the center, giving the impression of a bite mark. The rash evolves to form the typical "Christmas tree" pattern, but this may progress after the patient is initially examined. Tinea corporis demonstrates a typical circular pattern with an erythematous area and central clearing; however, the gap typically found in bite marks is not present. Granuloma annulare can present in a variety of colorations from skin tone to erythematous or violaceous papules that form an annular pattern. Differentiating a bite mark from these annular and arc-like lesions can be challenging. Often, the patient's history may be vague and unhelpful. An important distinction is that bite marks are usually nonscaly and often have teeth marks.[22]

A bite wound may be the only manifestation of child abuse, and in one study of bite mark victim demographics, approximately one-third of all the bite mark cases were classified as child abuse.[4] Identification of an adult bite mark (determined by intercanine distance) on a child is pathognomonic for abuse.[12] Otherwise, a mismatch in the child's history and physical exam should increase the practitioner's index of suspicion for abuse.

There are, however, skin conditions common to children that should not be misdiagnosed as bite marks. Some of the more common conditions include Mongolian spots, erythema multiforme, and Henoch-Schonlein purpura (HSP). Mongolian spots can be mistaken for bruises in babies of African American, American Indian, Asian, and Latino heritage. Mongolian spots are differentiated by their indistinct borders, lack of inflammation, and failure to progress through color or size changes.

Erythema multiforme can be confused with bruising given its rapidity of onset. Typically, annular lesions appear on the palms, soles, and extensor surfaces (but can be anywhere) and progressively develop a ringlike configuration with central clearing. Erythema multiforme usually results from drug sensitivity or infections such as herpes simplex and Mycoplasma.

HSP is characterized by a palpable purpura on the buttocks, arms, and legs with associated gastrointestinal and arthritic complaints. HSP is typically diagnosed in a child of 2 to 7 years of age. When considering the possibility of a bite wound on a child, the practitioner should also be aware of cultural treatments such as dry or wet cupping that may produce similar skin changes and not misdiagnose these folk remedies as child abuse.[23]

EVIDENCE COLLECTION

Once a bite mark has been identified, evidence should be collected to facilitate any potential forensic investigation. The most qualified person for this job is a forensic odontologist. When these specialists are not available, acute care providers are responsible for the collection of evidence. The types of physical evidence needed primarily include salivary DNA samples and photographic records, but may also incorporate dental moulds.

The American Board of Forensic Odontologists (ABFO) recommends a double swab technique for use in the collection of saliva from the injury site. The first swab should be covered completely in sterile water, and then rolled over the skin while moving it in a circular pattern for 7–10 seconds. That swab is put aside to air-dry at room temperature. Immediately thereafter, a second dry swab is used to collect all of the moisture remaining on the skin from the first swab. Both swabs are then air-dried for at least 30 minutes or stored in a sterile container that allows air circulation. Never store the swabs in an airtight container. Room temperature samples must be submitted within 6 hours. If this is not possible, store them in a refrigerator, not a freezer. If the bite was inflicted through clothing, the clothing should be secured for DNA analysis. A control DNA sample from the victim, usually in the form of blood, should be obtained for comparison.[1,24]

Salivary sample processing and the markers by which an attacker is identified have changed greatly over the years. Previously, chemical methods of matching the victim's wound to an assailant were used to test for drugs, inorganic ions, and polymorphic proteins or enzymes. However, the results of these tests were extremely sensitive to degradation. For these reasons, DNA identification has largely replaced these methods.[8]

Although more stable in sufficient quantities, DNA in saliva on victims' skin after bite infliction must be collected in timely manner. Delays in sampling the bite site can lead to lower yields of DNA because a substantial amount of DNA is lost to degradation between 5 and 24 hours after the bite. The concentration of DNA recovered between 24 and 48 hours remains stable, although at a significantly decreased level.[25]

Once collected, salivary DNA is amplified using polymerase chain reaction (PCR) techniques and processed to look at short tandem repeats (STRs) or, more recently, mitochondrial DNA.[24,26–28] Use of DNA technology allows for the identification of individuals based on their unique DNA sequence (with the exception of an identical twin). Many governments worldwide have begun collecting DNA profiles from criminals and crime scenes, similar to the practice of fingerprinting. The goal is to establish an improved means of matching a perpetrator of violent crime to the victim and any previous victims.[28–30]

Following salivary collection, photographic documentation of the bite mark is the next step in evidence collection. Again, a forensic odontologist or someone trained in photographic documentation of bite wounds would be the most appropriate person to perform this role. When these specialists are not available, the acute care provider may obtain photographic evidence. Orientation (relative body location) and close-up photographs should be taken with either a high-quality digital or conventional camera. (Chapter 7 provides more information on forensic photography.) Pictures should always be taken at right angles to the wound. A right angle scale, ideally an American Board of Forensic Odontologists (ABFO) scale No. 2 (see Figure 8-2), and circular reference (e.g., coin) should be used in photographs.[31] Position the scale next to and in the same plane as the wound to minimize distortion and to allow accurate analysis of the wound later. This can prove difficult if the bite mark is on a curved surface. For these wounds, separate photographs for each angle of the curve should be taken. Pictures should be taken both with and without the scale so as to ensure that wound evidence is not obscured by the scale.[1,9,11,32]

Alternate photographic techniques are also available to further elucidate injury patterns not seen with the naked eye. Because of the limitations of the human eye, wounds appear differently in black-and-white, UV, and IR photographs, as compared with color photographs. Because each of these mediums produces different images, pictures should be taken in each format. Interestingly, ultraviolet light only penetrates a few microns into the skin, so imaging by UV light will yield very detailed pictures of the surface injury. Conversely, infrared penetrates up to 3 mm into the skin and produces an image of the damage below the surface. Both of these techniques require special light sources, filters, and films to obtain. Accordingly, they are less likely to be performed unless someone skilled in forensic photography is available.[1,33]

Photographic evidence is challenging to obtain. Even when photographs of bites are obtained by a trained forensic odontologist, these data can still be of little use in criminal investigations if the photographer is inexperienced or out of practice.[34] When photos are of sufficient quality, photocopied overlays are used to provide accurate matching with the correct bite mould.[35]

The final piece of evidence that needs to be collected, if possible, is an impression of the wound. This, however, is not something within the purview of the emergency medicine practitioner. The person performing this procedure needs to be familiar with dental casting and the materials used. A physician from the maxillofacial unit of the hospital may be able to help with this service. Care must be taken to preserve the natural contour of the area to be casted. If the wound is suspected of being self-inflicted, a dental mould of the victim should be preformed.[1,7]

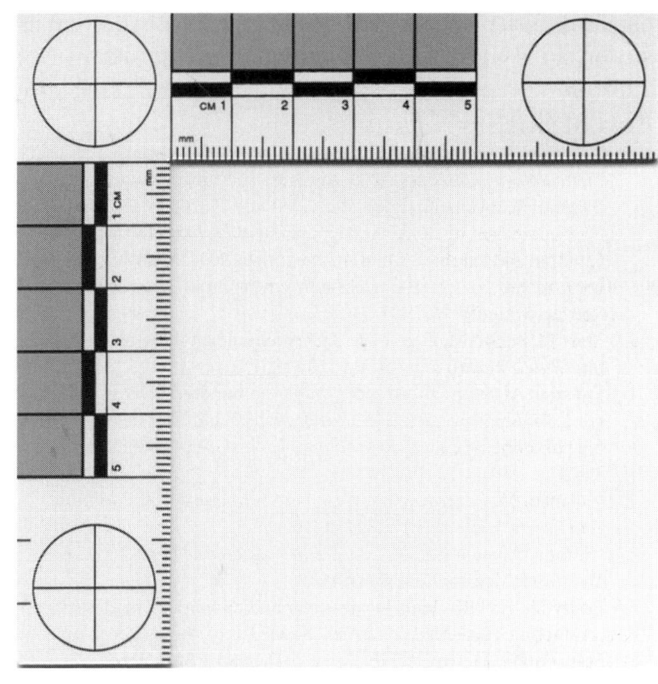

FIGURE 8-2 **American Board of Forensic Odontologists scale No. 2.**

DOCUMENTATION

The American Board of Forensic Odontologists emphasizes the accurate and complete documentation of a bite mark. When describing the bite mark location, the practitioner should focus on the anatomic location, surface contour, and tissue characteristics (e.g., tissue mobility/stability, elasticity). Description of the bite mark itself should include severity, shape, color, size, and any injuries such as abrasions, contusions, or avulsions. Any unusual conditions or three-dimensional characteristics of the wound should also be documented.[1,7,9] If uncertainty or insufficient evidence exists regarding the cause of the skin markings, the term "suggestive" should be used to describe the possible bite mark. If the skin markings were clearly not caused by a bite, the practitioner should appropriately document that the wound is "not a bite mark."[1]

Age or speculation regarding the age of the bite mark, based on the color of the contusion or skin condition, should not be made. Although most bite wounds initially trend in color from red (after immediate bite infliction) to a blue/purple, and then to green and yellow, there are too many factors (e.g., depth, natural pigmentation, gender, menstrual cycle, specific tissue characteristics, metabolic rate, drugs, observer interpretation of color, and ambient light) associated with the rate at which these changes occur to accurately place the time of the bite.[36]

In addition to thorough documentation, if the bite mark is part of a criminal act, it must be reported to the proper law enforcement agency.[37]

TREATMENT

Although the overall treatment of bite marks is beyond the focus of this chapter, treatment as it pertains to the forensics of bite wounds merits some discussion. The ABFO recommends evaluation of the bite mark site repeatedly over time including taking photographs because some characteristics will appear or change, thereby making a positive identification possible.[1] Therefore, prevention of infection and alteration of the site is important to the criminal case as well as to the victim. There is not a consensus, however, on the use of antibiotics for bite wounds. Most human bites are polymicrobial with alphahemolytic streptococci, staphylococci, and *Eikenella corrodens* as the most common microbes.[5,13,38]

Wound care appears to be the most effective treatment for nonhand wounds and should include irrigation and debridement of devitalized tissue. These procedures do not necessarily alter the bite mark and its forensic value. Prophylactic antibiotics should be administered for any hand, foot, or genital bite or any bite to an immunocompromised individual or any bite near a prosthetic joint. Use of prophylactic antibiotics may also be judiciously prescribed in the case of severe bite wounds.[38] Wounds involving the metacarpophalangial (MCP) joint, however, need to be evaluated by a hand surgeon for tendon rupture, X-rayed, and antibiotics need to be administered because of the risk of intra-articular infection.[5,38]

CONCLUSION

Bite marks, when part of a criminal act, can serve as valuable forensic data. Acute care providers will likely evaluate patients with bite marks during their career and should be knowledgeable about identification of these wounds and the collection of forensic data from them. Several medical conditions exist that resemble human bites and the medical practitioner should carefully discern these conditions from human bite marks. Once a human bite has been identified, salivary DNA and photographic evidence needs to be collected. If additional expertise is available, a mould of the bite mark may also be obtained. Last, proper wound care is imperative to prevent infection of the bite mark and distortion of forensic data.

REFERENCES

1. American Board of Forensic Odontology. *ABFO Bitemark Methodology Guidelines*. 2006. Available at: http://www.abfo.org/Bitemark%20Guidelines.doc. Retrieved July 25, 2008.
2. US Department of Health and Human Services, Administration for Children and Families. *Child Maltreatment 2004*. Available at: http://www.acf.hhs.gov/programs/cb/pubs/cm04/ http://www.acf.dhhs.gov. Retrieved August 15, 2007.
3. Marr JS, Beck AM, Lugo JA Jr. An epidemiologic study of the human bite. *Public Health Rep.* 1979; 94:514–521.
4. Freeman AJ, Senn DR, Arendt DM. Seven hundred seventy eight bite marks: analysis by anatomic location, victim and biter demographics, type of crime, and legal disposition. *J Forensic Sci.* 2005;50:1436–1443.
5. Callaham M. Controversies in antibiotic choices for bite wounds. *Ann Emerg Med.* 1988;17:1321–1330.
6. Cottone JA, Standish SM, eds. *Outline of Forensic Dentistry.* Chicago: Year Book Medical Publishers; 1982.
7. Pretty IA, Hall RC. Forensic dentistry and human bite marks: issues for doctors. *Hosp Med.* 2002;63:476–482.
8. Stimson PG, Mertz CA, eds. *Forensic Dentistry.* Boca Raton, Fla: CRC Press; 1997.
9. Bell K. Identification and documentation of bite marks. *J Emerg Nurs.* 2000;26:628–630.
10. Smock WS. Forensic emergency medicine. In: Marx JA, Hockberger RS, Walls RM, et al, eds. *Rosen's Emergency Medicine: Concepts and Clinical Practice.* 6th ed. Philadelphia, Pa: Mosby; 2006: 952–968.
11. Kellogg N, Committee on Child Abuse and Neglect. Oral and dental aspects of child abuse and neglect. *Pediatrics.* 2005;116:1565–1568.
12. Kini N, Lazoritz S. Evaluation for possible physical or sexual abuse. *Pediatr Clin North Am.* 1998;45:205–219.
13. Goldstein EJ. Bite wounds and infection. *Clin Infect Dis.* 1992;14:633–638.
14. Griego RD, Rosen T, Orengo IF, et al. Dog, cat, and human bites: a review. *J Am Acad Dermatol.* 1995;33:1019–1029.
15. Fallouji MA. Traumatic love bites. *Br J Surg.* 1990;77:100–101.
16. Harvey W. *Dental Identification and Forensic Odontology.* London: Henry Kimpton; 1976.
17. Lowry TMcG. The surgical treatment of human bites. *Ann Surg.* 1936;104:1103–1106.
18. Spiers RF. Prevention of human bite infections. *Surg Gynecol Obstet.* 1941;72:619–621.
19. Sweet D, Pretty IA. A look at forensic dentistry—Part 2: teeth as weapons of violence—identification of bitemark perpetrators. *Br Dent J.* 2001;190:415–418.
20. Vale GL, Noguchi TT. Anatomical distribution of human bite marks in a series of 67 cases. *J Forensic Sci.* 1983;28:61–69.
21. Pretty IA, Sweet D. Anatomic location of bitemarks and associated findings in 101 cases from the United States. *J Forensic Sci.* 2000;45:812–814.
22. Gold MH, Roenigk HH, Smith ES, et al. Human bite marks: differential diagnosis. *Clin Pediatr.* 1989;28:329–331.
23. Mudd SS, Findlay JS. The cutaneous manifestations and common mimickers of physical child abuse. *J Pediatr Health Care.* 2004;18:123–129.
24. Sweet D, Lorente M, Lorente JA, et al. An improved method to recover saliva from human skin: the double swab technique. *J Forensic Sci.* 1997;42:320–322.
25. Sweet D, Lorente JA, Valenzuela A, et al. PCR-based DNA typing of saliva satins recovered from human skin. *J Forensic Sci.* 1997;42:447–451.
26. Anzai-Kanto E, Hirata MH, Hirata RD, et al. DNA extraction from human saliva deposited on skin and its use in forensic identification procedures. *Pesqui Odontol Bras.* 2005;19:216–222.
27. Committee on DNA Technology in Forensic Science, National Research Council. *DNA Technology in Forensic Science.* Washington, DC: National Academy Press; 1992.
28. Varsha. DNA fingerprinting in the criminal justice system: an overview. *DNA Cell Biol.* 2006;25:181–188.
29. Federal Bureau of Investigation, US Department of Justice. CODIS. Available at: http://www.fbi.gov/hq/lab/html/codis1.htm. Retrieved July 25, 2008.
30. Johnson P, Williams R, Martin P. Genetics and forensics: making the national DNA database. *Sci Stud.* 2003;16:22–37.
31. Hyzer WG, Krauss TC. The bite mark standard reference scale—ABFO No. 2. *J Forensic Sci.* 1988;33:498–506.
32. Rothwell BR. Bite marks in forensic dentistry. *JADA.* 1995;126:223–232.
33. Wright FD. Photography in bite mark and patterned injury documentation—Part 1. *J Forensic Sci.* 1998;43:877–880.
34. McNamee AH, Sweet D. Adherence of forensic odontologists to the ABFO guidelines for victim evidence collection. *J Forensic Sci.* 2003;48:382–385.
35. Kouble RF, Craig GT. A comparison between direct and indirect methods available for human bite mark analysis. *J Forensic Sci.* 2004;49:111–118.
36. Dailey JC, Bowers CM. Aging of bitemarks: a literature review. *J Forensic Sci.* 1997;42:792–795.
37. Koegh S, Callaham MC. Bites and injuries inflicted by domestic animals. In: Auerbach PS, ed. *Wilderness Medicine.* 4th ed. St. Louis, Mo: Mosby; 2001.
38. Myers JP. Bite wound infections. *Burr Infect Dis Rep.* 2003;5:416–425.

9 Forensic Documentation

Ralph Riviello, MD, MS, FACEP, FAAEM

INTRODUCTION

One important tool the forensic examiner or emergency medicine clinician/nurse has at his or her disposal is documentation. The proper documentation of the history, physical exam, and evidence retrieved is an important part of the care a crime victim receives in the emergency department. Improper, inadequate, and incomplete documentation can lead to difficulties in prosecution, evidence handling, and may deny the victim a positive criminal justice outcome. A chart review of trauma cases by Carmona and Prince found poor, improper, or inadequate documentation in 70% of cases.[1] They cited lack of education as the primary reason for documentation failure.

Documentation failure is often caused by lack of training, inattention to detail, patient's condition, excessive workload of personnel, and lack of photographic resources. The time when the patient arrives in the emergency department (ED) is often the only chance for medical practitioners to document wounds and injuries accurately. This is important because wounds change over time and can be altered by medical procedures, treatments, and interventions.

HISTORY

All attempts should be made to document as thorough a history as possible. This is often limited by the patient's condition and need for life-saving medical intervention. History may come from other sources as well, including family members, emergency medical services personnel, police, and nursing home records. Sometimes the history is extremely limited.

The history should attempt to document accurately the who, what, where, when, and how of what happened. This information not only helps investigators, especially if the patient dies from injuries prior to police questioning, but also helps the medical personnel caring for the patient to focus their attention on potential injuries and problems. Whenever possible, the history should be taken down in the patient's own words. Any statements made by the victim about the incident should be recorded word for word and enclosed in quotation marks so that others reviewing the chart can see that these are the words spoken by the patient. Direct quotations of the patient's words also are potentially important later in court proceedings.

All documentation should be clear, concise, and legible. Standard documentation practices apply to forensic documentation as well. Some departments use standardized forensic examination documentation forms. A classic example is the forensic medical reports/charts used for sexual assault survivors. Departments may choose to create special forms to be used for other crime/accident victims to document the history and exam. In most cases, however, the standard ED chart should suffice.

PHYSICAL EXAM

The physical exam should also be clearly and concisely documented. Injuries should be well documented and described in terms of location, type of injury, unique characteristics, and presence of forensic evidence. Wounds should be described in a sequence, for example, starting at the patient's head and proceeding downward. Other strategies include describing wounds from front to back and from proximal to distal. Use correct terminology and accepted abbreviations when documenting injuries and findings.

The location of the injury should be documented as specifically as possible. Use landmarks to reference wound locations. Some landmarks include midline of the body, the notch at the top of the sternum, the centerline of a limb, and the top of the head. For example, it is much easier to understand and visualize "a stab wound, second intercostal space, midclavicular line, left chest 2 cm from the left sternal border" versus "a stab wound to the left chest." Body map diagrams and anatomic charts are very helpful to record injuries on. They are fast, accurate, and help prevent right/left errors. The body map chart should include written descriptions of the injuries, as well, once again being as specific as possible (Figures 9-1, 9-2, 9-3). The face of a clock is often used to describe the angulations or inclination of a wound or injury. It is commonly used to describe injuries of the external genitalia in rape exams but can also be applied to other body parts.

Describe the type of injury as specifically as possible. Describe its shape, dimension, and associated characteristics. Photodocumentation is helpful but does not replace a well-written chart. Use a ruler to measure and document the size and dimensions of all wounds. Physicians often incorrectly estimate the size of wounds.[2] Accurate wound dimensions can be very important in matching a weapon to the wound it caused. A sketch of unique wounds can be made.

Any evidence found in a wound or on the body of a victim should be thoroughly documented. The location of where the evidence was collected from, the time of collection, and the name of the person who collected it should be documented. The chain of custody must be maintained. The name and badge number of the officer receiving the evidence should also be recorded. The specifics of evidence collection in the ED are discussed in Chapter 4 .

INJURY-SPECIFIC DOCUMENTATION

The next section will review injury-specific guidelines for documentation. All documentation should conform to the standard and acceptable practices at one's own institutions and jurisdictions.

Blunt and Sharp Injuries

Once again, it is important to document exact wound characteristics. This includes location, size, shape, and unique characteristics. Some characteristics to look for are shape of the wound, paired wounds, wound directionality, associated injuries, and physical evidence present.

Wounds should be assessed for *patterned injury*. A patterned injury is one that has features or configuration indicative of the object(s) or surface(s) that produced it.[3] It can be an imprint of clothing, car grille, clothes iron, or tool. Accurate measurements and descriptions of these patterned injuries are necessary. Photographic documentation can be critical for these injuries.

Chapter 11 describes the different types of sharp force injuries. It is important to use proper terminology when describing these wounds: *cut* versus *incised wound* versus *stab wound* versus *slice* versus *slash*. Other important clues from the history and wound can be used to describe hesitation wounds and defensive wounds, and these should be taken into consideration when documenting them. When describing stab wounds, it is helpful to describe the presence of an associated contusion with the wound indicating injury from the weapon handle such as a knife guard or ice pick.

Blunt force injuries, both intentional and unintentional, are encountered in emergency departments every day. Blunt force injuries range from abrasions to contusions, to lacerations (tears) and fractures. Chapter 10 describes the characteristics of these injuries. It is important to remember that a laceration is caused by a blunt object whereas a sharp object produces cuts, incisions, or incised wounds. These terms are often confused and used interchangeably, but forensically they are clearly different and must be used correctly.

Another documentation error occurs with contusions. Never attempt to predict the age of a bruise based on color. Many factors are related to bruise characteristics and

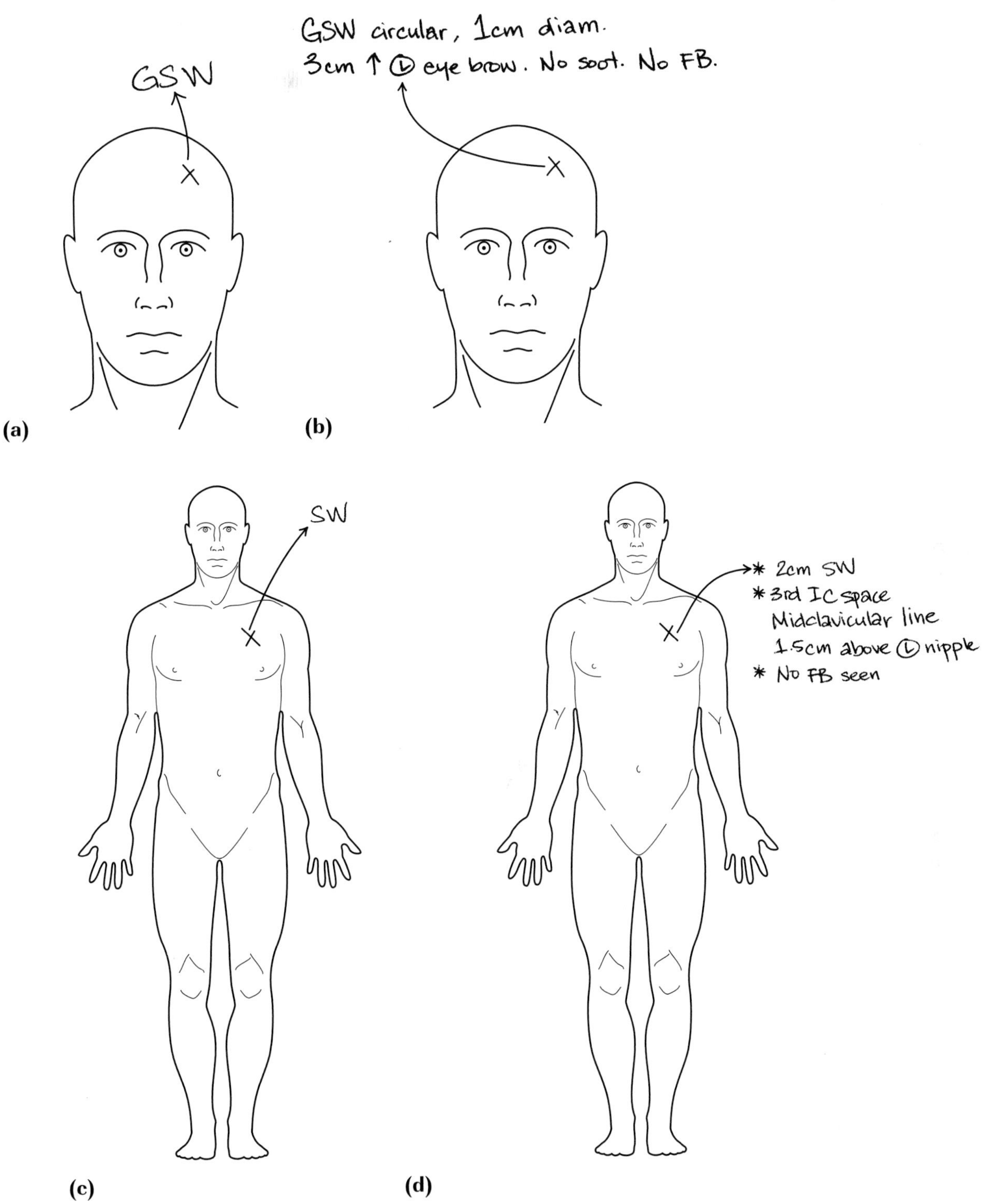

FIGURE 9-1 **Documentation using body diagrams: (a) incomplete information; (b) more complete documentation and description of wound; (c) incomplete information; (d) more complete description of wound.**

healing. Attempting to date a bruise/contusion is difficult and should be stated with great caution.[3] It is better not to attempt to date a bruise but rather to describe the characteristics of the bruise in terms of precise location, exact size, color, and pattern. Color photography is extremely useful in documenting bruises.

Firearm Injuries

Firearm injuries account for a significant number of victims in the ED, especially urban trauma centers. Often these patients are critically injured and require immediate resuscitative procedures and operative intervention. It is important to realize that proper forensic documentation also plays an

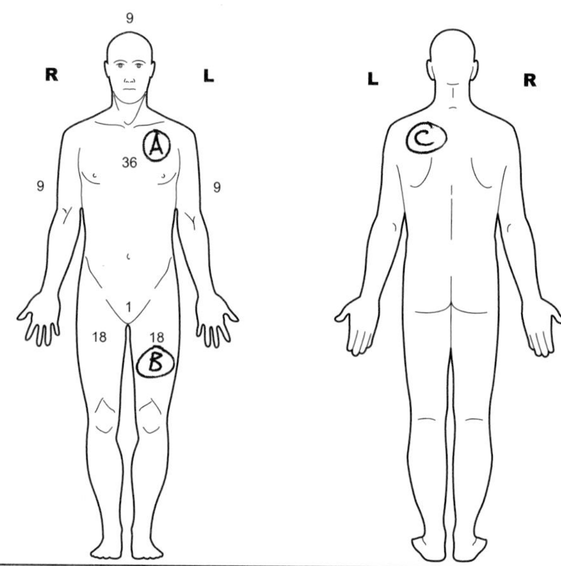

LEGEND: Types of Findings ☐ Findings ☐ No Findings ☐ Additional copies of this page attached

AB	Abrasion	DS	Dry Secretion	IN	Induration	OI	Other Injury (describe)	TA	Tooth Avulsed
BI	Bite	EC	Ecchymosis (bruise)	IW	Incised Wound	PE	Petechiae	TD	Tooth Decay
BU	Burn	ER	Erythema (redness)	LA	Laceration	PS	Potential Saliva	TF	Tooth Fractured
CS	Control Swab	FB	Foreign Body	MS	Moist Secretion	SI	Suction Injuries	TM	Tooth Missing
DE	Debris	F/H	Fiber/Hair	OF	Other Foreign Materials (describe)	SW	Swelling	V/S	Vegetation/Soil
DF	Deformity	FT	Frenulum Torn			TE	Tenderness		

Locator #	Type	Description	Locator #	Type	Description
A	IW	4cm; 3rd IC space; edge is 1cm	C	BI	5 x 4.5 cm; ⊕ ecchymosis & petechiae;
		from sternum.			purple & red in color
B	EC	2cm circular; purple in color;			
		∅ patterned			

FIGURE 9-2 **Alternative method of body diagram documentation.**

important role. Some important documentation tips are as follows:

1. Accurately describe the wound location. Use body map diagrams and photos whenever possible.
2. Accurately describe the wound dimensions. Use a ruler to measure the wound.
3. Describe the presence or absence of any gunpowder residue or soot around the wound or on the clothing.
4. *Never* describe a wound as an entrance or exit wound. Use the general term *gunshot wound*, and then describe the wound.
5. Document the presence or absence of a muzzle stamp, muzzle imprint, or barrel abrasion—these are outlines of the end of the gun.
6. *Never* document the caliber of the bullet, but include description of the wound's appearance and/or the bullet's size/appearance on a radiograph.
7. If radiographs are taken, thoroughly document injuries seen and characteristics of bullets if present. The description should include location of the bullet on the X-ray relative to landmarks, whether or not the bullet is intact or fragmented, and the injuries present.
8. Document any evidence recovered from bullet wounds including location, type of evidence, the collector, and the receiving officer.
9. Document any specific characteristics of the bullet or the presence of any adherent material to the bullet.
10. Document the condition of clothing the victim is wearing and package it according to accepted procedure.
11. Document any other materials recovered from the victim such as drugs, drug paraphernalia, weapons, and so forth.

Bite Marks

Document bite marks for location and size whenever possible. Describe characteristics of the bitemark in regards to the presence of petechiae, abrasions, contusions, erythema, ecchymosis, indentation, and laceration. Measurements may be taken. Bite marks are best documented by using photography and an ABFO ruler.

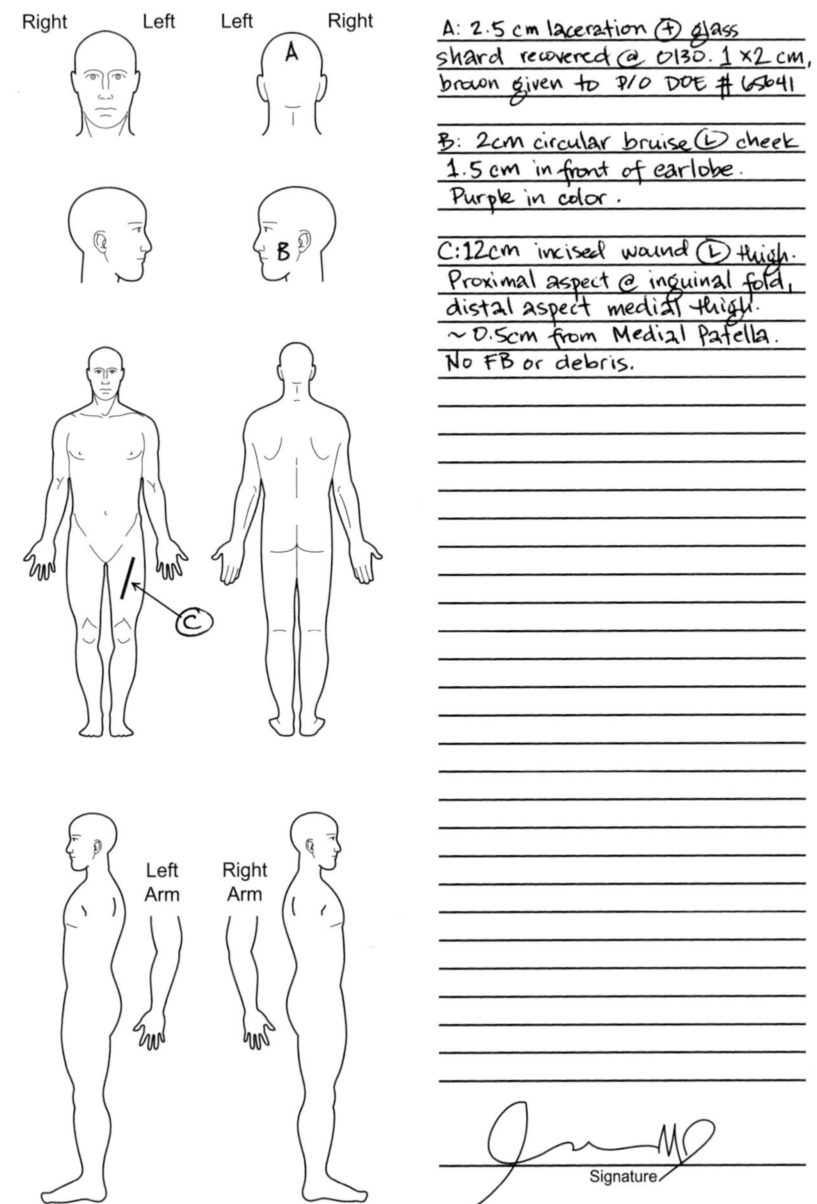

Right
Left
Left
Right
A
B
C
Left Arm
Right Arm
A: 2.5 cm laceration (+) glass
shard recovered @ 0130. 1 x 2 cm,
brown given to P/O DOE # 65641
B: 2cm circular bruise (L) cheek
1.5 cm in front of earlobe.
Purple in color.
C: 12cm incised wound (L) thigh.
Proximal aspect @ inguinal fold,
distal aspect medial thigh.
~0.5cm from Medial Patella.
No FB or debris.
Signature

FIGURE 9-3 **Another example of documentation using body diagram maps.**

Motor Vehicle Injuries

Motor vehicle–related trauma is very common, and victims most often seek care in the ED. Oftentimes, forensic questions arise related to the accident, such as, "Who was driving?" "Were drugs and alcohol involved?" "What injuries are present?" "Who was the hit-and-run driver?" The emergency or forensic clinician can play a crucial role in answering these questions. Some guidelines for documentation in motor vehicle injuries include the following:

1. Take a thorough history of the accident from the victim, EMS personnel, and police.
2. Thoroughly document all injuries with regards to location, pattern, directionality, and characteristics. Important motor vehicle–specific patterns include the seat belt, steering wheel, airbag, airbag covers, window cranks, dashboard components, rearview mirror, radio knobs, and window glass. When confronted with a seat belt injury, be sure to document its directionality because this can help to determine the victim's position in the vehicle at the time of the accident. For example, if the victim's seat belt injury goes from right shoulder to left upper abdomen, then that person can be excluded as the driver because the driver's injury should go from left to right (see Figure 9-4).
3. Document the presence or absence of "dicing injuries," which are multiple tiny, often L-shaped lacerations caused by shattering of the tempered glass from side and rear windows of cars. The location of these dicing injuries may also assist in locating a person's position in the vehicle.

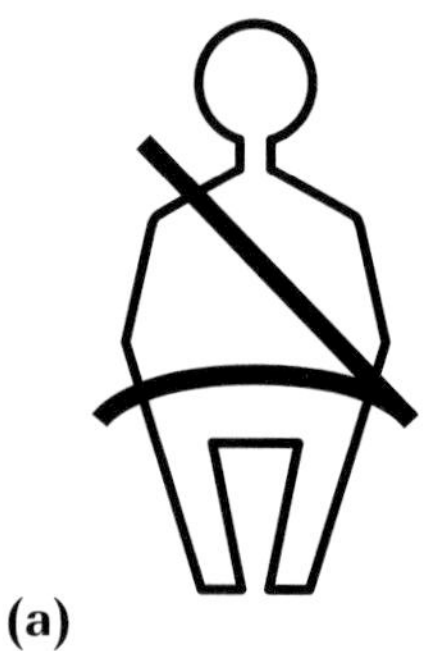
(a)

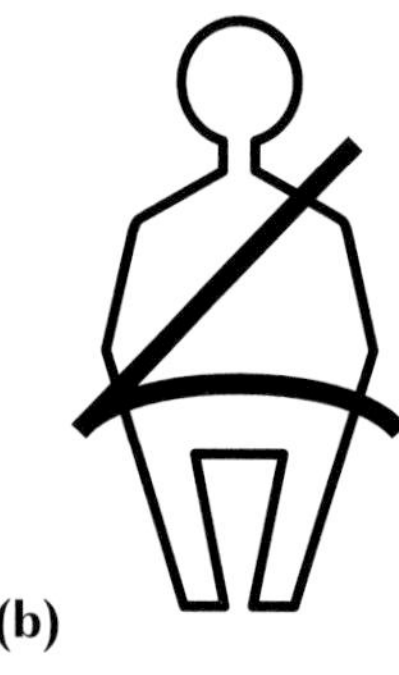
(b)

FIGURE 9-4 **Injury orientation in patients with seat belt sign: (a) people sitting on passenger side of vehicle; (b) people sitting on driver side of vehicle.**

4. Look for trace evidence in wounds and document its description, location, and how it was handled.
5. In pedestrian–vehicle injury, thoroughly document location and presence of wounds and injury.
6. Patterned injuries from tires and radiator grilles may be present. Document them for size and location. Photographs can be helpful.
7. Trace evidence from wounds might include automobile parts, vehicle glass, oil, and paint chips. They should be documented and handled as evidence.
8. In pedestrian–vehicle injury, consider documenting the height of bumper injuries, measured from the heel and including the height of the shoe. These measurements can later be compared with the bumper height to determine whether or not the vehicle was braking at the time of impact. Braking causes the front end of the vehicle to dip, thus causing a discrepancy between the bumper injury height and actual bumper height. These measurements should be taken before surgical repair of injuries.
9. In pedestrian–vehicle injury, document the direction of wedge fractures of the tibia in bumper injuries. The tip of the wedge points in the direction of impact and is opposite the side of impact.

INTERPERSONAL VIOLENCE: CHILD ABUSE, INTERPERSONAL VIOLENCE, AND ELDER ABUSE

Victims of interpersonal violence are often seen in the ED. Sometimes their victimization is obvious; other times it can be very subtle. When caring for these patients, documentation is an important tool in aiding the victim. Use the following guidelines to collect usable evidence:

1. Be as specific as possible with the history. Document exactly what the victim says. Remember, you may need to use other sources of information especially for children and the elderly.
2. Document any inconsistencies in the patient's story and in other people's account of the incident, especially when they are discrepant with each other.
3. Thoroughly document all injuries seen. Remember, there may be multiple injuries in various stages of healing. Accurately measure and describe each injury, paying special attention to wound color and characteristics.
4. Remember to look for patterned injuries.
5. The use of body diagrams and photographs can be extremely helpful.
6. Document any conversations you have with law enforcement or adult and child protective services. Record the name of the individual you spoke to and the time of the conversation. Remember to complete any regulatory forms as required by state or local law.

CONCLUSION

Clear, concise, accurate, and precise documentation is crucial in forensic emergency medicine. Unfortunately, documentation is often done quickly and improperly, especially in the midst of treating a critically injured patient. Patient care always takes precedence, but medical practitioners should make a conscious effort to document each case as thoroughly as possible. Multiple forms of documentation can be used including written descriptions, body diagrams, and photographs. The proper documentation of a case can help the victim have a very positive legal outcome, whereas the opposite is also true.

REFERENCES

1. Carmona R, Prince K. Trauma and forensic medicine. *J Trauma.* 1989;29(9):1222–1225.
2. Lemanski M, Smithline H, Blank FS, Henneman PL. Accuracy of laceration length estimation. *Am J Emerg Med.* 2005;23(7):920–921.
3. Smock WS. Forensic emergency medicine. In Olshaker JS, Jackson MC, Smock WS, eds. *Forensic Emergency Medicine.* Philadelphia, Pa: Lippincott Williams & Wilkins; 2001:63–84.

SUGGESTED READING

Olshaker JS, Jackson MC, Smock WS, eds. *Forensic Emergency Medicine.* 2nd ed. Philadelphia, Pa: Lippincott Williams & Wilkins; 2007.

Lynch VA, ed. *Forensic Nursing.* St. Louis, Mo: Elsevier Mosby; 2006.

DiMaio VJM. *Gunshot Wounds: Practical Aspects of Firearms, Ballistics, and Forensic Techniques.* 2nd ed. Boca Raton, Fla: CRC Press; 1999.

10 Blunt Force Trauma

Paul Ko, MD, and Christine Dang, MD

INTRODUCTION

B*lunt trauma* is the physical bodily damage caused by blunt force. This force could arise from any or all of three causes: impact, as in a fall from height; a blunt object; or a physical attack. *Blunt force trauma* is a subset of blunt trauma and refers to injuries caused by a physical attack.

When patients are brought to the hospital for care, the emergency department physician is the first physician to care for them. It is therefore essential that the physician is able to describe the wound accurately, assess and treat the multiple injuries that may have been sustained, and use the correct terminology in the documentation of the patient's injury. The latter is important in assisting the crime scene investigator and the criminal justice system to find and try the perpetrator as well as for the physician who delivers the follow-up care to the patient. This chapter focuses on the different mechanisms, injury patterns, injury detection, and crime and forensic aspects of blunt force trauma.

TERMINOLOGY

There is little difference between the definition of a wound and an injury. *Stedman's Concise Medical Dictionary* defines *injury* as "damage, harm or loss particularly when the result of external force." *Wound* is defined as "trauma to any tissues of the body, especially which was caused by physical means and with interruption of continuity."[1] In some legal systems, however, a slight distinction is made, with a *wound* arising from an intentional or purposeful action whereas an *injury* implies the possibility of an accidental cause.[2]

It should be briefly mentioned that in forensics there is also a small difference between an instrument and a weapon. A *weapon* is an object whose primary purpose is to injure, destroy, or harm. An *instrument* is an object whose primary purpose is something other than injury but that is used in an offensive or defensive manner.[3]

DOCUMENTATION

It is extremely important to describe what is seen in the emergency department patient accurately because this department is one of the first places the wound is seen. Emergency department physicians are often guilty of illegible writing and brief, scant description of the wounds they treat. As a result, when these accounts appear in court, the true appearance of these wounds is lost, and perpetrators can be released and physicians could be potentially prosecuted for negligence.

Information that needs to be included in the description of the wound includes type, location, dimensions, and direction of the wound or injury[2,3] because these are the aspects that can credit or discredit the allegations and circumstances presented in court. Formats that can help relate wound descriptions include body diagrams, clock face orientation for angulation or inclination of the wound, description of the wound in a logical progressive sequence (i.e., head to toe or front to back), use of easy and consistent landmarks when possible, use of nationally or internationally standard abbreviations, and a notation for incidental findings that could be misinterpreted as an oversight if not documented (such as birthmarks).[2,3] Full descriptions of pattern injuries, along with sketches or photographs, are also extremely vital to forensic evidence collection.

CLASSIFICATION OF WOUNDS

Wounds can be divided into four main types: abrasions, contusions, lacerations, and fractures. This classification applies to all types of wounds, including those caused by strangling, shooting, and blasts.

Abrasions

Abrasions are the most superficial type of trauma. Other terms that are often used include *scrape, graze,* or *scratch.* Abrasions occur when the superficial layer of the skin is damaged, removed, or destroyed via a sliding and/or compressive force. They are confined to the cuticle or epidermis and do not penetrate the dermis, making these types of injuries less likely to bleed.[2] Wounds with bleeding components that emergency department physicians document as "abrasions" have entered the dermis and ruptured some of the small blood vessels in the dermal papillae located under the epidermal surface.

Abrasions occur when an object strikes the skin or when the body hits a stationary surface. They can be further broken down into four types of abrasions: scrape, graze, impact, and patterned.

Scrape abrasions, sometimes called brush abrasions, include linear abrasions, sliding abrasions, and dragging abrasions. Linear abrasions are simple straight scratches, as seen in cat scratches. Sliding abrasions are typically seen on the lower extremities of a pedestrian after being struck by a motor vehicle (see Figure 10-1). Dragging abrasions are those formed on the skin after it is pulled along a surface, and they can be antemortem or postmortem.[2,4]

Grazes are brush burn abrasions that are wide and cover a large surface area on the body, usually the back, knees, or

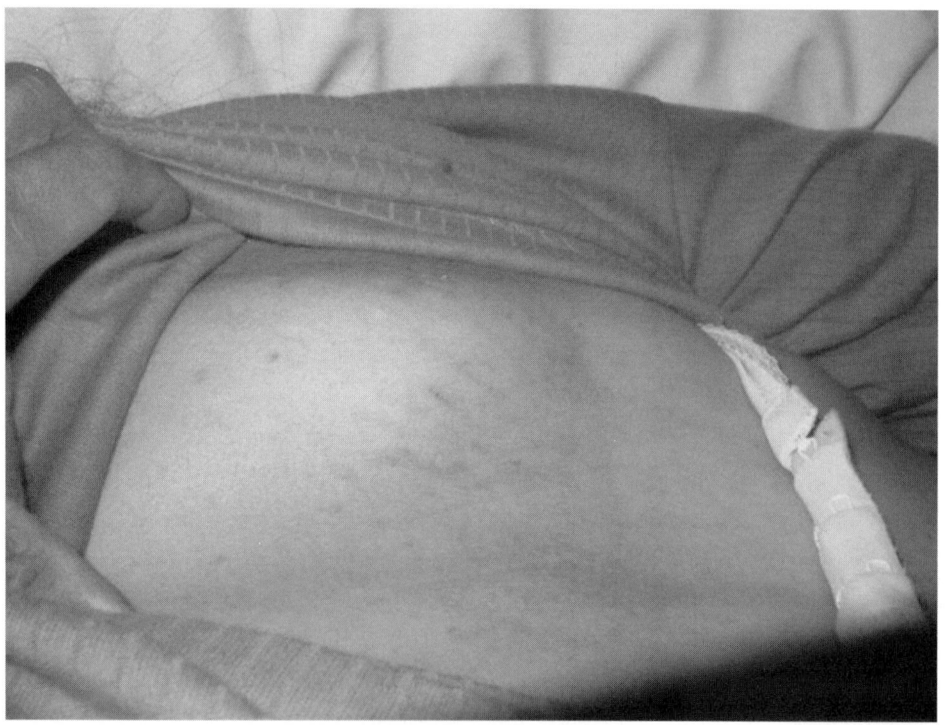

FIGURE 10-1 **Sliding abrasion. This picture is from the back of an intoxicated patient who was pushed to the ground and beaten. Notice the scraping-like pattern on her back where she presumably hit the ground and slid.**

elbows.[2–4] These generally occur secondary to motorcycle accidents when the body is hurled across a rough surface after being struck or when the victim falls to the ground with a sliding motion, as when children fall off their bicycles onto the pavement (see Figure 10-2). Upon further inspection, the injury may appear to be multiple linear abrasions running in parallel when there is direct skin-to-surface contact. When clothing covers the skin surface, there may be no discrete linear marks, but instead an erythematous, excoriated area of skin, like that obtained in the childhood game of Indian rug burn.

Impact abrasions occur when the delivery of force is perpendicular to the skin surface, resulting in the skin being crushed against a bony surface.[4] These occur when the body hits the ground with a certain degree of force and can be seen perimortem or postmortem. Patterned abrasions are a type of impact abrasions where there is a definitive imprint on the underlying skin, such as bite marks, belt marks, and button holes (see Figures 10-3 and 10-4).

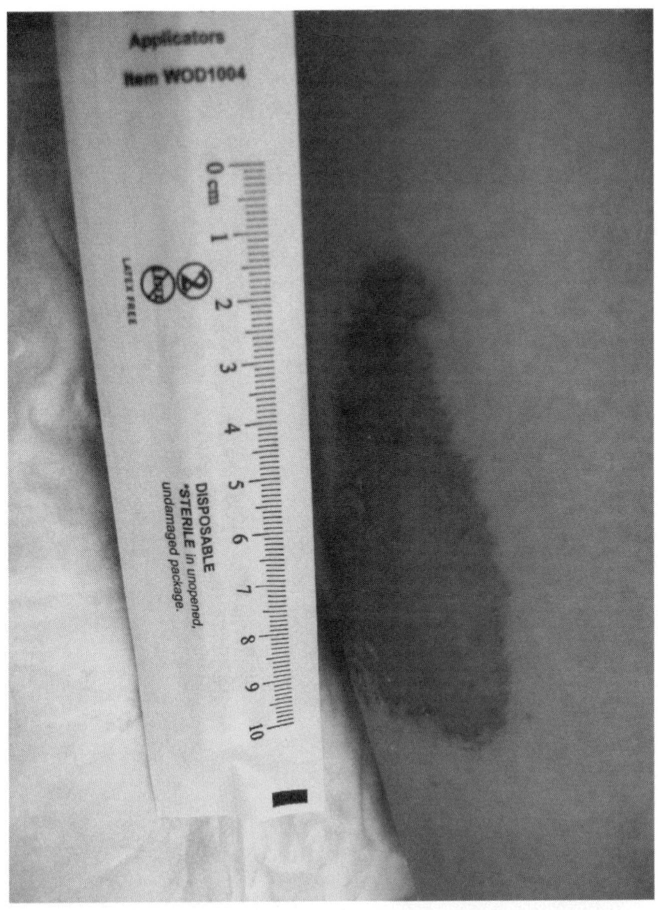

FIGURE 10-2 **Graze. This photo shows an example of a graze type wound, or brush burn abrasion. This injury, on the patient's forearm, occurred within hours after the patient fell off of his moped onto the pavement. See Color Plate 3.**

There are four stages of healing for abrasions that occur in a predictable and reproducible manner.[4] It is important to remember that although the timeline is consistent, the exact time that each change occurs is different for each person based on preexisting physical and medical conditions, location of the injury, and secondary infection. Stage 1 is scab formation, which occurs when fibrin, serum, and red blood cells accumulate on the abrasion surface. By 18 hours post injury, polymorphonuclear cells will have infiltrated the underlying area of the injury and collagen may stain abnormally in the area of injury. It is this collagen that causes abrasions to darken, usually first at the edges, and then in more shallow areas of the wound.

Stage 2 is epithelial regeneration, occurring at the edge of the abrasion and in hair follicles usually between 30 and 72 hours post injury. Stage 3 is subepidermal granulation, becoming prominent during days 5 to 8 post injury and most prominent at days 9 to 12 post injury, after there is epithelial covering of the abrasion. Events that occur include prominent perivascular infiltration and chronic inflammation, and epithelium thickening with new keratin.

Stage 4 is regression, starting day 12 post injury. The epithelium begins to thin and become atrophic. With new collagen fibers, dermal vascularity decreases and a definite basement membrane becomes present. It is important to note that postmortem abrasions dry and darken secondary to the lack of blood circulation or body movement. This may lead to false interpretation of the injury as a burn or bruise.

Although abrasions are superficial and rarely fatal wounds, they provide some of the most important and vital forensic

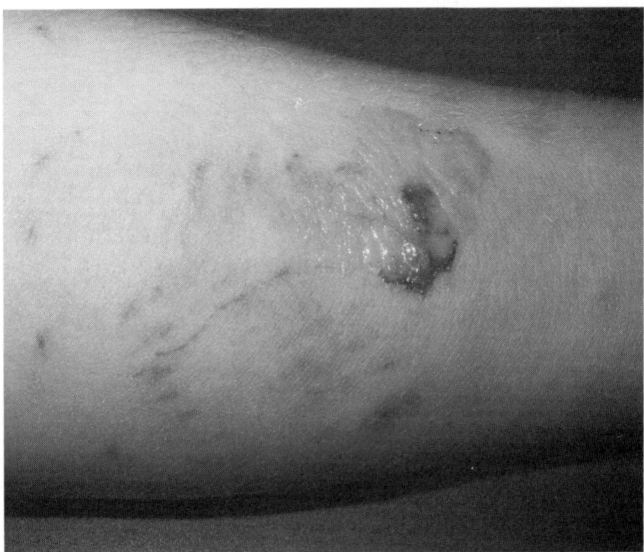

FIGURE 10-3 **Patterned abrasion. This photo shows an example of a dog bite on the forearm of a young child. This wound occurred 3 days prior to the photograph being taken. The oval-round shape of the bite can be seen where the dog bit the arm. The sheen on the skin is from a topical antibiotic ointment applied to the wound by the child's mother.**

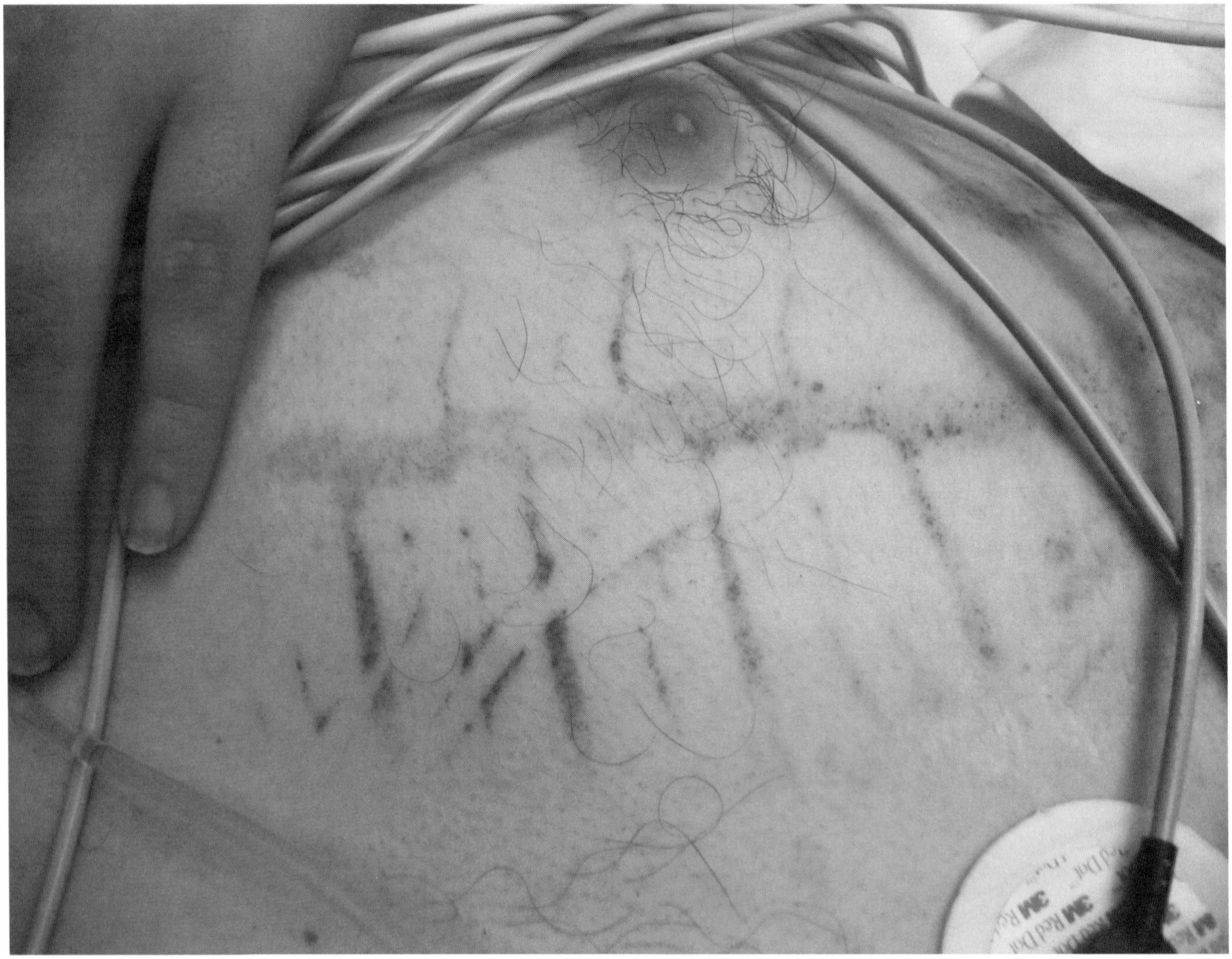

FIGURE 10-4 (*above*) Patterned abrasion. This photo shows an example of tire marks on the chest of the patient. The patient was struck and run over by a motorized vehicle. The strength of the impact left tire track impressions on the patient. See Color Plate 4.

FIGURE 10-5 (*right*) Patterned abrasion-contusion. This photo shows the letters *SRS*, which stand for supplemental restraint system. The patient was the driver in a single-vehicle accident. The airbag deployed and struck her hand, leaving the imprint on the dorsum of her hand. See Color Plate 5.

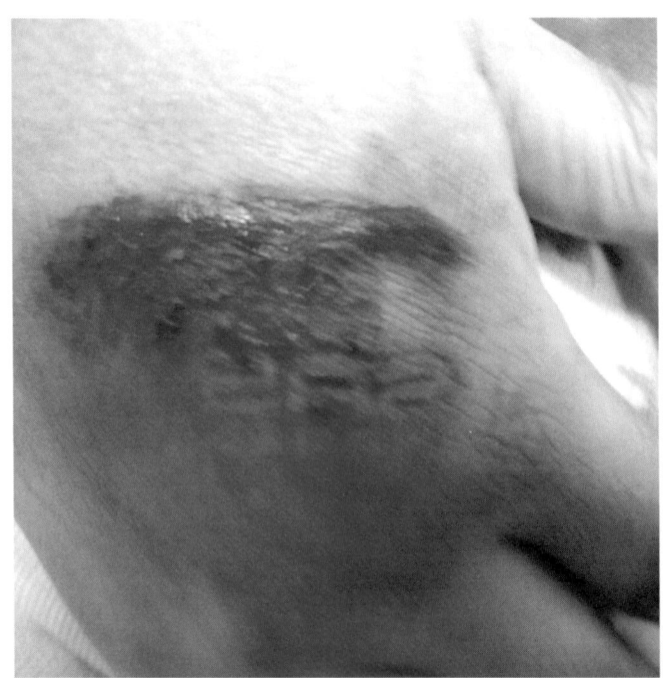

information by demarcating the exact point of contact. They can reveal the directional vector of the force applied to cause the abrasion in addition to characteristic patterns. Two vectors are involved with blunt trauma, an inward pressure and a longitudinal pressure. Epidermal tissue is displaced toward the distal (final) end of a sliding abrasion injury, occasionally leaving ragged tags and fragments (see Figure 10-5). In addition to accurate and descriptive written documentation of the wound, photographic documentation with a ruler to indicate scale should be performed to assist with forensic presentation of evidence in court.

Contusions

Contusions, in reference to blunt trauma, are also called bruises and occur when there is hemorrhage (leakage of blood) into the soft tissues after the application of blunt force.[2–4] This occurs when soft tissue is distorted, blood vessels are torn, and extravasation occurs. Capillaries, small veins, and arterioles are typically the vessels injured; however, larger vessels may also bleed, which leads to a more rapid accumulation of blood and occasionally a hematoma formation. There are three divisions of contusions: patterned bruises, bruises, and hematomas.[4] They oftentimes occur in conjunction with one another or with abrasions and lacerations.

When contusions occur intradermally in the skin surface itself, patterned bruises arise, such as finger impression from forceful gripping or tire treads on skin surfaces (see Figures 10-4 and 10-5). The area of hemorrhage occurs immediately under the epidermis in the uppermost dermal layer. Bruises occur beneath the skin, in the dermal layer. Extravasation occurs in the fascial planes, spreading outward along the path of least resistance, thus not leaving the pattern of the causative object and sometimes creating contusions that do not necessarily correspond to the location of direct impact. Examples of these include basilar skull fractures where blood pools behind and below the ear (Battle's sign) and/or periorbitally (raccoon sign). Hematomas are focal collections of blood within an area of contusion, oftentimes deep seated, such as in the internal organs.[3,4]

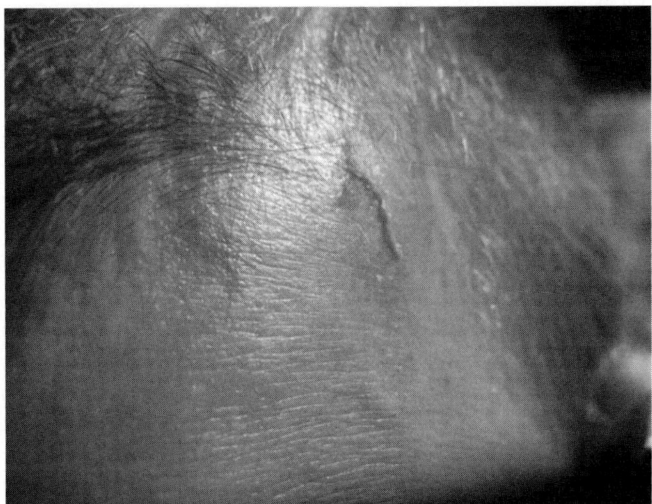

FIGURE 10-6 **Sliding abrasion with directionality. This wound was caused by the sharp edge of a car door hitting the patient in the forehead. Note the raised skin edge on the abrasion indicating that the door hit the patient more medially on the forehead, and then slid laterally.**

The extent and severity of contusions depend on multiple factors including the amount of force applied; the structure, type, location, and vascularity of the tissue injured; age and gender of the victim; and physical and medical condition of the victim.[2–4] Internal organ damage occurs with sudden, severe, forceful blunt trauma impact to the abdomen and chest. Depending on the severity of the force applied, external bruising may not even appear on the external skin surface. Loose, lax, and soft tissues such as those areas with copious subcutaneous fat bruise more easily than firm, supported tissue.[2–4]

Contusions are caused by blood vessel extravasation; areas that are highly vascularized tend to bruise more easily than those that are less vascularized. Therefore, obese individuals tend to bruise more easily than muscular individuals do. Location also plays a factor because of circulatory effect and gravity. The two extremes of age—the young and the elderly—both bruise easily. It is important to note that minor blunt trauma may produce senile ecchymoses on the upper extremities of the elderly, often appearing with multiple hypopigmented scars that may persist for a long time. Women bruise more easily than men do.[4] Easy bruising also occurs in individuals with clotting and bleeding dyscrasias, such as leukemia and von Willebrand's disease; individuals on blood thinners or antiplatelet agents; individuals on medications that have antiplatelet activity as a nonprimary mechanism of action (selective serotonin reuptake inhibitors); as well as individuals who have cirrhosis.[3]

Like abrasions, contusions may demonstrate patterns that can suggest causation. Two parallel lines of bruises with an unaffected area between them ("railway line") indicate the impact of a rod-like instrument.[2] The area of impact of the instrument compresses and empties the underlying blood vessels so that they do not extravasate. In contrast, the edges are stretched, tearing the blood vessels and leaving two distinct lines of hemorrhage. Other examples of patterned contusions include knuckles from a fist injury, pinching bruises on the arm when grabbed by the thumb and forefingers, and circumferential bruising around wrists and ankles from being restrained.

As contusions heal, they go through a consistent and predictable color change progression.[2–4] As with abrasions, although the progression occurs predictably, the exact time that the changes occur is different for each person depending on their preexisting medical and physical conditions. Therefore, although it is vital to include the color or colors of the contusion when describing it, it is important not to offer an opinion on the age of the contusion based on color because two contusions might occur simultaneously but have two different times to resolution.

Contusions initially may be red, purple, or dark blue, secondary to the color of oxygenated blood, from the arterial side of the circulation. They may appear dark blue because blue light reflects more easily than does red light, which penetrates more deeply. This usually occurs within minutes to hours after impact. The next stage is green, dark yellow, or brown, like the ripening of a banana, secondary to the breakdown of hemoglobin (see Figure 10-7). The last stage is pale yellow as the coloration fades. Resolution may be as short as 72 hours to as long as several months.

In terms of forensics, there are a few important details to remember. First, when photographing the contusion, color photography works best and it is important to include a color scale in the photograph. Second, although two simultaneously occurring contusions may heal at different rates, if there are markedly different colors in the same person, it is relatively safe to assume they were inflicted at different times. The only caveat to this is if the wounds were inflicted with very different severities. Third, contusions are very difficult to inflict postmortem.[2] These may occur within hours after death and only with the application of severe force. Postmortem bruising typically appears in the skin and/or soft tissue over bony prominences.[2,4] Interpretation of these bruises as antemortem or postmortem can be extremely challenging because even the presence of polymorphonuclear cells could result from mechanical disruption of blood vessels and not as one of the vital reactions to the injury. Last, skin tone can camouflage contusions, especially in dark-skinned or heavily tanned individuals.[3,4]

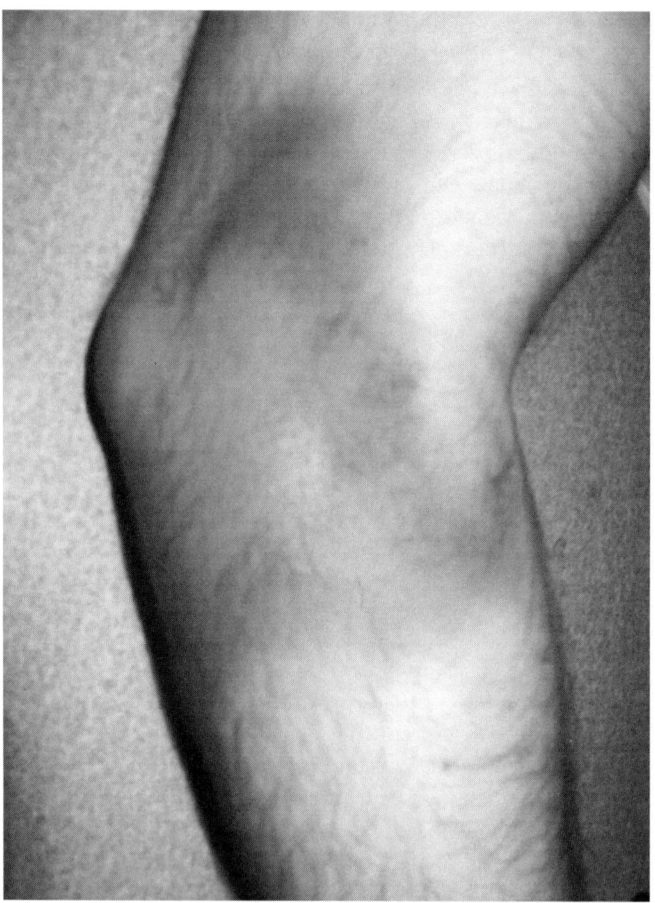

FIGURE 10-7 **Contusion. This photo shows a bruise in the second stage of healing. This wound to the elbow region was caused by another person's arm or foot—it was obtained during a Judo class. See Color Plate 6.**

Lacerations

Lacerations can be one of the more dangerous types of blunt trauma. Other names for them include gashes or tears. Lacerations should be differentiated from cuts or incised wounds: the difference lies in the mechanism of action that produces the injury. Lacerations are blunt force injuries leading to soft tissue defects as a result of tearing, shearing, crushing, or avulsion.[2–4] Incised wounds are usually produced by sharp objects.[2,3] The difference in the mechanism of injury also accounts for the usual irregular and ragged-edge appearance of lacerations that is formed by strands of bridging tissue within the wound. This is a key feature of lacerations: they contain tissue bridges within the wound. In contrast, incised wounds have a sharp, clearly delineated edge, which makes wound approximation easier.

Emergency physicians tend to use the term *laceration* to describe any cut in the skin; forensically speaking, this is inaccurate. The term *laceration* should be reserved for those injuries associated with a blunt force mechanism, whereas the term *incised wound* should be used to describe injuries associated with a sharp-force mechanism. For example, if someone is struck in the head with a glass bottle, the resulting wound is a laceration. If a person took a piece of the broken glass and injured someone with the sharp edge, it is an incised wound.

Lacerations in the skin are full-thickness injuries, accounting for the profuse bleeding that occurs after the injury.[2] Because the skin breaks as a result of overstretching, lacerations usually occur in areas overlying bony prominences because the skin and soft tissue there are usually more fixed and less likely to move when stressed.[2,4] Lacerations can also occur in internal organs as a result of blunt trauma. As mentioned before with contusions, severe blunt injuries to the chest or abdomen can result in internal organ hematomas; they may also result in aorta or organ laceration. These lacerations also tend to occur in areas of decreased mobility.[3,4] Organs that are often lacerated after motor vehicle collisions include the liver, spleen, and kidney.

As with abrasions, lacerations may indicate the direction of force applied and occasionally the type of object used. *Trapdoor* lacerations are those avulsion injuries that occur in which an inverted U- or V-shaped flap of skin remains attached at its upper margin.[3] When present, the direction of the force is from the skin flap (beveled, angled edge) toward the undermined edge. These are seen in frontal impact injuries such motor vehicle injuries. One such case was seen when a restrained driver was wearing a visor with an attached cell phone clip that caused a very large trapdoor laceration across his forehead when his head went forward into the steering column. Slender, elongated objects (such as lead pipes and broomsticks or mop handles) produce linear or elongated lacerations.[4] Blows to the head also tend to produce similar appearing wounds.

Forensically, there are a few details to remember. Lacerations will often have abrasions and contusions accompanying them on the outer wound margin. Examination of wound edges with a dissecting microscope or magnifying lens frequently shows foreign material such as dirt, grass, paint chips, or fabric fibers, which can be collected for trace evidence.[4] These small bits of evidence are very important because they can help identify the object that caused the wound and also the locale in which the wound occurred. Last, lacerations caused by angulated objects over bony prominences may result in linear injuries without bridging tissue and may be mistaken for incised wounds. Inspection with a lens will show the area of crushing and bruising around the wound edge as well as tissue strands intact and crossing deeper in the wound. In incised wounds, these tissue strands would be cleanly and completely cut throughout the depth of the wound.

Fractures

Fractures are a break in the bone and/or cartilage that result from direct or indirect trauma.[3,4] Direct trauma is divided into three types of fractures: focal (tapping), crush, and penetrating.[4] These categories are based on the amount of force applied and the size of the affected area. Indirect trauma results from force that is applied at a remote site and has six associated types of fractures: traction; angulation; rotational; vertical compression; angulation and compression; and angulation, rotation, and compression.[4]

Focal fractures occur when a small force impacts a small area. They are usually transverse and occur in regions where two bones lie adjacent to one another, such as in the forearm and lower leg. Crush fractures occur when a large force hits a large area. They are usually comminuted, broken into several pieces, and have accompanying contusions. Penetrating fractures occur when a great force hits a small area, as in gunshot wounds. Traction fractures occur when bone is pulled apart. Angulation fractures occur as a result of bones being bent until they are unable to sustain the tension and snap. These usually result in transverse fractures. Rotational fractures occur when bone is twisted, producing a spiral fracture. These are seen in skiers who fall, as well as children who are abused. Vertical compression fractures occur in long bones and result, as the name implies, from vertical compression of the bone. These can be seen in jumpers from certain heights and result in oblique fractures. They produce T-shaped fractures at the distal end of the femur. Angulation and compression fractures are curved fractures as opposed to transverse fractures.[4]

SPECIFIC BLUNT TRAUMA INJURIES

This section reviews specific types of blunt force injuries that may occur. Particular attention will be paid to unique injuries and injury patterns. Of course, with any blunt force injury, nothing is exact.

Punching and Kicking

Punching injuries occur when force is applied with a clenched fist, usually to the upper part of the body.[2] Abrasions and contusions are the usual wounds created by punching; lacerations can occur over bony prominences or in the oral cavity. Punching to the chest and abdomen can result in internal organ damage if the force is strong enough, especially in children.

Kicking injuries occur when force is applied with a foot, bare or shoed, and can occur anywhere on the body.[2] These injuries usually occur to the knees and below when both victim and assailant are upright; kicking tends to continue after the victim has fallen to the ground, and it is often accompanied with stomping or heel grinding. Abrasions, contusions, lacerations, and fractures all can occur. Injuries from kicking tend to be more severe than punching injuries are because the lower leg can deliver more force than the clenched fist can, especially when aided by the weight and hardness of a shoe or boot toe.

Common sites of injuries are the face, neck, chest, abdomen, and perineum. Abrasions, contusions, and lacerations are common on all parts of the body, but fractures typically occur on the face (nose, zygoma, maxilla, and mandible). Kicking of the neck may lead to compression or contusions of the pharynx and/or larynx, leading to airway obstruction and subsequent death. Bleeding from facial and jaw trauma may also lead to airway obstruction and intracranial injuries.

Bites

Bite marks tend to leave a characteristic pattern wound that can be any combination of abrasion, contusion, and laceration. They tend to occur in sexual assaults, child abuse, sports-related injuries, and physical fights.[2,4] They often appear as a pair of curved contusions or abrasions in mirror opposition to one another. Documentation should include a photograph with a scale or a detailed scaled sketch. For forensic collection, bite marks may be gently rubbed with saline, and then swabbed with a dry cotton swab. Both the saline rubbed gauze and the dry cotton swab should be air dried, placed in sterile tubes, and then sent for DNA analysis. If possible, a latex or silicone rubber dental impression or cast of the mark should be made as well.[2,4] Management of bite wounds include tetanus prophylaxis, irrigation and cleaning of the wounds, and appropriate antibiotic coverage depending on source of bite (e.g., humans, cats, dogs, and so forth). Bites to the hand and face need to be observed closely and may need to be admitted for IV antibiotics because of the high risk of infection.

Blunt Chest Trauma: Rib and Sternal Fractures

Rib fractures may occur from blunt trauma in three forms, based on mechanism: therapeutic, direct, and indirect.[4] Therapeutic rib fractures may occur during cardiopulmonary resuscitation and are usually seen in the elderly. As aging occurs, bones become more brittle and less pliable. As a result, when chest compressions are applied, fractures are more likely to occur in the elderly than in children or young adults.[2,4] These injuries are typically left sided, although bilateral and right-sided fractures can and do occur, and they can be accompanied by sternal fractures, mediastinal and substernal hemorrhages, and pneumothorax, secondary to puncture of lung from the fractured rib.

Rib fractures can also occur from direct trauma to the chest wall.[2,4] These tend to occur directly below the point of impact and can be simple, displaced, or compound. Simple rib fractures are isolated rib fractures in a single rib. Displaced rib fractures are those fractures in which the fragments are separated and unaligned. Compound fractures are those fractures that perforate the skin, creating an open track down to the bone.[4] Depending on the location of rib fracture, there may be associated underlying injuries. For example, fractures of ribs 1–3 often are accompanied by severe injuries to the trachea and great vessels of the superior chest (aorta, superior vena cava, and subclavian vein), whereas fractures of ribs 10–12 are often accompanied by splenic, diaphragmatic, and liver injuries.[4,5]

Rib fractures that occur from indirect trauma occur secondary to general compression of the chest (as opposed to localized compression in cardiopulmonary resuscitation).[4] When the direction of the compression is anterior to posterior, as when a piece of heavy machinery is dropped onto the front of a person, lateral rib fractures occur. When the direction of the compression is posterior to anterior, fractures occur near the spine. Finally, when the direction of the compression is laterally applied, rib fractures occur near the spine and the sternum. Facial petechiae may be seen especially when the compressive force is caused by a large, heavy object (traumatic asphyxia).

Complications of rib fractures that occur include flail chest, hemothorax, pneumothorax, hemopneumothorax, pneumonia, and laceration of the heart.[2,4,5] Flail chest occurs when three or more consecutive ribs are fractured in at least two places on the same side of the chest, resulting in chest wall instability.[1] The fractures tend to occur both anteriorly and posteriorly, are extensive (ribs 2–9), and are bilateral. The patient with flail chest has paradoxical respiratory movement of the injured segment (chest collapse with inspiration and expansion with expiration), which leads to significant respiratory difficulty. Cardiovascular instability may also occur as a result of decreased venous return to the right atrium. Lacerations of the underlying intercostal vessels may lead to hemothorax, whereas lacerations of the lung parenchyma may lead to pneumothorax or hemopneumothorax. Pneumonia is a late complication that may be from splinting for the pain. Severe rib fractures may lacerate the heart and lead to cardiovascular compromise and instability. Air embolisms may also occur from rib fractures.

Sternal fractures are caused by high-impact direct blunt trauma, applied in an anterior to posterior direction.[4] They tend to be transverse and occur on the body of the sternum. Cardiopulmonary resuscitation would cause fractures in the midlevel body of the sternum at the third or fourth interspace, depending on where the pressure was applied.

The emergency and trauma physician must have a high index of suspicion for such chest injuries given the mechanism of the trauma (e.g., high-impact motor vehicle crash with direct chest trauma against the steering wheel). The clinical examination in conjunction with imaging (chest X-ray, computed tomography scan of the chest) is essential in diagnosing thoracic injuries quickly. In cases of hemothorax and pneumothorax, immediate chest tube placement is indicated.[5] For significant rib fracture and chest wall injuries, pulmonary contusion may not be evident on the initial imaging studies because it often lags behind. These patients must be observed closely, often in an ICU setting, and significant analgesia is needed (such as an epidural, regional nerve blocks, patient controlled analgesia [PCA] pumps) to prevent secondary complications and infections.

Cardiac Injuries

Cardiac injuries occur from direct or indirect application of force, deceleration, compression of the heart between the sternum and the spinal column, blast injury, or any combination of the preceding mechanisms.[4] The nature and extent of injury are determined by severity of localized trauma and the heart cycle at the time of injury.

Myocardial contusions, or contusions to the middle layer of the heart, occur from severe direct trauma to the heart, typically applied anteriorly to the thorax.[4,5] The anterior ventricles or the intraventricular septum are usually affected, unless the heart is driven against the posterior column, and then posterior contusions can result.[4] These injuries may simulate myocardial infarct, leading to electrocardiogram changes and/or elevated cardiac enzymes.[4,5] Typically, there is external evidence of trauma (such as contusions) on the anterior chest wall when myocardial contusions occur. It should be noted that if open thoracotomy is performed with manual cardiac massage, areas of subendocardial hemorrhage may occur, and these should not be mistaken for antemortem contusions.[4]

Myocardial lacerations may occur if the heart is filled with blood at the time of impact.[4] These lacerations may occur anywhere in the heart: ventricles, atria, valves, papillary muscles, or septa. Cardiac tamponade occurs in the presence of cardiac laceration without pericardial laceration. Death results with as little as 150 cc of intrapericardial hemorrhage from the progressive external compression of the heart and subsequent inadequate filling. Cardiac valve laceration occurs approximately in 5% of cases, with the mitral valve being the one most commonly lacerated.[4]

Cardiac concussions occur after a sudden, forceful impact to the midanterior chest wall.[4] This injury is also known as *commotio cordis* and can occur in a sudden acceleration–deceleration motor vehicle accident[4] or from direct chest trauma such as while engaging in various sports activities.[6–9] This injury needs to be differentiated from a cardiac contusion, or *contusio cordis,* where there is actual myocardial tissue damage resulting in medical complications or death.[6] *Commotio cordis* results from low-impact blunt trauma to the chest wall, as opposed to *contusio cordis,* which results from high impact. Commotio cordis occurs more often in young athletes,[6,7] but has occurred in young nonathletes engaging in non-sports-related activities. Items that have struck the chest wall to result in this injury include baseballs, softballs, hockey sticks and pucks, lacrosse sticks and balls, cricket balls, soccer balls, tennis balls, a hollow plastic bat, a circular plastic sledding saucer, closed or open fists, the head of a pet dog, an elbow, a knee, a shoulder, a forearm.[8]

The US Commotio Cordis Registry reports the median age seen in *commotio cordis* as 14 years,[6] with the oldest person being 44 years.[8] Although substernal hemorrhage and sternal fractures can accompany this injury,[4] there is generally no microscopic or gross cardiac damage.[4,6–9] Death, when it occurs, is caused by ventricular fibrillation,[4,6–9] or asystole.[4,8] Other cardiac rhythms seen include ventricular tachycardia, bradyarrhythmias, idioventricular rhythm, and complete heart block.[8] Although the pathophysiology of *commotio cordis* is not completely understood, it is generally believed that the cardiac dysrhythmia is produced by a blow to the chest wall, directly over the area of the heart.[6,9] Another important finding is that the development of ventricular fibrillation (the most common cause of mortality) requires that the impact occurs 10 to 30 milliseconds before the peak of the T wave in the cardiac cycle.[6] The young are more susceptible to *commotio cordis* because their chest walls are more compliant, allowing for greater transmission of energy to the myocardium.[6,9]

Aortic injuries, as mentioned earlier, tend to be lacerations.[4,5] They tend to occur from motor vehicle accidents, either from frontal or lateral impact. They most commonly occur in the descending thoracic aorta, just distal to the origin of the left subclavian artery. There is decreased mobility of the aorta in this area, and when there is sudden acceleration–deceleration of the automobile, the heart and great vessels are forcefully pulled from the anchored descending aorta and aortic arch resulting in incomplete or complete transverse lacerations. Sudden compression of a blood-filled heart can lead to increased intra-aortic pressure and result in bursting lacerations of the aortic arch or root and/or the ascending aorta.[4] A false aneurysm may develop from nontransmural lacerations. These typically occur in the intima. Erosion through the vessel wall may lead to delayed hemorrhage or false aneurismal formation, or even post-traumatic aortic dissections. These injuries may stabilize or rupture.

In cases where cardiac injuries are suspected, bedside ultrasound (Focused Assessment Sonography in Trauma, or FAST) and/or echocardiogram is often indicated.[5,10] When cardiac tamponade is suspected (jugular venous distension, muffled heart sounds, hypotension), an emergent bedside pericardiocentesis is often necessary to relieve the tamponade, and ultimately a pericardial window performed in the operating room is necessary. In most such cardiac injuries, transfer to a facility with cardiothoracic surgery availability is necessary for definitive care.

Diaphragmatic Injuries

Blunt trauma to the lower anterior chest can lead to diaphragmatic rupture and/or laceration. They may occur in any location on the diaphragm and are typically associated with rib fractures and intrathoracic or intra-abdominal organ injury. Displacement of left-sided intra-abdominal organs (stomach, spleen, intestine) into the thoracic cavity may occur. The posterolateral left hemidiaphragm is the area most commonly injured.[4,5] These injuries are often missed on chest X-ray and might only be seen on CT of the chest.

Pulmonary Injuries

As mentioned under rib fractures, pneumothorax, hemothorax, and hemopneumothorax may occur from chest wall trauma. A tension pneumothorax may occur from a simple pneumothorax and can rapidly lead to severe cardiac complications if not quickly decompressed. Pulmonary contusions and lacerations may result from sudden blunt force applied to the chest, usually occurring when the glottis is closed at the time of impact. Simple pulmonary contusions may heal within a few days or take months depending on the severity of the injury. Preexisting pulmonary disease (e.g., sarcoidosis, emphysema, tuberculosis) predisposes the lung to injury, and less force can cause damage that would not be caused in an otherwise healthy, elastic lung.

BLUNT FORCE INJURIES TO THE ABDOMEN AND GENITALIA

Blunt force applied to the anterior or lateral abdomen may result in intra-abdominal organ damage. Some of these injuries occur as a result of compression against the rigid lumbar spine, which protrudes into the abdominal cavity, acting as a sharp instrument.[2] The severity of the injury depends on the force of the impact, size of the impact and object delivering the impact, the organ involved, and preexisting physical and medical condition of the victim. Solid organs such as the liver and spleen rupture and lacerate more easily than do hollow organs such as the intestines. As mentioned in the section titled "Lacerations" earlier in this chapter, fixed organs are more easily injured than mobile organs are. Organs that are distended or enlarged (full bladder, swollen spleen secondary to infection from mononucleosis, malaria, typhoid, leukemia, or hemophilia) also are injured more frequently than hollow organs are. It is important to remember that there may be no external signs of abdominal injury when there is intra-abdominal injury present.

Hepatic injuries may be classified as transscapular (involving both capsule and parenchyma) and subscapular (involving only the parenchyma).[4] Preexisting liver disease may also make the liver more likely to be injured in blunt trauma. Most injuries occur in the right lobe on the domed surfaces. Subcapsular hematomas may resolve without incident or rupture leading to fatal intraperitoneal hemorrhage. Concomitant injuries to the hepatic vasculature may also occur. Capsular lacerations occurred at 27 to 34 ft-lb of force.[4] Rupture and pulpification of the liver and disruption of only the tributaries of hepatic vasculature and bile duct are reported to occur at 285 to 360 ft-lb of force.[4]

Splenic injuries occur when force is applied to the left upper quadrant of the abdomen or the left lateral wall of the chest. Splenic injuries run the gamut from superficial capsular lacerations to pulpification and disintegration. As with the liver, subcapsular hematomas may also form. Contusions may result in splenic infarct from splenic vein or artery thrombosis.

Pancreatic injuries occur when severe, direct force is applied to the upper mid abdomen or there is massive abdominal trauma. Injuries do not occur often because of the pancreas's retroperitoneal location in the abdomen. The body of the pancreas is injured when it is crushed against the vertebral column.[4,5] Lacerations and contusions can both occur. Lacerations result in chemical peritonitis and mesenteric fat necrosis resulting from the leakage of exocrine secretions into the peritoneum. Esophageal rupture secondary to trauma is rare and occurs in the setting of massive blunt trauma, as from a motor vehicle accident. Stomach laceration, contusion, or rupture may occur with severe enough blunt trauma, typically when the stomach is distended secondary to food. Small bowel injuries may occur, and contusions, perforations, or transections can occur.[4] Perforation, as sequela of contusion, may be seen if there is significant devitalization of tissue. Most often, if the small bowel injury occurs, the area of the ligament of Treitz by the duodenojejunal flexure is injured because the small bowel is immobile and fixed at that point. This can be seen in the blunt trauma from bicycle handlebar injury to the abdomen. Jejunal and ileal injury may occur with severe blunt force trauma. Mesenteric injury may occur, and when involving a large mesenteric vessel (typically artery), massive intraperitoneal hemorrhage can lead to death. Large bowel injuries may range from contusions to lacerations to transaction.[4] These occur infrequently because of the location of the large bowel in the abdomen, as well as its nature of being a hollow viscous organ. When there is fecal impaction or volvulus, however, colonic distention occurs, making large bowel rupture more likely when blunt trauma is applied.

The imaging study often used to diagnose such abdominal injuries from blunt trauma is computed tomography (CT). CT better evaluates injuries to the liver and spleen than injuries to the pancreas, bowel, stomach, or diaphragm.[5,10] Oral contrast administration for CT is not essential for aiding in the diagnosis of blunt abdominal injury.[10–12] CT should be performed only in the hemodynamically stable patient. Diagnostic peritoneal lavage (DPL) or FAST can be performed bedside to look for hemoperitoneum in patients with unstable vital signs in whom you may be concerned of an intra-abdominal injury. However, these two modalities are not able to diagnose retroperitoneal injuries.[5,10] Prompt evaluation by a trauma surgeon is necessary if such abdominal injuries are suspected because many of these patients need prompt and emergent exploratory laparotomy in the operating room.

Renal injuries are uncommon in blunt trauma and typically occur when force is applied laterally (at the flanks) or when there is trauma from a fall from height.[4,5] When injury does occur, it usually is in the form of a contusion, although small transverse lacerations may be present, leading to insignificant bleeding. As with pancreatic injuries, blunt trauma applied to the kidneys may lead to renal artery thrombosis and multiple renal infarcts. Associated or independent adrenal gland injury (laceration, contusion, or rupture) may also occur when the impact is directed in the vicinity of the kidneys.

Bladder rupture is possible in blunt force trauma, especially when the bladder is distended with urine and rises above the symphysis pubis. Extraperitoneal bladder rupture occurs in a nondistended or slightly distended bladder and is associated with pelvic fractures or abdominal trauma that is directed downward into the pelvis. Intraperitoneal bladder rupture occurs in a distended bladder, usually occurring in the superior or posterior aspect of the bladder because the bladder is pushed against the sacrum. Complications of bladder rupture include hemorrhage leading to shock and death or sepsis, peritonitis, and ascending renal infections. It is important to rule out urethral and bladder injuries prior to placement of Foley catheters in the trauma patient with any evidence of such injuries (e.g., scrotal hematoma, blood at the urethral meatus, or high-riding prostate). A retrograde urethrogram (RUG) and CT urethrogram or cystogram are imaging studies to perform in ruling out genitourinary (GU) injuries.

External male genitalia injuries ranging from abrasions, lacerations, contusions, to subtotal and total amputations may occur from blunt trauma to the area. Scrotal hematomas may or may not occur. Internal male genitalia injuries include contusion and lacerations, resulting in testicular hematomas and/or interstitial hemorrhage. In extremely rare cases, trauma to the scrotal region may cause cardiac asystole and immediate death from simultaneous hypervagal stimulation.[4] If there is suspected genitalia injury in the absence of external injury, further imaging with ultrasound or intravenous pyelogram (IVP) may be indicated.[4,5] External female genitalia injuries including abrasions, lacerations, and contusions may result from blunt force, usually in association with sexual assault. Internal female genitalia injury is less likely to occur in the nonpregnant state.

ORTHOPEDIC INJURIES

A general description of fractures was previously discussed. This section deals with specific bone fractures, including spinal, pelvic, and extremity fractures.

Spinal Fractures

Vertebral column fractures are usually caused by indirect blunt trauma, except in the cases of gunshot wounds.[4] Mobility is greatest in the cervical region, least in the thoracic region, and intermediate in the lumbar region. The most common spinal fracture is an anterior compression fracture, usually occurring at or near the thoracic/lumbar junction.[4] Thoracic spine transection may occur in falls from heights or severe motor vehicle accidents.[2]

Pelvic fractures are caused by direct or indirect trauma. Both require a large amount of force, and indirect trauma is caused when the force is applied to the lower extremities. Pelvic fractures may be divided into three types: open-book, lateral compression, and vertical shear.[4] Open-book fractures occur when there is compression in the anterior to posterior direction, separating the symphysis pubis. Lateral compression fractures occur when lateral force is applied to the iliac crest or the femoral head. These lead to pubic rami fractures, either ipsilaterally, contralaterally, or bilaterally when the force is applied to the iliac crest, and acetabular fractures combined with ipsilateral pelvic rami fractures when the force is applied to the femoral head. Vertical shear fractures occur when severe vertical force is applied that results in hemipelvis displacement. There is anterior disruption of symphysis pubis and/or pubic rami with gross posterior disruption of the sacroiliac joints with adjacent sacral or ilial fractures. The most common complication of pelvic fractures is severe intraperitoneal and retroperitoneal hemorrhage,[4,5] with mortality ranging from 5–20%.[4]

EXTREMITY INJURIES

Extremity injuries caused by blunt force trauma may result in any combination of abrasions, contusions, lacerations, and fractures. The different types of fractures include bumper fractures, ankle fractures, patellar fractures, femoral fractures, humeral fractures, radial or ulnar fractures, and metacarpal fractures.[4] Bumper fractures are produced by the front end of a moving vehicle that strikes a standing individual. Patellar and femoral fractures also may occur from a moving vehicle. All three of these types of fractures are discussed further in Chapter 14 on motor vehicle accidents.

Upper extremity injuries occur from motor vehicular accidents, falls, or assaults. They can be divided into defensive and offensive wounds. Defensive wounds tend to result in abrasions, contusions, and lacerations on the posterior aspect of the hands and forearms and fractures of the phalanges.[2,4] Offensive wounds result in abrasions and contusions of the knuckles and fractures of the metacarpals.[4]

Complications of lower extremity injuries include hemorrhagic shock from massive soft tissue crush injury and/or large artery laceration, pulmonary embolism, fat embolism (manifesting 24 to 48 hours after the injury occurs), infection, and rhabdomyolysis. Complications of upper extremity injuries include infection and exsanguinations if a major vessel is involved.

BLUNT FORCE TRAUMA TO THE HEAD

Blunt force trauma to the head can cause abrasions, contusions, lacerations, and fractures. The presence and extent of skull fractures depend on the severity of the blow, the instrument or weapon that impacts the head, the amount and thickness of the hair around the impact site, the thickness of scalp at the impact site, the thickness and shape of the skull at the impact site, and the age of the victim. If the skull hits a hard surface, 33–75 ft-lb of energy is required to cause a single linear skull fracture.[4] If the skull hits a soft surface, 268–581 ft-lb of energy is required to produce the same skull fracture.[4] Skull fractures begin at the impact site and radiate outward. Depressed skull fractures occur from high-velocity impact, driving skull fragments inward.[2,4] Linear skull fractures occur from flat impact and commonly run down the temporoparietal plates but may run along the base of the skull.[2,4] When both bases are involved, the floor of the skull may separate, creating the "hinge fracture" seen in motor vehicle accidents.[2]

Intracranial hemorrhages or hematomas may also result from blunt trauma. These include epidural hematomas, subdural hematomas, subarachnoid hemorrhages, and intracerebral hemorrhages.[2,4] Epidural hematomas, bleeding in the potential space between the skull and the dura,[1,4] result from trauma caused by falls or from a motor vehicle accident. The middle meningeal artery is involved, and 90–95% of cases have a fracture present at the site of impact, which is usually the squamous portion of the temporal bone.[4]

Subdural hematomas, bleeding between the dura and the arachnoid membranes,[1] from blunt trauma occur mainly from falls or assaults. They are usually caused by shearing/tearing forces as seen in acceleration–deceleration injuries.[2,4] They may be on the ipsilateral or contralateral side of the impact site and may or may not be accompanied by other cerebral injuries or skull fractures.

Subarachnoid hemorrhage, bleeding between the arachnoid and pia mater,[1] is the most common intracranial finding after blunt head trauma. These injuries may be caused by force applied to the lateral neck, leading to vertebral artery damage.[2,4] Intracerebral hemorrhages and/or hematomas tend to be located in the frontal and temporal regions and are usually associated with skull fractures.

Cerebral contusions occur from falls or from trauma to a stationary head. There are different types of cerebral contusions: coup (occurring at the site of impact), countercoup (occurring on the side opposite to the site of impact), fracture (resulting from an overlying fracture), intermediary coup (when deep brain structures hemorrhage), gliding (usually occurring in the dorsal surfaces of the frontal lobe), and herniation (resulting from herniation of brain matter through the foramen magnum).[4]

CONCLUSION

Blunt force injuries are commonly seen in the ED. Proper evaluation, documentation, and management are essential for proper medical care as well as forensic care of the patient. Clinicians should carefully document all wounds seen and consider using photographic documentation.

REFERENCES

1. *Stedman's Concise Medical Dictionary for the Health Professions.* 4th ed. Version 2.0. Philadelphia, Pa: Lippincott Williams & Wilkins; 2001.
2. Knight B. The examination of wounds and regional injuries. In: *Simpson's Forensic Medicine.* 11th ed. New York, NY: Oxford University Press; 1997:44–64.
3. Besant-Matthews PE. Blunt and sharp injuries. In: Lynch VA, ed. *Forensic Nursing.* St Louis, Mo: Elsevier; 2006:189–200.
4. DiMaio VJM, Dana SE. Blunt force injury. In: *Handbook of Forensic Pathology.* 2nd ed. Boca Raton, Fla: CRC Press; 2007:73–106.
5. American College of Surgeons Committee on Trauma. *Advanced Trauma Life Support for Doctors.* 7th ed. Chicago, Ill: American College of Surgeons; 2004.
6. Madias C, Maron BJ, Weinstock J, Estes NAM, Link MS. Commotio cordis—sudden cardiac death with chest wall impact. [Review] *J Cardiovasc Electrophysiol.* 2007;18(1):115–122.
7. Maron BJ, Poliac LC, Kaplan JA, Mueller FO. Blunt impact to the chest leading to sudden death from cardiac arrest during sports activities. *N Engl J Med.* 1995;333:337–342.
8. Maron BJ, Gohman TE, Kyle SB, Estes NAM, Link MS. Clinical profile and spectrum of commotio cordis. *JAMA.* 2002;287:1142–1146.

9. Geddes LA, Roeder RA. Evolution of our knowledge of sudden death due to commotio cordis. *Ann Emerg Med.* 2005;23:67–75.
10. ACEP Clinical Policies Committee. Clinical policy: critical issues in the evaluation of adult patients presenting to the emergency department with acute blunt abdominal trauma. *Ann Emerg Med.* 2004;43(2):278–290.
11. Tsang BD, Panacek EA, Brant WE, et al. Effect of oral contrast administration for abdominal tomography in the evaluation of acute blunt trauma. *Ann Emerg Med.* 1997;30(1):7–13.
12. Shreve WS, Knotts FB, Siders RW, et al. Retrospective analysis of the adequacy of oral contrast material for computed tomography scans in trauma patients. *Am J Surg.* 1999;178(1):14–17.

11 | Sharp Force Injury

Marianne Hamel, MD, PhD, FCAP

INTRODUCTION

Intentionally or unintentionally, emergency department physicians serve as front-line agents in the practice of forensic medicine. Although the examination and treatment of sharp force injury in the emergency department naturally focuses on restoring the health of the patient, the application of the basic principles of forensic medicine—particularly those concerning wound identification, documentation, evidence collection and preservation, and photography—contribute both to the ease of criminal investigation, if warranted, and to the ability of the treating physician to offer a medicolegal opinion, if called upon to do so. Emergency departments are prepared to handle a vast variety of injuries, but standardized protocols mandating thorough documentation and careful evidence collection in cases of sharp force injury serve both the patient and the medical community well.

ANATOMY OF A KNIFE

Single-edged knives are composed of a grip; a guard, meant to protect the bearer's hand from the blade; a ricasso, an unsharpened portion of the blade adjacent to the grip with two squared-off edges; a blade, which has both squared-off and sharp edges; and a point (Figure 11-1). The unsharpened portion of the knife opposite from the blade is referred to as the spine. Double-edged knives have, of course, two cutting surfaces, and serrated knives have a crenulated cutting surface meant for sawing.

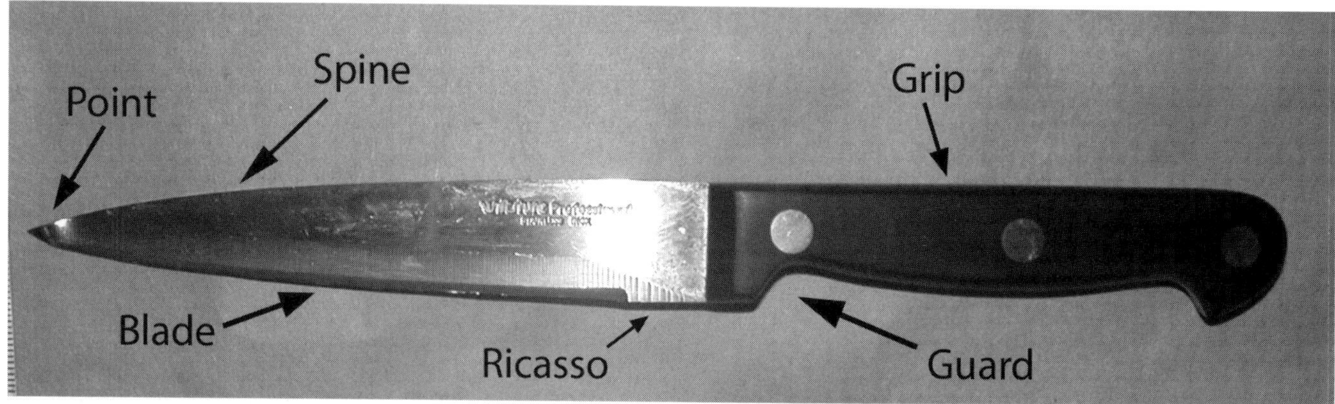

FIGURE 11-1 **A knife is composed of a grip, a guard, a ricasso, a blade, a point, and a spine.**

Stab Wounds

Correct interpretation of both the pattern and the morphology of stab wounds contributes to the differentiation between accidental, homicidal, and suicidal injuries. A comparison should be made between the history offered by the victim and the conclusions that can be drawn from the victim's wounds; discrepancies between the two invite further investigation.

Careful examination of a stab wound offers information about the shape of the blade. Wounds inflicted with a single-edged weapon have a blunted end and a pointed end (Figure 11-2); wounds inflicted with a double-edged knife have two sharp ends. Wounds from serrated-edge knives cannot be reliably differentiated from those of straight-bladed weapons unless drawn across the skin to produce multiple, parallel superficial lesions.

Stab wounds may gape depending on their relationship to the cleavage lines of Langer, which are delineated by the orientation of connective fibers in the dermis. Wounds oriented parallel to the lines of Langer remain relatively approximated; those perpendicular tend to gape widely, potentially leading to an incorrect interpretation of the characteristics of the weapon (Figure 11-3). Skin elasticity should also be taken into consideration when examining a wound because dermal laxity can somewhat increase or decrease the size of a wound in relation to the blade that caused it. Gaping wounds must be reapproximated to estimate the maximum width of the blade and to determine whether the weapon was single- or double-edged (Figure 11-4).

A collar of contusion or abrasion injury may surround a wound from a completely inserted weapon as a result of contact with the knife guard or fist holding the weapon. If the weapon is inserted at an oblique angle to the skin, the contusion or abrasion may be present at only one end of the wound. Additionally, rotational force (i.e., the movement of perpetrator or victim in relation to the knife) may produce asymmetrical or oddly shaped wounds. Single stab wounds may overlie more than one wound track because of repositioning of the blade after incomplete removal of the knife.

Knives that remain *in situ* at examination should be removed with minimal handling of the grip and guard. If

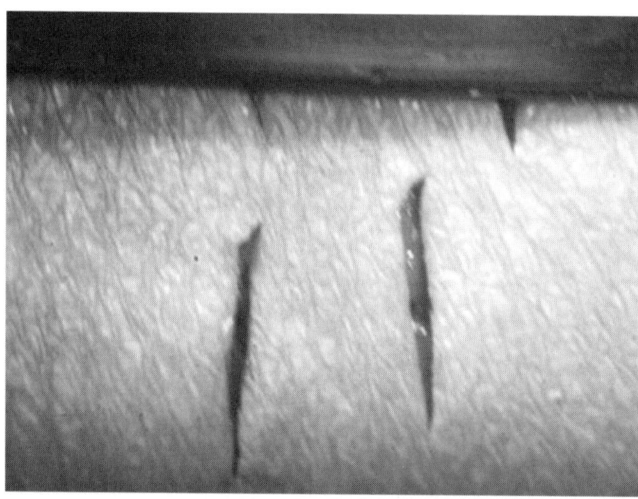

FIGURE 11-2 **Single-edged wounds have both blunted and sharp ends.**

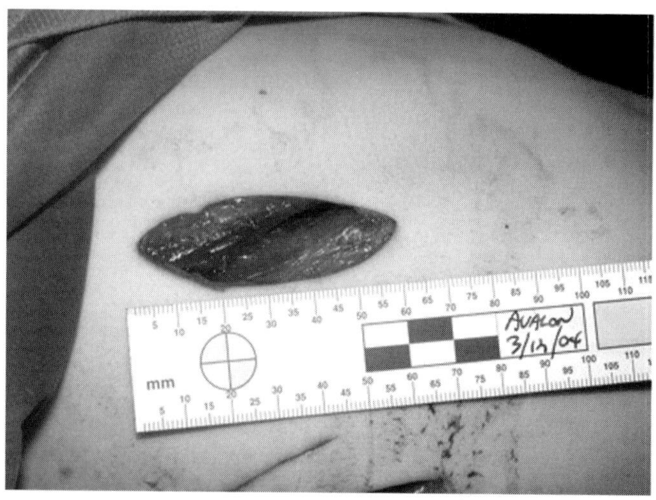

FIGURE 11-3 **Wounds can gape and distort the interpretation of weapon characteristics.**

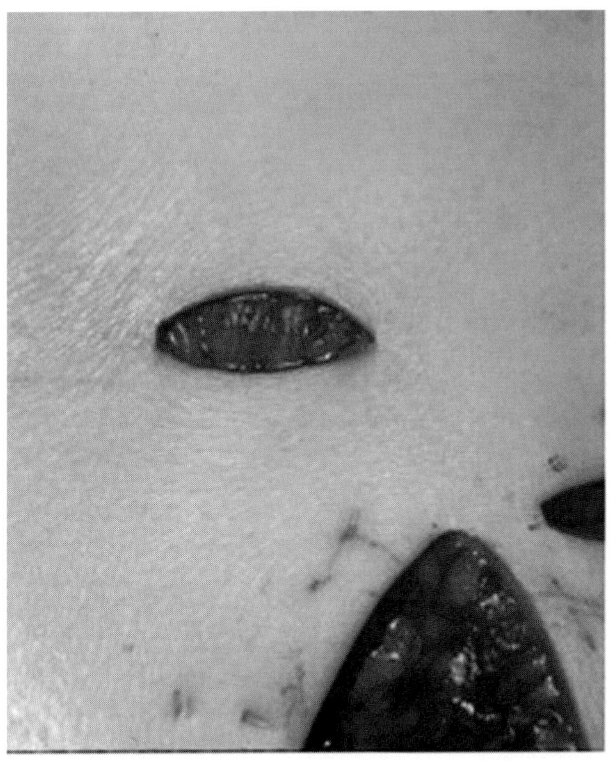

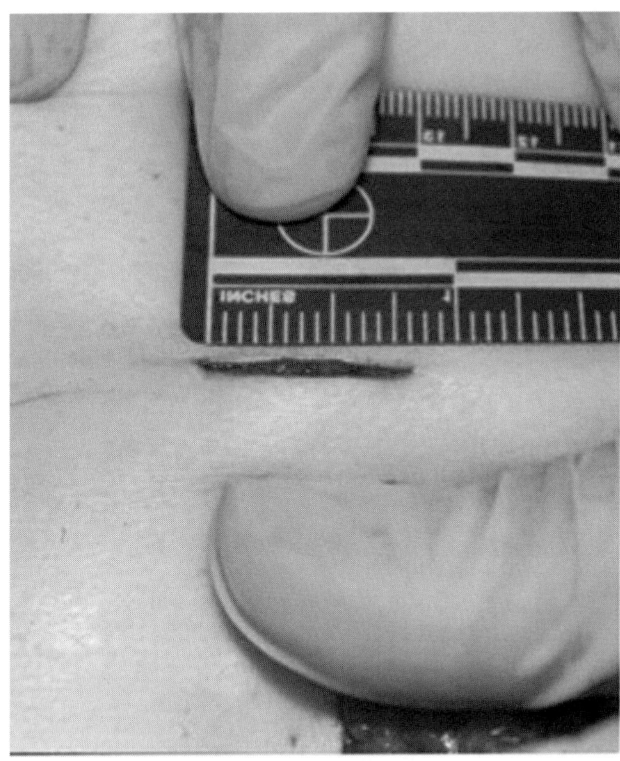

FIGURE 11-4 **Gaping wounds should be reapproximated to estimate the width of the blade.**

appropriate, the knife should be placed in an evidence bag and turned over to authorities after removal. Embedded blade fragments identified on radiographs should be extracted, if possible, and retained for comparison with potential weapons.

Incised Wounds

Incised wounds have a greater length than depth and can be differentiated from lacerations by a lack of tissue bridging. Tissue bridging results from the application of blunt force that overcomes the elasticity of the skin; as a result, the skin splits while underlying structures such as vessels, nerves, and connective tissue visibly span the wound. Unlike stab wounds, the depth and morphology of incised wounds provide no information about the weapon[1] or the directionality of the assault.

OTHER WEAPONS

Although knife injuries are common, wounds from other implements are regularly treated in the emergency department. Recognition of common pattern injuries can assist in evaluation of the history offered by the victim.

Assault with a standard screwdriver leaves slit-like wounds that are indistinguishable from those caused by a knife with a narrow, thick blade. Phillips head screwdrivers leave roughly circular wounds with abraded margins (Figure 11-5).

Injuries inflicted with scissors are notable for two patterns: a nearly square notched wound, caused by closed scissors; and paired wounds, the result of assault with an open pair of scissors (Figure 11-6).

Injuries from broken bottles are generally grouped and are notable for the varied size and depth of the wounds.[2]

CHOP INJURIES

Chop wounds combine the crushing traits of blunt force injury with the incisive qualities of sharp force injury. Typical weapons are heavy with a cutting edge, such as machetes, propellers, cleavers, lawnmower blades, or axes, and produce gaping wounds, often associated with chipping or fracture of underlying bone (Figure 11-7).[2] Radiating fractures and avulsion of a wedge-shaped bone fragment are characteristic of axe injuries.[3]

SELF-INFLICTED INJURIES

Suicide by sharp force injury makes up 2–3% of completed suicide attempts, most commonly through the use of knives and razor blades. The presence or absence of hesitation marks, perforation of clothing, and defensive injuries has been touted as a reliable indicator of homicidal or suicidal intent.

Reliable differentiation between sharp force injury by an assailant and self-inflicted injury can often be aided by the presence of hesitation marks. Hesitation marks are multiple, relatively superficial incisions often found adjacent and parallel to a deeper, more serious wound (Figure 11-8). The presence of hesitation marks suggests that the wound is self-inflicted, and such wounds were noted in 77% of cases of sharp force injury suicides in a 2000 case series.[4] Hesitation marks are more common in cases with multifocal injuries.[5] Perforation of clothing has also been suggested as a reliable indicator of homicidal intent; however, the same study

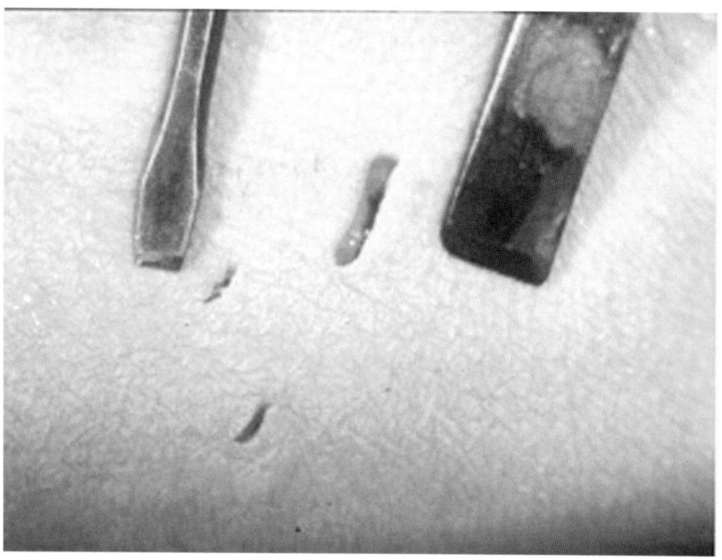

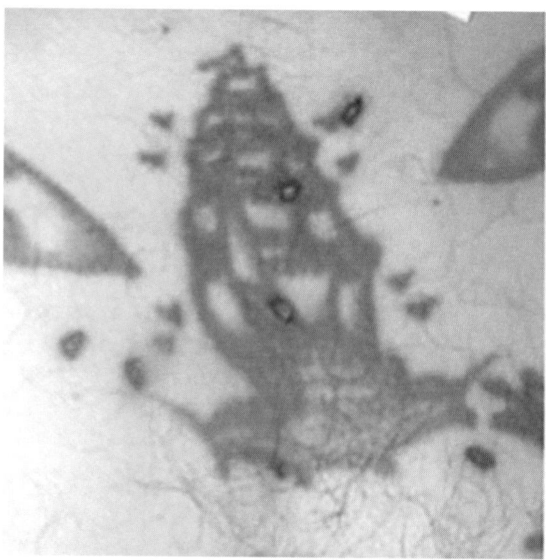

FIGURE 11-5 Standard screwdrivers leave slit-like wounds that are indistinguishable from those caused by a knife with a narrow, thick blade (*left*), whereas Phillips head screwdrivers leave roughly circular wounds with abraded margins (*right*).

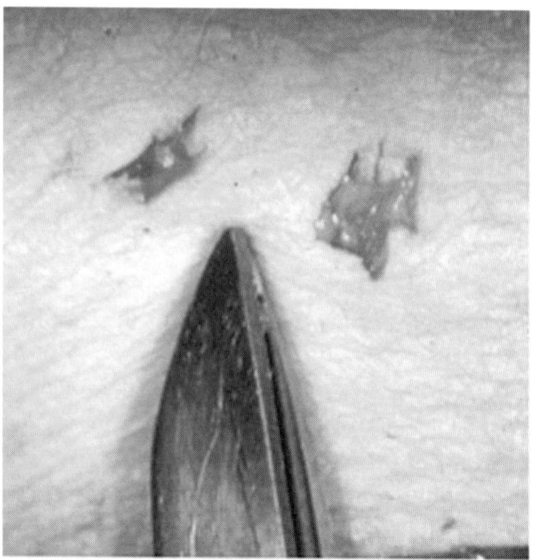

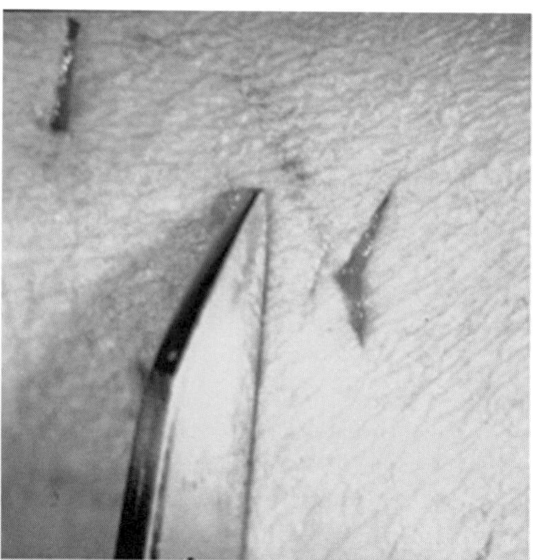

FIGURE 11-6 Closed scissors (*left*) produce squared-off notched wounds, whereas attacks with open scissors (*right*) cause paired wounds.

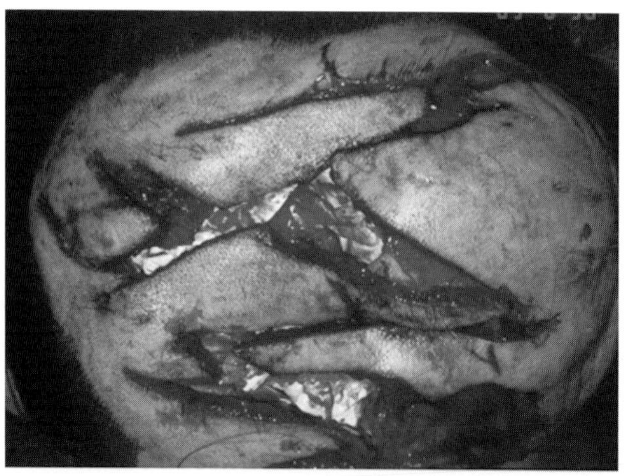

FIGURE 11-7 Chop wounds combine the crushing traits of blunt force injury with the incisive qualities of sharp force injury.

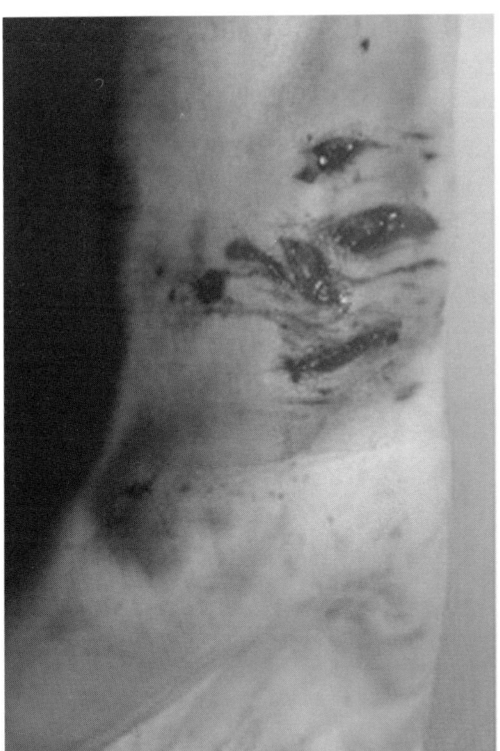

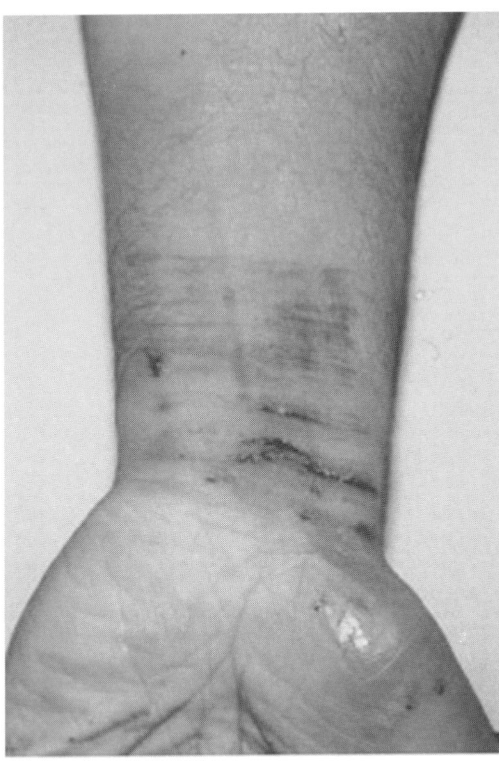

FIGURE 11-8
Hesitation marks are superficial self-inflicted cuts parallel to a more serious wound.

demonstrated that removal of clothing before self-injury was an unreliable sign of suicide. Suicide attempts involving razor blades (particularly those that are double-edged) often result in superficial digital wounds that may be mistaken for defensive injuries,[4] and cuts to the fingers should be interpreted with caution in such cases.

Healed scars from previous self-injury are common in patients who attempt or complete suicide by sharp force (Figure 11-9).

DEFENSIVE INJURIES

Defensive injuries are defined as nonfatal wounds to the upper extremities acquired in an attempt to ward off sharp force injury. Injuries are most commonly seen on the palms and flexor surfaces of the hands after attempts to grasp the blade and can also be seen on the ulnar aspects and extensor surfaces of forearms and the upper arms (Figure 11-10). However, it should be noted that hand wounds may instead represent unintentionally self-inflicted injuries on the part of the perpetrator.[6]

Defensive injuries on the feet or legs may result from an attempt to ward off attack from a reclining position and are suggestive of sexual assault. Consequently, lower extremity sharp force injuries in women should prompt emergency department staff to obtain oral, anal, and vaginal swabs to ascertain the presence of semen.[2]

EVIDENCE HANDLING AND DOCUMENTATION

Although patient care is, of course, the primary concern in the emergency department, minor efforts by first responders to preserve evidence can have a major impact on the ease and quality of forensic investigation. Documentation of injuries should be complete, accurate, and performed at the time of the patient's presentation. Wound descriptions should include a measurement of the injury, distance from landmark structures (i.e., distance from the umbilicus or top of the head), and a characterization of the wound edges and the surrounding tissue. Documentation of cuts and tears in overlying clothing and the relative position of clothing damage to injury is helpful.[7] Sharp force injuries and withdrawn weapons should be photographed at the time of treatment, and a small ruler should be placed in the photographic field for accurate size comparison.

Wounds produced in the course of diagnosis or therapeutic intervention (chest tubes, drains, laparotomy incisions) should be clearly documented; if the patient expires, all evidence of medical intervention (such as defibrillator pads, endotracheal tubes, and intravenous lines) should be left in place. Therapeutic incisions should be kept distinct from those of sharp force injury, if possible.

Though defects in clothing offer a tempting site through which to initiate the removal of clothing with scissors, the tears should instead be preserved for comparison with the injury.[8] Each item of removed clothing should be collected in a paper bag to avoid transfer of evidence or blood from one garment to another and should be set aside for examination by police or the medical examiner. Plastic bags should be avoided for the collection or storage of evidentiary clothing because trapped humidity promotes mildew growth.

CONCLUSION

Standardized protocols concerning wound identification, documentation, evidence collection and preservation, and photography are the mainstay of the practice of

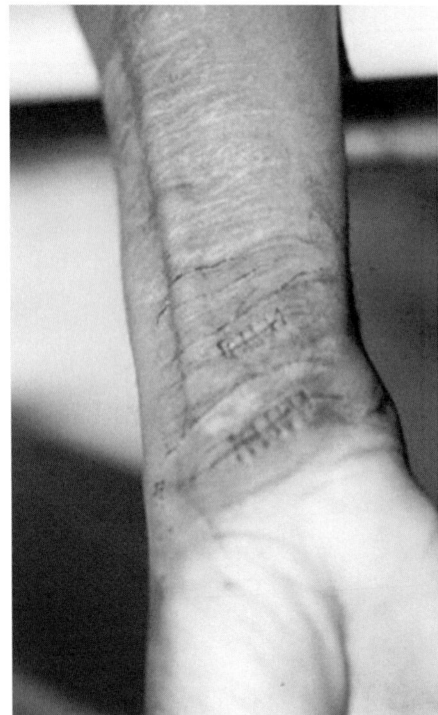

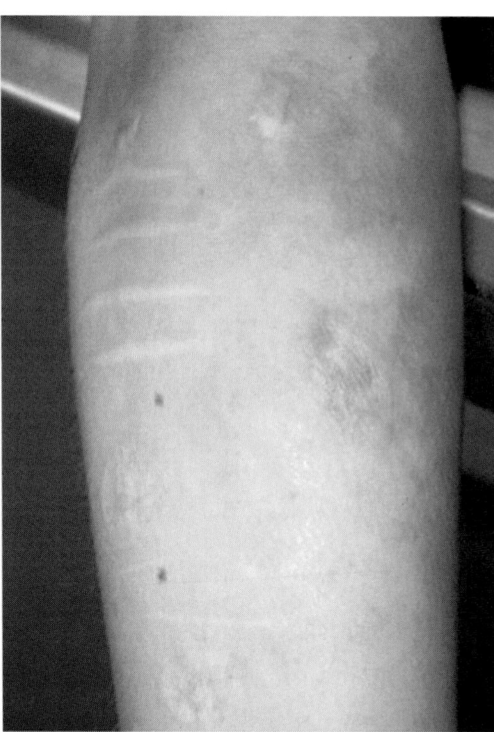

FIGURE 11-9 **Cases of self-inflicted injury often demonstrate scars from previous sharp force injury.**

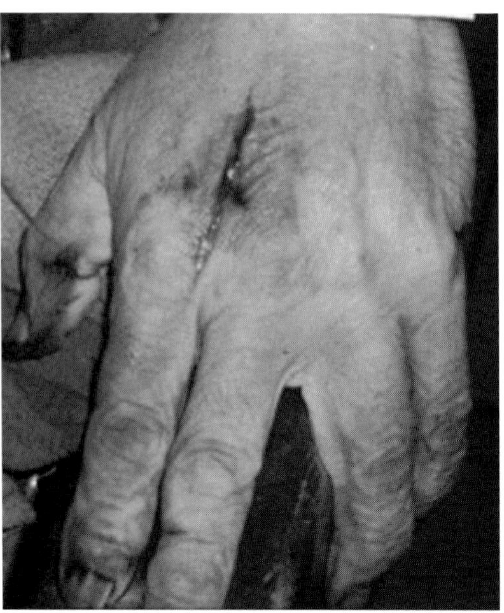

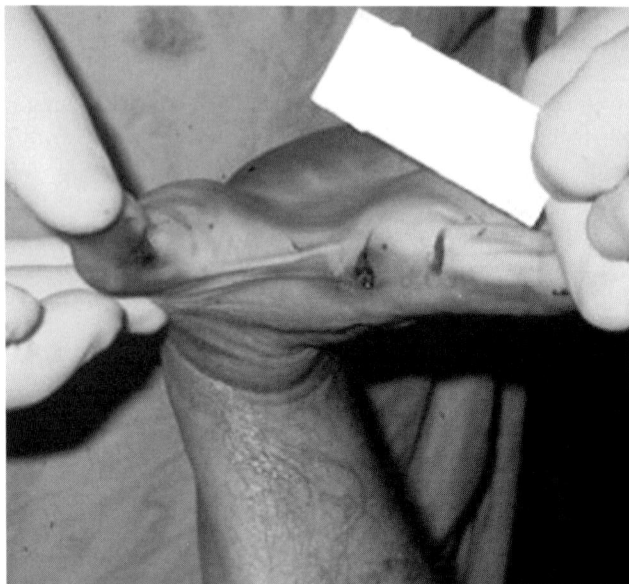

FIGURE 11-10 **Defensive wounds result from a victim's attempt to grasp the attacker's blade or ward off blows.**

forensic emergency medicine, especially with regard to sharp force injury.

REFERENCES

1. DiMaio VJ, DiMaio D. *Forensic Pathology.* 2nd ed. Boca Raton, Fla: CRC Press; 2001.
2. Spitz WU. *Medicolegal Investigation of Death.* 3rd ed. Springfield, Ill: Charles C Thomas; 1993.
3. Humphrey JH, Hutchinson DL. Macroscopic characteristics of hacking trauma. *J Forensic Sci.* 2001;46(2):228–233.
4. Karger B, Niemeyer J, Brinkmann B. Suicides by sharp force: typical and atypical features. *Int J Legal Med.* 2000;113:259–262.
5. Byard RW, Klitte Å, Gilbert JD, James RA. Clinicopathologic features of fatal self-inflicted incised and stab wounds. *Am J Forensic Med Pathol.* 2002;23(1):15–18.
6. Schmidt U, Pollak S. Sharp force injury in clinical forensic medicine—findings in victims and perpetrators. *Forensic Sci Int.* 2006;159:113–118.
7. Paul DM. The general principles of clinical forensic medicine and the place of forensic medicine in a modern society. *Yale J Biol Med.* 1977;50:405–417.
8. Mittleman RE. Preserving evidence in the emergency department. *Am J Nurs.* 1983;83(12):1652–1656.

12 Firearms

Ralph Riviello, MD, MS, FACEP, FAAEM

INTRODUCTION

Firearm injuries are commonly seen in the emergency department. Some basic understanding of the weapons, ammunition, and injuring mechanisms can help medical personnel in caring for victims. In addition, several important forensic principles and practices come into play when treating victims of firearm injury.

ANATOMY OF WEAPONS

Five general categories of firearms can produce injury that will be seen in the ED. They are handguns, rifles, shotguns, submachine guns, and machine guns.

Handguns

The revolver is the most common type of handgun in the United States (see Figure 12-1). Revolvers contain a revolving cylinder that contains several chambers, each of which holds one bullet. The cylinder is mechanically rotated to align each chamber with the chamber and firing pin. Revolvers may be further divided into the way in which the cylinder moves to be loaded. These include the swingout, break-top, and solid-frame (uses a loading gate to load the cylinder). Revolvers are also designated as single action or double action. In single-action revolvers, the hammer must be cocked manually each time the weapon is to be fired. Cocking the hammer rotates the cylinder to align the chamber with the barrel and firing pin. When pressure is applied to the trigger, the hammer releases and the weapon discharges. With double-action revolvers, continuous pressure on the trigger rotates the cylinder, aligns the chamber with the barrel, and cocks and then releases the hammer, firing the weapon.

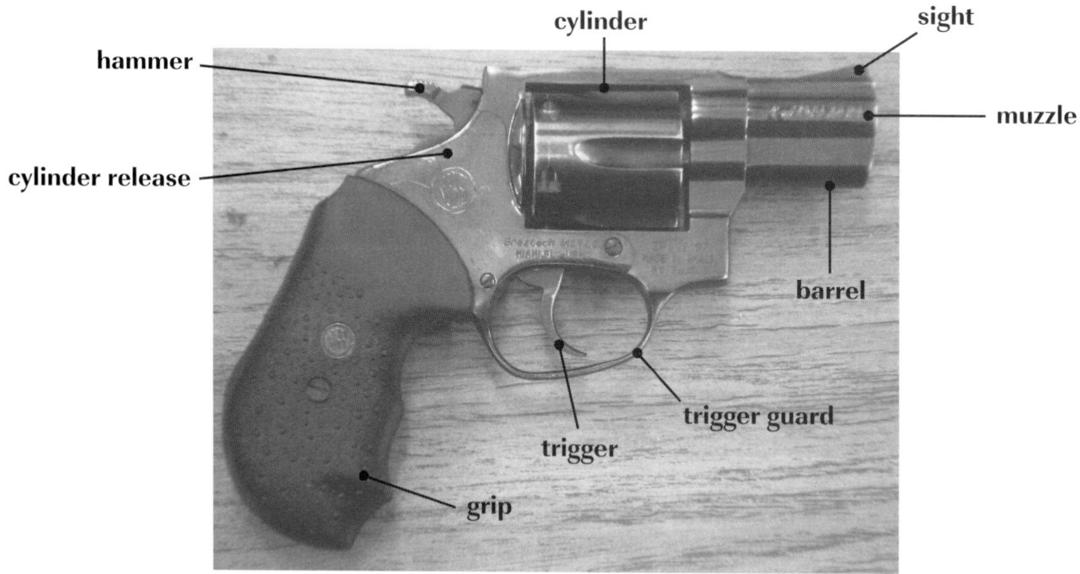

FIGURE 12-1 **Parts of a revolver.**

The other commonly used handgun is the autoloading or automatic pistol (see Figure 12-2). These are often referred to as automatics or pistols. For autoloading pistols, the trigger must be pulled for every shot fired. The cartridges are stored in a removable magazine in the grip of the pistol. Most people refer to the cartridge as a clip. Cartridges can hold different numbers of bullets. Common automatic pistols include the Sig-Sauer, Intratec Tec 9, Beretta, Glock, and Colt. The mechanism by which the pistol operates varies for each automatic weapon. Automatic pistols have at least one manually operated safety device that, when used, locks the firing mechanism and prevents the weapon from firing. Automatic

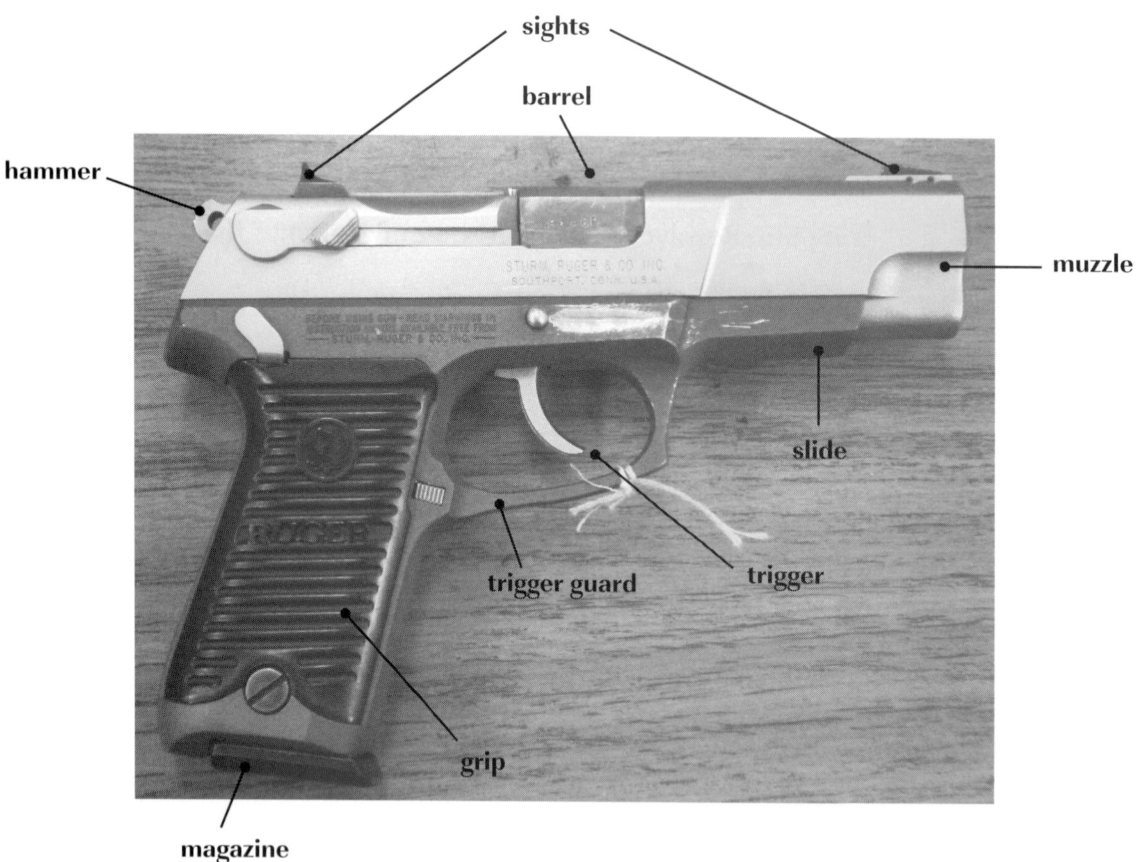

FIGURE 12-2 **Parts of a semi-automatic handgun.**

pistols have become popular weapons because of the number of bullets that can be fired at a relatively fast rate.

Rifles

A rifle is a firearm with a rifled barrel (described later) that is designed to be shot from the shoulder (see Figure 12-3). US federal law requires rifles to have a minimum barrel length of 16 inches. The types of rifles commonly available are single shot, lever action, bolt action, and auto loading. These distinctions describe how the weapon ejects and loads a cartridge to be fired. A fully automatic rifle is one that, when the trigger is pulled, initiates a cycle of events that is repeated until all the ammunition is used or the trigger is released. Fully automatic weapons are only used by the military and police organizations.

An assault rifle is a rifle that is auto loading, has a large-capacity (more than 20 rounds) detachable magazine, is capable of full-automatic fire, and fires an intermediate rifle cartridge. All four criteria must be satisfied for it to be considered an assault rifle. A common misconception about assault rifles is that the wounds they cause are more severe than those caused by other rifles. This is not true. In fact, the wounds are less severe than those produced by almost all hunting rifles. The severity of a wound is determined by the amount of kinetic energy transferred to the body. The intermediate cartridges used in assault rifles possess significantly less kinetic energy, and most ammunition used in these weapons is encased in a shell of copper alloy (full metal jacket).

Shotguns

A shotgun is also designed to be fired from the shoulder. It has a smooth bore and is designed to fire multiple pellets. US federal regulations require shotguns to have a minimum barrel length of 18 inches. A shotgun may have one or two barrels, and the barrels may be on top of each other (over-under) or side by side (double barrel). Other classifications include single shot, bolt action, lever action, pump action, and auto loading.

Submachine Guns/Machine Pistols

A submachine gun or machine pistol is a weapon that can be fired from either the shoulder and/or the hip. It has fully automatic fire, has a rifled barrel, and fires pistol ammunition.

Machine Guns

A machine gun is a weapon that is capable of full-automatic firing, and it fires rifle ammunition. Most machine guns have the ammunition fed by belts. They are capable of firing a large number of bullets at a very rapid speed.

RIFLING

The barrels of rifles, handguns, and submachine guns are rifled. This means that spiral grooves have been cut the length of the interior of the barrel. Rifling consists of these grooves and the metal left behind between the grooves, the lands. Rifling gives a rotational spin to the bullet as it travels through the air, preventing it from tumbling end over end. The direction of the rifling can be right (clockwise) or left (counterclockwise). In the United States, the Colt Company is the only major company that uses a left-hand twist.

Rifling imparts a number of markings onto the bullet. These are called class characteristics. They may help identify the make and model of the gun from which the bullet was fired. The characteristics are number, diameter, and width of lands and grooves; depth of grooves; direction of rifling twist; and degree of twist. These characteristics can also be used to compare bullets to each other in an attempt to link crimes together.

Other imperfections on the surfaces of the lands and grooves can produce individual characteristics. No two barrels produce the same markings on a bullet. These individual characteristics are unique to the weapon that fired the bullet and cannot belong to any other. They are as individual and identifying as fingerprints. Also, the magazine, firing pin, extractor, ejector, and breech face of a weapon may impart class and individual characteristics to a cartridge case or primer.

WEAPON CALIBER

In the United States, the caliber of a rifle or handgun represents the diameter of the bore, measured from land to land. This measurement is the diameter of the barrel before the grooves were cut. In reality, caliber may be given in terms of

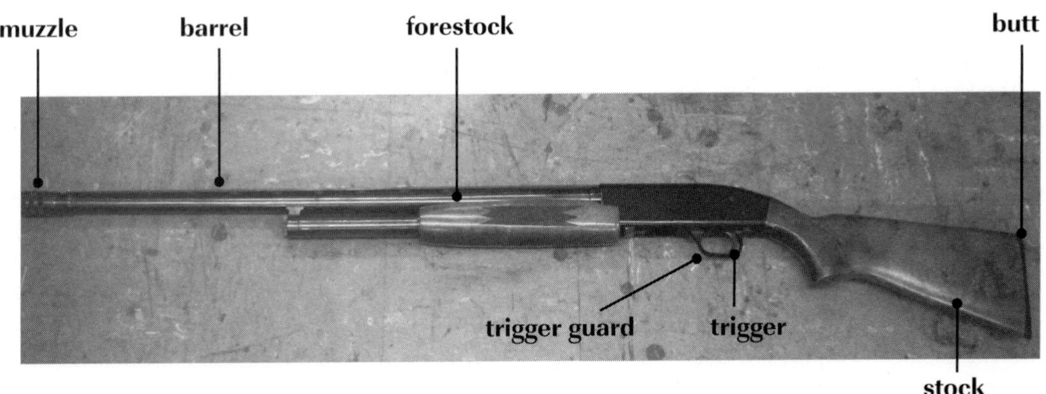

FIGURE 12-3 **Parts of a rifle.**

bullet, land, or groove diameter. The caliber specifications in the US system are neither accurate nor consistent. In the US system, a decimal point is used in the caliber designation and the measurement is made in inches.

The European system for cartridge designation is more thorough and uses the metric system. The cartridge is clearly identified by giving both the bullet diameter and the case length as well as type of cartridge case (R, rimmed; SR, semirimmed; RB, rebated; and B, belted).

The caliber of a shotgun is referred to as gauge. The term *gauge* actually refers to the number of lead balls of a given bore diameter that make up a pound. So, *12-gauge* means that it takes 12 of the lead balls to make one pound.

AMMUNITION

A cartridge, which is what is loaded into the weapon, consists of several parts. These include the following:

- A cartridge case
- A primer
- Propellant (gunpowder)
- A bullet or projectile

Cartridge Cases

Cartridge cases are typically made of brass but may be composed of steel or aluminum. The cartridge expands and seals the chamber against the rearward escape of gases when the cartridge is fired. The brass cartridge, after it expands in the chamber, will spring back to approximately its original size and make the case easy to extract. Cartridges can come in a variety of shapes including straight, bottleneck, and tapered. The cartridges are classified according to the configuration of their bases: rimmed, semirimmed, belted, rebated, and rimless. Almost all cartridges have headstamps on their bases. The headstamp consists of a series of letters, numbers, symbols, and/or trade names. The caliber may be designated as well. Headstamps can be unreliable indicators of the caliber of the cartridge case because the case may have been reformed to another caliber.

Cartridge cases are automatically or manually (in revolvers) expelled from the weapon after it is fired. These fired cartridge cases (FCCs) can be recovered at crime scenes and may contain identifiable fingerprints. Sometimes shooting victims come to the emergency department with these cartridges on their body or intermingled with their clothing. Cartridges are valuable forensic evidence; they should be collected in such a way as to preserve any fingerprints and ballistics markings present, and then should be turned over to law enforcement.

Primer

The primer is what ignites the propellant. In general, when a weapon is fired, the firing pin strikes the center of the primer cup, compresses the primer composition between the cup and the anvil, and causes the composition to explode. The flame passes through the flash holes into the cartridge case, and then ignites the propellant. Primer compounds were originally made of fulminate or mercury. Currently, all US-manufactured primers are nonmercury and noncorrosive. Compounds used include lead styphnate, barium nitrate, and antimony sulfide. The detection of these compounds constitutes the basis for tests to determine whether someone has fired a firearm.

Propellant

Originally, the propellant was made of black powder (charcoal, sulfur, and potassium nitrate). When it burns, black powder produces a large amount of solid residues that appear as white smoke. Currently, smokeless powder is used in almost all ammunition. It is converted completely into gaseous products and does not leave a significant residue in the bore of the weapon.

Bullet

The bullet is the part of the cartridge that leaves the muzzle of the gun when it is fired. Currently, bullets fall into two categories, lead and metal jacketed. Lead bullets are made out of lead with added antimony and/or tin to make the bullet harder. Some may be covered with a thin coating of copper or copper alloy. It helps to harden and lubricate the bullet. Lead bullets come in four configurations: roundnose, wadcutter, hollow point, and semiwadcutter.

Jacketed ammunition is used in semiautomatic pistols to prevent lead deposits on the ramp and in the chamber leading to gun jams. Jacketed bullets have a lead or steel core covered by an outside jacket of gilding metal (copper and zinc), gilding metal-clad steel, cupro-nickel, or aluminum. The jacketed bullet may have a full metal jacket or partial metal jacket. Partial metal jacket bullets have the metal jacket open at the tip of the bullet, exposing the lead core. These bullets can be further classified as soft point and hollow point. Semijacketed hollow point bullets have a cavity in the tip of the bullet.

Bullets can often be recovered from victims when they present to the ED. Bullets may fall out of wounds or be encountered at the time of surgery or wound exploration. The forensic importance of bullets cannot be stressed enough. Bullets should be removed using a gloved hand or with plastic or rubber-tipped instruments so as to protect the markings on the bullet and not introduce new extraneous markings from metal instruments. Bullets should not be dropped into metal bowls or basins for the same reason.

Also, the person recovering the bullet should never use a surgical instrument to "mark" the bullet or carve their initials into it for future identification. The way to identify recovered bullets properly in the future is to have a well-documented chain of custody maintained. Bullets can be placed into a coin envelope or a padded container (such as a specimen container) to be turned over to law enforcement. It is not necessary to clean the bullet of any debris or body tissue that may adhere to it because valuable forensic trace evidence may be lost in doing so. Any other materials (clothing, paint chips, drywall, etc.) that may be found in a wound tract or body cavity should be handled in the same way.

Shotgun Ammunition

Shotgun shells contain several parts:

- The case (plastic or paper)
- A thin brass or brass-coated steel head
- A primer
- Powder
- Paper, cardboard, composition, or plastic wads
- Lead shot

The case holds the primer, powder, wad, and pellets or slug. The primer compound explodes when struck by the firing pin and ignites the powder. The powder burns and creates gas to move the wad and shot down and out of the barrel. The wad protects the shot and/or barrel and seals the gas behind the shot charge. The lead shot is usually referred to as shotgun pellets. It falls into two general categories, birdshot used to kill birds and small game, and buckshot used for larger game. The smaller the shot number, the greater the pellet diameter is. So, a No. 12 birdshot has a diameter of 0.05 inches, whereas No. 4 birdshot has a diameter 0.13 inches and weighs almost 20 times as much (11 mg versus 210 mg).

Shotgun slugs are used for deer and bear hunting. Slugs are large and weigh more than shot. Slugs also exhibit a rapid loss of velocity after firing. However, shotgun slugs can produce massive internal injuries. Some slugs may also flatten in the body or break into a few large pieces. Even if loaded with birdshot, at close range, the shotgun is the most destructive of all small firearms. The severity and lethality of a shotgun wound depend on the number of pellets entering the body, the organs struck, and the amount of tissue destruction. The pellets, slug, and wad are traditional evidence that may be recovered from a victim in the ED.

GUNSHOT WOUND CLASSIFICATION

Gunshot wounds are described as perforating or penetrating. Penetrating wounds occur when the bullet enters the body but does not exit. In perforating wounds, the bullet passes completely through the object. There are four categories of wounds: contact, near-contact, intermediate, and distant (see Figure 12-4).

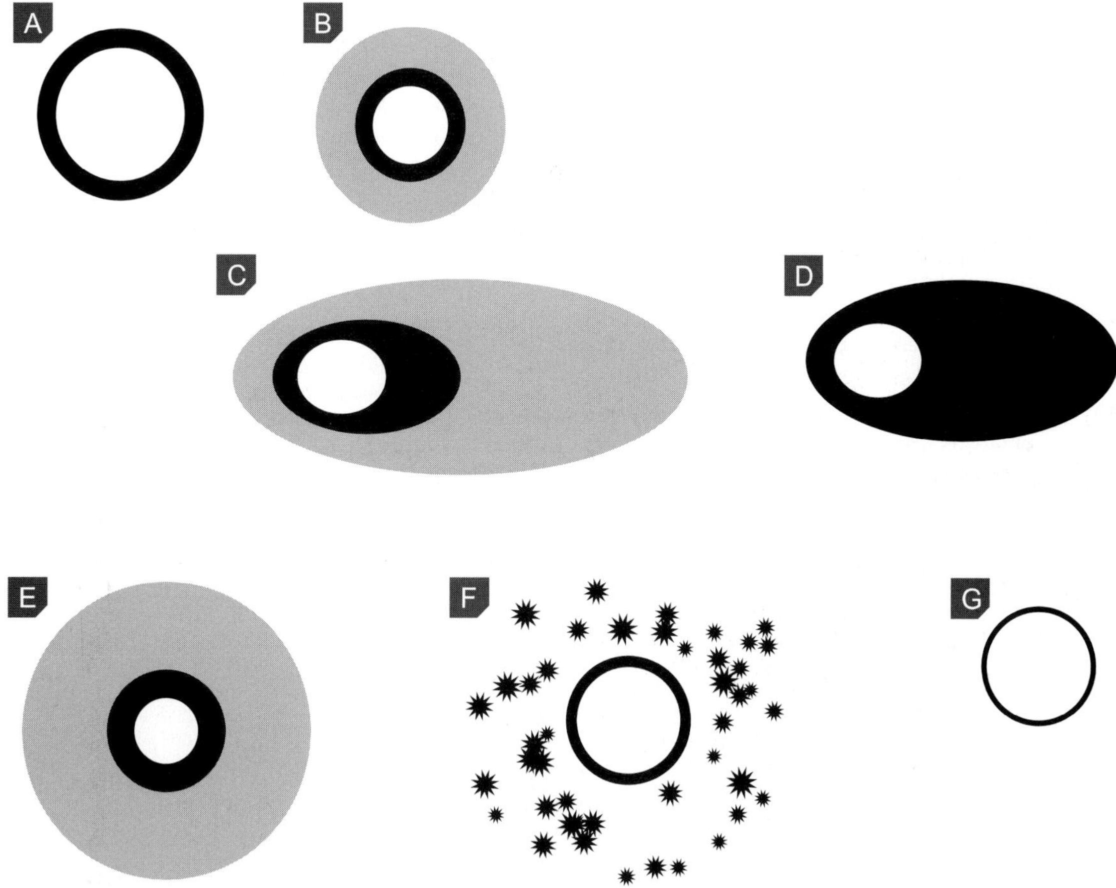

FIGURE 12-4 **Characteristics of gunshot wounds: (a) hard-contact wound with blackened seared margins; (b) loose-contact wound with soot deposited in a zone around the entrance; (c) angled-contact wound with seared blackened zone of skin on opposite side of wound from muzzle pointing the way the gun was directed (soot is also present); (d) incomplete-contact wound; (e) near-contact wound with a wide zone of powder soot overlying seared black skin; (f) intermediate-contact wound with powder tattooing; and (g) distant wound with only the bullet wound.**

In contact wounds, the muzzle of the weapon is held against the surface of the body when the weapon is fired. There are many other subclassifications of contact wounds. Hard-contact wounds occur when the weapon is held "hard" against the skin surface so that the skin envelops the muzzle. In these wounds, the edges of the entrance are seared by the hot gases of combustion and blackened by soot. The soot tends to be embedded in the seared skin and cannot be removed. Oftentimes, a muzzle stamp may be present. This is a patterned wound around or near the entrance wound caused by heating of the muzzle. The muzzle stamp may be characteristic for a particular weapon.

Loose-contact wounds occur when the muzzle is held against the skin lightly. Soot is deposited in a zone around the entrance wound and can be easily wiped away. Unburned grains of powder may also be deposited on the skin. If the weapon is loosely held at an angle to the skin, an angled-contact or incomplete-contact wound is made. This can result in an eccentrically arranged pattern of soot around the entrance.

Near-contact wounds are in between contact wounds and intermediate-range wounds. Their appearance overlaps between the two as well. In general, in near-contact wounds, the weapon is held a short distance from the skin. The distance is so short that the powder grains cannot disperse and mark the skin, producing tattooing. Near-contact wounds generally consist of an entrance wound surrounded by a wide zone of powder soot overlying seared, blackened skin.

Intermediate-range wounds occur when the muzzle is held away from the body but close enough that powder grains expelled from the muzzle produce powder tattooing. Thus, the hallmark feature of intermediate-range wounds is powder tattooing. Tattooing is numerous reddish-brown to orange-red punctate lesions surrounding the entrance wound.

Distant wounds are characterized by only the presence of the entrance wound and any marks made by the bullet. There is no soot, powder, or tattooing.

Knowing these characteristics of gunshot wounds is important because the appearance of the wound changes over time, mostly because of surgical intervention. Wounds should be described as precisely as possible, and whether there is any soot, tattooing, or a muzzle stamp present should be documented.

CONCLUSION

This chapter discusses firearms and the wounds they can inflict. Following are some forensic guidelines for dealing with firearm-related incidents:

1. Do not cut through bullet holes in clothing.
2. Store all clothing in paper bags.
3. Use paper bags to bag the hands of shooting victims if requested to do so by law enforcement.
4. Any recovered cartridges should be handled with gloves, placed in an evidence container, and turned over to law enforcement.
5. Any recovered bullets should be handled with gloves or plastic or rubber-tipped instruments. Bullets should never be marked or placed in a metal container.
6. It is unnecessary to remove biological tissue from bullets.
7. Cartridges and bullets should be placed in envelopes or in a gauze-lined specimen containers before they are given to the police.
8. Save and package any debris recovered from gunshot wounds or their tracks.
9. Never describe wounds as entrance or exits.
10. Never guess the caliber of the bullet by the size of the entrance wound or by the bullet size on an X-ray.
11. Maintain a well-documented chain of custody for any evidence recovered.

SUGGESTED READING

DiMaio VJM. *Gunshot Wounds: Practical Aspects of Firearms, Ballistics, and Forensic Techniques.* 2nd ed. Boca Raton, Fla: CRC Press; 1999.

Lynch VA, ed. *Forensic Nursing.* St. Louis, Mo: Elsevier Mosby; 2006.

Olshaker JS, Jackson MC, Smock WS, eds. *Forensic Emergency Medicine.* 2nd ed. Philadelphia, Pa: Lippincott Williams & Wilkins; 2007.

13 | Gunshot/Shotgun Injuries

Ronald F. Sing, DO, FACS, and J. Michael Sullivan, MD

INTRODUCTION

Annually, approximately 100,000 persons are victims of gunshot wounds in the United States. Up to one-third of these injuries result in a mortality.[1] Whether intentional (violence-related) or unintentional, the circumstances surrounding these injuries are not always clear and are not the priority of the treating physician. The forensic considerations of firearm injuries should never impede the undertaking of appropriate medical care to the victim (patient).

That being said, all firearm injuries have potential criminal implications, and all physicians involved in the care of patients can help or significantly hinder any forensic investigation. Inaccurate documentation resulting from a lack of understanding of the mechanisms of firearms and ballistics has potential to influence future criminal proceedings. Clinical experience in the treatment of gunshot wounds does not confer expertise in wound ballistics or forensic science. More than a decade ago, Collins and Lantz demonstrated that trauma specialists (trauma surgeons, emergency physicians, and neurosurgeons) err in classifying gunshot wounds (classifying wounds as entrance or exit wounds) more than 50% of the time![2]

The greatest contribution clinical physicians can make to a forensic investigation is clear and objective documentation. This is most pronounced when, during the course of evaluation/treatment, wounds and injuries are altered, such as when wounds are debrided. It is the objective of this chapter to provide a fundamental understanding of the mechanisms of firearm injuries and their forensic considerations. Important concepts to be discussed include internal ballistics, external ballistics, and terminal ballistics (see Table 13-1). Simply, these terms refer to the behavior of the bullet in the gun barrel, in flight, and in the target, respectively.

TABLE 13-1 **Terminology**

Internal Ballistics:	what happens to the bullet within the gun
External Ballistics:	what happens to the bullet during its flight
Terminal Ballistics:	what happens when the bullet strikes the target

INTERNAL BALLISTICS

The bullet is propelled down the gun barrel by the rapid expansion of gases caused by the burning (explosion) of the propellant (gunpowder). As the bullet leaves the barrel, these gases continue to expand, expelling flame and many burning and burned particles of gunpowder as well as material derived from the gun barrel and bullet itself. This cloud of material is called gunshot residue. This residue not only exits the end of the gun barrel but also is expelled through the small spaces between the cylinder and the gun barrel (revolvers) and the slide of pistols as the empty cartridge is ejected (see Figure 13-1).

The forensic consideration of internal ballistics is twofold: (1) the residue of the burned gunpowder is deposited onto the hand of the shooter (unless wearing gloves), and (2) the particles and gases that follow the bullet out of the barrel travel only a few feet. They can impact the target (victim) and leave characteristic marks on the target if the shot occurs within a short distance (see the sections titled "Terminal Ballistics" and "Morphology of Gunshot Wounds" later in this chapter).

Gunshot residue on the hands can be rapidly identified by crime scene investigation officers using commercially available gunshot residue analysis kits. Because it dissipates quickly in the first hour after a shot or shots were fired, gunshot residue can be indiscernible within several hours. By avoiding direct contact with the hands of a victim, officers can avoid potential contamination. In addition, placing paper bags (plastic bags tend to increase sweating and runoff of residue) over the hands can increase the time in which residue can be detected. This may not be feasible in a critically injured patient who requires intravenous access (hands) and rapid transport to the operating room. To reiterate, it is the physician's responsibility to treat the patient, not perform a forensic investigation to determine whether a close-range gunshot wound to the head is self-inflicted. However, the physician can assist in this investigation by not interfering with evidence if at all possible.

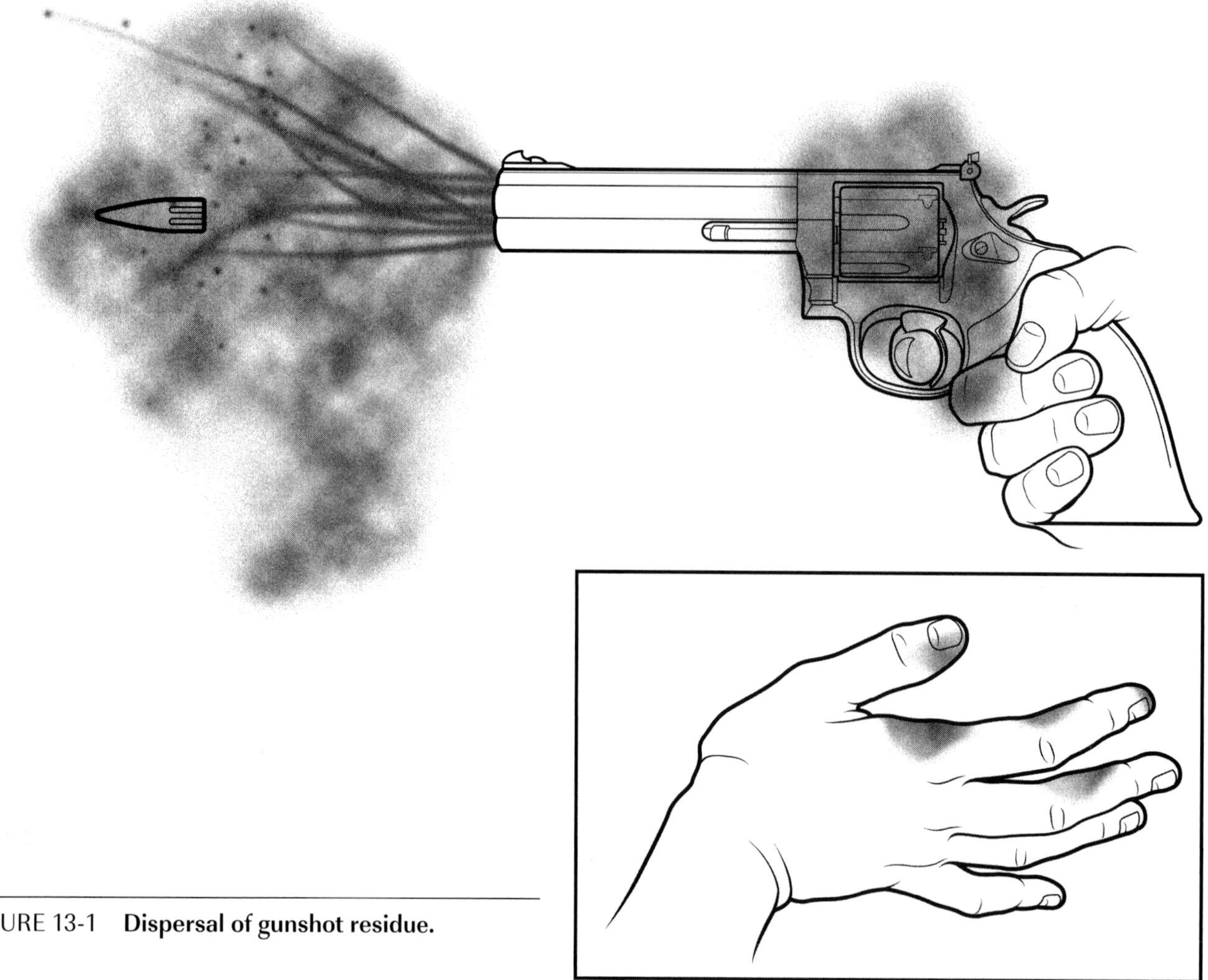

FIGURE 13-1 **Dispersal of gunshot residue.**

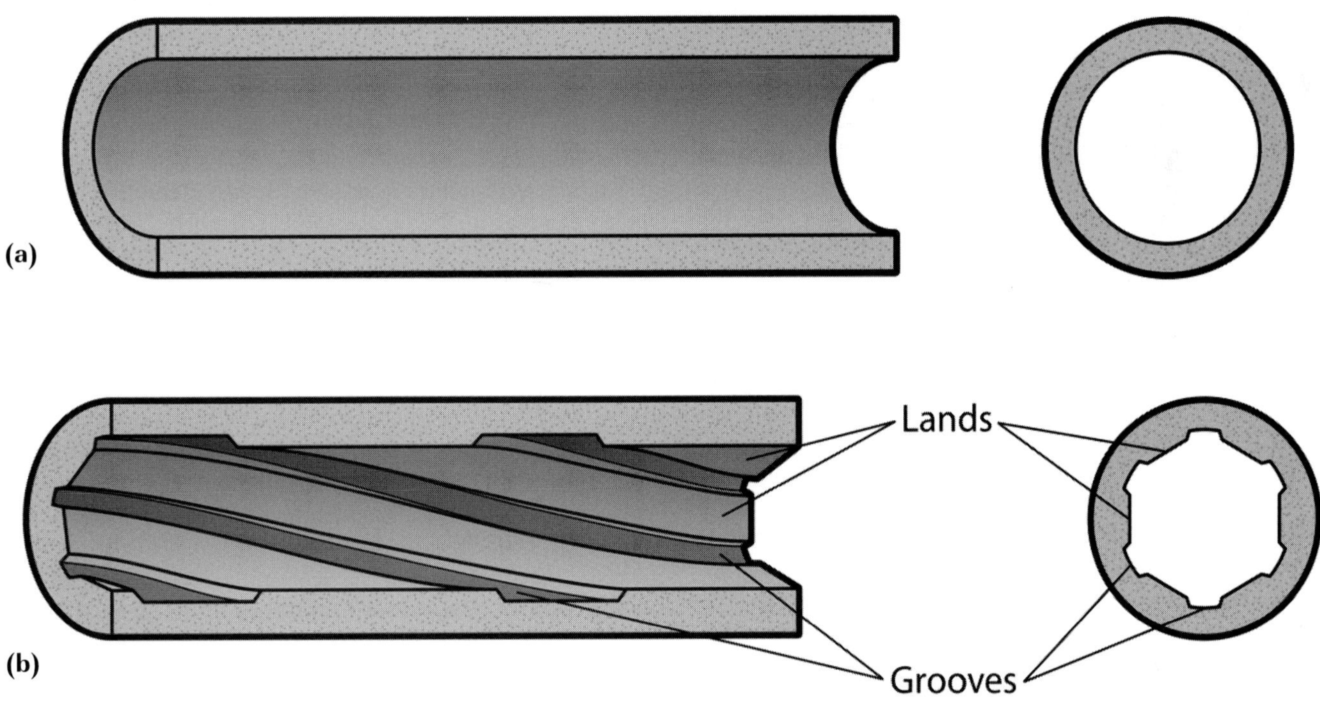

FIGURE 13-2 **(a) Smooth bore and (b) rifled gun barrels.**

As the bullet travels down the barrel, it comes in contact with twisting grooves of the gun barrel. These grooves are called rifling and cause the bullet to spin, which greatly increases the stability of the bullet as it travels through the air. The nongrooved areas of the barrel are called lands. Few modern firearms (with the exception of shotguns) are without rifling grooves (see Figure 13-2). This rifling imparts grooves on the bullet called toolmarks. Unless these grooves are deformed or obliterated from ricochet or the bullet striking the target (e.g., bone), these grooves are unique to the particular weapon that fired the bullet. The grooves have forensic importance because they are useful in determining that a bullet was fired from a particular weapon by comparing the toolmarks of a different bullet fired from the same weapon (see Figure 13-3).

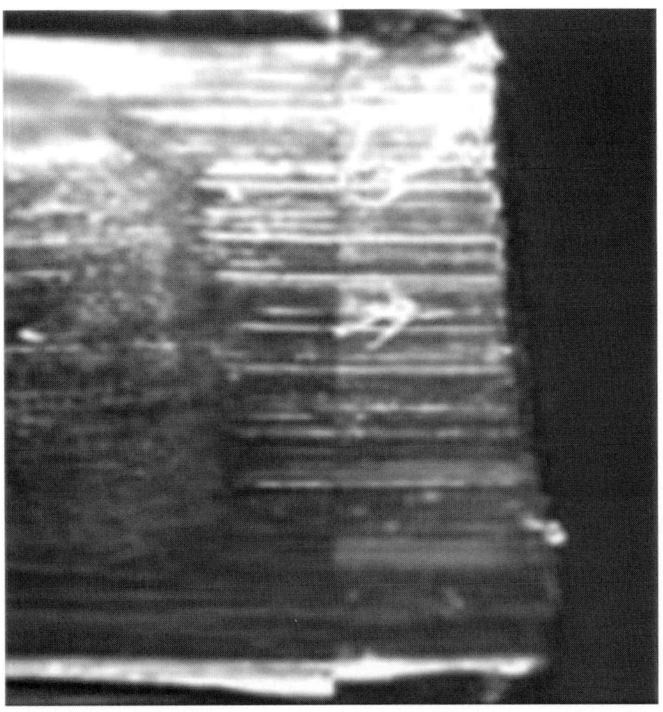

FIGURE 13-3 **Toolmark comparison.**

When removing bullets from patients, physicians can alter these grooves by forcibly grasping or manipulating the bullets with metallic instruments such as forceps and hemostats. Plastic forceps are useful but not always available to the clinician. Rubber shods can be easily made by cutting sections of a red rubber catheter to cover the ends of a hemostat or Kelly clamp (see Figure 13-4). Once the bullet is removed, it is important not to wash the bullet, but to place it into a plastic specimen container. Washing the bullet can remove particulate matter that may be useful in a criminal investigation. For example, paint or plaster from drywall may be imbedded in the bullet if the bullet passed through a wall prior to striking the victim. A chain of custody of the bullet must be maintained. The chain of custody is a form signed by each person who takes possession of the bullet until it is delivered to the police or crime scene detective (see Figure 13-5).

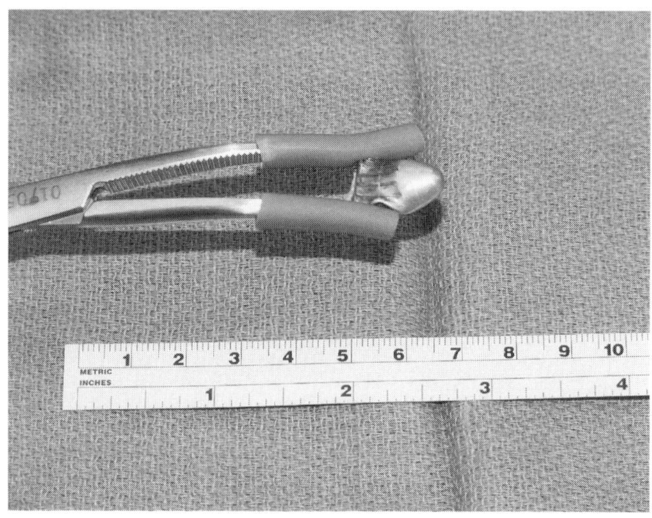

FIGURE 13-4 **(*above*) Rubber-shodded hemostat used to extract a bullet from a patient. See Color Plate 7.**

Confusion frequently arises as to which jurisdiction (sheriff or police department) is ultimately responsible for the bullet. The jurisdiction responsible is usually county specific to where the incident occurred, not where the patient is eventually treated. It is not unusual for a gunshot victim to be taken to a trauma center in another county. Specimens may be temporarily stored in a lockbox with the last medical personnel in the chain of custody maintaining control of the key.

EXTERNAL BALLISTICS

Misconceptions regarding wounding potential (terminal ballistics) come from incorrect theories regarding the physics of external ballistics. It is a commonly held belief that the kinetic energy (KE) of a bullet ($KE = \frac{1}{2}\text{ mass} \times \text{velocity}^2$) is the primary influence on the wounding potential of bullets. Whereas doubling the mass of a bullet doubles the KE, doubling the velocity of a bullet quadruples the KE. The concept is that this energy is released into the tissues causing "significant damage" beyond the diameter of the bullet. This has led to the use of the term *high velocity* (arbitrarily defined

FIGURE 13-5 **(*below*) Chain of custody form.**

[PATIENT LABEL]

CHAIN OF CUSTODY

All items listed are labeled and sealed

Name: ______________________________

To: ______________________________ Title/Badge # ______________

Date: ____________ Time: ____________

Signature: ______________________ / ______________________

Name: ______________________________

To: ______________________________ Title/Badge # ______________

Date: ____________ Time: ____________

Signature: ______________________ / ______________________

Name: ______________________

To: ______________________________ Title/Badge # ______________

Date: ____________ Time: ____________

Signature: ______________________ / ______________________

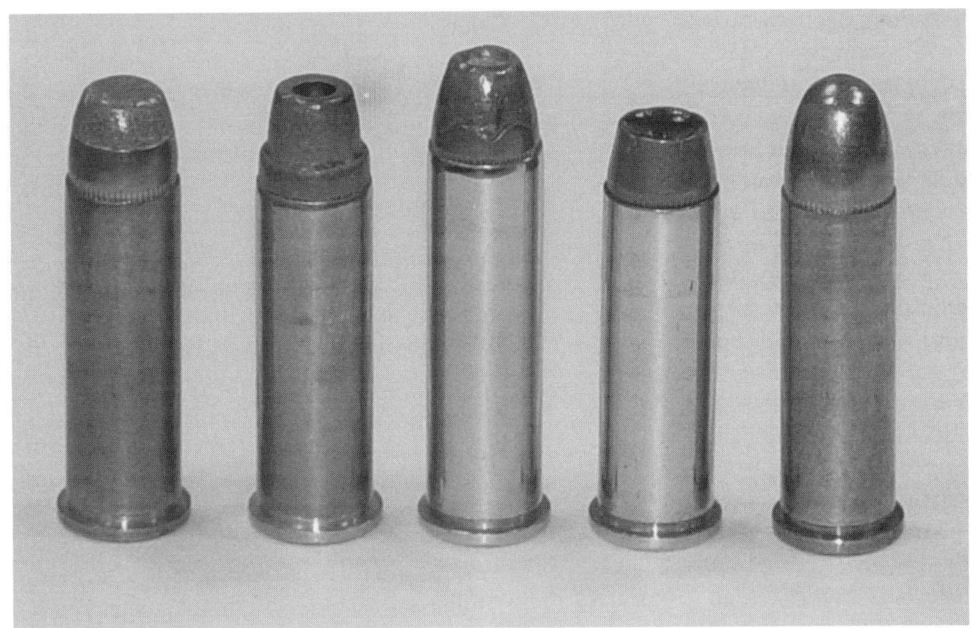

FIGURE 13-6 **Bullet designs: (*left to right*) partially jacketed wadcutter, unjacketed hollow point, partially jacketed hollow point, frangible round, full metal jacket.**

as greater than 2,000 feet per second) as creating "devastating" wounds. High-velocity weapons are characteristically long guns (rifles), whereas most handguns are considered low velocity.

For example, a standard 115-grain 9-mm handgun bullet travels at 360 meters per second resulting in 484 joules of energy. The much smaller 60-grain 5.56-mm NATO round (fired by the M-16 military rifle) travels at 800 meters per second and results in 1,700 joules of energy. Wounding and the wounding potential of bullets, however, are multifactorial and involve aspects of internal, external, and terminal ballistics. A physician description of a wound being caused by a high-velocity weapon can easily be erroneous. The forensic issues relevant to clinical physicians should be focused on describing the morphology of the wounds and injuries.

TERMINAL BALLISTICS

Several factors affect the wounding potential of bullets; kinetic energy is one factor. Additional factors are the type of bullet, its physical properties, its actions within the target, and finally, the type of tissue the bullet encounters. There are four basic bullet designs with many varieties of modifications: the full metal jacket (FMJ), the hollow point, wadcutters, and frangible bullets (see Figure 13-6). The characteristics of the bullet's design can predispose it to change its orientation, deform, or fragment.

The full metal jacket bullet is a lead bullet fully encased in a hard metallic cover. This type of bullet maintains its shape unless it strikes hard objects such asphalt, brick, or metal. Bone deforms a FMJ bullet to a lesser extent.

Hollow point bullets can have an almost complete or partial metal jacket, with the nose of uncovered lead with the tip hollowed out. The technology behind this design causes the projectile to change its shape after it strikes the target. As the bullet strikes its victim and travels through the body, tissue is pushed into this hollowed-out space. Radial forces are imparted into the lead as the projectile travels deeper into the tissues, causing it to expand in diameter and thus causing a larger wound than its original diameter.

The wadcutter is a cylindrical projectile with a flat nose commonly used in target shooting. This shape cuts circular holes into paper targets as opposed to rips caused by more conical-shaped bullets. These bullets may or may not have a metal jacket and tend to deform significantly as they travel through tissue. The deformation of the bullet may increase its diameter, thus increasing the diameter of the wound (similar to the hollow point concept).

Frangible bullets are bullets composed of hybrid materials initially designed to reduce lead exposure at target shooting ranges. The materials used are also designed to fragment upon hitting the target, eliminating ricochet hazards. Frangible ammunition is also thought to have potential benefit in urban environments and is used by some law enforcement agencies and is marketed to the public for personal defense. Some of these designs actually use small lead shot covered by a thin metal jacket. As the bullet strikes the target, it fragments, releasing the small shot, that is, multiple projectiles. The proposed benefits are the decrease in the risk to bystanders from ricochets, from passing through a wall and striking a bystander (frangible bullets rapidly disintegrate or fragment), and overpenetration (bullet passing through the target and striking a bystander). By not passing through the target, all of the kinetic energy is released into the target, thus causing greater tissue damage. It has not been proven that these bullets lead to greater lethality or greater tissue destruction. By also being lighter than conventional bullets, they have higher muzzle velocities and therefore greater kinetic energy. This ammunition is 4 to 10 times as expensive as conventional ammunition. There is little experience with this type of ammunition in civilian gunshot incidents.

Yaw can greatly affect the wounding potential of a bullet. Yaw refers to rotation of the bullet about a vertical axis. As a bullet turns sideways within tissue, its cross-sectional area is greatly increased, causing greater drag and thus cavitation. The depth at which the yaw occurs has great influence on the extent of tissue damage that occurs. For example, the notorious AK-47 military bullet (7.62 × 39 mm) is more stable in tissue than other military bullets are and commonly causes no greater wounds than common handgun bullets of much less KE, especially through muscle.[3] However, any deflection of the bullet can cause it to yaw quickly, thus causing more drag within the tissues and causing greatly increased cavitation (compared with slower handgun bullets) and tissue damage.

Different tissues vary in their response to gunshot wounds. Skin, muscle, lung, and bowel are relatively pliable and demonstrate minimal effects of the shearing forces caused by bullets as they traverse the tissue. Solid organs (liver and kidney) are less elastic and can show increased wounding beyond the permanent track of the bullet's path.[4] Bullets striking bone have the most dramatic wounding effects. Whereas a high-velocity bullet can strike through a thigh (skin and muscle) leaving a relatively minor wound, a common handgun bullet striking a femur can cause significant injury. A bullet striking the bone imparts a significant amount of its KE into the bone (rather than dissipating throughout a soft tissue track or exiting the victim). This can cause the bone and the bullet to fragment, sending secondary missiles in a variety of directions. The fragments cause their own path of tissue destruction, and the result is a much greater area of injury than the diameter of the bullet. It is easy to understand how designating whether the bullet that made a wound is high or low velocity can be confused.

A bullet's metal jacket is significantly less dense than its lead core. Partially jacketed bullets can separate (jacket from the lead) as they travel through tissue, essentially resulting in two separate missiles. Partial jackets frequently separate when striking bone (see Figure 13-7). For example, tangential gunshot wounds to the head can leave two separate wounds and can easily be misinterpreted as occurring from two separate gunshots. As the bullet strikes the skull, the impact separates the bullet from the jacket. Because the lead has greater density and mass as it travels into the skull, the lesser mass of the metal jacket is deflected off the skull and exits the scalp, creating the second wound.

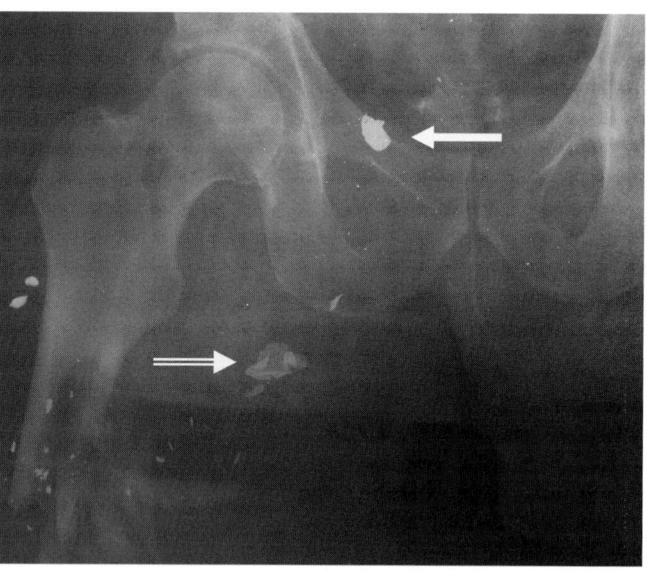

FIGURE 13-7 **Bullet separated from metal jacket. Lead bullet (solid arrow), metal jacket (hollow arrow).**

MORPHOLOGY OF GUNSHOT WOUNDS

Several factors can affect the appearance of gunshot wounds. As stated previously, the morphologic description of gunshot wounds can be the most important contribution of the clinical physician to a forensic investigation. Although there are some distinguishing characteristics of entrance wounds and exit wounds, they are not always clear-cut; therefore, describing wounds as *entrance* or *exit* should be avoided.

Straight-on entrance wounds can have a circular ring (marginal or annular abrasion ring) caused by abrasion of the skin as the bullet stretches the skin as it strikes (Figure 13-8). This ring may be overlaid by a gray ring from soot and/or lubricant that was present on the bullet and deposited on the skin as the bullet passed through the skin. Oblique entry leads to an elliptical wound and often has eccentric marginal abrasion. Exit wound morphology is extremely variable and is dependent on the shape and orientation of the bullet as it exits the skin. A wound from a yawed bullet or an expanded hollow point can appear jagged on the edges or stellate (Figure 13-9), whereas a full metal jacket bullet can have a slit-like exit wound (Figure 13-10).

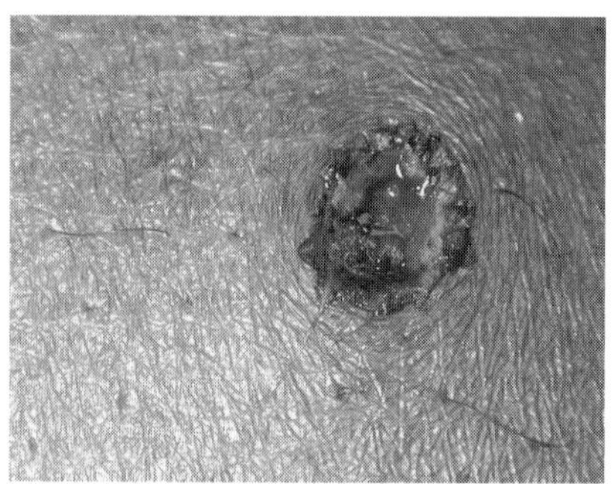

FIGURE 13-8 **Entrance gunshot wound with annular abrasion ring. See Color Plate 8.**

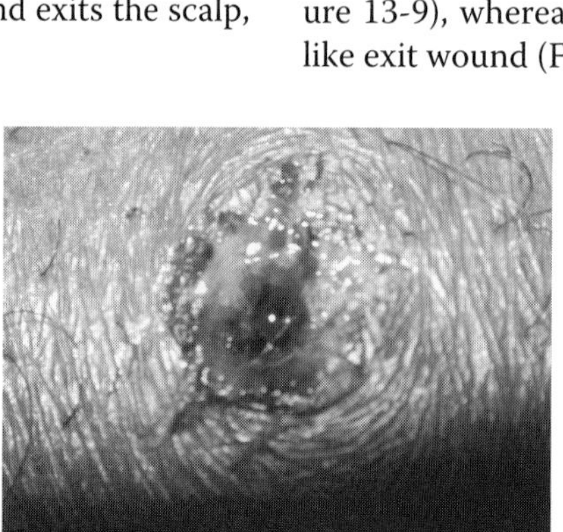

FIGURE 13-9 **Gunshot wound with jagged edges. See Color Plate 9.**

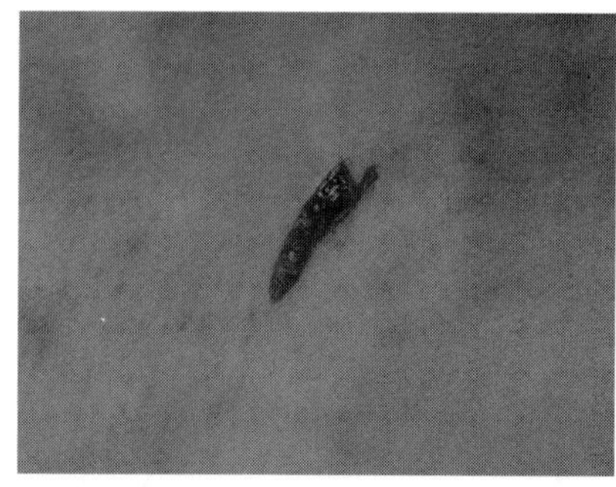

FIGURE 13-10 **Gunshot wound with slit-like exit. See Color Plate 10.**

The distance of the weapon from the victim *can* greatly affect the morphology of a gunshot wound (Figure 13-11). If the gun is in contact with the victim, the weapon might actually leave an imprint of the barrel on the victim, which is called a contact wound. In contact wounds of the head (or very close range gunshots), gas propellant combustion will enter subcutaneous tissue and cause expansion and tearing of the skin and subcutis, resulting in a stellate wound. These wounds are commonly misclassified as exit wounds. Wounds occurring from up to several feet away may show tattooing of the skin from gunshot powder particles being expelled from the barrel (Figure 13-12). Because of the low mass of the gunshot powder particles, they rapidly dissipate after just a few feet. After this distance is passed, the wounds are a result of the bullet itself. It is important to note that clothing will easily stop gunshot residue unless the weapon is in direct contact with the victim; therefore, a close-range wound through clothes will have the same appearance as a wound made from greater distances. Thus, the clothes themselves have forensic importance.

As part of the primary survey of Advanced Trauma Life Support,[5] the *E* for exposure involves rapidly removing the clothes of the victim to allow for a total body physical examination. In many situations, this involves cutting the clothes off the patient. If possible, the medical staff should try to avoid cutting directly through gunshot holes or even near holes. This may be difficult to impossible in the heat of the moment with unstable patients. However, short-range gunshots leave residue, and the blast from near-contact shots can char and even melt small areas of synthetic materials such as polyester. Clothes removed from victims should be handled as little as possible so as to preserve any evidence. Optimally, the clothes should be laid on a flat surface and folded or rolled with a layer of paper or plastic to avoid cross-contaminating one area of clothes with another. It is important for the nursing and ancillary staff of the emergency department, operating rooms, and other departments of the hospital to have a basic understanding of evidence collection and the chain of evidence.

The radiologic observations regarding bullets should also be described objectively. The caliber of a bullet seen on X-ray is easily over- or underestimated as a result of the magnification artifact inherent in plain film X-rays. Fortunately, X-rays are hard-copy evidence and easily rebuked by forensic experts if misinterpreted by clinical physicians. Mark gunshot wounds with paper clips prior to diagnostic X-rays. Using electrocardiogram leads should be discouraged because they can appear as bullets themselves. It has been our practice to place closed paper clips on anterior wounds and open paper clips on posterior wounds. This is clinically helpful in determining bullet trajectories. Bullets travel in predictable trajectories, mostly straight, unless deflected by bone. Slower-moving bullets can travel curvilinear along tissue planes, but bullets do not bounce around. Confusion often occurs during laparotomy when the internal injuries may not be in line with the bullet trajectories. It is important to realize that the orientation of internal organs may shift somewhat depending on the position of the patient when shot compared with the patient's position when examined or operated on; for example, a patient may be shot in a standing position but operated on in a supine position.

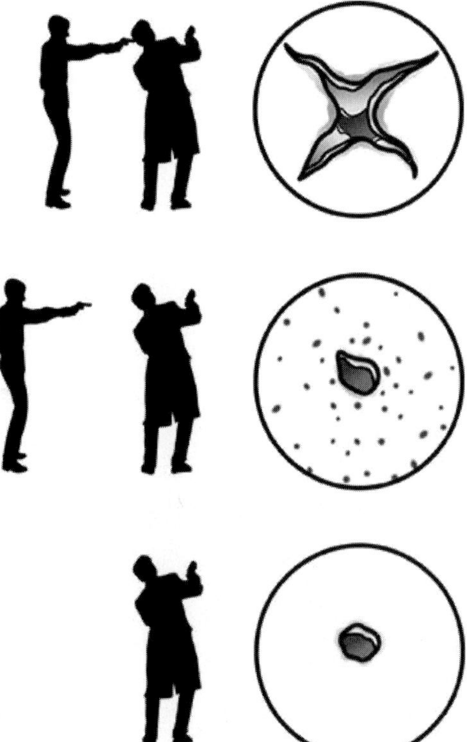

FIGURE 13-11 (*left*) Potential effect of the distance of the shooter from the victim in gunshot wounds.

FIGURE 13-12 (*below*) Tattooing caused by close-range gunshot wound. See Color Plate 11.

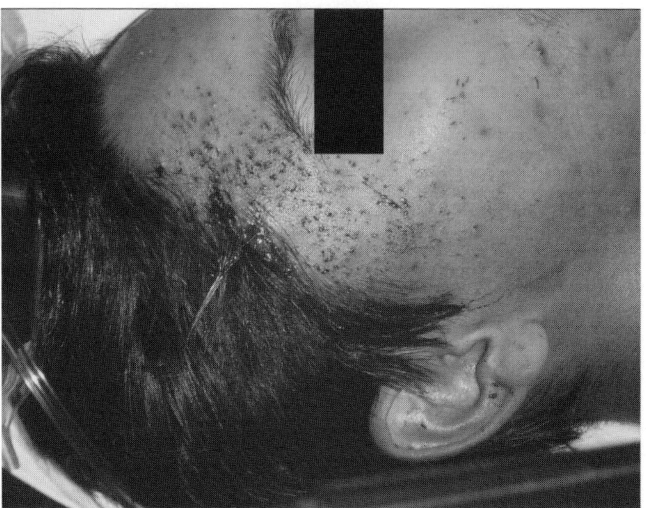

SHOTGUN WOUNDS

Shotguns are prevalent worldwide and are legal in many countries that have prohibited the ownership of rifles and handguns. The severity of wounds produced by these weapons can be devastating. Ammunition for shotguns is referred to as shotgun shells or, when there is a single projectile, shotgun slugs. The nomenclature for both the barrel size of the weapon (defined as *gauge* rather than *caliber*) and the projectiles (*shot*, defined by size and weight) is archaic. A 12-gauge shotgun was originally defined as the barrel size required to fit a 1/12-lb round ball of lead, 20-gauge is a 1/20-lb ball of lead, and so forth. Shot is essentially pellets of varying sizes further categorized as birdshot or buckshot. Birdshot pellet size is indicated by a number ranging from 12 (0.05 in) to 2 (0.15 in). The amount of shot contained in a shotgun shell is determined by the gauge (size) of the gun. Buckshot ranges from 000 or "triple aught" (0.36 in) to number 4 (0.24 in) projectiles.[6] A 12-gauge shotgun shooting 000 buckshot (6 pellets per shotgun shell) essentially shoots six .38 caliber bullets at once.

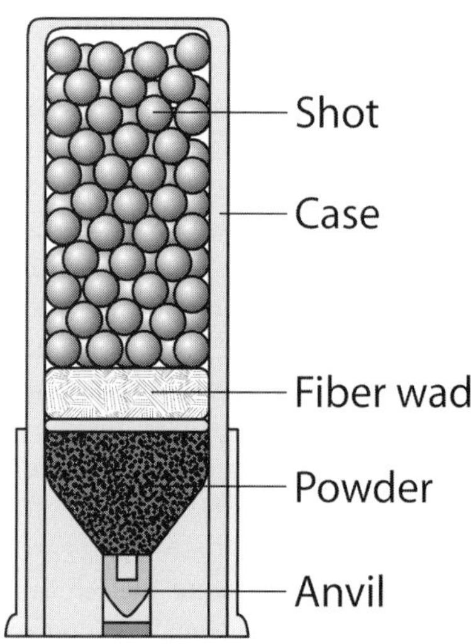

FIGURE 13-13 **Shotgun shell.**

Shotgun shells consist of a casing (usually plastic) to house the projectiles (shot or slug).[6] (See Figure 13-13.) The projectiles are separated from the gunpowder by a wad or wadding, which pushes the projectiles out en masse as the gunpowder explodes, also protecting the shot from deformation as it travels down the gun barrel. The wad can be made of textile fiber or plastic, or the shotgun shell can have two separate wads, one being an over-powder wad (fiber) and the second encasing the shot as it travels down the barrel (plastic cup). Of low mass, the wadding is shot out the end of the gun barrel with the projectiles and can travel several feet. The wadding is commonly embedded in close-range shotgun wounds (Figure 13-14). Clinically, in addition to any accessible shot, the wadding needs to be removed as part of the surgical debridement of shotgun wounds to avoid infection from this foreign body. Forensically, the wadding can be identified to a particular brand of shotgun ammunition and should be handled like any evidence using a chain of custody form. The shotgun pellets are less specific evidence, but

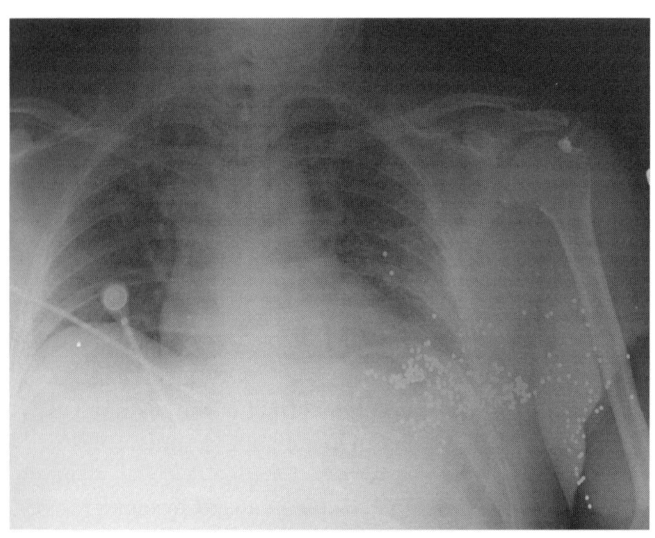

(a)

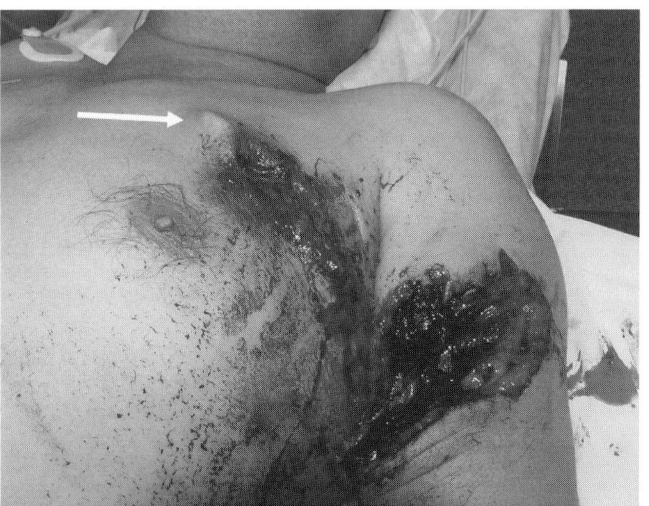

(b)

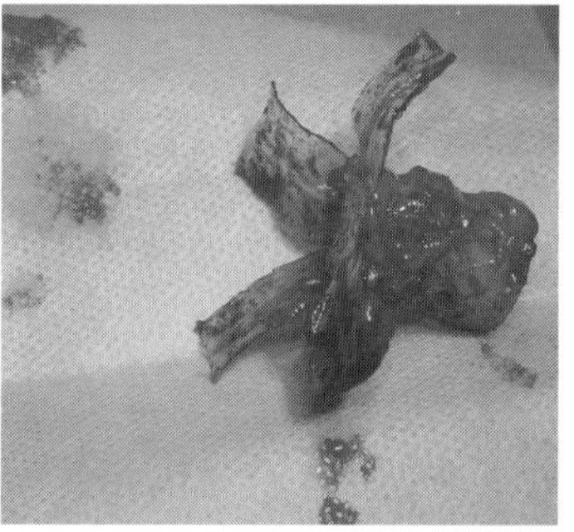

(c)

FIGURE 13-14 **Close-range shotgun wound: (a) chest X-ray demonstrating multiple birdshot pellets; (b) tissue destruction obvious (arrow points to wadding embedded in wound); (c) wadding removed from patient. See Color Plate 12 for 13-14 (b) and (c).**

much like knowing the caliber of a bullet, knowing the size of shot is helpful in a criminal investigation.

Shot is round and delivered without spin and therefore is much less stable in flight compared with bullets. The round shape leads to a rapid deceleration of the projectiles; thus, the effective range of shotguns is much less than that of handguns or rifles. Once the shot has left the gun barrel, the shot begins to disperse. The spread of shot is called the shot pattern and is variable owing to several factors: distance, gun barrel length, and choke. The farther from the gun barrel, the wider the shot disperses. Fired from longer barrels, shot maintains a straighter alignment for longer distances. A constriction device called a choke can be inserted in the end of a shotgun barrel. Different chokes and their settings can narrow or expand the shot pattern. These variables make it difficult to determine the distance of the patient from the weapon based on the shot pattern.

CONCLUSION

The clinical physician can do much to assist with a forensic investigation of gunshot wounds without losing focus on the care of a patient. The handling and collection of evidence (bullets, clothes, etc.) should not interfere with good patient care. Although the necessary treatment of the patient can alter or even destroy evidence, clear and objective documentation of wounds and injuries is not only helpful in an investigation, it is good clinical practice.

ACKNOWLEDGMENTS

The authors wish to thank Roger Thompson and Patty Lavins of the Charlotte-Mecklenburg Police Crime Laboratory, and Peter Gilchrist, the Mecklenburg County District Attorney, for their assistance in the preparation of this chapter.

REFERENCES

1. National Center for Injury Prevention and Control. WISQARS Injury Mortality Report, 2005 US Firearms Deaths and Rates. Available at: http://www.cdc.gov/ncipc/wisqars/default.htm. Accessed August 25, 2008.
2. Collins KA, Lantz PE. Interpretation of fatal, multiple, and exiting gunshot wounds by trauma specialists. *J Forensic Sci.* 1994;39:94–99.
3. Fackler ML, Malinowski JA, Hoxie SW, Jason A. Wounding effects of the AK-47 rifle used by Patrick Purdy in the Stockton, California, schoolyard shooting of January 17, 1989. *Am J Forensic Med Path.* 1990;11:185–189.
4. Fackler ML. Gunshot wound review. *Ann Emerg Med.* 1996;28:194–203.
5. American College of Surgeons Committee on Trauma. *Advanced Trauma Life Support.* 7th ed. Chicago, Ill: American College of Surgeons; 2006.
6. Ordog GJ, Wasserberger J, Balasubramaniam S. Shotgun wound ballistics. *J Trauma.* 1988;28:624–631.

14 | Mechanisms of Injury Related to Motor Vehicle Crashes

Edward T. Dickinson, MD, FACEP

INTRODUCTION

The fundamental vernacular change in the past decade from motor vehicle *accident* (MVA) to motor vehicle *crash* (MVC) represents more than mere semantics. It serves to reinforce the concept that vehicles crash for a reason, not by random chance. Speeds unsafe for conditions, failure to yield, and impairment of drivers with distractions and the effects of ethanol and other drugs are common catalysts for collisions that produce traumatic injuries related to motor vehicles.

ESSENTIAL PRINCIPLES OF PHYSICS

Several fundamental laws of physics are particularly relevant to the mechanisms of injury related to motor vehicle crashes. Foremost among these physical realities is that energy cannot be destroyed. Thus, the energy of a vehicle traveling at 70 miles per hour that suddenly comes to a stop as it strikes an immovable 100-year-old oak tree does not simply dissipate into thin air. Rather, the energy is transferred back through the vehicle, resulting in vehicular deformity and occupant injury as the energy passes through the vehicle and its occupant. It is also critical to understand that the magnitude of energy involved in MVCs is a result of both the speed and the mass of the vehicle(s). However, because energy is equal to 1/2 mass × velocity^2, it is the speed at which an object is traveling that is far more important than its mass.

Of equal relevance is Newton's first law of physics, which states that an object in motion will remain in motion traveling in a straight line until acted upon by an outside force, and an object at rest will remain at rest. In the setting of an MVC, this law explains the reality that fixed objects (such as a bridge abutment) usually "win" in collisions and cars traveling at high speeds often exhibit remarkable aerobatics after impact before ultimately coming to a rest.

MECHANISMS OF INJURY AS A TRIAGE TOOL

Mechanisms of injury are widely used as a component of prehospital triage of trauma for the victims of motor vehicle crashes. The list of mechanisms of injury established by the American College of Surgeons (ACS) Committee on Trauma forms the basis for most trauma triage protocols encountered in both prehospital and hospital-based emergency care (see Table 14-1).[1]

In general, mechanism of injury (MOI) must be linked with anatomic and physiologic criteria to have value as a trauma triage predictor of serious injury.[2–4] In one study, however, Esposito identified prolonged prehospital time, death of another occupant in the same vehicle, and a pedestrian being struck at greater than 20 mph (32 km/hr) as "high yield" for identifying major trauma victims, even when used as a single criterion.[3] The remainder of the ACS's MOIs listed are in fact anecdotal, but based on clinical experience and the sound premise that the greater the energy involved in a trauma, the greater propensity for serious injury.

VEHICLE RESTRAINT AND SAFETY SYSTEMS

Crash data clearly demonstrate that vehicle restraint and safety systems, specifically seat belts and airbags, are responsible for a profound reduction in the morbidity and mortality of patients involved in MVCs. The majority of the data has been generated by the insurance industry and the National Highway Traffic Safety Administration (NHTSA) of the federal Department of Transportation. Paradoxically, these vehicle restraint and safety systems themselves can result in their own specific mechanisms of injury that are side effects of their interface with crash victims.

TABLE 14-1 **American College of Surgeons Committee on Trauma: Trauma Center Triage Guidelines Based on Mechanism of Injury**

Ejection from automobile
Death in same passenger compartment
Extrication time > 20 minutes
Falls > 20 feet
Vehicle rollover
High-speed auto crash
Auto-pedestrian/auto-bicycle with significant impact
Pedestrian thrown or runover
Motorcycle crash > 20 mph

Seat belts have long been associated with a complex of injuries often referred to as the "seat belt syndrome."[5] In its classic presentation, the syndrome represents a triad of injury to the abdominal organs, the mesentery, and a Chance fracture of the upper lumbar spine (see Figure 14-1). Although this complex of injuries was originally described in the setting of lap-belt-only mechanisms (Figure 14-2), it remains a viable clinical entity in the age of integrated seat belt systems that include lap and shoulder restraints (Figure 14-3). The clinical finding of linear ecchymosis or erythema across the abdominal wall in the MVC patient demands that a meticulous evaluation for seat belt syndrome injuries be initiated.[6] Computed tomography (CT) scan of the abdomen—although the mainstay of radiologic evaluation in these patients—has historically been reported to miss both subtle visceral injuries as well as Chance-type lumbar fracture.[7]

More recent literature has found the augmentation of CT images with a lateral scout image of the spine has greatly increased the sensitivity of the CT scan for detecting seat-belt-related injuries.[8]

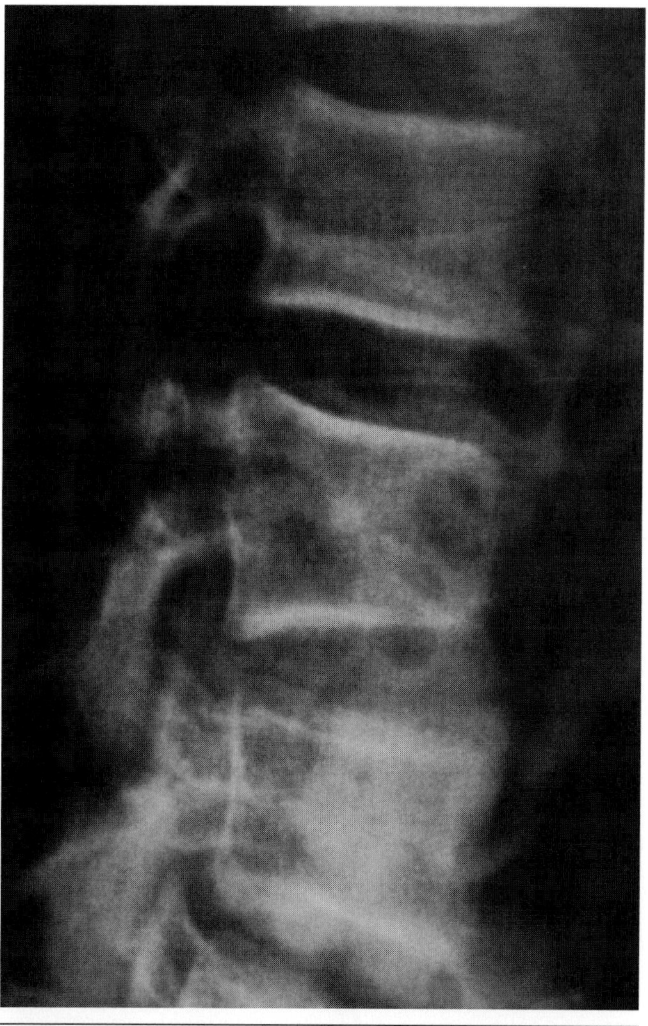

FIGURE 14-1 **Chance fracture of second lumbar vertebra resulting from lap belt injury.**

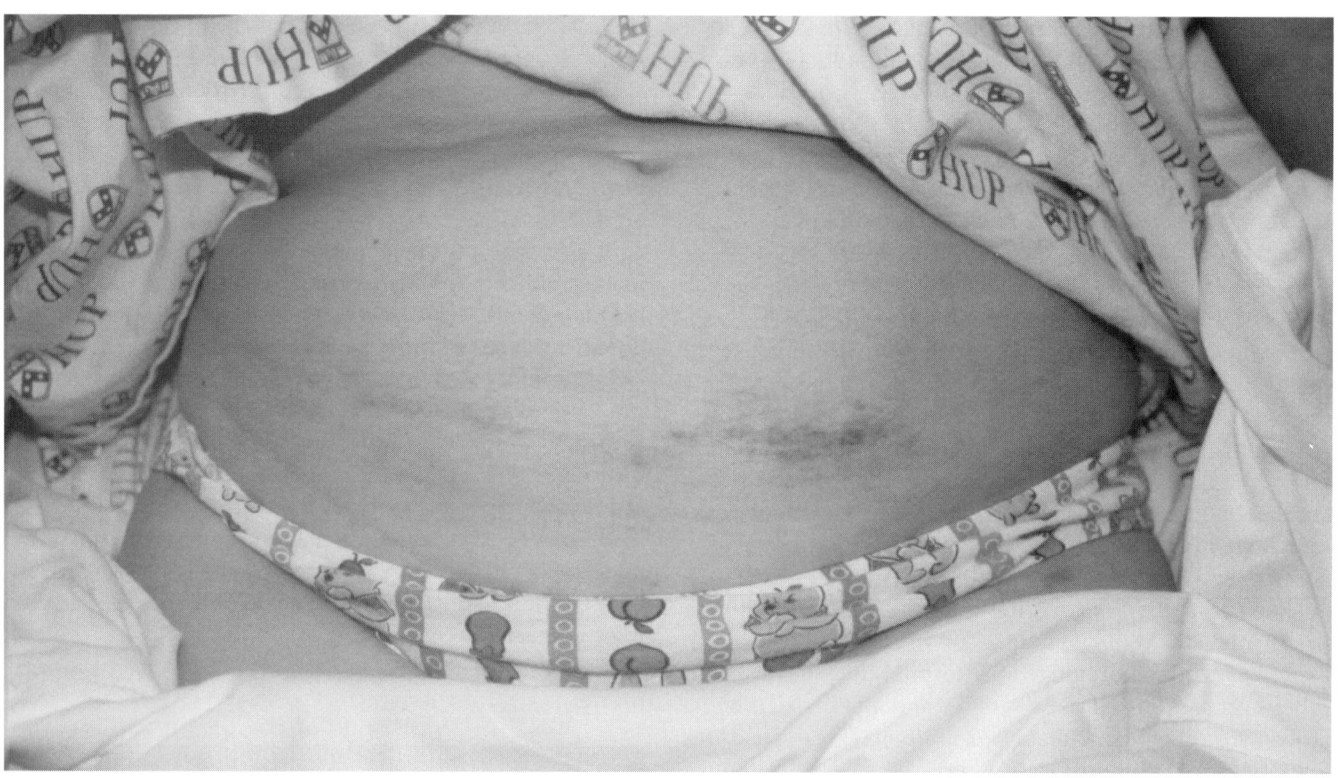

FIGURE 14-2 Abdominal linear ecchymosis resulting from lap belt injury.

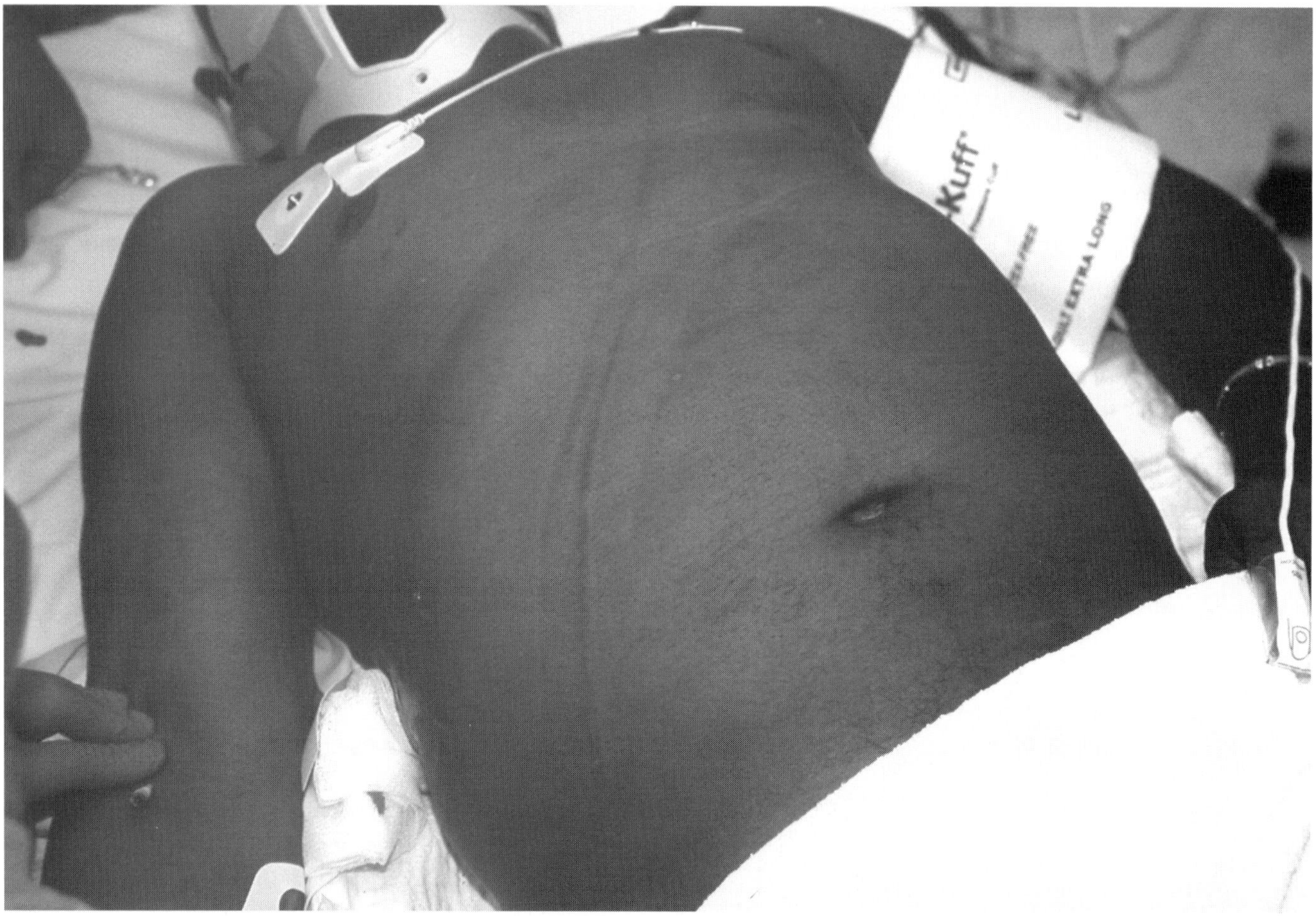

FIGURE 14-3 Abdominal and chest linear ecchymosis from driver's side combined lap and shoulder belts. See Color Plate 13.

AIRBAG-RELATED INJURIES

In 1998, NHTSA estimated that the inclusion of dual frontal airbags in all cars and light trucks, along with two-thirds of the population using seat belts, would result in approximately 3,000 lives being saved per year. Since 1991, the Special Crash Investigation (SCI) program at NHTSA has tracked airbag-related fatalities in MVCs. In the last decade, SCI has expanded its surveillance to include life-threatening injuries that are the result of airbag deployments. As of 2003, the SCI has accumulated a total of 227 confirmed cases where deployment of the driver or passenger side airbag resulted in a fatal injury to an occupant in a minor-to-moderate severity crash.[9] Sixty-one percent (141) of the fatalities were children, of whom 119 were not in rear-facing child safety seats (RFCSSs) and 22 were infants in RFCSSs. The high incidents of pediatric fatalities, especially those that have occurred in RFCSSs, resulted in a national initiative to place children in the back seat of vehicles and revised NHTSA regulations that allow for deactivation of the front passenger side airbag when this is not possible.

Throughout the body of airbag-related morbidity and mortality investigation data there is one consistent theme: much of the trauma would have been avoided if proper restraints (and common sense) had been in use at the time of the crashes. Nowhere is this more evident than in the case of forward-facing child fatalities where more than 50% of the patients were unbelted and approximately 20% were seated on the laps of another passenger. Fortunately, the incidents of both pediatric- and adult-related airbag fatalities in the United States have progressively declined since the late 1990s.

FRONTAL IMPACTS

Frontal impacts (often referred to as "head-ons") are an extremely common MVC mechanism. Frontal impact is the most common mechanism in single-car crashes, which are often the result of inattentive driving or falling asleep at the wheel, which results in driving into fixed or more slowly moving objects. In addition, frontal impacts are almost always a component of multiple-vehicle crashes. For example, when a car is struck from behind or in its side, the other vehicle that struck the vehicle has in fact sustained a frontal impact as part of the crash.

The basic physics of the frontal impact crash is sudden, sequential deceleration of the vehicle and the occupant(s) (see Figure 14-4). In frontal impacts, conceptually a rapid sequential cascade of decelerations take place beginning with the exterior surface of the vehicle striking an object and rapidly decelerating to a stop, followed by the surface of the occupant's body striking the interior surface of the vehicle (dash, steering wheel, airbag, and/or seat belt), followed by the body's internal organs coming to a sudden stop. Traumatic injuries are the result of the latter two impacts. Impacts to the interior surface of the vehicle can result in either penetrating (see Figure 14-5) or blunt injuries. Sudden deceleration of the internal organs has been classically associated with transection-type injuries such as aortic disruption.[10] However, more recent data have challenged the concept that aortic transections are simply the result of deceleration forces alone.[11]

For unrestrained occupants, blunt injuries are often determined by their path of travel as the vehicle decelerates beneath them. The two generic paths are described as either "down and under" the dash (see Figure 14-6) or "up and over" (or sometimes even out by ejection) the dash (see Figure 14-7). The down and under pathway can yield injuries to the knee, femur, and the classic posterior hip dislocation (see Figure 14-8). The up and over pathway can result in abdominal injuries, blunt chest trauma from steering wheel impact, and head and neck injuries from windshield or roof impacts.

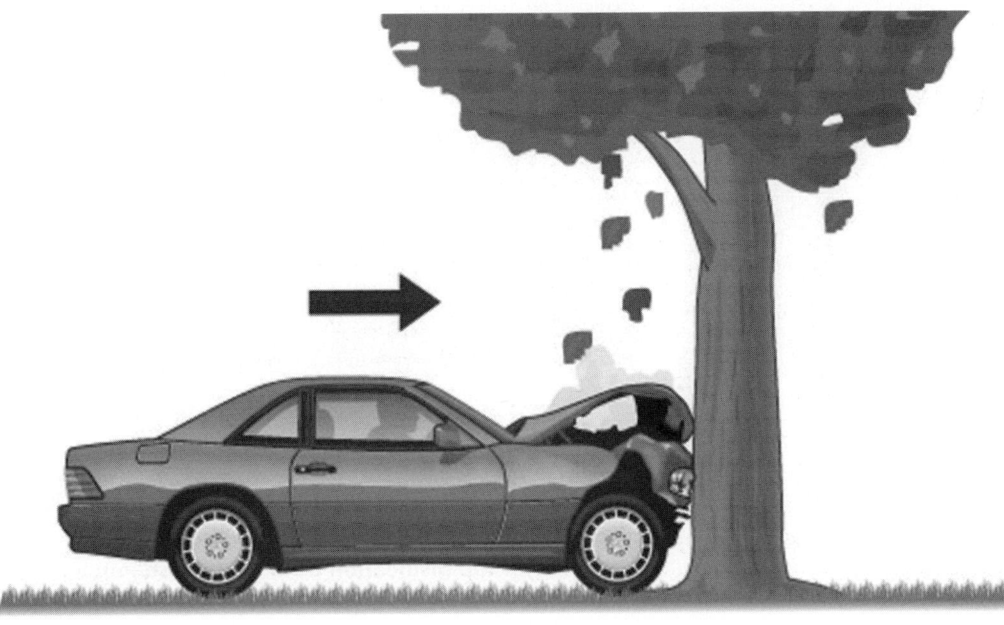

FIGURE 14-4 **Sudden deceleration in frontal impact.**

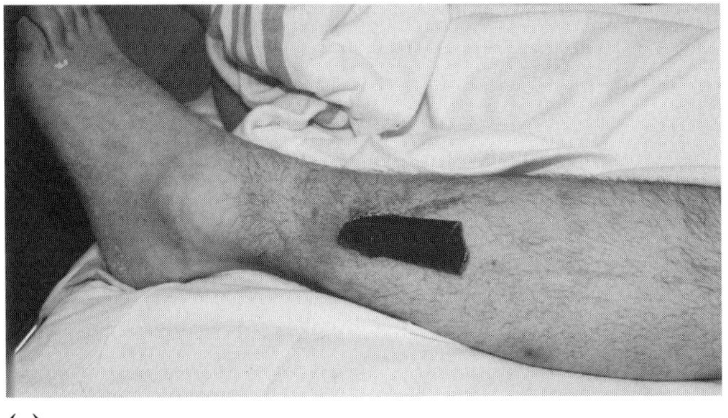

(a)

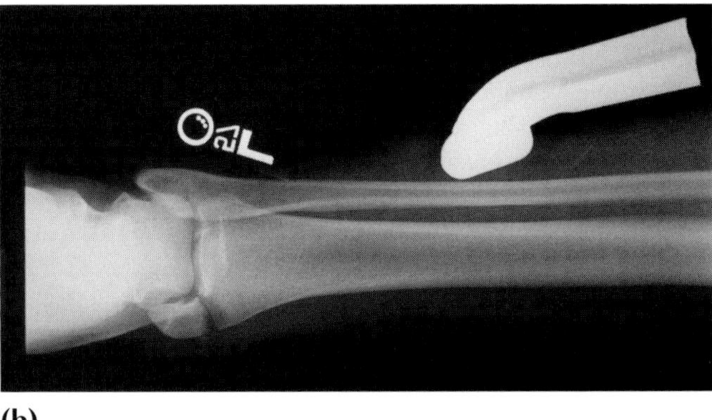

(b)

FIGURE 14-5 Penetrating injury: (a) impaled brake pedal in lower leg; (b) radiograph of impaled brake pedal. Note contralateral malleolar fracture. See Color Plate 14 for 14-5 (a).

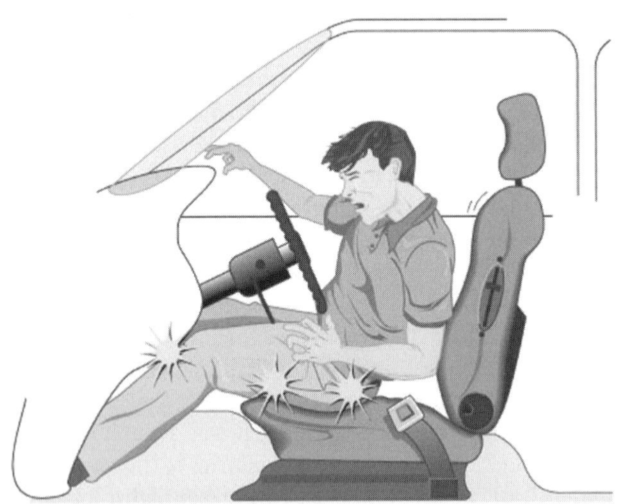

FIGURE 14-6 Down and under pathway in frontal impact.

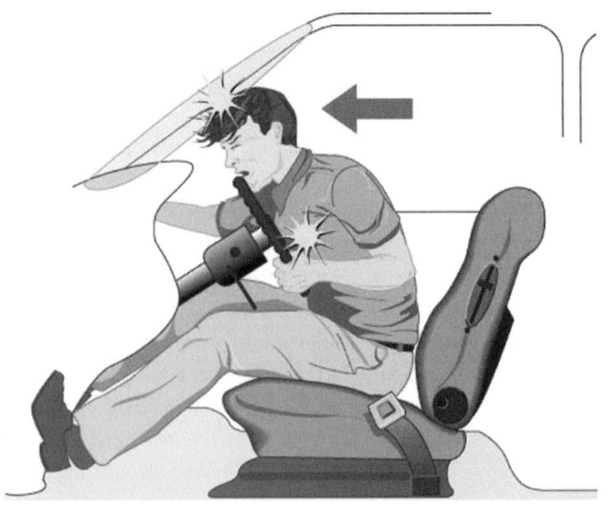

FIGURE 14-7 Up and over pathway in frontal impact.

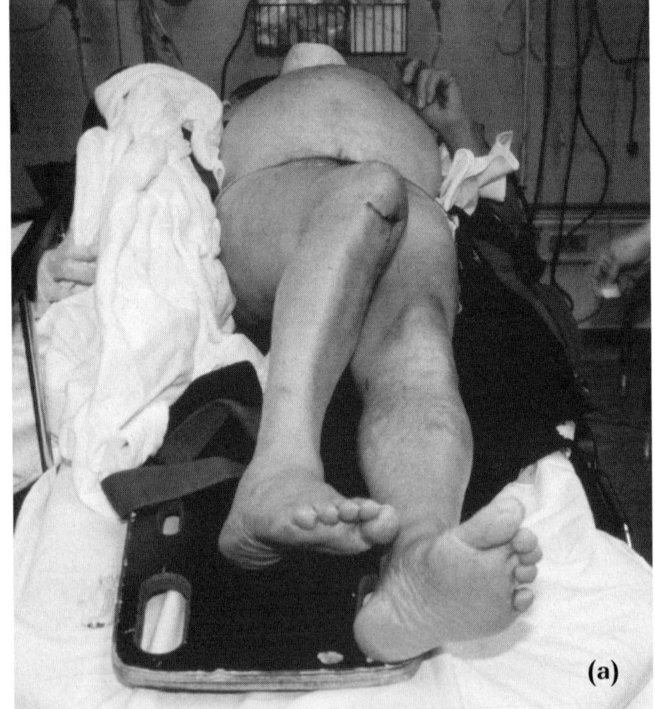

(a)

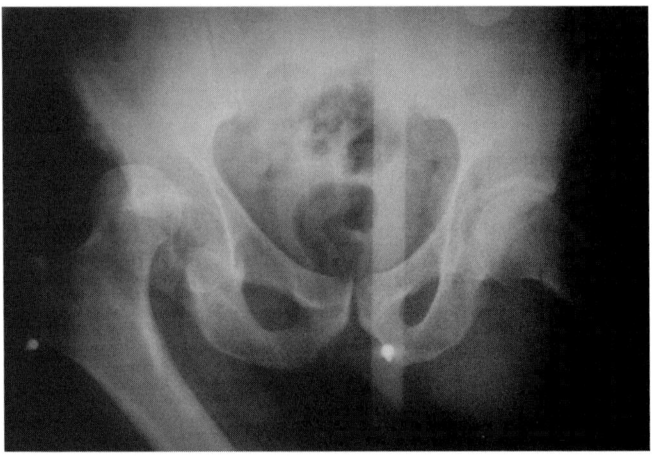

(b)

FIGURE 14-8 Results of down and under pathway: (a) posterior hip dislocation from dashboard impact (note anterior knee laceration); (b) radiograph of a left posterior hip dislocation.

REAR IMPACTS

The major physical force applied to occupants of a vehicle that is struck from behind by a faster moving vehicle is sudden acceleration of the vehicle "out from under" the occupants (Figure 14-9). The sudden acceleration commonly results in hyperextension of the patient's (or patients') cervical and lumbar spine. Vehicles struck from behind usually offer the vehicle's occupants relative safety because of the crush zone afforded by the vehicle's trunk, bed, and/or backseat. Despite this advantage, rear impact collisions can result in severe injuries. Two secondary mechanisms that can be particularly devastating in rear-end collisions are the failure of the seat to withstand the forces of the occupant being thrust backward, and the vehicle being sent forward into other impacts (sometimes called the "battering-ram" effect). Seat failure can result in ejection of the patient into the back seat or even out the rear window of the vehicle (Figure 14-10). The battering ram effect can result in severe frontal impacts (Figure 14-11).

SIDE IMPACTS

Side impact crash mechanisms are broadly divided into nearside and far-side impacts, relative to the patient's position within the car and the side of impact. Because side impacts allow for much less crush space (only the door) as compared to the larger crush spaces in frontal or rear impacts (the engine compartment and trunk, respectively), there is a high risk of injury in this mechanism, especially in nearside impacts where the only protection is the few inches of the door's width (Figure 14-12). The resultant impact displaces the torso and pelvis medially toward the center of the vehicle while the head and neck move laterally toward the outside of the vehicle as the body accelerates out beneath it (Figure 14-13).

Resultant skeletal injuries from high-energy side impacts include pelvic and rib fractures as well as neck injuries. Internal injuries from this mechanism may include bladder rupture (associated with pelvic compression), as well as splenic and liver injuries (from either direct lateral impact of the nearside door or when the front seat occupants are thrown into the center console, especially the stick shift, during far-side impacts). Horton has demonstrated that aortic transections are actually three times more common in side impact MVCs as compared to head-on collisions.[11] He found that the most common associated injury to aortic transection was rib fractures, thus hypothesizing that sudden chest compression likely results in a "water hammer" effect that when coupled with other crash forces results in the frequently fatal injury.

Because of the limited crush space afforded in side impact collisions, airbags that are activated by side impact collisions have become prevalent in motor vehicle safety design. Recent data from the Insurance Institute for Highway Safety have shown that occupants in cars with side impact airbags with head protection integration are 53% less likely to die in nearside collisions than those in cars without them.[12]

It is noteworthy that according to NHTSA data, a disproportionate number of nearside driver-side collisions occur in the elderly population when they attempt to make a left turn. Left-hand turns account for 33% of elderly crashes as compared to 11% in the younger cohort.[13]

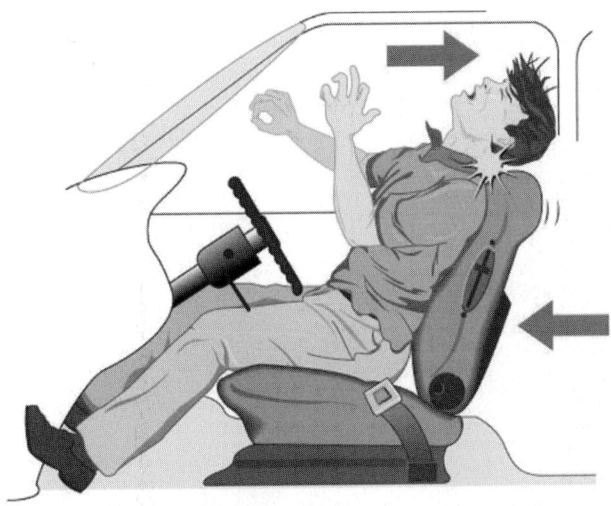

FIGURE 14-9 ***(above)*** **Sudden acceleration associated with a rear impact crash.**

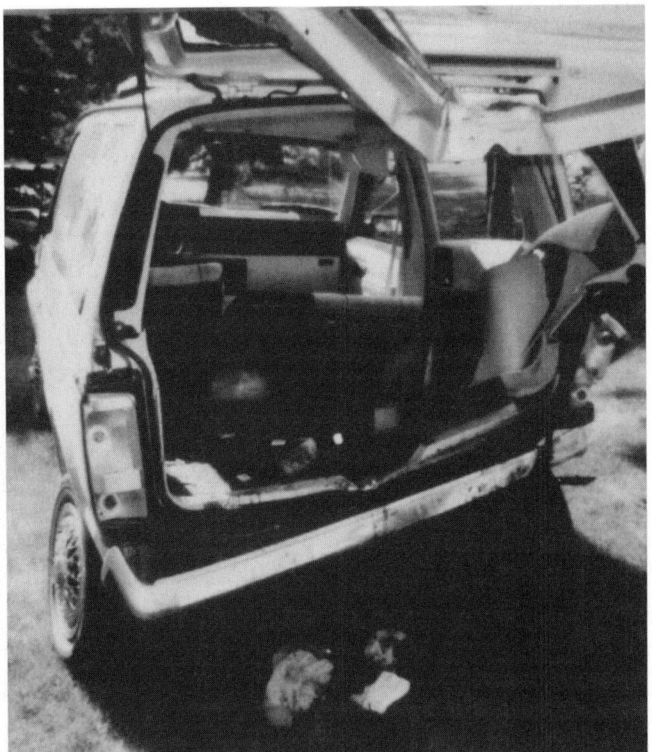

FIGURE 14-10 ***(right)*** **Seat failures in a rear impact collision resulting in ejection into the tailgate (note blood stains on bumper area from driver and passenger head impacts).**

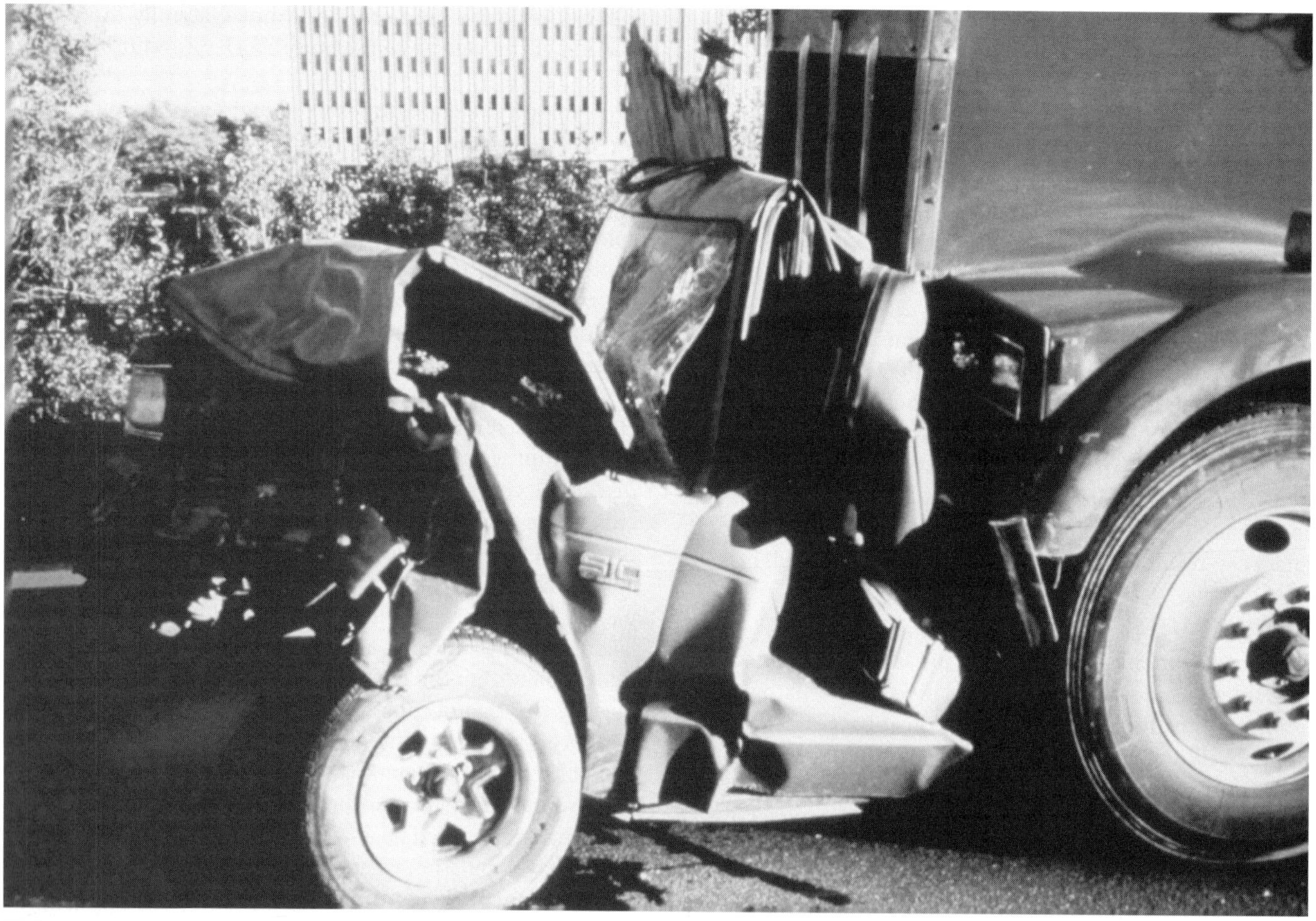

FIGURE 14-11 **Fatal battering-ram effect of a pickup truck initially rear-ended by a truck, and then propelled into multiple secondary frontal impacts.**

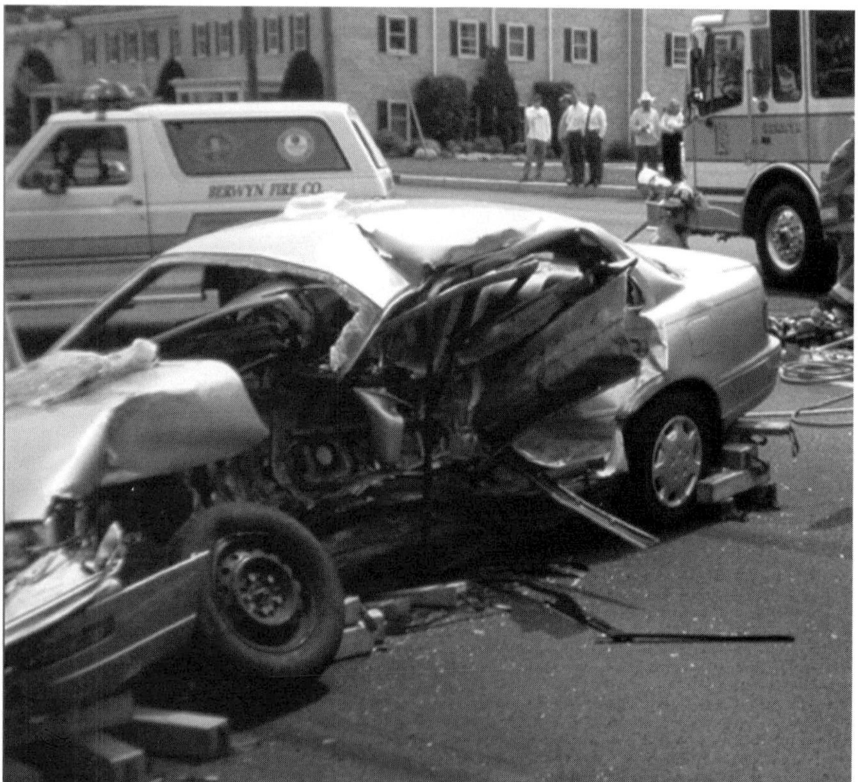

FIGURE 14-12 **(*left*) Fatal nearside impact collision.**

FIGURE 14-13 **(*below*) Nearside impact.**

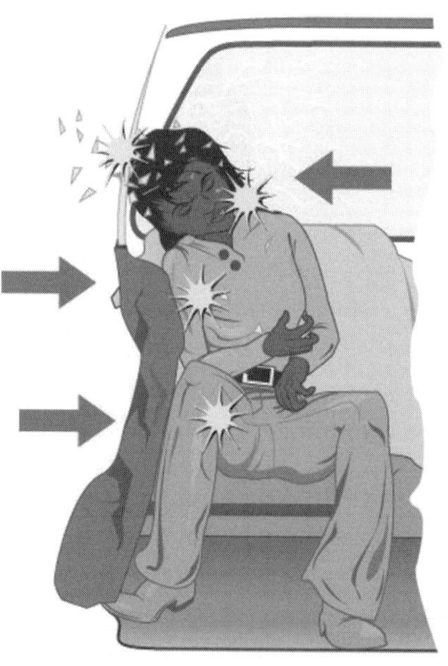

ROLLOVERS

In the United States, rollover crashes have now become the most lethal MVC mechanism of injury (Figure 14-14), closely paralleling the increased number of fatal sports utility vehicle (SUV) crashes that have more than doubled since 1990.[14] NHTSA data report almost 10,000 deaths from rollovers in 2000. Remarkably, these data demonstrate that three-quarters of the occupants killed were not wearing seat belts and two-thirds of them were completely ejected from the vehicle. Intuitively, and also based on these data, if the occupants are properly restrained by seat belts within the vehicle, the mortality of this mechanism is greatly reduced.

Some rollovers occur as the result of a vehicle rolling down an embankment or similar inclined plane. However, many rollovers are the result of sudden lateral motion of a vehicle coupled with a sudden increase in the coefficient of friction between the tires and the road surface (often the change from normal road surface to shoulder surface as a vehicle shifts) causing a lateral roll. Fast-moving sport utility vehicles, with their high center of gravity and large tires, are prime vehicles for rollovers as compared to more conventional sedans.

The morbidity and mortality of rollovers are greatly enhanced by not only ejection from the vehicle, but by protrusion of body parts in the crush/maceration zone created by the interface of the side window and the road surface. When limbs (usually the upper extremities) are exposed into this zone, amputations and near amputations with extensive tissue loss are often encountered. In Figure 14-15, note the extensive arm length loss caused by the large interface of the extremity with the pavement crush zone during vehicle rollover.

CAR VERSUS PEDESTRIAN IMPACTS

The impact of a motor vehicle and an unprotected pedestrian can produce devastating injuries. Traditionally, the impact of a car and a pedestrian produces a sequence of impacts that begins with lower extremity trauma from the bumper (Figure 14-16a) followed by hip and torso impact as the body is carried up onto the hood or windshield (Figure 14-16b). The third and final phase of this sequence is the pedestrian separating from the car and rolling to the ground where he or she could be struck by the wheels of the same or another passing car.

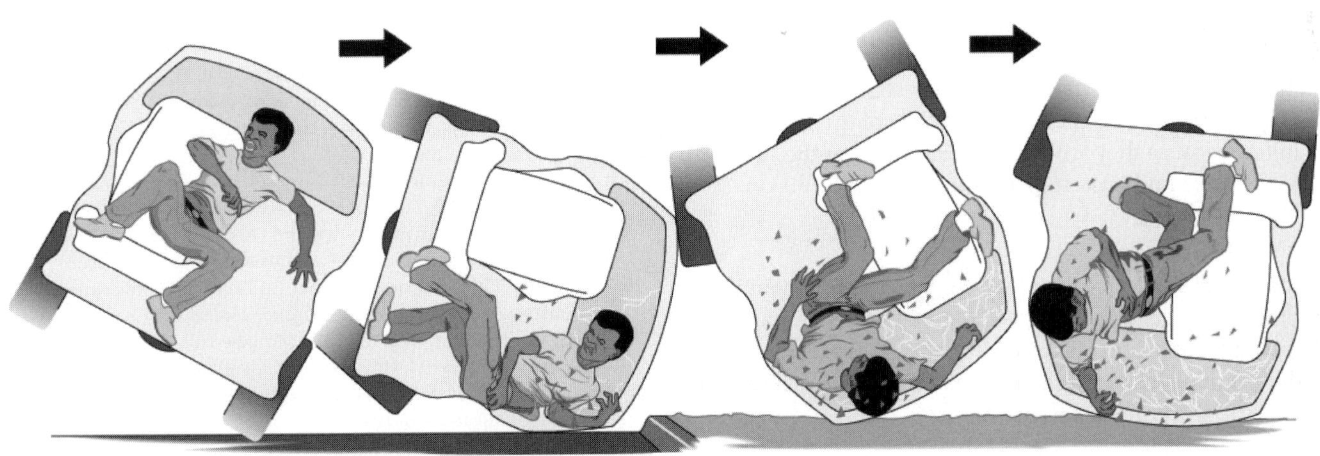

FIGURE 14-14 **Rollover MVC.**

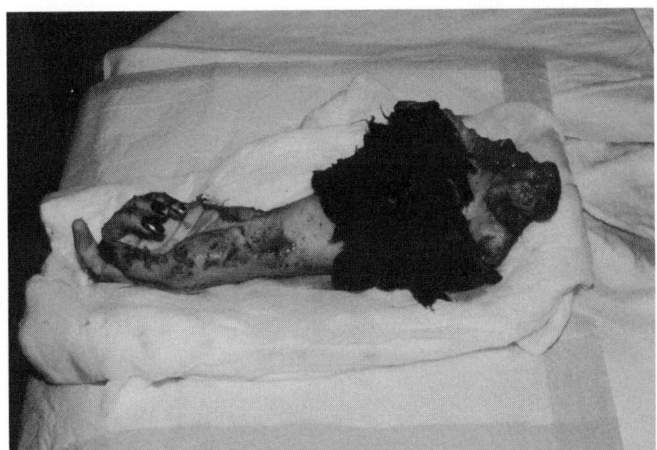

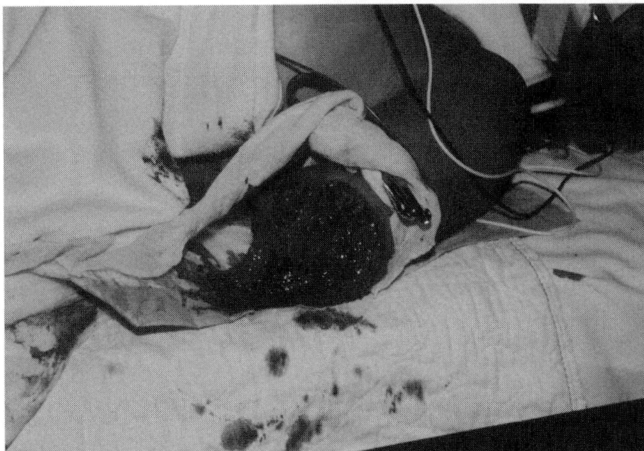

FIGURE 14-15 **Upper extremity amputation from rollover MVC.**

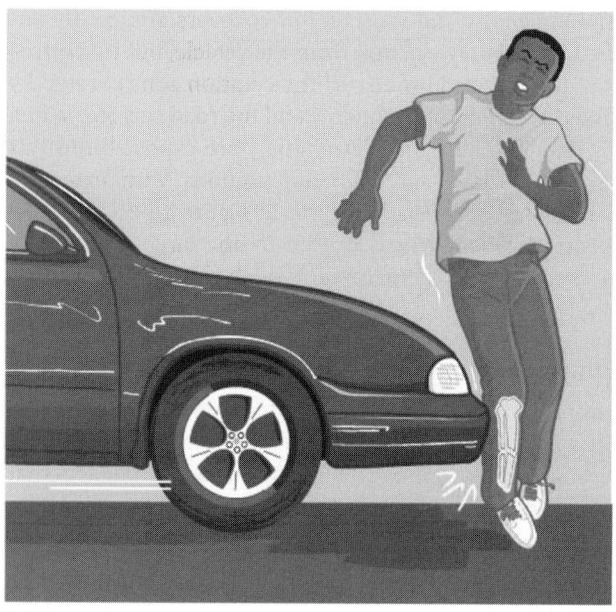
(a)

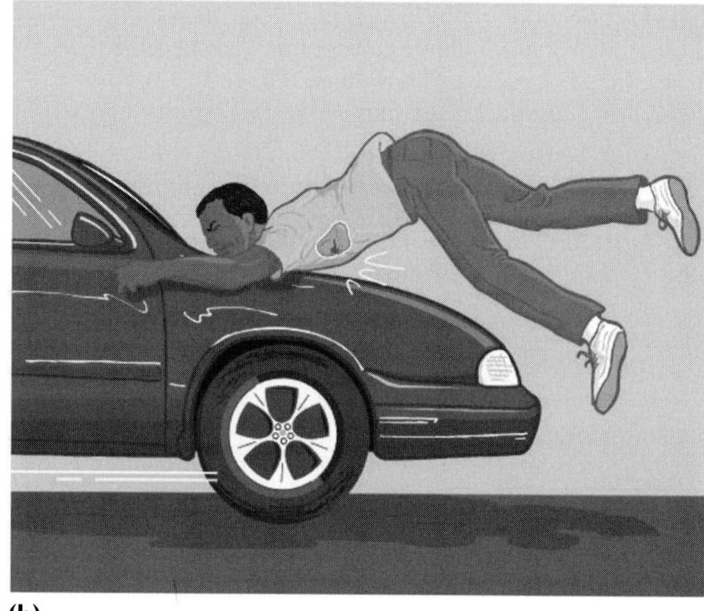
(b)

FIGURE 14-16 **Car versus pedestrian collision: (a) lower leg impact with bumper; (b) torso impact with hood.**

Epidemiologically, children and elders suffer a disproportionate incidence as the pedestrians in auto versus pedestrian collisions. Children are at the highest risk because of inattentive play near streets. Elder pedestrians' slower walking speeds may doom them to be victims of this mechanism of injury because they are unable to ambulate at the standard 4 ft/sec speed built into signaled crosswalks.[15]

CONCLUSION

Victims of motor vehicle crashes are frequently encountered in emergency departments and trauma centers. A basic understanding of mechanisms of injury can assist the physician in determining injuries and injury patterns and can direct the diagnostic work-up of the patient.

REFERENCES

1. American College of Surgeons Committee on Trauma. *Resources for Optimal Care of the Injured Patient.* Chicago, Ill: American College of Surgeons; 1999.
2. Simon BJ, Legere P, Emhoff T, et al. Vehicular trauma triage by mechanism: avoidance of unproductive evaluation. *J Trauma.* 1994;37(4):645–649.
3. Esposito TJ, Offner PJ, Jurkovich, GJ, et al. Do prehospital trauma center triage criteria identify major trauma victims? *Arch Surg.* 1995;130:171–176.
4. Shatney CH, Sensaki K. Trauma team activation for "mechanism of injury" blunt trauma victims: time for a change? *J Trauma.* 1994;37(2):275–282.
5. Garrett JW, Braunstein PW. The seat belt syndrome. *J Trauma.* May 1962;2:220–238.
6. American College of Surgeons Committee on Trauma. *Advanced Trauma Life Support for Doctors.* 7th ed. Chicago, Ill: American College of Surgeons; 2004.
7. Sivit CJ, Taylor KD, Newman DI, et al. Safety-belt injuries in children with lap-belt ecchymosis: CT findings in 61 patients. *Am J Roentgenol.* 1991;157:111–114.
8. Gestring ML, Gracias VH, Feliciano MA, et al. Evaluation of the lower spine following blunt trauma using abdominal computed tomography supplemented with lateral scanograms. *J Trauma.* 2002;53:9–14.
9. Kindelberger JC, Chidester AB, Ferguson E. *Air Bag Crash Investigations 2003.* National Highway Safety Administration Paper No. 299. Available at: http://www-nrd.nhtsa.dot.gov/pdf/nrd-01/esv/esv18/CD/Files/18ESV-000299.pdf. Accessed August 13, 2008.
10. Buchman TG, et al. Thoracic trauma. In: Tintinalli JE, American College of Emergency Physicians, eds. *Emergency Medicine: A Comprehensive Study Guide.* 6th ed. New York, NY: McGraw-Hill; 2004.
11. Horton TG, Cohn SM, Heid MP, et al. Identification of trauma patients at risk of thoracic aortic tear by mechanism of injury. *J Trauma.* 2000;48:1008–1013.
12. Insurance Institute for Highway Safety. *In Real-World Crashes, Side Airbags with Head Protection Are Saving Lives.* Arlington, Va: Insurance Institute for Highway Safety; August 2003. Available at: http://www.iihs.org/news/2003/iihs_news_082603.pdf. Accessed August 13, 2008.
13. American Medical Association, National Highway Traffic Safety Administration, US Department of Transportation. Chapter 1, Safety and the older driver: an overview. In: *Physicians' Guide to Accessing and Counseling Older Drivers.* National Highway Traffic Safety Administration Web site. Available at: http://www.nhtsa.dot.gov/people/injury/olddrive/OlderDriversBook/pages/Chapter1.html. Accessed August 13, 2008.
14. US Department of Transportation, National Highway Traffic Safety Administration. *Characteristics of Fatal Rollover Crashes.* Washington, DC: Department of Transportation; 2002. Available at: http://www-nrd.nhtsa.dot.gov/pdf/nrd-30/NCSA/Rpts/2002/809-438.pdf. Accessed August 13, 2008.
15. Schwab CW, Kauder DR. Trauma in the geriatric patient. *Arch Surg.* 1992;127:701–706.

15 | Sexual Assault

William M. Green, MD

INTRODUCTION

Few crimes in our society present greater challenge and complexity than does sexual assault. The sexual assault victim is often confronted by a terrifying array of threats, intimidation, and brutality. Physical injuries range from minor to life-threatening. The emotional impact may initially appear deceptively mild, but the inner turmoil and long-term sequelae are devastating and life-altering for many victims. For the community, sexual violence presents significant public safety and criminal justice concerns. Because sexual assault is such a multifaceted issue, a number of community agencies and disciplines will be involved.

One critical intersection is between the victim and the healthcare system. The individual who presents with the complaint of sexual assault has unique needs that go far beyond the traditional clinical encounter (Table 15-1). While in the healthcare arena, the person is more properly characterized as a sexual assault patient. The medical and emotional needs of the patient constitute one category of problems that must be addressed. Evaluation and management of acute medical issues get the highest priority. As medical condition permits, crisis intervention and emotional support can be initiated in parallel to medical care. The healthcare provider must be knowledgeable regarding the psychodynamics of sexual assault and the unique emotional disequilibrium it can create. Strategies for prophylaxis against sexually transmitted infections (including HIV) and potential pregnancy must be discussed and offered. Specific plans for follow-up (both medical and emotional) must be developed.

TABLE 15-1 **The Forensic Medical Approach to Sexual Assault: Two Sets of Needs**

Patient	Criminal Justice System
• Acute medical evaluation and treatment	• Focused medical and assault-related history
• Crisis intervention and emotional support	• Documentation of physical findings
• Prophylaxis against STDs and pregnancy	• Proper collection and handling of evidence
• Follow-up care for medical and emotional issues	• Interpretation of findings
	• Presentation of findings and expert opinion

Source: CCFMTC–California Clinical Forensic Medical Training Center.

The second main category of need that must be confronted is related to the criminal justice system. These tasks will fall outside the comfort zone and expertise of healthcare providers who have not had appropriate and specific training. The criminal justice system needs a focused medical and assault-related history. Pertinent physical findings must be identified and carefully documented. Evidence (both trace and biological) must be anticipated, identified, collected, packaged, preserved, and labeled in strict compliance with local crime laboratory policies and procedures. Law enforcement and the courts will require medical expertise in the interpretation of findings and will potentially need the formulation and presentation of expert medical opinion regarding the significance and relevance of the findings.

In essence, forensic medicine is the interface between the legal and medical systems. When a healthcare provider expands his or her role beyond traditional medical care and assumes the added responsibility of addressing the forensic needs of the criminal justice system, that provider is functioning as a forensic medical examiner. Along with professional colleagues from law enforcement and the crime laboratory, the forensic medical examiner plays a key role in meeting the fundamental forensic objective of providing an independent reconstruction of the events in question (Table 15-2). Ideally, the assembled evidence stands alone to recreate a scenario of the events that is indisputably accurate, scientifically sound, and objective. In a perfect circumstance, the reconstruction is robust enough to be independent of witness testimony. The forensic application of this objective that comes closest to this ideal is the use of DNA typing to establish the human source of tissue evidence.

Although DNA technology has had a staggering impact on identification issues, many other criminal justice problems have reconstructions that are less certain and are subject to contentious and controversial expert interpretation. The evaluation of sexual assault provides some excellent examples. Most of the time, a sexual assault has no independent witnesses. Many cases are distilled down to a "she said . . . he said" situation. Forensic evidence is often crucial for criminal justice decision making. There are three basic questions in a sexual assault case (Table 15-3). First, *did the sexual contact occur?* This is obviously a fundamental element of the crime and may be addressed by physical findings and/or biological evidence (especially sperm). The second question is: *if the sexual contact occurred, with whom?* Again, forensic evidence (especially DNA but also hair and trace evidence) may be helpful. The third question, *was the sexual contact consensual or nonconsensual?* does not rely on any identification evidence because sex between the parties is conceded. History and physical findings are the focus for this question.

TABLE 15-2 **Fundamental Forensic Objective**

Provide an independent reconstruction of the events in question that is:
• Accurate
• Scientifically sound
• Evidence-based
• Objective (does not rely on witness testimony)

Source: CCFMTC–California Clinical Forensic Medical Training Center.

TABLE 15-3 **Sexual Assault: Three Basic Forensic Questions**

• Did sexual contact occur?
• If contact occurred, with whom?
• Was the sexual contact consensual or non-consensual?

Source: CCFMTC–California Clinical Forensic Medical Training Center.

BASIC LEGAL ISSUES

The word *rape* derives from the Latin *rapere*, to take by force. The jurisprudence of sexual assault has its roots as a theft crime because women have historically been considered to be property without individual rights. The rapist "stole" the virginity of a father's daughter (which resulted in a lower dowry amount) or "stole" the sexual exclusivity of a husband's wife. In the latter scenario, the wife was presumed to be an accomplice in the "theft" and was also punished. This basic distrust of the female sexual assault victim is the centuries-old foundation for the "victim blaming" that tenaciously persists in the legal system and public opinion. More reform of sexual assault law has occurred in the last 40 years (largely spearheaded by the feminist movement of the 1970s) than in all of prior recorded history. Much has changed to more precisely define the crimes, to protect the victim at trial (rape shield statutes), and to hold the assailant accountable. Unfortunately, societal attitudes, myth, and misconception still shroud sexual assault and disadvantage its victims.

Every state (and the federal government) defines sex crimes in its own specific statutes. To generalize, sex crimes involve sexual touching or penetration of a body orifice (by an assailant body part or foreign object) "against the person's will" or "without consent." Means to overcome a person's will generally include force or violence, threat of immediate injury or death (the victim or another person), or threatening harm or retaliation in the future. Any "consent" obtained under these circumstances is invalid. The concept of consent to sexual contact may superficially seem straightforward, but when intertwined with traditional attitudes and beliefs, it becomes functionally quite complex. The California penal code (section 261.6) provides an example of a practical definition:

> Consent shall be defined to mean positive cooperation in act or attitude pursuant to an exercise of free will. The person must act freely and voluntarily and have knowledge of the nature of the act or transaction involved.

Other situations in which sex is accomplished without legal consent may not include elements of force or threat of violence. For example, sex with an individual below the legal age of consent is a crime (statutory rape or unlawful sexual intercourse), and the underage person's willingness to participate is immaterial. Consent may not be used as a defense. If a person is unconscious, intoxicated, or disabled (mentally or physically) to the point that he or she lacks the capacity to "exercise free will" or "understand the act involved," legal consent cannot be given.

PSYCHOLOGICAL IMPACT OF SEXUAL ASSAULT

Any person who survives a sexual assault has been through an unforgettable crisis that has the potential to create both immediate and long-term disruption in life. Victims almost universally report that the predominant emotion experienced during the assault was the fear of death. The violence and intimidation concomitant with the assault are often much more significant stressors than the sexual aspects. In general, the experience creates a sense of helplessness, intensifies conflicts about dependence and independence, and produces shame and guilt, which may lower self-esteem and hamper trusting relationships. Anxiety, feelings of vulnerability, and depression may be persistent problems. Victim responses vary depending on life stages, circumstances of the assault, preexisting emotional health, coping style, and resources for support.

The best known conceptual model describing victim reaction to sexual assault is the *rape trauma syndrome*,[1] which is a cluster of symptoms and responses (physical, emotional, and psychological) experienced by victims in the aftermath of the event. Although there is significant variation in duration, shock and disbelief are often the first responses once the victim is beyond the fear and danger of the assault. Depending on individual coping style, some victims may express their anxiety and distress openly with crying, agitation, restlessness, or garrulousness. Others may contain their emotions with a controlled style and appear outwardly calm or even indifferent. Regardless of external appearance, internally victims are churning with feelings of guilt, shame, embarrassment, betrayal, and powerlessness. Over time, the acute phase blends into a stage of outward adjustment (really pseudoadjustment) where denial is common and true feelings are suppressed. Victim activity and functioning may appear "back to normal" except for punctuations of anxiety, flashbacks, and fear. Depression, social constriction, and withdrawal may be subtle but are common and may persist indefinitely without effective therapy. The final stage, or integration phase, represents survivor acceptance of the assault as part of life and marks the incorporation of the crisis into the spectrum of other life experiences. Therapy and support are usually critical to achieve resolution.

The initial healthcare encounter after the assault may have a significant and far-reaching impact on victim recovery. If conducted in a sensitive and supportive way, the sexual assault forensic exam may be a first step toward healing. If done poorly, the exam could retraumatize the victim and compromise both recovery and victim participation in the criminal justice process. It is critical that the forensic medical examiner understand the psychodynamics of sexual assault and be prepared to respond with the appropriate support and crisis intervention.

The burgeoning of rape crisis resources throughout the country offers immeasurable hope and comfort for victims. In many communities, both law enforcement and forensic medical examiners routinely rely on trained rape crisis advocates to provide emotional support and accurate factual information for victims from the time of the initial crisis, during the forensic medical exam, and throughout the investigation and prosecution. The advocate's role is also to ensure that victims are treated with dignity and respect. They help explain and buffer against behaviors, attitudes, beliefs, traditions, regulations, or laws that may be perceived by the victim as unfair, unjust, or harmful. Most rape crisis centers provide acute and ongoing counseling and group support as well as assist in accessing other community resources. It is essential that the forensic medical examiner have a good working knowledge of local rape crisis resources and a strong working relationship with the advocates.

SEXUAL ASSAULT FORENSIC EXAMINATION

The sexual assault forensic examination (SAFE) is the cornerstone of the forensic evaluation and documentation of findings related to the sexual assault patient. From the forensic standpoint, the patient is a "walking crime scene" that must be "processed" in a meticulous, thorough, and standardized fashion. Obviously, the patient was also a witness to the crime and his or her history of events is a fundamental part of the forensic evaluation. It is essential that the SAFE be conducted and documented using a protocol with strictly defined policies and procedures. Thoroughness and consistency are prerequisite to the reliability and validity of the results and conclusions. The California protocol[2] is a good example of a complete system that includes detailed instructions for performing the SAFE and a dedicated form to facilitate proper documentation. The form and instructions are supported by a comprehensive manual.[3]

Because the clinical encounter with the sexual assault patient includes both a forensic component and a medical component, it is generally a best practice to have separate medical and forensic records. The forensic record (exemplified by the California protocol) is driven by strict policies and procedures and includes only medical information that has direct bearing on the evaluation of the alleged crime(s). The medical record (typically in the form of an emergency department medical record) includes all pertinent medical information necessary to evaluate, diagnose, and manage the patient's complaints and risks. Data that are needed for good medical care and documentation may be inappropriate or even potentially prejudicial if included on the forensic form. Examples include past medical history not relevant to current findings, mental health history, gynecological history, and medications.

Before the actual history and examination process begins, the examiner's first responsibility is to assess the patient's medical condition and stability. The medical screening exam should explore injury mechanisms and acute complaints. Preexisting medical conditions may require attention whether related to the assault or not. Vital signs and a screening physical exam are necessary for all patients. Urgent medical issues always trump forensic evaluation. When the patient is seriously ill or injured, the forensic medical examiner may work in parallel with the healthcare provider(s) addressing medical priorities. In this situation, a complete forensic exam is not possible, but the forensic medical examiner should document physical findings and collect as much evidence as possible without interfering with acute patient care.

After medical stability is ensured, the forensic examination process will be facilitated by attending to a few basic principles (Table 15-4). All individuals participating in the process should introduce themselves and describe their role. The examination environment should be safe and quiet. Privacy and confidentiality must be ensured. A busy emergency department will fail most of these criteria. The patient and any waiting family or friends should be given a realistic appraisal about the duration of the process (typically 2–4 hours). It is prudent for the forensic medical examiner to spend a few minutes alone with the patient to discuss the detailed and personal nature of the questions (e.g., past sexual history, drug/alcohol use) before the patient makes a decision to have a family member or friend be present for support during this part of the forensic process. Make the patient as comfortable as possible. This may require some flexibility. For example, if the patient is thirsty, the oral examination and swab collection could be done first. If at all possible, include a rape crisis advocate to help support and educate the patient. Obviously, all team members must understand and be sensitive to the emotional needs of the patient. A well-trained, experienced advocate can focus on those needs and comfort the patient, enabling other team members to direct their energies to the other tasks at hand.

TABLE 15-4 Sexual Assault Forensic Examination: Preliminary Issues

- All team members involved in the forensic examination process (examiner, advocate, law enforcement officer) should introduce themselves and explain their roles
- Provide a quiet, safe examination environment
- Ensure privacy and confidentiality
- Educate the patient and waiting family and friends about the duration of the process (often 2–4 hours)
- The forensic medical examiner should spend a few minutes alone with the patient to discuss the detailed nature of the questions before a decision is made about family/friend support during the history
- Address patient comfort needs
- Provide rape crisis advocacy

Source: CCFMTC–California Clinical Forensic Medical Training Center.

TABLE 15-5 Sexual Assault History: Basic Principles and Strategies

- Ask the questions in the same way and in the same order every time
- Use language the patient understands and assess comprehension
- Leave more emotionally charged questions to the end
- Explain the reasons for questions that could be perceived as judgmental
- Make no assumptions: ask every question every time
- Create an accepting environment and suppress bias

Source: CCFMTC–California Clinical Forensic Medical Training Center.

Sexual Assault History

The history of the events in question is a key part of the sexual assault forensic evaluation process. Understanding and adopting some basic interviewing principles and strategies promote quality and consistency (Table 15-5). Developing and following a routine in conducting the SAFE supports completeness and provides a usual and customary practice that can be relied upon later (e.g., in the courtroom) to substantiate thorough, high-quality work when independent recollection regarding the details of a specific case has faded over time. This routine begins with the history. Ask each question the same way and assess the patient's comprehension (especially important when discussing sexual acts and body parts). Leave the most difficult questions (drug/alcohol use, prior sexual history, sexual aspects of the assault) to the end of the interview process to allow trust and rapport to develop. Asking questions in the same order each time helps prevent omissions.

Explain why you are asking questions that could be perceived as judgmental (e.g., assault-related clothing, risk-taking behavior prior to the assault, past sexual history). It is imperative not to make assumptions about the history; to do so invites errors, omissions, and discrepancies. The best practice is to ask every question on the protocol to every patient in every exam. It is appropriate to start a list of questions with a disclaimer acknowledging that the examiner realizes not everything happened, but asking each question ensures completeness and promotes accuracy.

Creating an accepting atmosphere for the history is sometimes quite challenging but always important. No matter how seemingly implausible the scenario, it is the examiner's responsibility to record the history as presented. Clarifying responses and resolving obvious inconsistencies or discrepancies are always appropriate, but it is never the forensic medical examiner's role to determine credibility or veracity. The truthfulness of the patient will be addressed by the whole investigative process, and the ultimate determination belongs to the jury. A closely related issue is the necessity for the forensic medical examiner to suppress "gut feelings" or personal bias about the patient's account, personal characteristics, or behavior. Patients, especially recently traumatized patients, may be extremely sensitive to subtle innuendo or language that implies disbelief or a negative attitude. Sympathy and a "benefit of the doubt" approach are best.

Person Providing the History

Most of the time the history comes directly from the patient. If this history is facilitated or assisted by another individual (interpreter, translator, caregiver, etc.), that person must be documented so that if questions about patient comprehension versus quality of interpretation arise later, the original participants can supply clarification.

Pertinent Medical History

As discussed earlier, most historical medical information should be entered on the separate medical record, not the forensic record. The past medical history items that have a direct bearing on the forensic evaluation (and therefore belong in the forensic record) include any information that is necessary to properly interpret the current physical findings. For example, last menstrual period helps differentiate traumatic bleeding from a normal process. Preexisting injuries must be separated from injuries related to the assault. Medical conditions (e.g., vaginal infection), medications (e.g., blood thinners that may increase bruising), or recent treatments (e.g., recent freezing procedure to the cervix because of an abnormal Pap smear) that could potentially alter the interpretation of current findings must be documented.

Preassault Sexual Activity

The crime laboratory requires contextual information related to recent sexual contact to properly interpret DNA evidence recovered from swabs containing sperm. DNA left by a recent consensual partner must be differentiated from assailant DNA. Recent sexual activity must be documented (oral, vaginal, anal) and whether ejaculation occurred and whether the consensual partner used a condom. Controversy about the appropriate time frame for consensual inquiry exists, and maximum reported intervals for sperm recovery vary greatly among laboratories and depend on the body cavity involved.[4]

Drug/Alcohol Use Before and After the Assault

This area is controversial but must be objectively explored and documented. Voluntary alcohol and/or drug use are very common in the prelude to sexual assault, and it is not uncommon for a victim to self-medicate after the assault (and prior to the forensic exam) in an effort to cope with the stress of the event. Indications for obtaining blood alcohol and/or urine toxicology specimens vary from jurisdiction to jurisdiction. It is imperative that the patient be candid and accurate historically to prevent discrepancies between the history and the laboratory analysis. The impact of both the history and the lab tests may be very significant. Intoxication may affect the credibility of the history. Intoxication may be of sufficient magnitude to preclude the patient's ability to engage in the thought process required to legally grant consent. A clinical state of intoxication that is disproportionate to the historical information and laboratory analysis may support the suspicion of drug-facilitated sexual assault with a drug such as gamma hydroxybutyrate (GHB) that is difficult to recover.

Postassault Hygiene Activities

Depending on the sexual acts involved and the time frame, patient activity may significantly reduce the likelihood of evidence recovery. Oral recovery may be diminished after eating, drinking, gargling, or brushing the teeth. Urinating (and wiping) or douching may remove genital evidence. Defecating may reduce anorectal recovery. If the patient changed clothes after the assault, the original clothing should be sought and collected.

Three postassault activities have special evidence considerations. First, it is common following a vaginal penetration assault for the patient to "clean up" and wipe the genital region. The item used for the wipe may contain the best semen evidence available. Every patient should be questioned about this activity and the wiping item should be sought and collected. Second, if a tampon was in place at the time of the assault, it should be collected. If the patient removed it after the assault, it should be retrieved, if possible. And third, even if the patient changed clothes after the assault, any clean clothing nearest to the genital structures should be collected because gravity drainage may deposit evidence.

Assault-Related Signs and Symptoms

If the patient has any complaints related to assault-associated injury or activity (pain, bleeding, soreness, tenderness, etc.), these should be carefully documented. This information can help focus attention later in the history when injury mechanisms are described and again during the physical exam.

Vomiting during or after the assault may be related to injury, emotional upset, or the effects of drugs and/or alcohol. If vomitus is available, a sample should be obtained for the crime lab. Depending on the circumstances, medical attention to evaluate the cause of the vomiting may be indicated.

Any loss of memory or periods of unconsciousness must be thoroughly explored and documented. Obviously, contributory medical issues must be carefully evaluated and patient stability ensured. Because the quality and credibility of the history rest directly on the patient's memory of the events in question, any compromise of memory has a potentially significant impact. The documented history must reflect the patient's level of certainty for any information that falls below the "perfectly clear memory" standard. The integrity of the patient's memory (and the resultant history) may come under intense scrutiny in the courtroom, and the examiner must be prepared to provide detail as to how certain the patient was about all aspects of the history.

Date and Time of Assault

The time the assault occurred has important criminal justice implications (suspect alibi, timeline of events, victim corroboration, etc.). From a clinical forensic medicine perspective, the two most important aspects are when injuries occurred and when ejaculation happened. The interpretation of findings relative to both of these variables is time sensitive and requires the patient's best estimate of the time or, at minimum, the narrowest time frame.

Physical Surroundings of the Assault

The geographic location of the assault is a law enforcement responsibility. The forensic medical examiner needs to know what the patient's body (or clothing) directly contacted to anticipate potential trace evidence (sand, weeds, gravel, grease, fibers, etc.). Another consideration is the anticipation and interpretation of patterned injuries or skin findings that resulted from specific contact(s) at the scene.

Assailant(s)

The detailed description of the assailant(s) and the relationship to the patient is generally left to law enforcement. From a forensic standpoint, proper crime lab analysis and interpretation of some biological evidence may require knowing the gender and ethnicity of the donor. If multiple assailants were involved, the protocol must facilitate accurate documentation of "who did what."

Methods Employed by Assailant

This section provides the essential details of the contact between patient and assailant and documents the assailant's activities and behaviors that were employed to overcome the patient's will and accomplish the nonconsensual acts. A fundamental underlying principle in this section is the documentation of the mechanism(s) of injury. This may be done in a narrative format or using a checklist of methods (e.g., physical blows, grabbing, holding, restraints, burns, strangulation) with descriptions. The documentation must be complete and with sufficient detail to assess the consistency between this historical information and the physical exam findings. The relationship between mechanisms and findings (consistency, probability of association, and differential diagnosis) will be key in both the investigation and prosecution.

If threats were employed to subdue and control the patient, those must be specified. Using exact quotes (documented with quotation marks) of verbal threats helps substantiate the fear experienced by the patient. Threats to harm another person (e.g., child in the next room) or to retaliate in the future may also invalidate any consent so obtained. Nonverbal assailant behavior alone may be sufficiently intimidating to prevent resistance and gain compliance. Weapons that are alleged or brandished or assailant size and strength are common examples.

Drug-Facilitated Sexual Assault

The use of alcohol and/or drugs is another method that may be employed by the assailant to control the patient, prevent resistance, and impair the memory. The history of events is typically fragmented, vague, or absent. The documentation must specify the patient's level of certainty for any memories. Any information about potential substances, suspected or known, must be recorded. The timeline from last certain memory to next certain memory should be explored and documented. Blood and urine toxicology specimens should be obtained as soon as possible.

Injuries Sustained by the Assailant

If the patient is aware of any injuries to the assailant (either inflicted by the patient during the contact or by assailant behavior alone) or the possibility of assailant blood deposited anywhere, the details should be documented. This information may be helpful to law enforcement for identification purposes or may focus crime lab attention on evidence from the patient (e.g., fingernail scrapings) or from clothing.

Sexual Acts

This is the most difficult information to discuss for everyone involved in the examination and investigation. The nonconsensual acts are intensely personal, embarrassing, humiliating, and often degrading. The patient must understand that complete detail is needed to help uncover subtle physical findings and to ultimately charge the assailant with every illegal act.

Each question in this section has four potential responses. "Yes" and "no" are straightforward. "Attempted" must be explained because what the patient may interpret as incomplete might meet the legal definition of a chargeable act. For example, in California, forced oral copulation only requires contact, not penetration; if the patient turned her head and the penis only touched the lips or cheek, the patient might respond to this question with "he tried" while the district attorney could file the charge. "Unsure" is the fourth possible response. This is a completely legitimate answer because the patient may not be able to absolutely confirm or deny the occurrence of a given act. The reason(s) for the uncertainty should be documented.

Specific, separate questions should be asked about penetration of a body orifice (mouth, vagina, anus) by any object (penis, finger, foreign body). Any foreign object that was used should be described. The patient's impression about ejaculation (in a body cavity and/or on the surface of the body or clothing) should be recorded. Any other sexual touching by either party (fondling, masturbation, etc.) should be described in sufficient detail to facilitate charging decisions by the prosecutor.

Oral contact has special consideration. Biting may produce indentations, abrasions, ecchymoses, or incised wounds that, when properly documented (forensic photographs, dental castings), can provide very precise identification of the bite inflictor. All oral contact (biting, licking, kissing, etc.) has the added potential of saliva transfer. The detection of saliva alone may be important corroboration of the history of oral contact. In addition, saliva contains cells shed from the salivary glands and ducts that provide the potential for DNA analysis and specific identification of the saliva donor.

The history should conclude with an open-ended question to capture any missing information (e.g., "Did anything else happen that we haven't already discussed?"). This last question may yield additional details of the assault that may be unusual or particularly degrading. Providing a gentle reminder about the necessity for thoroughness and candor along with the acknowledgment of how difficult and embarrassing these questions is prudent.

PHYSICAL EXAMINATION AND EVIDENCE COLLECTION

As previously discussed, the sexual assault forensic examination must be driven by strictly defined policies and procedures. Nowhere is this concept more critical than in the performance and documentation of the physical examination and evidence collection. Attention to detail is mandatory and the burden on the forensic medical examiner is significant. Many "downstream" interpretations and decisions by the crime lab, law enforcement, and prosecution will depend on the assumption that the exam was thorough and accurate and the evidence was handled competently and in rigid compliance with the local protocol. The forensic medical examiner must know and carefully follow the protocol, and also must understand and be prepared to explain the scientific and forensic foundation for the protocol component parts. The examiner should anticipate a very high level of scrutiny by the criminal justice process.

The entire system for evidence management (anticipation, recognition, collection, packaging, labeling, documentation, and transport) must be developed in conjunction with the local crime laboratory. A standardized rape evidence kit containing all supplies and material needed for evidence management should be constructed. Chain of custody details must be addressed. Some types of evidence may require special handling and/or transport. Examples include drying of swabs and slides, wet clothing, and liquid biological fluids (blood, urine, vomitus, used condoms, used tampons, etc.).

The examination and evidence collection process should be structured to minimize the loss of evidence. Time delays compromise evidence recovery because of degradation or drainage. Sperm quickly becomes nonmotile after ejaculation. Patient activity may diminish recovery because evidence is washed away, brushed or wiped off, swallowed, or flushed down the toilet. The forensic medical examiner may contribute to the problem by failing to collect all available evidence or by giving the crime lab a sample too small for adequate analysis. All of these potential pitfalls can be prevented by thorough and expeditious evidence collection procedures. Anyone who interacts with the patient before the forensic exam (9-1-1 dispatch, rape crisis hotline, law enforcement, hospital triage) should be trained about the risks of losing evidence and advise the patient accordingly.

Evidence contamination is a huge issue and especially problematic with the ultrasensitive evaluation of DNA. Contamination can occur between or among the forensic medical examiner, the patient, the examination environment, and other items of evidence. The protocol (developed in cooperation with the local crime lab) should specify practices and techniques to prevent contamination. For example, the swab drying box should be cleaned (a 10% bleach solution works well) before and after each use. Only evidence from a single patient should be handled at the same time and in the same exam area. The exam environment must be thoroughly cleaned between forensic patients. Glove changing by the examiner must be frequent enough to ensure that contamination did not occur from one activity to the next. If the examiner coughs, sneezes, or even talks over evidence, examiner DNA may be picked up by the crime lab. Many criminalists prefer examiners wear a surgical mask during evidence handling.

SYSTEMATIC FORENSIC APPROACH TO THE PATIENT

These next sections will take you through the forensic evaluation of the sexually assaulted patient step by step. Some procedures listed may not be applicable to all jurisdictions.

Medical Screening Exam and Vital Signs

The medical screening exam (MSE) to identify urgent medical needs and to ensure patient stability is best done when the patient interacts with the first qualified health professional. If the MSE has not yet occurred, it may be performed as the first portion of the physical exam. Traditional vital signs (temperature, pulse, respirations, blood pressure) should be documented. Any abnormalities should be appropriately addressed or explained. Blood pressure and pulse elevations may normalize by simply repeating them later in the process.

Time Frames

It is useful to document the times of the various components of the sexual assault forensic examination. These time frames help nonmedical or nonforensic individuals better understand the detail and complexity of the process. These data may also be useful programmatically for resource utilization and allocation (forensic medical examiner time, use of facility time, etc.) and for quality assurance purposes. The most important times to note include time of patient arrival, time that the forensic medical examiner became directly involved, time the patient was discharged from the facility, and time the examiner finished the entire process. Documenting the time that evidence (especially potential biologic evidence) was obtained may be necessary for proper interpretation.

General Description of the Patient

It is useful to provide a brief description about what the patient was like at first presentation. The two components of this description are physical appearance and demeanor. A short sentence or a few phrases should be sufficient for each part. The terms used should be objective and descriptive rather than interpretative or conclusive. If properly constructed, these "word pictures" should provide an accurate image of how the patient looked and acted in the mind of the reader. It is also helpful to include a brief description of the patient's ability to give the history and cooperate with the examination.

Clothing

After patient stability and urgent medical needs have been addressed, the first evidentiary issue for the forensic medical examiner is the patient's clothing. If the patient has changed clothes after the assault, or if law enforcement has already collected the clothing worn during the assault, the examiner should collect the item of clothing nearest the genital structures (usually the underwear). Even if freshly laundered, gravity drainage of vaginal secretions or direct contact with the external genitalia may deposit valuable semen (or possibly saliva) evidence on the clean garment. If the patient is still wearing the assault-related clothes, those items must be inspected, collected, and packaged.

The crime lab will perform the detailed forensic evaluation of the clothing, but the examiner should obtain the clothing one item at a time as the patient disrobes and inspect it for moist stains (which require special drying and handling) and for damage consequent to the assault. The examiner can discuss the cause of the damage with the patient and document assault-related findings; the crime lab can only identify nonspecific damage. Each piece of clothing should be packaged separately to prevent contamination from one item to the next. The patient should disrobe over two drop sheets. The top one will catch any evidence that falls from the clothing and can be bindled (specifically folded and labeled). The bottom sheet protects the underside of the top sheet from floor contamination and is discarded after clothing collection. The examiner must have a method for labeling each item of clothing to be able to positively identify it later in court.

Body Surfaces Exam

The physical examination for the detection of injuries generally proceeds in parallel with evidence identification and collection. Typically, the forensic medical examiner follows the same sequence of activities and develops a system of usual and customary practice that promotes completeness and consistency. It is expected, however, that the examiner is a flexible problem solver who can appropriately adjust or customize the process as required by the specific issues in a given case. If any significant deviation from protocol is required, that deviation, and the reasons for it, should be documented.

The general sequence of the clinical/forensic examination begins with inspection. Any pertinent physical findings, injuries, or potential evidence are noted. Photographic documentation, using forensic technique, should follow inspection. Ideally, any visible evidence should be photographed in situ before it is collected. Any visible evidence can then be collected and managed using appropriate forensic technique. Scanning the region with an alternative light source (e.g., ultraviolet Wood's light) may reveal evidence (especially dried semen) not seen with plain light. Collection of any highlighted areas should proceed until the fluorescent stain is completely transferred from the body surface to the evidence swab. Any potential (nonvisible) evidence described during the patient history (saliva, semen, etc.) can be presumptively collected. This is a logical time to collect control swabs that are intended to be evidence-free and only contain "background" patient material. Control swabs should be obtained from the region of actual evidence collected but from an area without visible, historical, or Wood's-light-positive findings.

Palpation is necessary to identify areas of tenderness that may be the result of trauma but that appear normal. Patient history and clinical suspicion guide palpation. Any tender areas should be documented and the area reexamined in 2–3 days. If bruising has developed, forensic photographs should be taken.

This same basic clinical/forensic process is repeated regionally until the entire body surface has been evaluated. A complete body surface exam must include careful inspection of the scalp, all body hair, nostrils, ear canals, behind the ears, web spaces in between the fingers and toes, and within any skin folds or crevasses. After the scalp and hair are examined for findings, head hair reference samples are obtained. Usually, 20–30 hairs are obtained from various locations to cover the spectrum of length and color. Plucking provides more morphological characteristics but is uncomfortable for the patient. Although less than ideal, some crime labs allow reference hairs to be clipped close to the skin. The patient's reference hairs will be used for comparison to any evidence hairs potentially left by the assailant. Fingernail scrapings or clippings should be routinely obtained and packaged separately for each hand.

There are three components to the forensic documentation of findings. The first is a diagrammatic representation on body diagrams ("traumagrams"). The goal is to show a finding's size, shape, orientation, and location. The second part is a written description of each finding that includes the type of finding, size, color, texture, and other pertinent information (active bleeding, tenderness, etc.). Diagrammatic and written descriptions are needed for every finding, including nonvisible items such as control swabs, sampling based on history (e.g., potential saliva), and tenderness. In addition, all visible findings should include the third component, forensic photographs taken using specific techniques. Note that only forensically significant findings related to the event in question should be documented. So, unless acutely traumatized, scars, piercings, tattoos, preexisting skin lesions, and so forth should not be documented. An exception would be a non-acute skin finding that will appear in the photographs near an assault-related finding that might be misinterpreted as an acute finding.

Oral Cavity Examination

After the body surface examination is complete, attention is turned to body cavities. The mouth is routinely and carefully examined. Special focus is directed at the frenula, palate, gums, and buccal surfaces to search for subtle injury (abrasions, ecchymoses, petechiae, lacerations) that could result from forced oral copulation, a direct blow, or the assailant's hand over the patient's mouth. Photographic documentation and evidence collection follow using the standard sequence and techniques. The oral cavity should be sampled for potential semen if there is a history of completed or attempted oral copulation or if the patient's history is uncertain. Typically, two evidence swabs are used to obtain material from under the tongue, behind the upper incisors, the tonsilar fossae, and the buccal sulci. Dental floss may be used to obtain evidence from between the teeth.

Genital Examination

Obviously, the genital exam is frequently a critical component of the sexual assault forensic examination. Many cases pivot on findings and evidence found in this region. The same systematic forensic approach as previously described is applied here. The forensic examiner must be familiar with the pertinent anatomy (see Figure 15-1). Some additional techniques and enhancements are also employed. As always, thorough and meticulous attention to the details of inspection, forensic photography, evidence management, and documentation are mandatory.

After the usual process of regional inspection, forensic photography, evidence collection, and Wood's light scanning, the pubic hair is examined. Any crusted secretions or adherent evidence is clipped out in total. A drop sheet is placed under the patient (seated on the edge of the exam table) and on top of the clean sheet or paper that covers the exam table. The pubic hair is then brushed with a comb or brush (supplied in the rape evidence kit). Any loose fibers, hairs, debris, and so forth will be trapped in the comb/brush or fall onto the drop sheet. The comb/brush is placed on the drop sheet, which is then bindled and labeled. Pubic hair reference samples (20–30, preferably plucked) are then harvested.

The external genital structures are then inspected again using one or more enhancement techniques. The first enhancement, magnification, has become the standard of care in the sexual assault forensic examination. Traditionally, the colposcope, developed in gynecology to assess the cervix after an abnormal Pap smear, has been used to provide a good light source, stereoscopic magnification, and photographic capability. Use of magnification has significantly improved the detection threshold for genital microtrauma. Unfortunately, this improvement in detection has brought controversies in interpretation of findings because consensual sexual activity can also result in genital microtrauma.

The second enhancement technique, use of toluidine blue dye, is not as universally applied as magnification. It,

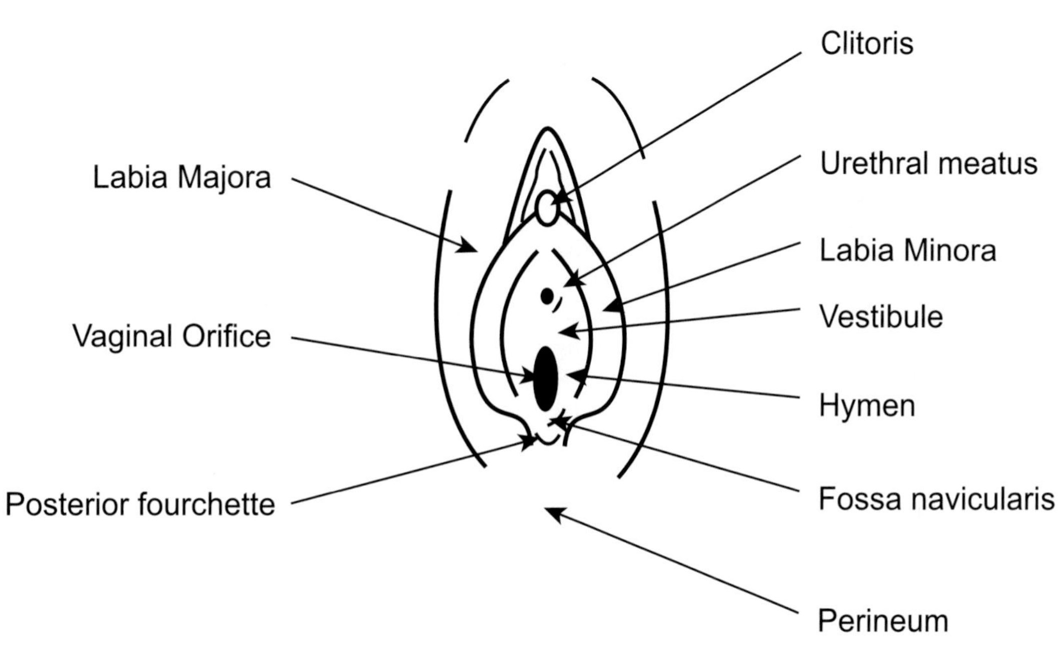

FIGURE 15-1 **External female genital structures.**

too, improves detection but generates controversy. Toluidine blue is selectively taken up by cell nuclei. To get to the nuclei, cell membranes must be ruptured. From this perspective, toluidine blue has been used to detect and highlight traumatic injuries. Unfortunately, nontraumatic (and non-assault related) inflammation and infection can also cause positive intake. Residual dye (especially in skin folds and creases) may be misinterpreted as traumatic intake. Another problem is that vaginal speculum insertion has been reported to create toluidine blue–positive microabrasions. If toluidine blue dye is used, it must be applied before the underlying tissue is manipulated or instrumented.

After all examination and collection tasks for the external genital structures are complete, the vagina and cervix are examined and sampled. A vaginal speculum (preferably water moistened) is inserted. The vaginal walls and cervix are inspected for injury and evidence in the usual fashion. If a foreign body is present (e.g., condom, tampon, diaphragm), it should be removed and packaged. The colposcope (or other magnification instrument) is used for magnified inspection and photodocumentation. Vaginal or cervical injury is uncommon and usually the result of foreign body penetration. Blunt trauma injury from penile penetration alone is unusual in patients between puberty and menopause. Misinterpretation of the colposcopic appearance of the cervix may be problematic. Unless the forensic medical examiner is trained and experienced in the traditional application of colposcopy for the analysis of cervical pathology, normal or nontraumatic findings may be wrongly ascribed to blunt force trauma. If blunt force injury is suspected, it is essential that the patient be reexamined in 1 to 2 weeks (preferably by the same examiner using the same colposcope). The exam and follow-up photos can then be reviewed in conjunction with an expert knowledgeable in cervical pathology.

The next phase is sampling the vaginal pool for semen. Typically, four swabs are placed into the posterior fornix (most dependent part of the vaginal canal in the standard pelvic exam position) and allowed to uniformly absorb any secretions that have pooled there. When the swabs are removed, one is used to prepare a dry mount slide for the crime lab. A second swab should be used to prepare a wet mount slide that the forensic medical examiner will examine for the presence of motile sperm. Sperm lose motility rapidly on the slide, so it must be examined within 10 minutes of preparation. This important forensic analysis must be mastered by the forensic medical examiner because it will be the only opportunity to identify motility, which narrows the potential time frame of deposition.[4]

Anorectal Examination

The external perianal and anal structures and the anal canal (visible with manual traction) should be routinely examined in every sexual assault patient. Any physical findings and/or evidence should be handled in the usual fashion. An internal inspection (using an anoscope) may be indicated for either medical or forensic reasons. If the patient reports rectal bleeding, rectal pain, foreign body insertion, or has external injuries, medical evaluation must be performed to exclude significant injury. If there is a history of attempted or completed anorectal penetration, or if the patient cannot reliably deny a rectal act, anoscopy is also needed to obtain rectal swabs for potential semen or other evidence. The possibility of vaginally deposited evidence leaking out of the vagina over the perineum and being collected on an anal/rectal swab risks the misinterpretation of primary anorectal deposition. The anoscopic collection of rectal swabs from undisturbed rectal mucosa above the tip of the instrument helps mitigate the contamination issue. Any visible anoscopic finding (injury or evidence) should be photographed and documented using standard technique.

SUMMARY AND ACCOUNTABILITY

The final portion of the sexual assault forensic examination is the documentation of evidence collected, procedures performed, and all personnel involved in the exam or evidence management. The system for management and distribution of evidence will vary by jurisdiction, but the record must always reflect who collected each item, when it was collected, and where it went. Documentation must adhere to the local chain of custody standard.

Clothing may go to the police evidence facility. Some clothing (usually the underwear) may be included in the rape evidence kit. Any trace evidence collected, any swabs obtained, or dry mount slides prepared should be individually documented. If a vaginal wet mount was done, the time it was prepared, the time it was interpreted, and the name of the interpreter should be noted. If blood and/or urine was collected for toxicology or blood alcohol, documentation should include the time the specimens were obtained. All reference specimens should be individually documented. The details regarding any forensic imaging should include the equipment used and the number of images taken. If any pictures were taken with magnification, the power of the magnification should be recorded. Any enhancement techniques or special exam procedures should be listed or described. The names of all personnel involved in the sexual assault forensic examination process and their role(s) (history, exam, evidence collection, assistance, etc.) should be clearly recorded. Similarly, all individuals taking custody of evidence items (clothing, rape evidence kit, reference samples, toxicologic specimens, etc.) should be individually documented, and the record should indicate the date and time of transfer and the destination of the items.

DEBRIEFING

After completing the history, physical examination, and evidence management, the forensic medical examiner needs to finish the encounter with both law enforcement and the patient. If law enforcement is still present (or has returned to take custody of the evidence), it is helpful for the examiner to briefly summarize the pertinent findings, review the evidence collected, discuss any new information regarding potential evidence still at the scene, and discuss any recommended forensic follow-up. Forensic follow-up may include reexamination and photography of developing injuries or subsequent "wellness photos" to clarify nonspecific findings that may or may not be acute.

The forensic medical examiner should discuss several issues with the patient at the end of the process. Validating the patient's response to events and offering positive feedback about his or her role in the forensic medical examination process may support the first steps in healing. Any detected injuries should be discussed in regards to clinical significance, treatment recommendations, expected course, and follow-up. Reassurance about physical health concerns is a high priority for most sexual assault patients. If not already addressed, strategies to prevent sexually transmitted infections and emergency contraception must be offered. Logistics and safety planning must be addressed. Follow-up for counseling and mental health needs are frequently facilitated by the rape crisis advocate. If forensic follow-up is needed, the patient should understand why and how that happens. All questions should be answered and detailed written information given. Instructions about home care and any "when to return" precautions must be included. All follow-up care instructions (medical, emotional, forensic) should be detailed and include phone numbers for scheduling and questions.

EXTRAGENITAL INJURIES

The trauma of sexual assault frequently produces injuries. The reported incidence of injuries outside the anogenital region varies from 23% to 85%.[5–9] Factors influencing this wide variability include examiner training and experience, injury definition, time frames, and study population. The classification of injury severity also varies, but, in general, severe injuries (requiring hospitalization) are found in only 1–2% of sexual assault patients. Moderate injuries (requiring evaluation and emergency department treatment) account for 2–17% of cases whereas the remainder (and vast majority) are minor, self-limited, and generally need only basic wound care. Some patients have no injuries at all.

Extragenital injuries may play a very significant role in the investigation and prosecution of a case. Injuries may corroborate the use of force and provide consistency between the history and the physical findings. Some injuries (especially pattern injuries) may give very specific information about the mechanism of the injury and the events in question. Both direct assailant activity and victim resistance may produce traumatic findings. Extragenital injuries may render a defense of consent difficult, illogical, or even impossible.

When an injury is detected on physical exam, the forensic medical examiner should ask how and when it happened and whether it is related to the assault. The mechanism of injury should be explored and documented. Correct forensic injury classification and definitions should always be applied. As always, documentation of any traumatic finding should include a diagrammatic representation, a written description, and forensic imaging.

Most of the injuries sustained during sexual assault are to the result of blunt force trauma. Blunt force may produce (singly or in combination) abrasions (scrape or impact) or contusions (ecchymoses, petechiae, hematoma). Sharp force injury (stab, incised, or chop wounds) are less common but not infrequent. Bites may involve multiple mechanisms with the teeth creating blunt and/or incised wounds related to the dental arches with additional suction producing an ecchymosis between the dental arches (suction ecchymosis or "hickey"). Burns are an infrequent, but potentially serious, mechanism. Burning mechanisms include not only thermal injury but also chemical and electrical etiologies. Detailed discussion about injury mechanisms and characteristics is found in Chapters 10, 11, and 13.

Three points about extragenital injuries in the context of sexual assault deserve emphasis. First, analyzing the mechanism and the appearance of a traumatic finding may reveal patterning. Both blunt and sharp force wounds may provide information (sometimes very specific) about how the injury was caused or the nature of the injuring object. Interposed clothing or jewelry may stamp an image into the skin when blunt force is applied. The injuring object itself may leave wounds that identify the object. If available, the imprinted or injuring object should be photographed next to the wound to demonstrate the correlation.

The second point for emphasis is a caution about the age dating of bruises. A body of older literature suggests that an analysis of the various colors of a bruise can provide an accurate time frame for determining when the injury occurred.[10–13] Unfortunately, better methodology has invalidated most of these color-based determinations. The only characteristic that stands up to scientific scrutiny is that the color yellow does not appear until the wound is at least 18 hours old.[14,15]

The third point is a cautionary note about the interpretation of subjective and nonspecific findings. Tenderness is the subjective perception of discomfort produced by palpation or pressure. There may be no corresponding visible finding. A contusion may be tender hours to days before subcutaneous bleeding becomes visible. Erythema is increased superficial capillary dilatation and congestion. This nonspecific response may be from trauma but may also be produced by infection, inflammation, allergic response, thermal injury, or autonomic response. Erythema may also be a stable normal variant of dermal appearance. Likewise, swelling is another nonspecific finding that may be related to recent trauma but may have nontraumatic etiologies. What appears to be swelling may actually be a stable, normal variant. The mandatory approach to subjective and nonspecific findings is a follow-up evaluation before the final interpretation or determination of forensic significance.

ANOGENITAL INJURIES

The detection, characterization, and documentation of anogenital injuries are critical parts of the sexual assault forensic examination. Unfortunately, considerable mythology and controversy revolve around anogenital injury in the context of sexual assault. A number of factors contribute to the problem. The wide variation in examiner education, training, clinical experience, and expert oversight raises legitimate concern about the accuracy of finding identification and the credibility of interpretation. Pertinent scientific and forensic literature is limited and contains numerous flaws. Significant methodologic variations (exam techniques, injury classification, inclusion of nonspecific findings, spectrum of examiner competence, etc.) make comparisons between studies problematic and often invalid. To compound the issue, training and even testimony have relied upon misinterpretation and inappropriate use of the existing literature.

Published rates of anogenital injury vary widely from 16% to well more than 80%.[6,7,9,16–21] It is important to note that nearly all the reported injury data come from series of patients who present complaining of sexual assault. Very limited information has been published regarding findings identified in the subset of presenting patients for whom a legal outcome (conviction or guilty plea) is known and hence provides some corroboration of the history.

VISUALIZING INJURIES

Most early studies on genital injuries used only gross visualization and standard pelvic examination techniques, and injury rates were usually low. Adjunct examination methods (primarily developed in the pediatric sexual abuse arena) may uncover subtle injuries that standard exam technique could miss. Labial separation and traction, knee–chest position, use of moistened swabs to carefully manipulate genital tissue, and hymenal examination using a vaginally inserted Foley catheter or large swab are all techniques that have been adapted for use in the sexual assault forensic examination of adults and adolescents.

The use of toluidine blue dye to stain cell nuclei enhanced the detection of genital injuries up to 56%.[20,22] The use of magnification (primarily the colposcope) brought the most dramatic increases in injury detection rates, with one study reporting 87% of sexual assault patients having positive findings.[23] The application of colposcopy for adult/adolescent sexual assault forensic examination is becoming the standard of care.

Injury Sites and Severity

Any anogenital structure can be injured as a consequence of sexual assault. The number of anogenital injury sites varies from none to multiple.

The posterior fourchette and fossa navicularis (usually considered as a single anatomic region) are the most frequently injured sites. This is probably because of, in part, the underlying common perineal tendon, which does not stretch or flex so that when blunt trauma (e.g., penis or finger) is applied, the overlying tissue is more likely to be damaged. The labia minora and hymen are the next most common sites of injury. Damage to other external structures (vestibule, periurethral area, perineum, and labia majora) is not uncommon. Internal structures (vaginal walls and cervix) are injured much less frequently. Blunt force vaginal trauma from penile or digital penetration has been reported (mainly in elderly and "first coitus" patients) but is very uncommon. Documented blunt force cervical trauma is rare and requires clinical expertise and serial follow-up examinations to confirm.

Depending on the object, foreign body penetration may produce blunt force and/or sharp force injury. Digital penetration is more likely to create sharp force trauma from an incising or avulsing fingernail mechanism. Structures at greatest risk for fingernail damage include posterior fourchette and fossa navicularis, perineum, labia minora, vaginal walls, and cervix.[24] Serious anogenital injury (requiring repair and/or hospital admission) is very uncommon and probably more related to foreign object use.

AGE AND SEXUAL EXPERIENCE

One group found that adolescents sustain genital injury at a higher rate (83%) than do adults (64%), but all experienced the same type of injuries.[25] Postmenopausal women sustain significantly more genital injuries than do their menstruating counterparts.[26–28] This is quite logical considering the dryness, friability, and decreased elasticity that occurs in genital tissues after menopause. A number of investigators found that virgins had a higher genital injury rate than patients with prior sexual experience.[17,18,25,29] Hymenal injuries are more common in sexual assault patients without prior sexual experience and include ecchymoses, abrasions, and lacerations (partial or complete). There are many enduring myths and misconceptions about the hymen. It is essential to note that first coitus does not result in any hymenal injury in a significant percentage of patients. Tampon use, sports, and prior pelvic examination do not cause hymen injury.[30]

OTHER FACTORS POTENTIALLY RELATED TO GENITAL INJURY

Despite many beliefs to the contrary, the relationship between the sexual assault patient and assailant has minimal (and probably not statistically significant) influence on whether or not injuries occur. Between two-thirds and three-quarters of patients know their assailant. These relationships cover the spectrum from vague acquaintance to spouse. Some investigations have found a slightly higher genital injury rate in stranger assaults[31,32] and others have not.[33] Data about sexual assault patient alcohol use and genital injury are compromised because most studies have relied on retrospective self-reporting about level of intoxication. Adolescents may have a slightly higher genital injury rate when intoxicated (81% vs. 73%), but adults do not.[33,34] One large study (using gross visualization only) looked at genital injury in pregnant patients and found a significantly lower rate (5% vs. 21%) when compared to nonpregnant controls.[35] There was no difference between early and late gestation. One multicountry study using colposcopy following consensual intercourse has suggested that smoking may make vaginal epithelium more vulnerable to trauma.[36]

A number of other factors have been thought to influence the presence, absence, or severity of genital injury from sexual assault, but only intuition and conventional wisdom have been used to support conclusions. Coital position, genital size, extrinsic lubrication, multiple assailants, multiple events, and male sexual dysfunction all probably have some impact on the generation or lack of genital injuries, but none of these issues has been adequately studied scientifically. Likewise, medical conditions such as inflammation and infection or medications such as anticoagulants and steroids are known to generally reduce tissue vitality and lower the injury threshold, but studies specifically related to sexual assault trauma have not been done. Rigorous scientific inquiry needs to be applied to move from speculation and generalization to truly informed opinions and conclusions.

CONSENT VERSUS NONCONSENT

One of the most difficult, contentious, and misunderstood aspects of the sexual assault forensic examination is the application of genital injury findings in determining the presence or absence of consent. This complicated issue presents multiple challenges related to the scientific literature, human physiology, and the role of the examiner in the legal process.

In an ideal world, there would be a robust scientific knowledge base that could be used to analyze the genital injuries in any given sexual assault case and determine, definitively and conclusively, whether the last sexual contact was consensual or nonconsensual. The jobs of all involved would certainly be easier with such a forensic gold standard test. Unfortunately, the medical and forensic literature in this area is limited and much of it contains serious methodological flaws. Most published series that describe genital findings are gathered from patients who give a history of sexual assault rather than from the subset for which a legal outcome (conviction or guilty plea) is known, which would offer important corroboration for interpreting the findings. Variations in exam methodologies and examiner experience, inclusion criteria for "consenting control" patients, and the inclusion of nonspecific findings with traumatic injuries all compromise the validity and reliability of the results and conclusions. All studies have reported a significant minority of sexual assault patients who have no genital injuries. Conversely, all studies using consensual control patients have found some who have findings of traumatic intercourse.

At this point, the only general conclusions that can be drawn from the literature are that genital injuries can occur in both consensual and nonconsensual intercourse and a normal genital exam is not uncommon in patients who report sexual assault. It is also fair to conclude that genital injuries are more common in adults who report sexual assault than in consensual controls. Two studies focused on adolescents[22,25] found much less difference in genital injury rates between assault patients and controls. It may be statistically possible to separate a group of sexual assault patients from a group of consensual controls, but too much overlap exists to reliably place any single individual in one group or the other.

Another significant problem area related to genital injuries and the consent determination is the mythology that has developed about the role of the human sexual response. The concept of the human sexual response (HSR) emerged from the pioneering work of Masters and Johnson in the 1960s.[37] It is a sequence of physical and physiologic changes that occur in response to stimulation (cognitive, affective, and/or tactile). It classically has four phases: excitation, plateau, orgasm, and resolution. Unfortunately, a very simplistic application of this process has taken root in the conventional wisdom about genital injury and consent/nonconsent. This theory suggests that in consent the HSR is invoked and injuries will not occur, and, conversely, in nonconsent there will be no HSR and injuries will occur. Not even the flawed sexual assault literature supports this view.

A very comprehensive review of this subject found that subjective sexual arousal and perceptions of physical response may not correlate.[38] Tactile stimulation in women produces a strong response regardless of whether it is related to sexual activity. The first response to any stimulation is engorgement of genital blood vessels with resultant vaginal enlargement and lubrication via transudation. In the final analysis, it must be stressed that the forensic medical examiner cannot formulate any conclusions about causal relationships among sexual response, consent, and genital injury.

The third troubling aspect of genital injuries and the determination of consent to sexual activity revolves around the role of the forensic medical examiner in the criminal justice process. Expectations from law enforcement and the prosecution have sometimes pressured examiners to be more definitive about the absence of consent than is scientifically reasonable. Not only is this scientifically unsound, but it also risks invading the province of the jury regarding the "ultimate issue of fact."[39] In essence, determining the ultimate issue equates to the examiner making the "diagnosis" of rape. Deciding the ultimate issue is the role of the jury, not the examiner.

Anorectal Injuries

Attempted or completed anal penetration in the context of sexual assault frequently causes injury (Table 15-6).[16,18,21,40] These injuries are of obvious forensic significance but may also pose serious medical risk as well. Just as with genital

TABLE 15-6 **Anal Injuries**

Study	Hillman (1990)	Slaughter (1997)	Adams (2001)	Hilden (2005)
Gender	M	F	F	F
Injury Rate	57%	56%	61%	56%
Both males and females who report anal penetration sustain injuries at a similar rate				

Source: CCFMTC–California Clinical Forensic Medical Training Center.

injuries, it is important to note that a significant minority of patients reporting a nonconsensual anorectal act have normal exams.

Absence of Genital Injuries

As previously discussed, all studies that describe genital injuries in patients who report sexual assault include individuals who do not have documented traumatic findings. This lack of detected injury may have other causes besides the fact that some sexual assault patients do not sustain injuries. It is clear that examination methodologies and enhancements affect injury detection. Variation in examiner training and experience may result in subtle injuries not being appreciated. Other factors such as extrinsic lubrication or patient compliance with assailant demands may play a role as well.

Assessment and Conclusions

The forensic medical examiner's final task in conducting the sexual assault forensic examination is an assessment of the findings. Opinions about the form and scope of this assessment vary widely from one jurisdiction to the next. Some protocols relieve the examiner of any interpretive burden and omit assessment altogether in favor of a criminal justice determination. Others may push the ultimate issue envelope and ask the examiner to commit to a spectrum of alternatives that stratify a range of probabilities. The California protocol[2] offers an example of a middle-ground approach.

The California protocol asks the examiner to answer two questions at the conclusion of the exam. The first is a yes or no question as to whether there are positive physical findings. Positive physical findings include any injury related to the assault, tenderness, a wet mount exam that revealed sperm, the collection of any trace evidence, or any Wood's lamp–positive findings. Note that trace evidence and Wood's lamp–highlighted areas may ultimately be found to have nothing to do with the assault at all. At this point in the process, however, they are categorized as positive findings with significance to be determined later.

The second question is a deceptively simple determination as to whether the history is consistent or inconsistent with the exam findings. The fundamental issue is really whether or not it is *possible* for the findings (or lack of findings) to have resulted from the history as given. To determine that the history and findings are inconsistent is essentially proving the negative. Such a determination indicates that it is medically *impossible* to associate the history and findings. This is beyond an assessment that the findings are unlikely or the association of history and findings improbable. It is also not the examiner's gut feeling "polygraph" of the patient's credibility or veracity. The incongruence of history and findings should be extreme to find them inconsistent.

To find the association consistent indicates only that a possibility of association exists. This is the highest level of certainty to which the examiner can opine. It is not diagnostic certainty and neither does it prove or confirm the history. It is anticipated that the investigative and prosecutorial process will explore the probability of association between history and findings and this exploration will be tailored to the specific facts in each case. This probability discussion presents significant challenges for the forensic medical examiner. The examiner's opinion will rest upon general clinical experience, specific forensic training and experience, and knowledge of the pertinent medical, forensic, and scientific literature.

CONCLUSION

The forensic medical examiner cannot determine whether rape occurred or whether consent was absent; both rape and consent are legal principles, not medical diagnoses. The jury has the responsibility to determine the accuracy and credibility of the history. The examiner can describe any objective findings related to recent trauma or recent sexual contact. The examiner may also discuss opinions about the probability of associations between historical aspects and observed physical findings, but determining the ultimate issue of fact, that is, whether rape occurred, belongs solely to the jury.

REFERENCES

1. Burgess A, Holstrom L. Rape trauma syndrome. *Am J Psychiat.* 1974;131:981–986.
2. State of California Governor's Office of Emergency Services. Forms and instructions. Forensic Medical Report: Acute (<72 Hours) Adult/Adolescent Sexual Assault Examination. Available at: http://www.ccfmtc.org/pdf/oes_forms/oes_923_form.pdf and http://www.ccfmtc.org/pdf/oes_forms/oes_923_Instructions.pdf. Accessed August 13, 2008.
3. Davis G, Office of Criminal Justice Planning. *California Medical Protocol for Examination of Sexual Assault and Child Sexual Abuse Victims.* January 2001. Available at: http://www.ccfmtc.org/pdf/oes_forms/oes_923-950_Protocol.pdf. Accessed August 13, 2008.
4. Green WM. Clinical forensic medicine sexual assault and semen persistence. In: Siegel JA, Knupfer GC, Saukko PJ, eds. *Encyclopedia of Forensic Sciences.* London: Academic Press; 2001.
5. Hayman CR, et al. Rape in the District of Columbia. *Am J of Obstet and Gynecol.* 1972;113(1):91–97.
6. Solola A, et al. Rape: management in a non-institutional setting. *Obstet and Gynecol.* 1983;61(3):373–378.
7. Tintinalli JE, Hoelzer M. Clinical findings and legal resolution in sexual assault. *Ann Emerg Med.* 1985;14(5):447–453.
8. Pentilla A, Karhumen PJ. Mediocolegal findings among rape victims. *Med Law.* 1990;9(1):725–737.
9. Bowyer L, Dalton ME. Female victims of rape and their genital injuries. *Br J Obstet Gynaecol.* 1997;104(5):617–620.
10. Wilson EF. Estimation of the age of cutaneous contusions in child abuse. *Pediatrics.* 1977;60:750–752.
11. Polson CJ, Gee DJ. *The Essentials of Forensic Medicine.* 3rd ed. Vol. 109. Oxford, England: Pergamon Press; 1973.
12. Glaister J, Rentoul E. *Medical Jurisprudence and Toxicology.* 12th ed. Vol. 234. Edinburgh: E&S Livingston; 1966.
13. Camps FE. Refresher course for general practitioners interpretation of wounds. *Br Med J.* 1952;2:770–772.
14. Langolis NEL, Gresham GA. The aging of bruises: a review and study of the color changes with time. *Forensic Sci Int.* 1991;50:227–238.
15. Schwartz AJ, Ricci LR. How accurately can bruises be aged in abused children? Literature review and synthesis. *Pediatrics.* 1996;97:254–257.
16. Adams JA, Girardin B, et al. Adolescent sexual assault: documentation of acute injuries using photo-colposcopy. *J Pediatr Adolesc Gynecol.* 2001;14(4):175–180.

17. Biggs M, Stermac LE, et al. Genital injuries following sexual assault of women with and without prior sexual intercourse experience. *CMAJ.* 1998;159(1):33–37.
18. Hilden M, Schei B, et al. Genitoanal injury in adult female victims of sexual assault. *Forensic Sci Int.* 2005;154(2–3):200–205.
19. Jones JS, Rossman L, et al. Comparative analysis of adult versus adolescent sexual assault: epidemiology and patterns of anogenital injury. *Acad Emerg Med.* 2003;10(8):872–877.
20. Lauber AA, Souma ML. Use of toluidine blue for documentation of traumatic intercourse. *Obstet Gynecol.* 1982;60(5):644–648.
21. Slaughter L, Brown CR, et al. Patterns of genital injury in female sexual assault victims. *Am J Obstet Gynecol.* 1997;176(3):609–616.
22. McCauley J, Gorman RL, et al. Toluidine blue in the detection of perineal lacerations in pediatric and adolescent sexual abuse victims. *Pediatrics.* 1986;78(6):1039–1043.
23. Slaughter L, Brown CRV. Cervical findings in rape victims. *Am J Obstet Gynecol.* 1991;164:528–529.
24. Rossman L, Jones JS, et al. Genital trauma associated with forced digital penetration. *Am J Emerg Med.* 2004;22(2):101–104.
25. Jones JS, Rossman L, et al. Anogenital injuries in adolescents after consensual sexual intercourse. *Acad Emerg Med.* 2003;10(12):1378–1383.
26. Cartwright PS. Factors that correlate with injury sustained by survivors of sexual assault. *Obstet Gynecol.* 1987;70(1):44–46.
27. Ramin SM, et al. Sexual assault in postmenopausal women. *Obstet Gynecol.* 1992;80(5):860–864.
28. Burgess AW, Hanrahan NP, Baker T. Forensic markers in elder female sexual abuse cases. *Clin Geriatric Med.* 2005;21(2):399–412.
29. White C, McLean I. Adolescent complainants of sexual assault; injury patterns in virgin and non-virgin groups. *J Clin Forensic Med.* 2006;13(4):172–180.
30. Emans SJ, Woods ER, et al. Hymenal findings in adolescent women: impact of tampon use and consensual sexual activity. *J Pediatr.* 1994;125(1):153–160.
31. Jones JS, Wynn BN, Kroeze B, Dunnuck E, Rossman L. Comparison of sexual assaults by strangers versus known assailants in a community-based population. *Am J Emerg Med.* 2004;22:454–459.
32. Stermac LE, DuMont JA, Kalemba V. Comparison of sexual assaults by strangers and known assailants in an urban population of women. *CMAJ.* 1995;153:1089–1094.
33. Lindsay S. A retrospective case review from two sexual assault programs in San Diego. Unpublished doctoral dissertation; 1998. University of California, San Diego.
34. Testa M, Vanzile-Tamsen C, Livingston JA. The role of victim and perpetrator intoxication on sexual assault outcomes. *J Studies Alcohol.* 2004;65:320–329.
35. Satin AJ, et al. Sexual assault in pregnancy. *Obstet Gynecol.* 1991;77:710-714.
36. Fraser IS, et al. Variations in vaginal epithelial surface appearance determined by colposcopic inspection in healthy, sexually active women. *Hum Reprod.* 1999;14(8):1974–1978.
37. Masters W, Johnson V. *Human Sexual Response.* Boston: Little, Brown; 1966.
38. Gaffney DA. On the female sexual response; injury and consent and the Virginia case. *Sex Assault Rep.* 2001;4(6):81–96.
39. Gilson JA. The Virginia Supreme Court case: forensic nursing comes of age. *On The Edge.* 2002;8(2):1–13.
40. Hillman RN, O'Mara N, et al. Adult male victims of sexual assault: an underdiagnosed condition. *Int J STD AIDS.* 1991;2(1):22–24.

16 | Interpersonal Violence

Janelle Martin, MD

INTRODUCTION

Domestic violence, more recently referred to as intimate partner violence, is the willful intimidation, assault, battery, sexual assault, and other abusive behavior perpetrated by one intimate partner against another. These behaviors may occur alone or in combination and may occur sporadically or on a more regular basis. Intimate partner violence is part of a systematic pattern of control and dominance and often results in physical injury, psychological trauma, and death. This violence is a pattern of coercive behaviors used by a competent individual to maintain control over another individual. It reaches individuals in every community and makes no allowance for age, educational background, nationality, race, religion, or socioeconomic status. Intimate partner violence has a significant influence on the clinical practice of emergency medicine, and in the past, that significance has too often been ignored.

This chapter discusses forensic evidence of injuries resulting from intimate partner violence. Forms of physical violence can include choking, hitting, kicking, punching, pushing, shoving, slapping, restraining, and strangulation. The violence may escalate into assault with deadly weapons, including guns, knives, and moving vehicles, as well as weapons of opportunity, such as tools or household items.

PREVALENCE OF INTIMATE PARTNER VIOLENCE

Although it is difficult to estimate accurately the prevalence of intimate partner violence, the numbers range from 960,000 to 3 million incidents of violence against a current or former boyfriend, girlfriend, or spouse per year in the United States.[1] The difficulty in obtaining accurate numbers lies with the varying degrees of reporting, affected mainly by the social stigma that is associated with the label of an intimate partner violence victim. Generally speaking, only about 50% of intimate partner violence is actually reported to the police.[2] Despite this, nearly one-third of American women do report being physically or sexually abused by a boyfriend or husband in their lifetime.[1] Internationally, about 33% of women report being the victim of intimate partner violence at least once during their lifetime.[1]

Estimates show that 1.3 million women are victims of a physical assault by an intimate partner each year.[3] In 2001, 588,490 women in the United States were the victims of nonfatal incidents of intimate partner violence involving former or current boyfriends, girlfriends, or spouses of the victim.[1] A higher percentage of women are treated in emergency departments for injuries inflicted by an intimate partner than for those inflicted by a stranger.

BEHAVIORAL PATHOLOGY

The behavioral pathology of domestic violence is often referred to as the *cycle of violence*, and it consists of three components. The first component is a period of tension building, and during this period the victim often tries to be compliant and cooperative to avoid violence. The second component is the explosive and acute violence stage during which the violence occurs. The final stage is characterized by a lack of tension, sometimes called the loving respite, the reconciliation stage, or the honeymoon phase. During this phase, the batterer may be contrite and demonstrate particularly loving behavior.

One of the most dangerous times for a victim of intimate partner violence is during attempts to leave the violent relationship. Women who are only separated from their husbands are more likely to suffer from violent injuries than those who are divorced. A large percentage of intimate partner assaults reported to law enforcement occur after the separation of the couple. Women are more likely to be murdered as a result of a violent relationship during very specific points in the relationship, including when attempting to leave the relationship or when reporting abuse. Of all women murdered as a result of intimate partner violence, 60% of those homicides occurred when the women left or were attempting to leave the relationship.[4]

IMPACT ON SOCIETY

In addition to loss of life, intimate partner violence has a huge economic impact on society, including loss of productivity, loss of lifetime earnings, and direct healthcare expenses. The healthcare cost annually is more than $5.8 billion, with $4.1 billion for direct medical and mental healthcare expenses.[3] After adding the cost of police response, direct property loss, and the criminal justice system, the cost grows significantly.

MORBIDITY AND MORTALITY ASSOCIATED WITH INTIMATE PARTNER VIOLENCE

Physical as well as psychological abuse is associated with multiple health disorders, including sexually transmitted diseases and gastrointestinal disorder. Injuries from intimate partner violence can also result in time off of work and lost work, leading to increasing stress and depression for the victim. Intimate partner violence victims tend toward somatization disorders, presenting with multiple, vague physical complaints, but little in the way of objective findings. They can display chronic pain syndromes, insomnia, night terrors, and suicidal tendencies.

Various negative health behaviors are associated with intimate partner violence, including substance abuse and high-risk sexual behaviors. Women who have been abused are more likely to suffer from alcohol and drug dependency than are women who are not the victims of intimate partner violence. Fifty-six percent of female victims are diagnosed with psychiatric disorders, including anxiety and depression.[3] Post-traumatic stress disorder is also prominent among the more severely abused; it is sometimes associated with flashbacks, dissociation, and multiple personality disorders. Twenty-five percent of women who attempt suicide have been the victims of intimate partner violence.[3]

Many studies have looked at the morbidity and mortality of intimate partner violence and have found that a home in which anyone has been the victim of violence is more than four times more likely to be the scene of a homicide than is a violence-free home. A study in Maryland showed that homicide was the leading cause of death for pregnant women.[2]

Intimate Partner Violence During Pregnancy

Pregnant women who suffer from intimate partner violence represent a special population of victims. The incidence of intimate partner violence during pregnancy is higher than the incidence of more commonly known complications such as gestational diabetes and preeclampsia. Each year, 324,000 women are abused during their pregnancy by an intimate partner.[3] Various studies estimate that between 4% and 20% of all pregnant women are abused a least once during their pregnancy.[3] Unplanned pregnancy also significantly raises the risk of intimate partner violence.

Intimate partner violence during pregnancy increases the risk of complications during pregnancy, including raising the incidence of low-birth-weight infants by 400% and the risk of miscarriage by 200%.[1] In addition, rates of depression, substance abuse, and suicide attempts are increased among mothers who are the victims of intimate partner violence. Several clues may point the clinician to intimate partner violence within this special population, including delayed prenatal care and inconsistent reports of injuries. Noncompliance behaviors, such as skipping appointments and not taking medications, can also lead a clinician toward the diagnosis of intimate partner violence.

VICTIM DEMOGRAPHICS

Intimate partner violence victims are predominately referred to as female, but we need to acknowledge that this is not always the case and males may be the victims of intimate partner violence as well. It should, however, be recognized that females make up the larger percentage of intimate partner violence victims, approximately 73%, and 1 in 4 women will experience intimate partner violence at least once during their lifetime.[3] Females make up 84% of spousal violence victims and 86% of the victims of violent acts by a significant other.[3] When comparing violent crimes against females and males, 20% of violent crime against women is attributed to intimate partner violence and 3% of violent crime against men is attributed to intimate partner violence.[1] In 1999, intimate partner homicide accounted for 32% of murders of females[3] and 4% of murders of males.[5] In 2000, more than 1,200 women and more than 400 men were killed by their intimate partners.[1]

Statistically, females between the ages of 20 and 24 years are at the greatest risk for intimate partner violence.[3] The rate of homicide as a result of intimate partner violence remains the highest in females between the ages of 16 and 24 years.[2]

There is some variation of intimate partner violence among ethnic groups and a recent survey found higher rates of intimate partner violence among African American, Alaska Native, and American Indian populations. Lower rates of intimate partner violence were found among Asian and Pacific Islander populations.[2]

Intimate partner violence has a significant impact on the practice of emergency medicine healthcare professionals regardless of whether these practitioners choose to recognize or ignore its impact on the patient population.

Of all women seeking care in emergency departments, between 22% and 35% of them are victims of intimate partner violence.[3] More than 33% of women treated in emergency departments for violent injuries were injured by their intimate partners,[1] and intimate partner violence is the leading cause of injury in women.[4] At least 42% of women who are abused sustain physical injuries during their most recent assault.[3] Less than one-fifth of victims reporting an injury from intimate partner violence sought medical treatment following the injury.[3] A large percentage of female victims of intimate partner violence present to an emergency department with chief complaints other than those directly related to the injuries sustained as a result of the intimate partner violence.

Women who are the victims of intimate partner violence are six to eight times more likely to seek out healthcare services than are women who are not abused. Forty-five percent of intimate partner homicide victims had visited an emergency department within 2 years of their deaths. A recent study shows that 37% of battered women admitted abuse to their healthcare provider and began the first steps of healing.[3] Between 70% and 81% of survivors of intimate partner violence reported that they wanted their healthcare providers to ask them about abuse privately during an appointment.[3]

Healthcare-Seeking Behavior of Victims

When victims of intimate partner violence were asked where they would go for help and support after a violent incident, 14% of the victims stated they would go to a hospital. A study in the Northeast found that 95% of female victims of intimate partner violence sought medical care at least 5 times per year and that 27% of victims sought care more than 20 times per year.[2]

SCREENING FOR INTIMATE PARTNER VIOLENCE

Studies have shown that direct questioning can reveal more admissions to intimate partner violence than written questionnaires can. However, only 10% of primary care providers routinely screen for domestic violence during initial visits and only 9% screen during routine visits. Studies show that a 2-minute screening session for intimate partner violence is sufficient to increase the safety of pregnant women.[3]

Many national groups have published recommendations regarding the screening process for intimate partner violence. The American College of Physicians recommends routine screening for intimate partner violence in the emergency department when women present with traumatic injuries. The Joint Commission on Accreditation of Healthcare Organizations recommends that all emergency departments use protocols for identifying the victims of intimate partner violence. The American College of Obstetricians and Gynecologists and the American Medical Association have guidelines recommending that all physicians screen all pregnant women for intimate partner violence. The American College of Emergency Physicians has published a policy statement acknowledging the prevalence of intimate partner violence among emergency department patient populations. It emphasizes the importance of identification and assessment for intimate partner violence and the need for training programs to detect, diagnose, and intervene in intimate partner violence.[6] In addition, the United States Congress passed a Violence Against Women Act in 1994 that points to the importance of this issue. The US Department of Justice has established the Office on Violence Against Women, which serves to coordinate national efforts directed toward the study, prevention, and treatment of intimate partner violence.

CARE, INTERVENTION, AND REPORTING

Health professionals have a responsibility to patients to do no harm and to provide care. That care may, at times, include physical protection and involvement of the appropriate authorities. Mandatory reporting of child abuse is consistent throughout the United States; however, reporting violence between or directed toward competent adults varies between states. In most states, violence with deadly weapons, including guns and knives, is an incident that must be reported.[6]

Healthcare providers have many opportunities to intervene in situations involving intimate partner violence. When there is no direct request for assistance or direct report of violence, many factors can deter healthcare providers from intervening. Among those factors is a general tolerance of violence, both personally and within society. Other factors that come into play are more personal, including sex bias, a personal history of abuse, and personal views of family life norms. Professional factors may also play a part, such as time restraints, particularly within the emergency department, in addition to inadequate skills, and professional relationships with victims or abusers. Many clinicians are unsure of institutional and government policies regarding intervention and reporting and may fear legal factors including litigation.

Many barriers to recognizing and addressing intimate partner violence exist. Healthcare providers must address their personal views, such as views of norms of family life and possibly personal history of abuse. Other factors also come into play, including blaming the victims or disapproving of the victim's decisions or circumstances surrounding the situation. Healthcare providers often fail to question individuals secondary to preconceived notions of typical or classic victim profiles. There is also the concern for privacy of adults who are competent to make their own decisions and choices.

GATHERING FORENSIC EVIDENCE

Second only to the medical care of the patient is the gathering of forensic evidence. This gathering of evidence from the victim of intimate partner violence necessitates the exam of the whole person. Many victims may attempt to conceal the signs of abuse with hair, makeup, jewelry, or clothing. This attempted concealment of injuries emphasizes the importance of examining all areas of the body only after the victim has changed into a hospital gown.

The physical examination of the victim of intimate partner violence must begin as all other patient examinations begin, first with vital signs and evaluation of the airway, breathing, and circulation. Then, care must be taken to complete a thorough visual examination of the patient to assess for new and old abrasions, burns, ecchymoses, fractures, and scarring. The exam must include an abdominal exam to assess for internal injuries as well as a chest and back exam to check for rib fractures. An ear, nose, and throat exam will evaluate for broken or missing teeth as well as lacerations or contusions.

Characteristic Types of Injuries

Several characteristic injuries stem from intimate partner violence and healthcare provider awareness of those injuries can enable appropriate care for patients to be provided as well as appropriate forensic evidence to be gathered. These injuries may include cigarette burns, fingernail scratches, human bites, and rope burns or welts (Table 16-1). Pattern injuries are commonly seen with intimate partner violence. Pattern injuries are marks or designs imprinted on the epithelium and corresponding with the weapon or instrument used to cause the injury. The location of injuries may also be characteristic, such as trunk injuries and bilateral injures to the extremities.

TABLE 16-1 **Characteristic Injuries of Intimate Partner Violence Victims**

- Cigarette burns
- Hot water burns
- Fingernail scratches
- Fingertip contusions
- Human bites
- Ligature strangulation
- Rope burns or welts

Blunt force trauma to the skin is the cause of the most common violent injury, which is the contusion. Parallel contusions with central clearing are consistent with assault from linear objects. Slap marks are usually seen only with circular or oval areas of erythema or bruising, but occasionally the delineation of the digits can also be seen. Contusions circular in shape and averaging a size of 1 cm in diameter are consistent with fingertip pressure. These are often found on the medial aspect of the upper arms or thighs; both of these areas of the body are normally protected. These contusions usually occur as the result of grabbing the arms with a large degree of force. Other pattern contusions may result from impact of baseball bats, belts, buckles, combs, cords, and fly swatters. Shoes can also leave imprints of the soles or heels when the victim is kicked or stomped. Careful attention must be paid to each contusion to identify possible patterns.

Several factors must be considered during the evaluation of the development of a contusion. These factors include the amount of force applied to the skin as well as the vascular supply of that area of the skin. It is important to note that bruises of identical age and cause may not develop at the same rate on two separate individuals. Generally speaking, red, blue, purple, or black colors may develop in contusions any time from 1 hour after the assault until the resolution of the injury. Any yellow color ensures the contusion is older than 18 hours. Yellow, brown, and green bruising usually points toward an older injury; however, any further, more specific aging qualification based on color is not reliable. Multiple bruises of various ages and locations can be clues leading to the diagnosis of intimate partner violence.

Fingernail markings occur in three different types. The impression marks appear as a result of the fingernail cutting into the skin, making a comma or semicircle impression. Actual scratch marks are linear; they may be superficial or deep and may be as narrow or as wide as the fingernail. Scratches by female assailants are usually more severe than those by male assailants, usually because of the longer length of the nails. Claw marks occur when the skin is undermined; these are deeper and can appear in groupings or scattered about the body.

Bite marks are an additional injury pattern seen with intimate partner violence. They may be difficult to recognize, but bite marks can be identified because of semicircular contusions or abrasions, as well as markings from individual teeth.

Another type of injury often seen with intimate partner violence is strangulation, of which there are three forms: ligature, hanging, and manual. All three result in compression and possible closure of the trachea and carotid arteries. Ligature strangulation is defined as strangulation with a cordlike object, including telephone cords, ropes, belts, and clothing items. Manual strangulation is done with the hands or forearms, and occasionally with feet or lower extremities when standing or kneeling on the victim's throat.

Medical complaints include dysphonia, aphonia, dysphagia, odynophagia, dyspnea, apnea, and hyperventilation. Some studies report death up to 36 hours after initial presentations of strangulation with relatively mild complaints, presumably resulting from respiratory decompensation.[2] Petechiae are seen with strangulation and are most pronounced with ligature strangulation. Petechiae are commonly seen in the conjunctiva and periorbital regions, but may be seen anywhere above the area of constriction.

Abrasions and scratches may be seen with strangulation injuries, usually as a result of the victim's fingernails used in an attempt to ward off the assault. A single visible contusion is usually the result of the assailant's thumb, whereas ligature marks may be patterned according to the object used. Careful attention must be paid to these patterns to identify the braided pattern of a rope or clothesline or the wavelike pattern of a telephone cord. Differentiation between strangulation by ligature or by hanging can be made by the angle of the impression. With ligature strangulation, the patterns are generally horizontal and often result in a fracture of the hyoid bone. With strangulation by hanging, the patterns are vertical and teardrop shaped. They are often above the thyroid cartilage and the hyoid bone is usually spared.

Thermal injuries can often be identified by the pattern of the injury. Common patterns are those of cigarette burns and burns from household appliances, such as clothing irons, curling irons, and hair dryers. Hot water immersion injuries are identified by the distinct delineation between healthy skin and that of the thermal injury. This clear demarcation is seen only when a person is restrained in the hot water. The automatic response to accidental exposure to hot water is to withdraw from the exposure, which causes an uneven thermal injury without the clear demarcation.

Sprains and fractures are additional common injuries seen among the victims of intimate partner violence. Evaluation of each individual must be completed, including assessment of ecchymoses, instability, stiffness, swelling, and tenderness. Also included in the exam must be range of motion and weight-bearing ability.

Distribution of Injuries

The distribution of injuries resulting from intimate partner violence varies, but up to 50% of injuries are to the head and neck. Injuries are also commonly central in location, often referred to as the *bathing suit pattern*. This includes areas usually covered or hidden with clothing, primarily the chest, breast, abdomen, buttocks, and genitals. Victims of intimate partner violence are 13 times more likely to have injuries in these areas than are victims of unintentional trauma.[4] The location of injuries may also represent a defensive posture. Injuries to the distal upper extremities, including contusions, fractures, and sprains, may be sustained while attempting to deflect blows. Injuries may also be seen on the soles, sustained while attempting to kick away the assailant. Injuries to the back, buttocks, and the back of the head, neck, and legs can occur when the victim is curled into a fetal position or crouched on the floor.

TABLE 16-2 **Medical Documentation of Intimate Partner Violence Victims**

- What body part injured
- How body part injured
- What weapons used
- How weapons used
- When incident occurred
- Where incident occurred
- Who inflicted the injury
- Relationship to batterer

Although the incidence of acute injuries secondary to intimate partner violence as the primary cause of presentation to an emergency department is not remarkably high, it remains a significant comorbidity of emergency department patients. In a Denver, Colorado, study, it was estimated that acute injury stemming from intimate partner violence was about 2%. Also in that study, 10–15% of women stated that they believed that intimate partner violence contributed to the illness that caused them to seek medical attention in the emergency department that day.[7]

Documentation of Forensic Evidence

The collection of forensic evidence culminates with clear documentation and recording of each individual injury. The records should clearly state exactly what the patient reported, including which body parts were injured, how the body parts were injured, what weapons were used, and how they were used, as well as when and where the violent incident took place (Table 16-2). The history should also include the identity of the batterer, the relationship to the victim, and as much information about the batterer as possible, including the address, phone number, and date of birth.

It is advisable to use the exact words of the patient as much as possible. It is recommended that a body map as well as color photographs be utilized to record all injuries. Each patient chart should include a full body photograph that includes the face as well as photographs of each individual injury. Standard recommendations are for at least two photographs of each injury, incorporating at least two views of each injury. A ruler and some form of patient identification should be used with each individual injury photograph. A consent form for the photographs should be signed by the patient and placed with the chart.

CONCLUSION

Of utmost importance in the emergency department is clinician recognition and diagnosis of intimate partner violence. To begin the process of recognition, medical practitioners must first acknowledge the existence of intimate partner violence within all populations; there is no subset of patient population that is free from this violence. Practitioners must also rid themselves of all personal bias and open their minds to screen for intimate partner violence. Practitioners have three responsibilities to patients who are the victims of intimate partner violence: first, to diagnose intimate partner violence; second, to provide medical care; and third, to provide support and resources to the victims and ultimately, the survivors of intimate partner violence.

REFERENCES

1. Family Violence Prevention Fund. Domestic violence is a serious, widespread social problem in America. Available at: http://www.endabuse.org/resources/lists. Accessed January 15, 2008.
2. Burnett LB, Adler J. Domestic violence. eMedicine. 2006. Available at: http://www.emedicine.com/EMERG/topic153.htm. Accessed January 15, 2008.
3. National Coalition Against Domestic Violence. Healthcare and domestic violence. 2005. Available at: http://www.ncadv.org/files/healthcare.pdf. Accessed January 15, 2008.
4. Fulton D. Recognition and documentation of domestic violence in the clinical setting. *Crit Care Nurs Quart.* 2000;23:26–34.
5. Liebschultz JM, Frayne SM, Saxe GN, eds. *Violence Against Women: Physician's Guide to Identification and Management.* Philadelphia, Pa: American College of Physicians; 2003.
6. American College of Emergency Physicians Public Health and Injury Prevention Committee. Domestic family violence. 2007. American College of Emergency Physicians, Dallas, TX. Available at www.acep.org/practices.aspx?id=29184. Accessed January 15, 2008.
7. Abbott J. Injuries and illnesses of domestic violence. *Ann Emerg Med.* 19997;29:781.

SUGGESTED READING

Haywood Y, Scott J, eds. Domestic violence. *Emerg Med Clin North Am.* 1999;17:567–737.

Shadigian E. Partner violence. In: Pearlman MD, Tintinalli JE, eds. *Emergency Care of the Woman.* New York, NY: McGraw-Hill; 1998:577–588.

Silman JS. Diagnosing, screening and counseling for domestic violence. *UpToDate.* 2008. Available at: http://www.uptodate.com.

Sisley A, Jacobs LM, Poole G, Campbell S, Eposito T. Violence in America: a public health crisis—domestic violence. *J Trauma.* 1999;46:1105–1112.

Krasnoff M, Moscarti R. Domestic violence screening and referral can be effective. *Ann Emerg Med.* 2002;40:485–492.

Earl BJ, Omori M, Fenton P. Contusions. eMedicine. 2005. Available at: http://www.emedicine.com/sports/TOPIC28.htm. Accessed February 4, 2008.

Gremillion DH, Kanof EP. Overcoming barriers to physician involvement in identifying and referring victims of domestic violence. *Ann Emerg Med.* 1998;27:769–773.

Chescheir N. Violence against women: response from clinicians. *Ann Emerg Med.* 1996;27:766–768

Olson L, Anctil C, Fullerton L, Brillman J, Arbuckle J, Sklar D. Increasing emergency physician recognition of domestic violence. *Ann Emerg Med.* 1996;27:741–746.

Coonrod DV, Bay RC, Rowley BD, Del Mar NB, Gabriele L, Tessman RD, Chambliss LR. A randomized controlled study of brief interventions to teach residents about domestic violence. *Acad Med.* 2000;75:55–57.

Varvaro FF, Gesmond S. ED physician house staff response to training on domestic violence. *J Emerg Nurs.* 1997;23:17–22.

Verlander PM, Carson S. Improved identification and treatment toward victims of violence within a metropolitan area. *J Emerg Nurs.* 2003;29:421–422.

SoRelle R. ACEP's scientific assembly tackles gamut of issues. *Emerg Med News.* 2003;25:32.

Bacchus L, Mezey G, Bewley S. Experiences of seeking help from health professionals in a sample of women who experienced domestic violence. *Health Soc Care Community.* 2003;11:10–18.

Mezey G. Domestic violence in health settings. *Curr Opin Psychiatr.* 2001;14:543–547.

Ellis JM. Barriers to effective screening for domestic violence by registered nurses in the emergency department. *Crit Care Nurs Quart.* 1999;22:27–41.

Shea CA, Mahoney M, Lacy JM. Breaking through the barriers to domestic violence intervention. *Am J Nurs.* 1997;97:26–33.

Knight MA. Ethical debate: should doctors be more proactive as advocates for victims of violence? The police surgeon's view medical paternalism is unacceptable. *BMJ.* 1995;311:1620–1621.

Markowitz JR, Steer S, Garland M. Hospital-based interventions for intimate partner violence victims: a forensic nursing model. *J Emerg Nurs.* 2005;31:166–170.

Rhodes KV, Lauderdale DS, He T, et al. "Between me and the computer": increased detection of intimate partner violence using a computer questionnaire. *Ann Emerg Med.* 2002;40:476–484.

17 | Male Interpersonal Violence Overview

Mark Zwanger, MD

INTRODUCTION

Male interpersonal violence is an underreported medical condition that is often not recognized by medical practitioners. Although women are typically associated with the word *rape*, the male patient can also be a rape victim by either another man or a woman. To accommodate gender neutrality, the term *sexual assault* is commonly used with this terminology encompassing a broad spectrum of violent sexual acts. In the male patient, the types of acts included under *sexual assault* are the penetration of a male patient's mouth by a penis or tongue as well as the insertion into the anus of a tongue, penis, finger(s), or other objects.

Male sexual assaults occur for many of the same reasons that they occur with women and are usually not sexually motivated. Some of these reasons include control or power over others, acts of retaliation or retribution, issues related to violence or degradation, effects of drugs or alcohol, and unresolved sexual conflicts.[1]

The prevalence of male sexual assault is difficult to determine accurately. Studies suggest that anywhere from 2–10% of all rapes in the United States involve men as the victim.[1–7] In a 2006 publication by the US Department of Justice, it is estimated that 2.8 million men in the United States have been raped—this number would suggest that nearly 1 out of every 33 men has been a victim of a male sexual assault.[7] Most experts also acknowledge the possibility that this number could be underreported.

The US Department of Justice estimates that there were 366,460 rapes and sexual assaults annually from 1992 to 2000. Of this number, approximately 9,040 males were victims of a completed rape, 10,270 males were victims of an attempted rape, and 17,130 males were victims of other types of sexual assault. Six percent of all completed rapes were male victims, 9% of all attempted rapes involved male victims, and 11% of sexual assaults were directed against men as the victim.[2]

Many incorrectly believe that homosexual men are responsible for most male-to-male rapes when in reality the majority of men who rape other men are identified as heterosexual.[1,5,6,8,9] The victim's sexual orientation is also varied, with Reeves reporting that of male patients undergoing forensic examination for sexual assault, 30% were heterosexual, 34% were homosexual, and the remaining 36% did not provide a sexual orientation.[10]

In general, male victims of sexual assault are assaulted by a stranger almost as often as by an acquaintance; recent data, however, suggest that only 22.8% of male rapes are by strangers and that the assailant is an acquaintance most of the time. These acquaintances include family, friends, teachers, coworkers, or neighbors. A current or former intimate partner was involved in the rape of a male victim more than 9% of the time. Four percent of male sexual assault victims have been raped by a spouse or an ex-spouse, 3.7% by a current or former cohabiting partner, and 2.7% by a current or former date.[7]

Male victims tend to be young, single, and homeless. Often the victims have physical, psychiatric, or cognitive difficulties as well as involvement with alcohol, drugs, or other substance abuse.[11] The perpetrator was using drugs or alcohol 58.5% of the time whereas the victim was using drugs or alcohol 38.3% of the time. Almost 65% of the adult male rapes occurred in the victim's home.[7]

Male sexual assaults are often more violent than female assaults are, and weapons of violence are frequently involved.[11] Tiaden published that physical violence was reported in 34% of male sexual assaults with the perpetrator using a weapon 8% of the time. In 21% of these cases, the male victim thought that he or someone close to him would be seriously harmed or killed.[7]

The majority of sexual assault patients do not report their assault to the police. Tiaden notes that only 12% of adult male patients reported the rape to the police.[7] This lack of reporting of sexual assaults to the police is common for both injured as well as uninjured patients.[2]

DOMESTIC VIOLENCE

Most individuals think about male sexual assault and automatically assume the perpetrator was another male, possibly a stranger, an acquaintance, or friend. About 85% of the time, male victims are raped by another male; however, 18.2% of male victims report being raped by a female; in contrast less than 1% of female victims are raped by another female (total percentages are greater than 100% because some individuals are raped by both male and female assailants).[7]

US Department of Justice data for 1993–2001 document 691,710 nonfatal violent victimizations committed by current or former spouses, boyfriends, or girlfriends of the victims. The victims of these crimes of intimate partner violence are predominantly female, but 103,220 (15%) crimes were directed against men and included interpersonal violent acts such as rape, sexual assault, robbery, aggravated assault, and simple assault.[12]

The following bullets illustrate the prevalence of violence directed against men:

- In 2003, 10% (521,740) of violent crimes were committed by the victim's intimate partner. Women (19%) were victimized by intimate partners at a greater rate than were men (3%).[13]
- In 2003, 9% of murder victims were killed by their spouse or intimate partner. Seventy-nine percent of those victims were female and 21% were male.[14]
- Forty-four percent of the victims of lesbian, gay, bisexual, and transsexual (LGBT) domestic violence were men, 36% women, and 2% transgender. Gender identity was not recorded for 9%.[15]

The data on abuse of male husbands by wives or female spouses are limited. Because of societal biases, violence directed against male patients is likely to be very underreported and consequently overlooked by the healthcare provider. It is estimated that 1.5% of men are victims of domestic abuse by a female partner.[16]

Mechem published a much higher number, reporting that 12.6% of male patients interviewed in an emergency department setting had been victims of domestic violence committed by a female intimate partner during the prior year. They defined domestic violence to include both physical and sexual assaults. They also report that 7% of male patient victims were forced to have sex.[17]

In intimate relationships where domestic violence does occur, male victims frequently do not report the abuse because of embarrassment, self-image or self-esteem issues, a belief that they will be rejected by friends or family members, concerns that they will not be believed by police or healthcare workers, or concern that they will be ridiculed, made fun of, or belittled by commentary expecting that the male victim should have been stronger and more forceful. Police and healthcare workers often inject their own biases and query the male patient about what he did to cause the woman to hit him. These actions are all deterrents for a male patient to report a complaint of domestic abuse.[18,19] Some battered men are also concerned that they will end up being arrested and, in a twisted chain of events, end up accused of being the assailant if the police are involved. Mechem found that a minority of male victims contacted the police—only 19%.[17]

A variety of researchers have found that men and women tend to be equally physically abusive in relationships.[20,21] Herzberger found that the incidences of violent spousal abuse by men (27%) and women (24%) against a partner are actually very similar.[22] There also seems to be a double standard in which society is more accepting of a woman being the aggressor than a man. Burczyk and Standing's research indicates that there is less support and less sympathy for male victims of assault than there is for female victims.[23] According to Paul Szabo, a Justice Department survey of 60,000 individuals found that people believed a husband's stabbing his wife to death 40% worse than a wife stabbing her husband to death.[24]

Other biases that affect male sexual assault are based upon individual perceptions of sexual identity. Davies studied gender identity of perpetrator and victim and found that male participants regarded the female perpetrator in more favorable terms regardless of the victim's sexual orientation.[25] Victims also receive more blame if their sexual orientation suggests potential attraction to the perpetrator with gay men and heterosexual women more often blamed as victims when compared to lesbians or heterosexual men.[26]

There is also little information about men being assaulted by male partners who are in homosexual relationships, although some gay and lesbian organizations cite figures that 25% of gay and lesbian individuals suffer as victims of domestic violence. A recent study from Hong Kong indicates that gays and lesbians are 60% more likely to be battered by partners than are people in opposite-sex relationships.[27]

HEALTHCARE PROVIDER'S ROLE

The healthcare provider must examine and care for any life-threatening conditions first while assessing for physical injuries, providing emotional support, and offering a sensitive and supportive environment. The practitioner's role is also to provide information, answer questions that arise, offer counseling for emotional trauma, and in accordance with the local environment both document and obtain legal evidence for potential prosecution of the sexual assault.

Systems should be in place to deal empathetically, openly, and with expertise when collecting information, examining the patient, and providing appropriate follow-up needs for the assaulted patient. A multidisciplinary approach typically offers more complete care and includes emergency department physicians, nurses, social workers, and other individuals who can offer support and counseling; these latter individuals might include psychologists, counselors, chaplains, or community victim support groups.

Most male patients will feel embarrassed and reluctant to discuss a sexual assault and therefore will not be very forthcoming. Some male patients will feel that their masculinity has been tarnished or stripped away. It is the healthcare provider's responsibility to make the patient feel comfortable and to be supportive of the patient's needs. It is important to provide emotional support to the male patient who is a victim of a sexual assault while reassuring the patient that this does not change his sexual identity or gender identification should the question arise.

The medical evaluation of the male sexual assault patient follows similar protocols and guidelines used for the female sexual assault patient. Refer to Chapter 15 for more information about sexual examination collection and step-by-step basic examination guidelines. In general, the sexual assault evidence collection procedures are essentially the same for a male victim as for a female victim. In the male victim, more emphasis is placed on the anal examination. In addition, attention should be paid to obtaining possible fluid from the penis itself, especially when the perpetrator committed fellatio on the victim.

The following discussion provides information on the history and physical examination as related to the male sexual assault patient. The history should be taken in a private area and preferably alone. The healthcare provider should be sympathetic and, when interviewing the patient, allow the patient the opportunity to discuss issues of domestic abuse, interpersonal violence, unsafe environment, and/or details of this or other sexual assaults. Questions should initially be open ended, although direct questioning about physical, mental, or sexual abuse, violence, and safety should all be addressed.

The history of a sexual assault should be succinct while documenting pertinent information about when the event occurred, the use of force, complaints of physical abuse, use of drugs or alcohol, and the type of sexual contact. The male patient should be queried about oral and anal penile penetration and whether the assailant ejaculated in his mouth or rectum. What the victim did after the assault such as showering, defecating, changing clothing, and so forth should also be noted.

After the physician has determined the need for any life-saving treatments, the physical examination should closely inspect the anal and genital regions because sodomy is the most likely type of sexual assault on the male patient.[28] The examiner looks for signs of trauma over the patient's entire body, but particularly in the anogenital region because there may be evidence of bruising, redness, swelling, tenderness, tearing, fissures, and finger or tooth marks in this region. The anal sphincter may also be torn with decreased tone being present. Rectal injuries can appear as a linear tear from the anus into the rectum. Anoscopy or proctoscopy should be performed if bleeding or tears are noted. Anoscopy with toluidine blue can be used to detect injury. If there was oral penetration, the mouth is examined for cuts, soreness, swelling, gum tenderness, and bleeding as well.

The penis should be examined for bleeding or discharge. Swabs should be taken from the glans of the penis as well as along the shaft for possible DNA evidence. One alternative technique for the shaft of the penis is to use a moistened sterile 2 × 2 gauze pad. The pad is wiped along the entire shaft of the penis and allowed to air dry. A second pad is then wiped over the area and allowed to air dry. Both pads are then packaged in the rape kit and labeled.

The absence of any anal injury is a frequent finding and should not discount the history that the patient was sexually assaulted. McLean et al note that 18% of the patients they treated for male-on-male rape had anal injuries, but this statistic also indicates that the majority of the patients seen had no anal injury.[29] A recent Department of Justice report documents similar data with 16% of male rape victims suffering an injury during the attack.[7]

The sexual assault kit includes collecting for potential bodily fluids from the assailant that might be used as evidence in legal proceedings. It is therefore essential to maintain a chain of evidence for police. Rape kits should be collected according to local protocols and procedures.

Male patients should also be treated with prophylaxis for sexually transmitted infections. Because of increasing resistance, oral fluoroquinolones should not be used. When appropriate, HIV postexposure prophylaxis should be offered following the Centers for Disease Control and Prevention guidelines.

In general, most men are unlikely to use an emergency department for minor injuries such as cuts, abrasions, bruises, or contusions, but they might present for medical conditions. Because spousal abuse is frequently unrecognized and subsequently underreported, it is a good idea to ask screening questions of all patients who present to the emergency department about whether they are the victim of interpersonal violence or spousal abuse. Examiners should be suspicious if the partner of the abused answers questions or refuses to leave the victim alone. Explain to the patient that it is his right to be in a safe environment and work with social workers, police, or other government agencies for that goal.

SEQUELAE OF MALE SEXUAL ASSAULT

The victim of a sexual assault or an act of interpersonal violence may experience post-traumatic stress disorder symptoms. These symptoms can include reexperiencing the trauma or avoidance of similar trauma-related stimuli. Anger, irritability, sexual dysfunction, phobias, situational difficulties, sleeping disorders, depression, thoughts of self-harm, feelings of helplessness, and suicide are some of the symptoms that can manifest. Some male victims may develop a loss of their male identity, have confusion about their sexual orientation, or question their masculinity. Tiaden found that 25% of men who were raped needed mental health counseling, and 10% lost time from work.[7]

UNIQUE PATIENT POPULATIONS

The prison system is where many male sexual assaults occur. It is estimated that 140,000 prisoners are sexually abused annually in the United States.[30] Hensley published that 18% of prisoners reported inmate-on-inmate sexual threats, and 8.5% reported they had been sexually assaulted by another inmate while incarcerated.[31] Struckman-Johnson and Struckman-Johnson report similar statistics with 21% of male prisoners being coerced into having sex and 4% raped.[32] Within the prison environment, rape and sexual assaults again reflect the issues of power and control that these activities portray as well as the lack of opportunities for sexual activity with female companions.

The military is also a potential environment where unreported male sexual assaults may occur. Only a few reports of male violence in the armed forces exist, but there is a general perception that service members are less likely to report the crime because of possible retaliation. Martin found that 1.8% of men in the military report experiencing an attempted rape, but most of these encounters were before entering the military.[33]

PEDIATRIC MALE PATIENTS

Seventy percent of male victims are raped before their 18th birthday, and 48% of men are younger than age 12 when they are first raped.[7] De Jong reports that of the male pediatric patients who were sexually abused, 59% knew their assailants, who were frequently other relatives, and anal intercourse was attempted with 78% of the victims.[34]

When pediatric patients are seen in the emergency department with a complaint of rectal injury or trauma, sexual abuse should always be considered because Kadish et al. found that accidental injury to the anogenital area is uncommon in the pediatric population.[35] The most common physical findings in sexual abuse of male pediatric patients are the presence of rectal scars or skin tags (79%); localized venous engorgement (20%); sphincter dilation (18%); thickened, asymmetrical rectal folds (16%); and rectal lacerations/tears/abrasions (13%).[34]

CONCLUSION

Male interpersonal violence is underreported and underrecognized by healthcare personnel. Male victims are often embarrassed or ashamed that they were victimized. Emergency departments and sexual assault centers should have protocols in place to accommodate the medical, forensic, and psychological needs of male victims, especially victims of sexual assault.

REFERENCES

1. Groth AN, Burgess AW. Male rape: offenders and victims. *Am J Psychiatry.* 1980;137(7):806–810.
2. Rennison CM. Rape and sexual assault: reporting to the police and medical attention, 1992–2000. *Bureau of Justice Statistics Selected Findings.* August 2002; NCJ 194530. Available at: http://www.ojp.usdoj.gov/bjs/pub/pdf/rsarp00.pdf. Accessed August 13, 2008.
3. Kaufman A, Divasto P, Jackson R, et al. Male rape victims: noninstitutionalized assault. *Am J Psychiatry.* 1980;137(2):221–223.
4. Pesola GR, Westfal RE, Kuffner CA. Emergency department characteristics of male sexual assault. *Acad Emerg Med.* 1999;6:792–798.
5. Hillman R. Adult male victims of sexual assault: an underdiagnosed condition. *Int J STDs AIDS.* 1991;2:22–24.
6. Scarce M. Same-sex rape of male college students. *J Am College Health.* January 1997;45:171–173.
7. Tiaden P, Thoennes N. *Extent, Nature, and Consequences of Rape Victimization. Findings from the National Violence Against Women Survey.* Washington, DC: US Department of Justice; January 2006; NCJ 210346. Available at: http://www.ncjrs.gov/pdffiles1/nij/210346.pdf. Accessed August 13, 2008.
8. McMullen R. *Male Rape: Breaking the Silence on the Last Taboo.* London: Gay Men's Press; 1990.
9. Huckle PL. Male rape victims referred to a forensic psychiatric service. *Med Sci Law.* 1995;35:187–192.
10. Reeves I, Jawad R, Welch J. Risk of undiagnosed infection in men attending a sexual assault referral centre. *Sex Transm Infect.* 2004;80(6):524–525.
11. Stermac L, Del Bove G, Addison M. Stranger and acquaintance sexual assault of adult males. *J Interpers Violence.* 2004;19(8):901–915.
12. Rennison CM. Intimate partner violence, 1993–2001. *Bureau of Justice Statistics Crime Data Brief.* February 2003; NCJ 197838. Available at: http://www.ojp.usdoj.gov/bjs/pub/pdf/ipv01.pdf. Accessed August 13, 2008.

13. Catalno S. *Criminal Victimization, 2003*. Washington, DC: Bureau of Justice Statistics, US Department of Justice; 2004.
14. Federal Bureau of Investigation. *Crime in the United States, 2003*. Washington, DC: FBI, US Department of Justice; 2004.
15. National Coalition of Anti-Violence Programs. *Lesbian, Gay, Bisexual, and Transgender Domestic Violence: 2003 Supplement*. New York, NY: National Coalition of Anti-Violence Program; 2004.
16. Scott-Tilley D. Nursing interventions for domestic violence. *Am J Nurs*. 1999;99:24JJ–29JJ.
17. Mechem CC, Shofer FS, Reinhard SS, et al. History of domestic violence among male patients presenting to an urban emergency department. *Acad Emerg Med*. 1999;6(8):786–791.
18. Walker J, Archer J, Davies M. Most effects of rape on men: a descriptive analysis. *Arch Sex Behav*. 2005:34(1).
19. Mezey G, King M. The effects of sexual assault on men: a survey of 22 victims. *Psychol Med*. 1989:19(1):205–209.
20. Biller HB. The battered spouse may be male. *Brown Univ Child Adolescent Behav Letter*. 1995;1–3.
21. Strauss MA, Gelles RJ, Steinmetz SK. *Behind Closed Doors: Violence in American Families*. New York, NY: Doubleday; 1986.
22. Hertzberger S. Violence with the family. Boulder, Colo: Westview Press; 1996.
23. Burczyk K, Standing L. Attitudes towards rape victims: effects of victim status, sex of victim, and sex of rater. *Soc Behav Personality*. 1989;17(1):1–8.
24. Szabo P. Violence against men. In: Szabo P, ed. *Tragic Tolerance of Domestic Violence*. 1998:24–34. Available at: http://amen.ie/Downloads/26016.pdf. Accessed August 13, 2008.
25. Davies M, Pollard P, Archer J. Effects of perpetrator gender and victim sexuality on blame toward male victims of sexual assault. *J Soc Psychol*. June 2006;146(3):275–291.
26. Wakelin A, Long KM. Effects of victim gender and sexuality on attributions of blame to rape victims. *Sex Roles*. 2004;49:477–487.
27. Hong Kong News. Gays 60 percent more prone to domestic abuse: survey. February 15, 2007. Available at: http://www.hongkongnews.net/story/228408. Accessed March 15, 2008.
28. Standing Together Against Rape. Male victim of sexual assault. 2005. Available at: http://www.staralaska.com/scripts/malerape.asp. Accessed August 13, 2008.
29. McLean IA, Balding V, White C. Forensic medical aspects of male-on-male rape and sexual assault in greater Manchester. *Med Sci Law*. 2004;44(2):165–169.
30. Mariner J. No escape: male rape in US prisons. Human Rights Watch, 2001. Available at: http://www.hrw.org/reports/2001/prison/report.html. Accessed September 23, 2008.
31. Hensley C. Examining the characteristics of male assault targets in a southern maximum security prison. *J Interpersonal Violence*. 2005;20(6):667–679.
32. Struckman-Johnson C, Struckman-Johnson D. Sexual coercion rates in seven Midwestern prison facilities for men. *Prison J*. 200;80(4):379–390. Available at: http://www.justdetention.org/pdf/struckman.pdf. Accessed March 23, 2008.
33. Martin L, Rosen L, Durand DB, et al. Prevalence and timing of sexual assaults in a sample of male and female US Army soldiers. *Mil Med*. 1998;163(4):213–216.
34. De Jong AR, Emmett GA, Hervada AA. Epidemiologic factors in sexual abuse of boys. *Am J Dis Child*. 1982:136:990–993.
35. Kadish HA, Schunk JE, Britton H. Pediatric male rectal and genital trauma: accidental and nonaccidental injuries. *Pediatr Emerg Care*. 1998;14(2):95–98.

18 Physical Child Maltreatment

Raquel Mora, MD

INTRODUCTION

Child maltreatment has been in existence long before the symptoms were recognized by society—unfortunately, the medical community lagged even farther behind. The time of public awareness of child abuse to the extent of proposed action is marked in history by the pivotal story of Mary Ellen Wilson that took place in 1874.[1] Since that time, societal organizations and legal terminology were invented to care for these children. Not until the 1940s did Caffey enlighten the medical community through recognition of children with chronic subdural hematomas associated with multiple fractures in different stages of healing.[2] Though many of these children no doubt present to social service agencies, there are a staggering number of children who have met with the medical community whose condition of maltreatment went unnoticed before the allegations of abuse occurred.

The psychosocial nature of abuse lends to the likelihood of recurrence of the abuse unless the child is removed from the risk.[3,4] It wasn't until the 1960s after Kempe published "The Battered Child Syndrome" that states began implementing laws mandating the report of child abuse.[5] Though the laws began in the 1960s, the increases in reports began occurring in the 1980s possibly because of continued public education and increasing physician awareness. With this increase in reports came an increase in the number of unfounded or false accusations. This has swayed many physicians into making attempts to "investigate" the possibility of maltreatment from the bedside and reforming the suspicion into "possible innocence" of the parent. Unfortunately, this results in an increase in not reporting actual cases and heightens the risk of the child returning later with worse injuries or even death.

The studies done by Southall allowed for the dissolution of the myth "seemingly good parents" being associated with maltreatment.[6,7] It is the responsibility of the medical community to understand the limitations of the medical history, the physical examination, and the diagnostic procedures available. Screening methods are being investigated to capture the covert abuse cases while excluding the mimickers; however, none are proof enough for such reliability.[8] Though difficult for many physicians, it is acceptable to state uncertainty but still be able to protect the child with reports of concerns and allow the trained investigators to invalidate or substantiate the suspicion. The focus of this chapter is the medical evaluation in physical and neglectful child maltreatment.

EPIDEMIOLOGY

It is difficult to obtain the precise statistics for child maltreatment because of underreporting and variability of reporting in each state; however, national organizations have made considerable strides in developing incidence of child maltreatment throughout the United States. Each year there is an estimated national annual reporting of 3 million cases of child maltreatment from which a almost one-third are substantiated.[9] In 2003, the US Department of Health and Human Services Children's Bureau reported the incidence of maltreatment in artificial categories of maltreatment (many children that suffer from one aspect typically are subjected to one of the other forms as well): neglect (>60%), physical (20%), sexual (10%), emotional (5%), and other types (17%). More than half of the reported cases are reported by professionals: educators, medical, legal, and social services.

Though there is no uniform system for national reports of child maltreatment injuries and deaths, studies and current reports demonstrate children younger than 3 years old have the highest rates of victimization and make up the largest component of children who die as a result of maltreatment.[9,10] Although most national statistical compilations do not further stratify age of maltreatment, a few studies have demonstrated the highest rate of battering injury and/or neglect among infants to occur in the 0–5 months age range,[11–13] and this is the age range for which homicide is the leading cause of death.[14] It is estimated that 10% of children that present to the emergency department have been physically abused.[15] Table 18-1 reviews risk factors for abuse.

EVALUATION: HISTORY

Although the emergency department is not the ideal location for child maltreatment evaluation, this is often the site of the initial presentation. One of the important aspects to remember is the goal of the physician is to obtain sufficient history that can determine the course of medical evaluation for the patient.

Once the concern for maltreatment is present, it is important to discuss the matter individually with the caregivers. The inquiry begins with a synopsis of who, what, when, and where questions. It is important to keep these questions open ended (such as, "Can you tell us what happened?" or "How was your child injured?") so that the answers can be elaborated on by the person providing the information. It is additionally important to obtain as much information not only about the symptoms (last known time of normal mentation, time and sequential development of symptoms, etc.) but also regarding the biomechanics of the environment leading to the injury, such as the height of the fall, the number of stairs involved in the fall, the potential areas of impact the child may have sustained, and so forth.

Important is the question of developmental capability of the child. This can determine the plausible acts that the child can or cannot perform in relation to the injury. One study that evaluated trauma in children younger than 3 months old found the most common history offered was a fall from a bed or a couch, though most children younger than age 3 months cannot roll over.[16] From these answers, the suspicion or actual disclosure may unfold, but more important, the events can be compared to the injuries once the diagnostic studies are obtained to determine whether the mechanics are plausible in relation to the injuries sustained. If the concern for child maltreatment arises during the course of obtaining the history, it may be best for the medical personnel to allow the disclosure to continue until an opportunity occurs to discuss the situation apart from the child or other family members present.

Children are impressionable and often seek appropriate responses from caregivers. Thus, whenever possible, the history should be obtained separately from both the child and the caregiver. It is important not to introduce new vocabulary to the child's words or correct colloquial terms that the child may use for certain body parts. Typically, the medical examiner will confirm the area of reference the child is using by having the child point to or describe the area he or she is talking about. Additionally, the child should be asked open-ended questions or questions with more than yes or no answers to prevent leading questions.

If the caregiver can provide enough history to give sufficient information for a medical evaluation, there is often no need for the medical examiner to obtain further history from the child, especially if the child has limited verbal skills. Because it is likely that the child will be interviewed by the police or social services, if at all possible it is best to limit the frequency with which the child will need to recount the events.

Unfortunately, many instances of child maltreatment are not obvious in the presentation. In a study evaluating fractures of children younger than 3 years old, in the initial history in only 1 of the 52 cases of maltreatment did the parent state that the child was injured by an adult.[21] More than half of the presenting histories from caregivers were regarding an abnormality (seizure or difficulty with limb movement), one-quarter complained of falls, 10% stated the child was hit by an older child, and 6% stated the injury was self-inflicted. In a small number of cases, shaking in attempts to resuscitate was offered as a potential cause for injury.[22,23]

To make matters more complicated, a recent study demonstrated that no history of trauma in a child with head injury was highly specific for maltreatment.[24] Many behavioral signs and symptoms may arouse suspicion of maltreatment, such as lack of parental concern for the child's well-being, the

TABLE 18-1 **Risk Factors of Child Abuse**

Child factors
- Young age[16]
- Developmental handicaps
- Prematurity[17]
- Special needs child[18]
- Child in residential or foster care[19]

Caregiver factors
- Age of mother[13]
  - Younger than 19 years old with second or subsequent infant born
  - Maternal age younger than 17 years
  - No prenatal care[13]
- Stresses
  - After natural disaster[20]
  - Poverty/unemployment
  - Substance abuse
  - Domestic violence
  - Mental illness/developmental delay
- Parenting skills
  - Unrealistic developmental expectations of child
  - Poor impulse control

Discipline versus corporal punishment
- The laws that state which inflicted bruises may rise to criminal child abuse vary from state to state. Thus, it is recommended that physicians be aware of the criminal statutes and laws within their state of practice.

Environmental factors

Social factors

Inconsistent history
- Developmentally improbable
- Injury inconsistent with reported mechanism
- Historical alternates (story keeps changing)

parent describing or treating the child consistently in a negative manner, the child shrinking in the presence of parents or other adults, the child apparently lacking needed medical or general care, and so forth. In such instances, medical personnel may have a challenging time obtaining information. It is important to obtain as much information about the events surrounding and preceding the injury and/or symptoms prior to obtaining diagnostic studies because the findings may lead caregivers to offer "new" or "alternative" histories as potential injury patterns become revealed.

Though child services and legal organizations seek definitive yes or no answers from the medical community regarding the existence of potential for abusive injuries, there are in fact less-structured answers medical practitioners can offer. The answers lay in the presumption or suspicion of abuse being maintained as *highly suspicious for abuse, concerning for abuse,* and *less likely abuse* (i.e., likely accidental). The role of medical personnel is not to confirm the existence of maltreatment, but instead to report the suspicion to proper agencies and make attempts to ensure the child's safety.

With concern for abusive head injury, the timing of symptomatic events is important because the child is typically solely in the custody of the abuser immediately prior to the development of symptoms.[25,26] Most children with moderate to severe inflicted head injury become symptomatic immediately and exhibit depressed levels of consciousness, respiratory distress, apnea, and often seizures.[26,27] A head injury that affects the child's level of consciousness suggests diffuse as opposed to focal brain injury.[28,29] The timing of events from one symptom to another can vary, and prediction of the timing of events to death is currently not possible.[27]

Falls

Falls are one of the most common causes of nonfatal injuries to children; thus, it is understood that the history of fall is one of the most common explanations offered for presentation of injury in the emergency department. A majority of falls occur in children younger than 5 years of age, with a predominance in the summer months. Because the clinician must determine whether the injury is consistent with the mechanism, the question arises regarding the nature of the fall and whether the impact was sufficient enough to cause the injury and the severity of the injury.

Short falls (≤ 3 feet) from beds, couches, car seats, and bouncy seats (inappropriately placed) in infants have been shown in numerous studies to result in no serious sequelae.[30–39] Skull fractures may occur with a tendency for simple linear fractures, but can be depressed or complex.[40] These fractures are often without neurologic sequelae and infrequently associated with intracranial injury (up to 7%) or retinal hemorrhages (up to 9%).[27,30–33,35,41–48]

In evaluating stairway injuries in children, there is rarely injury to more than one body part, and life-threatening injuries do not commonly occur.[49–51] In 1988, more than 300 children who fell down steps were studied.[49] Most of the injuries involved the head and neck (more than 70%) with about one-quarter extremity injuries. None of the children suffered any life-threatening injuries.

Falls cause a small number of abdominal injuries (3%), and the severity is less than would be inflicted in a motor vehicle collision.[52]

Falls that have been associated with significant injury are walker related,[53,54] falls while the infant is in the arms of an adult,[50] bunk bed falls,[36,55] playground falls (regardless of height),[56] and falls from nonhousehold heights (one or more stories or ≥ 12 feet).[34,38,46,57–59] Skull fractures are common[43] and include a risk of mortality if these falls are associated with epidural hematomas, focal subdural with mass effect, or cervical fractures. Fortunately, given the number of children who experience these types of falls, these injuries are few in number but are frequently not fatal. Of note is that these injury patterns are not typically seen in inflicted pediatric head injury.

Acute Life-Threatening Events

An acute life-threatening event (ALTE) is characterized by combination of apnea, color change, marked change in muscle tone, choking, or gagging. Estimated incidence of ALTEs in children are between 0.5–3%,[60] and no cause will be found in half of these patients. Because abusive maneuvers may be performed to mimic ALTE (smothering, poisoning, shaken baby syndrome), child maltreatment is a potential etiology.[6,61,62] Recently dilated fundoscopy was shown to be a potential screening tool for retinal hemorrhage for the possibility of SBS in infants who present with ALTE.[60] Other findings that may be useful in the early diagnosis of inflicted ALTE are the presence of oral and/or nasal bleeding in association with the ALTE, positive family history of other sibling deaths, previous apnea, and age older than 6 months.[61]

Sudden Infant Death Syndrome

Sudden infant death syndrome (SIDS) cannot be differentiated from child maltreatment without an autopsy and a thorough investigation. SIDS is the sudden death of an infant under 1 year of age whose death remains unexplained after a complete autopsy and thorough investigation. SIDS peaks between 2–4 months of age, with 90% occurring by 6 months of age with a predominance in males.[63] It is estimated that infanticide among cases diagnosed as SIDS may occur up to 5%.[64,65] Suffocation, through smothering, is an uncommon form of child maltreatment and of child homicide; however, it can present with recurrent episodes of apnea or death, which may be erroneously diagnosed as SIDS.[61]

EVALUATION: OVERALL PHYSICAL EXAMINATION

The pediatric patient poses unique difficulties in determining the potential for injury. There is a constant state of growth from perinatal origins through infancy, adolescence, and finally into adulthood. Throughout each stage, structures mature at differing rates, and thus injury patterns and outcomes in various systems can vary from one age group to the next.[66] These developmental conditions are ever considered in the evaluation of pediatric injury and have led to the types of injuries, diagnostic modalities, and therapies stratified by age.

The child's emergent conditions should be addressed initially and resuscitative measures should be implemented immediately in the unstable or potentially unstable child. However, in the stable child, a different approach may be preferred. The examination should be performed in the usual manner from head to toe and not simply focused on the obvious injuries. Not only can a focus on the injuries cause increased anxiety in the child, but it may also lead to missing subtle findings on physical examination. The child should be completely disrobed (including removal of the diaper) to evaluate all areas of the scalp, eyes, oral cavity, thoracic and abdominal areas, skin, extremities, genitalia, and neurological status, complete with observed developmental capabilities.

Photographs should be obtained whenever possible and should not replace descriptive documentation. It is helpful to have a form of measurement in the pictures, such as a ruler or a penny (an object whose size is consistent), especially in close-up pictures.

EVALUATION: DIAGNOSTIC TESTING

Which types of diagnostic testing to perform are typically determined by the history and physical. A misleading history can result in an erroneous diagnostic pathway and thus an incorrect diagnosis. In cases of suspected child maltreatment, it is not uncommon to follow a diagnostic pathway that may differ from the complaint, but that ensures the child's occult medical, social, and legal needs are met.

Laboratory

No laboratory studies are pathognomonic for abuse; however, many studies are indicated to screen for organic disease and illness.

Alkaline Phosphatase

Elevations are usually caused by liver or bone sources; thus, this test has recently been evaluated for the potential of screening for bony injury in children. Currently, no guidelines exist for evaluating asymptomatic patients with abnormal levels.[67]

Coagulations Studies

In the presence of hematomas or bleeding when evaluating for abusive injury, many physicians obtain coagulation studies to determine preexisting conditions for potential risk for injury. Recently, elevated coagulation studies have been noted to occur as a complication of pediatric head injury and not as reflections of a previous condition. Thus, the serology is performed for screening for complications of consumptive coagulopathy (disseminated intravascular coagulopathy, or DIC) as a complication of head injury and is neither specific for abuse nor indicative of a preexisting hematologic condition.[68]

Lactate

The use of lactate as a marker for prognostic measures is not unique in trauma patients. The presence of lactate is associated with hypoxic-ischemic injuries within the body, and in patients with inflicted brain injury, elevated serial lactate levels have been shown to be a marker for worsening clinical outcomes than those with lower lactate levels.[69]

Liver/Pancreatic Enzymes

An increase in liver or pancreatic enzymes may suggest abdominal trauma[70,71]—even in the presence of a normal CT scan. Unfortunately, liver function levels can return to normal within 24–48 hours, and thus if there is a delay in care for a patient with intra-abdominal injury, the levels may not reflect the recent injury.[70]

Urinalysis

Hematuria is an important marker for renal and nonrenal injury in children. The abdominal physical examination with the urinalysis can detect 98% of all intra-abdominal injuries.[72]

Radiographic Studies

More than 80% of all identified child abuse cases in the United States are detected through radiographic testing.[73] In the symptomatic child or the child presenting with specific injury, there is little dilemma regarding the diagnostic workup. The question of whether to perform radiologic tests on the asymptomatic child with a normal examination but a suspicion for physical child maltreatment arises. Imaging for potential maltreatment not only identifies the extent of possible injury but may also lead to other diagnoses.[74–76]

X-Rays

In infants who present with fractures, more than half of the fractures are found to be caused by abuse or neglect,[16,77] and 80% of these are in infants 18 months of age or younger. In nonambulatory infants specifically (usually < 1 year old), up to 60% of fractures are inflicted.[25] Many of these fractures are not only multiple, but occult because they may lack overlying bruising or significant swelling.[75,78]

Though no radiographic findings are pathognomonic for abuse, some are highly suggestive of inflicted injury. In the nonverbal and often nonambulatory patient, the screening modality requires diversity because the localization of injury for such patients is not possible. Additionally, infants are found to have injuries in different stages of healing in different areas of the body, thus expanding the areas that require investigation.[21,79]

The skeletal survey consists of two views of all the bones of the patient's body. Additional oblique views are obtained for areas more difficult to visualize, such as the ribs, not of the "babygram" type (multiple areas on the same film).[76] Retrospective studies have determined the diagnostic yield for the skeletal survey is inversely related to age: the older the child, the less useful the survey.[80–86] Thus, the current recommendations are as follows: a skeletal survey should be performed in all cases of suspected abuse in children younger than 2 years old, and a skeletal survey should be used selectively in children 2–5 years of age. There is no role for a skeletal survey in the management of children older than 5 years.[76,87,88]

A skull X-ray is included, even when obtaining a head CT because the CT can miss small fractures in the axial plane.[88] In a child where the suspicion of maltreatment is present and an initial skeletal survey returns with or without findings, a follow-up skeletal survey 2 weeks after the initial may increase the diagnostic yield.[89] This improves the diagnosis multifold by confirming or refuting uncertain fractures as well as providing the potential for dating fractures.[90] Skull fractures are an exception because they do not go through the stages of healing that long bones do. A difficulty with fracture dating includes limited literary evidence for methods of radiographic dating.[91]

Bone Scintigraphy

Bone scintigraphy may be a useful adjunct to plain films because it can detect fractures missed on X-ray as a result of overlaying shadows (particularly rib fractures), spinal fracture, and diaphyseal fractures, and it can detect periosteal injuries from trauma without fractures.[75,88] Diaphyseal injury can occur when someone grabs the child's extremities (especially the humerus) and shakes, which can result in bowing or bending, and which may never show on plain film.[92] The use of bone scanning alone to screen for concerns of fractures related to abuse would only identify 20% of patients and thus is not recommended.[93,94] But to use both modalities as a screen would subject many children to unnecessary amounts of radiation. So, when used selectively with the skeletal survey, the sensitivity can be greatly increased.[95,96]

Limitations of scintigraphy include difficulty in detecting old fractures,[95,96] metaphyseal injuries (most common and suggestive inflicted skeletal injury found in infants), subtle spinal fractures, and linear skull fractures.[97] Additionally, bone scans may be positive within hours of an injury[98] and may remain positive for up to 1 year; thus, the bone scan has no role in the potential for fracture dating.

Computed Tomography

Computed tomography (CT) without contrast is very sensitive and thus is the emergency standard for the initial evaluation of acute bleeding.[88]

Occult head injury is not a rare occurrence in the pediatric patient. Without the complication of concern for inflicted trauma, the presence of a skull fracture with or without intracranial injury has been cited to occur in about 10% or more of children younger than 2 years old who undergo CT scanning for head injury.[99–102] The highest incidence of intracranial injury in these studies is found to occur in infants 1 year of age or younger. Up to 45% of children at the time of the initial neuroimaging will have radiologic evidence of prior intracranial injuries.[66]

The signs and symptoms sought for evaluation of significant injury (loss of consciousness, emesis, seizure) are often not present in nonfatal pediatric patients with intracranial hemorrhage with or without skull fractures.[41,42,96,99,101–105] In a recent study that examined 51 children younger than 2 years old with a suspicion of child maltreatment and no neurological findings, 16 were found to have skull fracture and/or intracranial injury.[106] Of these patients, the skeletal survey failed to identify 5 patients. Thus, the skeletal survey alone cannot be used as a screening modality for head injury in children younger than 2 years.

Currently, the common practice is for a head CT to accompany the skeletal survey (including skull X-rays) in children younger than 2 years old with suspicion of abuse. Additionally, the timing of events becomes of concern with possible inflicted cranial injury, and undue pressure can be placed on physicians to create a time line of injury. It is important to note that radiographic timing of cranial injuries remains imprecise.[107]

Abdominal injuries offer a different radiographic dilemma in the potentially abused child. The injuries include rupture of the liver and/or spleen, ruptured viscous, duodenal hematoma, mesenteric vascular injury, pancreatic injury, and renal trauma.[108] With solid organs as the most common injury, CT scan is the initial modality of choice not only because of the high specificity and sensitivity for these areas, but also because it allows grading of the injury that can determine management. However, a negative scan does not exclude the possibility of other injuries: ruptured viscous, duodenal hematoma, and pancreatic injury.

For the ruptured viscous, although plain films may show pneumoperitoneum, pneumatosis intestinalis, or portal venous gas, CT will demonstrate intraperitoneal air in only 33% of patients. Duodenal hematomas may present with obstructive symptoms (bilious vomiting) lending to initial imaging not with a CT but with an upper gastrointestinal series that would fully delineate the hematoma. For the pancreas, the CT scan may show normal pancreas, ascites, or possible pseudocyst.[109] In the presence of symptoms concerning for pancreatic injury, an ultrasound, which is noninvasive, can help identify such injury.

Magnetic Resonance Imaging

Magnetic resonance imaging (MRI) is more accurate for determination of fluid collection of differing ages,[110] intraparenchymal lesions (as occurs with shearing forces),[111,112] as well as early identification of infarction.[113] Additionally, certain aspects of the brain are better visualized with MRI, such as the posterior fossa.[114] A common practice is to follow up the initial noncontrast CT scan with an MRI within 5–7 days of the initial presentation because the MRI is more sensitive and able to detect subacute or chronic injury.[88] Some centers with significant MRI availability may rely solely on serial MRI evaluations as the imaging of choice.

Ultrasound

In abuse cases, ultrasound is a noninvasive and painless mode of adjunctive imaging that is useful in diagnosing rib injuries and subperiosteal hemorrhage, which is an early indication of fracture.[115] An additional use for ultrasound may be indicated when epiphyseal separations are suspected on plain films.[88]

In young neonates with open fontanelles, ultrasound may be an option for both short- and long-term results of inflicted injury; however, its limitations include the potential to miss small subdural hemorrhages, especially interhemispheric,[88] and thus it is not used exclusively as a diagnostic tool for evaluation of inflicted injuries.

INJURIES

The next sections will review commonly seen abuse injuries associated with various body parts and regions. It will review mechanism of injury and expected patterns and presentation of that injury.

Head

Myelination of neurons continues beyond the perinatal age into infancy. As a result, the injury patterns, findings, and outcomes differ within each pediatric age group. Head injury is the most common cause of mortality in victims of child maltreatment who are younger than 2 years of age.[90] About 80% of deaths resulting from traumatic brain injury in children younger than 2 years are the result of abusive head trauma. Traumatic brain injury is the leading cause of death in children younger than 4 years.[88] The presentation varies tremendously: neurologically asymptomatic, excessive crying, poor feeding, lethargy, seizures, apnea, or cardiac arrest. These children may present without apparent external signs of trauma (swelling, bruising, fractures).[22,23,27,106,116,117] The varied presentation and limitations of the physical exam should thus prompt consideration of child maltreatment in the absence of a reliable history.

The difficulty of diagnosing inflicted head injury has been demonstrated through missed cases of head injury[118] and missed cases of abuse.[43,119] One study found that almost 20% of head injuries in hospitalized children were the result of an inflicted injury. In the missed cases of abuse,[118] a concerning finding was that one-third of the children less than 3 years old with a final diagnosis of inflicted head injury made at least one prior visit to a physician at which time the diagnosis of child maltreatment was missed. The consequences noted by the authors was that almost one-third of those children were reinjured and four deaths occurred. In young children with vague symptoms, it is essential to perform a complete examination and to inquire about suspicious bruises on the head or face of infants.

In studies evaluating the outcome of inflicted head injury, one-third of victims die, one-third have severe disabilities (seizures, cerebral palsy, severe motor dysfunction, etc.), and one-third appear "normal" in the short term—however, they may have variable developmental difficulties in the long term (behavior, psychosocial, language, etc.).[120,121] Fatal inflicted head injury can occur in the older child as well; however, most occurs in children younger than 2 years old with the predominance occurring in those younger than 12 months of age.[122] This is likely because the developing skull and brain in children younger than the age of 5 years is especially vulnerable to shearing injuries.[27]

Shaken Baby Syndrome

Shaken baby syndrome (SBS) is commonly seen in infants younger than 15 months of age with a median age of 3 months. It occurs when the infant is held by the thorax and shaken. The initial presentation can be vague with complaints of lethargy, anorexia, irritability, respiratory distress, vomiting, "recent accident," seizure (up to 70% of patients), or even a history of "shaken to resuscitate." In 1972, Caffey[123] described shaken baby syndrome as the associated findings of retinal hemorrhages (up to 95%)[122] and subdural hematomas with minimal external signs of trauma (up to 35% have bruising), making the initial diagnosis difficult without the history of shaking. Other injuries may occur as well in isolation or with variations. However, no one finding is pathognomonic of SBS, thus caution should be exercised in diagnosing SBS with single findings. Likewise, the absence of other injuries or findings does not exclude the diagnosis of SBS.[124]

The mechanisms of injury include whiplash motions of the head and neck and the potential for a sudden impact injury as the infant is thrown against another object (typically a bed or sofa).[22,23] The acceleration–deceleration forces cause shearing of intracranial veins and cortical nerves, resulting in subdural hematomas (commonly interhemispheric), subarachnoid hemorrhage (16%), cerebral contusions, and edema (44%).[125–127] Each can occur in isolation or in combination.

SBS is one of the most common causes of subdural hemorrhage (SDH) in children younger than 2 years old.

Conversely, an acute SDH is the most common intracranial abnormality found in SBS, and it can occur in isolation or with other injuries.[107] The shaking motion may additionally cause retinal hemorrhages (seen in up to 95% of patients with SBS)[43] spinal fractures/hematomas/dislocations/cord injuries, rib fractures, and long bone metaphyseal fractures. Fractures are found in up to 50% of SBS cases.[14]

Shaking can be followed by sudden impact and may result in external signs of trauma, such as bruising, swelling, or fractures; however, in the absence of impact signs, shaking alone cannot be assumed because there may have been an impact that cannot be identified.[128] SBS has the highest mortality of all forms of physical abuse: up to 30% of victims die, and up to 70% of survivors have significant neurological disabilities.[121,129] Additionally, these children are being subjected to repetitive shaking events and/or other types of abuse, thus enhancing their poor prognosis.[130]

Intracranial Injuries

There are no intracranial injuries specific for abuse. However, different types and conditions predominate in nonaccidental versus accidental head injuries.

A spectrum of injury occurs in the head trauma of children, whether abusive or accidental. This spectrum is classified into primary versus secondary injury; focal versus diffuse injury; and acute versus chronic injury.[79,90,131,132] Primary injury, such as contusion and shearing injury (resulting in tearing of bridging veins), is a result of the immediate initial traumatic force. Secondary injury is the reactive events of the primary injury, such as swelling. Focal or contact injuries, which are more common in accidental trauma, are the result of linear or translational forces causing simple fractures, contusions, or epidural hematomas. Diffuse injury typically occurs in inflicted trauma as a result of shaking and shaking with impact that involves acceleration–deceleration forces. The resulting findings produce a variation of focal and diffuse injuries, such as subdural hemorrhage, shear injury, gliding contusions (focal hemorrhages between the gray and white matter commonly found in cases of diffuse axonal injury),[133] and retinal hemorrhages. Acute and chronic injuries also encompass a combination of the aforementioned forces and injuries leading to multiple types of intracranial hemorrhages and brain injuries.

Epidural Hemorrhage

For accidental head injury, the findings are typically the result of brief focal linear direct contact injuries that cause linear skull fractures, epidural hematomas, cortical contusions, or localized subdural hemorrhages.[132,134–136] Epidural hemorrhages are associated with falls and, though more common in older children, account for approximately 3% of intracranial injuries in infants.[137] Neonates as well are at risk for epidural hemorrhage from birth-related trauma, although it is rare (<2%) and often asymptomatic.[138]

Epidural hemorrhages, unlike other intracranial hemorrhages, are more commonly associated with skull fractures, though in infants (unlike in adults) they can occur in the absence of a fracture.[139] Epidural hemorrhage is rarely associated with nonaccidental head injury.[137,140] The "lucid interval" described in older children with intracranial hemorrhage is typically associated with epidurals; however, it occurs in less than one-third of cases.[25] Recent investigations of fatal head injuries have evaluated the possibility of a "lucid" interval occurring with intracranial injuries. The clinical presentation appears variable with the possibility of lucidity not exclusively with epidural hemorrhages.[46,56,141,142] Although some children may have been "lucid" on arrival, they were not asymptomatic and the lucidity is commonly short lived (minutes to hours).[56,141]

Subdural Hemorrhages

The findings noted in abusive head injury are commonly the result of an acute primary event with diffuse injury resulting in subdural hemorrhage (SDH) that is commonly interhemispheric.[4,110,121,122,131,136,143] An isolated subdural/subarachnoid hemorrhage is the only finding in less than 2% of fatal pediatric accidental head injury; however, the incidence is up to 98% if the fatal head injury is inflicted.[27]

Though not independently characteristic of abuse, SDHs can occur in up to 80% of nonfatal abusive head injury,[79,118,140,144,145] especially in the mechanism of shaken baby,[107,120,146] with a majority in children younger than 2 years old.[121] SDHs can be unilateral or more commonly bilateral and may be associated with a skull fracture, but the hemorrhage need not be on the same side as the fracture.[27] There is less incidence of SDH in accidental nonfatal injuries; however, the event is typically a major injury that is recounted in detail by the caregiver or witnesses to the event, such as a motor vehicle collision or fall from significant heights.[43,47,59,144,147]

SDH in the neonate can occur as a result of obstetric trauma, can be asymptomatic, and is commonly located in the posterior fossa.[137,146,148] Additionally, neonatal SDHs under these conditions tend to resolve within 4 weeks.[148]

SDHs are not solely the result of inflicted or traumatic head injury. Some conditions can be misdiagnosed as inflicted injury:

- Benign external hydrocephalus[149–152] (also called benign enlargement of the subarachnoid space, BESS) can develop SDH, and though it is cited in literature to be a rare occurrence in these children,[145] the prevalence has been suggested to be as high as 11%.[149] To further complicate distinguishing these patients from abusive injury patients, there is a case report of retinal hemorrhage with a subdural hemorrhage in a patient with BESS that was not inflicted[149]; however, it mimics the clinical picture of SBS.
- Glutaric aciduria type I[153] is a recessive metabolic disorder resulting in sudden encephalopathy at 6–18 months of age. These children additionally are at risk for subdural and retinal hemorrhages after minor head trauma—although the types of retinal hemorrhage tend to differ from that of inflicted head injury.
- Hemorrhagic disease of the newborn potentially occurs if the infant was not given vitamin K prophylactically

after birth and proceeds to be exclusively breast-fed.[154] Symptoms develop about 3–8 weeks of age; however, there is a case report of intracranial hemorrhage in a 10-month-old infant.

- Barlow's disease, otherwise known as infantile scurvy,[155] is rarely seen in the United States currently. It is caused by a deficiency of ascorbic acid and tends to occur with bottle-fed infants. Diagnostic testing is available via serology for whole blood histamine analysis or plasma analysis for ascorbic acid.

Table 18-2 lists the differential diagnosis of subdural hematoma in infants and children.[120,156]

Subarachnoid Hemorrhages

Subarachnoid hemorrhages (SAHs) are often found in the autopsies of premature infants.[137] Massive subarachnoid hemorrhages may occur with perinatal hypoxia, although this is very rare. Cerebral aneurysms are another potential cause, and another rare event.[162] With the older infant and young child, falls from heights tend to result in impact injuries that cause subarachnoid hemorrhages associated with impact skull fractures (depressed or comminuted), cortical contusions, or subdural hematomas.[146]

Mixed-Density Collections

To complicate matters, the CT findings of mixed-density extracerebral collections in an infant may give the appearance of a chronic subdural hematoma with rehemorrhage. In the presence of an acute SDH, rebleeding after a minor injury or spontaneous rebleeding from a preexisting chronic SDH should not be offered as an explanation.[27,107,122,163–167] The history of radiographic timing of SDHs has been extrapolated from adult and animal studies[146] but cannot be applied to children because the blood of an acute SDH in children is readily resolved or rapidly organized more completely and rapidly than in adults.[27,107,168,169] A child whose SDH organizes into a membrane at risk for rebleeding would likely be symptomatic before the time of rebleeding because of a preexisting brain abnormality.[27,169] Although this mixed-density finding occurs more commonly in inflicted head injury, it is not specific for abuse.[170] When subdural hemorrhages of mixed density are noted in children of nonaccidental head injury, the most common explanation has been repetitive episodes of head injury over time.[107,134–136]

Scalp

Scalp injury may be the only indication for head injury in the otherwise well-appearing child. The scalp injuries can appear as lacerations or hematomas of which there are two types: cephalohematoma (most common) and subgleal hematoma. The cephalohematoma is located under the periosteum, does not cross suture lines, and commonly occurs in the parietal or occipital regions. Approximately 25% of neonatal cephalohematomas are associated with skull fractures.[164] Subgleal hematomas (also known as caput succedaneum) are commonly the result of birth injuries resulting from forceps or vaginal canal narrowing, although an additional cause can be forceful hair pulling.[171] Also, subgleal hematomas can cross

TABLE 18-2 **Differential Diagnosis of Subdural Hematoma in Infants and Children**

Accidental versus inflicted trauma	**Hematologic condition**
• Shaken baby syndrome (SBS)	• Disseminated intravascular coagulation
• Major trauma[157]	• Hemophilia or other bleeding disorder
– Motor vehicle crash	• Leukemia
– Serious falls	• Sickle cell anemia
Neurosurgical complication	• Hemorrhagic disease of the newborn
Perinatal injury	• Idiopathic thrombocytopenia purpura
• Fetal[158]	**Metabolic disorder**
• Birth trauma	• Glutaric aciduria type I[153]
– SDH/SAH occurs in 30% of asymptomatic neonates during delivery[27]	• Galactosaemia
	• Menke's disease
	• Osteogenesis imperfecta[159]
Congenital malformation	**Vasculitis**
• Arteriovenous malformation	• Lead toxicity
• Aneurysm	• Moyamoya disease
– Rare with a predominant male:female ratio[160]	• Systemic lupus erythematosus
	• Kawasaki disease
• Arachnoid cysts[161]	**Infantile scurvy**
• Benign external hydrocephalus	**Radiation or chemotherapy effect**
Infection	**Tumor**
• Meningitis	
• Herpes simplex virus	

suture lines to the extent that the expansion may result in hypovolemia in infants. This can also result in recognizable patterns about the face and scalp such as Battle's sign or raccoon eyes.

Alopecia can be seen as a traumatic origin in children where a caregiver grabs or pulls the hair of the child. The scalp may be boggy with tenderness present and hair loss that is irregular and less complete than in classic alopecia areata.

RETINAL HEMORRHAGES AND OCULAR FINDINGS

Part of the physical examination includes the retinal exam, particularly in the infant with concern for head injury. Eye abnormalities are found in more than 40% of all child abuse cases[172]; specifically, in patients concerning for SBS, the incidence is higher (up to 95%).[122] Children with inflicted head injury are more likely to have retinal hemorrhages as opposed to children with accidental head injury, where the incidence of retinal hemorrhages is minimal to none.[66,173–175] Though the presence of retinal hemorrhage is not pathognomonic for child maltreatment, the existence strongly suggests intentional injury. The undilated fundoscopic exam can be limited or difficult, and 25% of cases will be missed when the exam is performed by someone other than an ophthalmologist; thus, a pediatric ophthalmologic consultation is recommended for these cases.[127,176]

It is not the presence of the hemorrhage but the type and location of the hemorrhage that raises concern for SBS. The location of the hemorrhage within the retina determines the appearance of the hemorrhage: superficial disruptions result in flame-shaped hemorrhages, deeper intraretinal hemorrhages appear as "dot and blot" hemorrhages, and the layered blood in the potential space of the retina and vitreous appears as "boat-shaped" preretinal hemorrhages.[177]

The description of retinal hemorrhages should be specific to assist with determination of cause and/or mechanism of injury. The number of hemorrhages present (few, moderate, too numerous to count), type (as described previously), pattern, and location (posterior pole, radiating from optic nerve, extending to the periphery, perivascular, random, focal, diffuse) should be included in the descriptions. The vitreous of young children is more adherent to the retina than in adults; thus, when the child is subjected to shaking, traumatic retinoscheisis can occur.[178] Specifically in pediatrics, this condition has been seen only in conditions concerning for SBS. Papilledema is a common cause of retinal hemorrhage, but is uncommon in children with SBS.[127] With the variations of retinal hemorrhage types and the fact that none are pathognomonic but are suggestive of abuse, it is important to describe the hemorrhage as much as possible in the hopes of further distinguishing between potentially inflicted and noninflicted mechanisms of hemorrhage. Disorders that mimic SBS through retinal hemorrhages can usually be distinguished by the retinal hemorrhage pattern, systemic symptoms, or serology testing.

Retinal hemorrhages occur in up to 80% of children with inflicted head injury.[35] Up to 95% of patients with shaken baby syndrome are found to have retinal hemorrhages.[122,179] However, the absence does not exclude shaken baby syndrome or other types of abuse as potential mechanisms of injury.[122] Of clinical importance is the association of retinal hemorrhage and subdural hematoma, which is useful in the presence of a minimally symptomatic child and is virtually diagnostic of abuse in the absence of a verifiable history.[177,180–183]

Recent studies have demonstrated the use of fundoscopic examination in children with ALTE with a potential for child abuse as an etiology for symptoms.[60] The retinopathy with SBS is as follows[184,185]:

- Multiple, bilateral[172] (but can be unilateral).[144,186–189]
- Have more than one layer of retinal involvement and extend to the periphery.[190]
- Located commonly where vitreous attaches to retina (ora serrata and in posterior portion near disk and macula).
- Vitreous hemorrhage.
- Associated with retinal detachments and retinal tears.[190]
- Optic nerve hemorrhage, although it is not specific for abuse.[27]
- Papilledema (< 8%).[127]
- Nonhemorrhagic ocular findings:
  - Retinoschisis and macular folds[178,191,192]
  - Described only in patients with SBS[193]
- Retinal hemorrhage cannot be dated.
- Though retinal hemorrhage is not pathognomonic for child maltreatment, the existence strongly suggests intentional injury.

Retinal hemorrhages occur in 3% of patients with accidental head injury.[120,174,175,194,195] Rarely do household falls result in retinal hemorrhage.[195] If hemorrhage occurs as a result of accidental injury, it is typically unilateral, few in number, focal, and located in the posterior pole in the superficial layers of the retina.[145,196]

Up to 50% of children have retinal hemorrhages following vaginal delivery.[197,198] Hemorrhages can be found after any delivery but are more common after spontaneous or forceps or vacuum use deliveries.[197–199] These are mainly flame-shaped (superficial) and resolve within 1–2 weeks.[197,198] There can be intraretinal hemorrhages (deeper), but these are rare and will resolve within about 6 weeks (usually 4 weeks).[184] In neonates with retinal hemorrhages, there does not appear to be an association with intracranial injury.[200] Additionally, there is no residual deficit in these neonates with retinal hemorrhages.

Resuscitation of a child whether at home, in the field, or in the hospital has been theorized to cause retinal hemorrhages. Studies over the last 20 years using both animal models and retrospective studies have shown that it is not common and the type of hemorrhage that results is not consistent with those from inflicted head injuries.[184,201–203.]

Other noninflicted causes of retinal hemorrhage include the following[200,204,205]:

- Infection (cytomegalovirus, *Rickettsia rickettsii*, falciparum malaria, bacterial endocarditis, sepsis, and meningitis). These conditions produce typical retinal injuries in geographical areas.

- Bleeding disorders. Even the most severe coagulopathies rarely cause severe retinal hemorrhages, and the presence of systemic symptoms would preclude the diagnosis.
- Osteogenesis imperfecta patient after minor injury.[206]
- Vasculopathies.[184] Vasculitis tends to cause a diagnostic perivascular pattern.
- Increased intracranial pressures or Valsalva maneuvers.
  - Elevated intracranial pressures may play a role in SBS, but further studies are needed.
  - Seizures to date have not been shown to cause retinal hemorrhage in infants.[207]
  - Severe cough or vomiting has not been shown to cause retinal hemorrhage in infants.[208,209]
- Aneurysm/AV malformation/arachnoid cysts.[210] Retinal hemorrhages rarely occur, but if present, they are few in number, intra- or periretinal, and confined to specific areas.

Retinal hemorrhages can take anywhere from 10 days to several months to resolve, depending on the severity.[120]

EARS

The ears are a common site for intentional injury through pinching, slapping, or boxing.[211] Chronic injury can result in pinnae deformity and sensorineural hearing deficits. The "tin ear" syndrome, described by Hanigan in 1987 consists of bruising of the ear associated with ipsilateral subdural hemorrhage with cerebral swelling and retinal hemorrhage.[212] The proposed mechanism for injury is caused by blunt trauma to the ear that results in rotational acceleration. Thus, bruising of the ear may warrant further investigation into the potential for abusive head injury.

ORAL AND DENTAL ASPECTS OF CHILD ABUSE

The most common site for inflicted oral injuries are the lips (54%), oral mucosa, teeth, gingival, and tongue.[213]

Tears of the upper or lower labial frenula in infants are highly suspicious for abuse, unlike in toddlers where this can be caused by a fall while the child has an object in the mouth.[214] This inflicted injury in infants is commonly caused by force feeding when the nipple of the bottle is jammed into the mouth.[215] This same mechanism can cause frenulum tears of the tongue. Forced oral sex in a child may also produce the same tears of the labial and lingual frenulum. Caution should be employed when considering midline defects as pathology because they may represent congenital defects instead.[216]

Lacerations or linear bruises around the corners of the mouth should raise suspicion of a gag injury.[217]

Esophageal injury is rare in child maltreatment and the morbidity is directly related to the time to diagnosis and treatment.[218] Fortunately, the mortality rate for children is significantly lower than for adults. With suspicion of esophageal perforation, a gastrograffin swallow is indicated followed by a barium swallow if the initial gastrograffin study is negative and suspicion for injury remains.

SKELETAL

Table 18-3 lists fractures that are suspicious for child abuse.

Skull fractures are found in 50% of children with inflicted intracranial injury[132]; however, unlike in adults, skull fracture is not frequently associated with fatal head injuries.[56] Overall the frequency of skull fractures is highest in infants younger than 2 years old, and fortunately the risk of intracranial injury is low.[219] To complicate matters, clinical methods are unreliable for detecting skull fractures, dating them, and correlating fractures to brain injury.

Many children with head injuries do not sustain skull fractures.[219] Soft tissue swelling is not a reliable predictor of the presence of a fracture because of the variability in presence of swelling, size, extension, and bruising.[35,220] Once a fracture is noted, it only partially correlates with intracranial injury because only up to 56% of brain injury patients are noted to have a skull fracture.[101,134,221–224] Likewise, children may sustain significant intracranial injuries without a skull fracture. Finally, dating skull fractures is difficult because they do not heal with the typical appearance of hard callus formation seen on plain X-rays or with staged healing on CT scan.

There are two types of skull fractures, simple and complex, each of which contains various subtypes.[146] A simple fracture is 2 mm or less in width, limited to one bone, does not violate suture lines, and extends in one direction (whether straight, jagged, or curved). A complex skull fracture can have a radial or stellate appearance. Comminuted fractures are circumferential and isolated. If there is an overlying scalp laceration, it is called a compound fracture. Wide, complex fractures are called diastatic. However, diastasis (splitting) of sutures can be misdiagnosed as a skull fracture and can happen within 24 hours of an event but is not considered as the primary injury because it is seen with all types of brain swelling before closure of sutures occurs.

Skull fractures as a result of accidental trauma occur at an incidence of up to 2% in mild–moderate impact mechanisms.[27,43] The fractures are typically linear, nondisplaced, unilateral, and parietally located.[30] Linear skull fractures may also be a complication of delivery in the neonate.[225] Unless there is an underlying epidural hematoma, these fractures are commonly benign.[140] Epidural hemorrhage commonly does not result in depressed consciousness. However, if bleeding continues, mental status will progressively decline.

If the skull fracture is the result of inflicted injury, it is more likely to be bilateral, comminuted, depressed, diastatic, wider than 3 mm, in a nonparietal location, violates suture lines, and associated with other injuries.[226–228] Though linear fractures predominate in accidental traumas and complex fractures tend to occur more in inflicted trauma, either fracture type can occur in either injury.[16,75,129] However, some of the characteristics more associated with inflicted injury are multiple fractures, bilateral, and crossing suture lines.[226]

Specifically occurring in infants are late sequelae that can be the result of skull fractures. One is a subepicranial cerebrospinal fluid hygroma where the fracture crosses the suture line and disrupts the arachnoid layer; this event typically resolves over time. The other is a leptomeningeal cyst where

TABLE 18-3 **Fractures Suspicious for Child Abuse**

- Fracture inconsistent with mechanism or no history provided
- Healing fractures; multiple, variable stages of healing
- Fracture in child younger than 1 year (nonambulatory)
- Complex skull fracture
- Rib fractures (posterior)
- Bilateral acute, symmetrical long bone fractures
- Femur fractures in child younger than 1 year
- Spiral fractures of the humerus
- Classic metaphyseal lesion (CML) = metaphyseal chip fractures
- Fractures of high-energy trauma without collaborating mechanism: sternum, first rib, spinous process, or scapulae

the contused brain swells and herniates through the dura tear of an enlarging skull, further separating the fracture margins. Infants who experience either of these sequelae can have neurologic symptoms (deficits or seizures) that require surgical intervention.

With the minimal soft tissue swelling that may occur in pediatric fractures, many skeletal injuries are found incidentally during a medical visit.[78] Once the skeletal injury is noted, the comparison with the mechanism offered in the history can help the physician decide whether the injury was inflicted or accidental.

There are five different types of fracture mechanisms[229]:

- Transverse: Trauma perpendicular to long axis of bone.
- Buckle/torus: Force along axis of bone (compressive/axial loading). This fracture type is unique to developing bone.
- Spiral: Twist or torque (Figure 18-1).
- Oblique: Combination of compressive force with rotation.
- Metaphyseal chips (Figure 18-2): Traction on extremity or violent shaking. This fracture type is unique to developing bone.

One of the suspicious findings for inflicted injury is a fracture in a child younger than 1 year of age. The force required for many of the fractures noted in this population is too great for a nonambulatory child to create him- or herself; thus, it is not surprising that more than 50% of fractures in this age group are inflicted.[77] In overall investigations of inflicted fractures, the majority are located in the diaphysis region (single, transverse)[230] of the femur, humerus, and tibia.[75,230] However, if the study is restricted to infants, the majority of inflicted fractures occur at the metaphyseal–epiphyseal regions.[231] This discrepancy is likely because of the age-related variation in injury patterns in the pediatric population. Of these sites, the metaphyseal–epiphyseal area is more suspicious for inflicted trauma.[75,143,230,232]

Multiple rib fractures are the most common bones fractured in abusive injury in infants younger than 3 years old.[86,233,234] However, they are difficult to identify radiographically when acute because visualization involves callus formation.[220,235] Rib fractures are associated with other injuries in

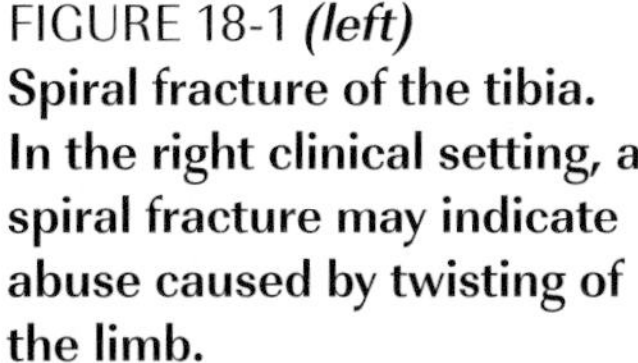

FIGURE 18-1 *(left)* **Spiral fracture of the tibia. In the right clinical setting, a spiral fracture may indicate abuse caused by twisting of the limb.**

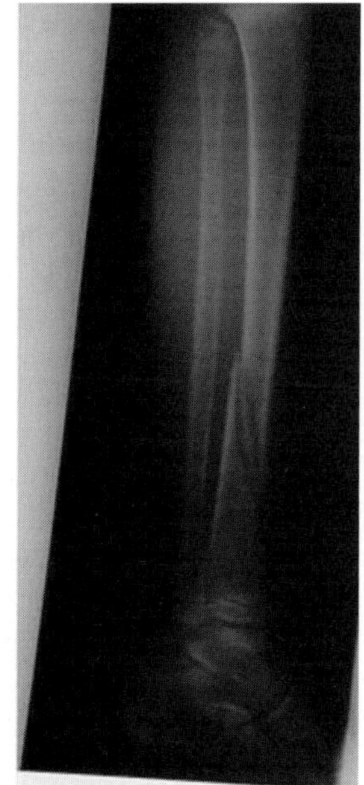

FIGURE 18-2 *(right)* **Metaphyseal chip fracture. This injury is highly suspicious for child abuse.**

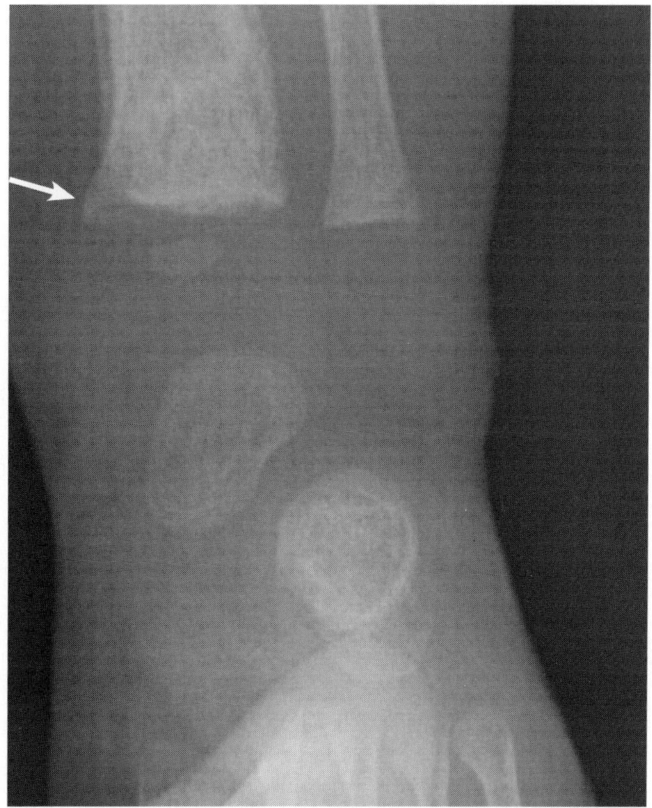

both fatal[236] and nonfatal inflicted injuries (up to 30%).[86,234] When inflicted, the location of the rib fractures tends to be posteriomedial and bilateral in addition to being multiple in number.[237] The mechanism for these injuries in infants tends to be squeezing by adult hands of the immature skeleton, which has significant plasticity. Noninflicted rib fractures can occur; however, they are uncommon and the fracture locations tend to be different from locations of inflicted injuries. Examples are as follows:

- Bone disease. There is a case report of a patient with osteogenesis imperfecta Type II who sustained no rib fractures after CPR.[238]
- Accidental/iatrogenic fractures resulting from cardiac surgery, struck by a vehicle, motor vehicle crash, birth injury, stairway fall in arms of adult, older sibling that fell onto infant.
- CPR (rarely if ever).[239–241]

Classic metaphyseal lesions (CMLs) were initially, erroneously noted in 1953 by Astley to occur in children with "fragile" metaphyseal bones. Caffey 5 years later correlated this finding with child maltreatment.[242] These fractures can appear as a "bucket handle" (metaphyseal fracture fragment projected at a craniocaudad angle producing a crescentic density) or "corner fracture" (metaphyseal fracture fragment as a triangular density adjacent to the corner of the metaphysic) depending on the view taken in plain radiographs.[81,231] However, the mechanism for either appearance is the same: shearing forces applied to immature spongiosa of the metaphysis that are produced by acceleration and deceleration (as seen in shaking), pulling, or twisting injury.[243,244] This injury occurs commonly bilaterally in the long bones (distal tibia, proximal femur, humerus). CMLs are found in up to 50% of abused children younger than 18 months of age and almost exclusively in children younger than 2 years old.[231,237,242,245]

Femur fractures in children younger than 1 year are suspicious for abuse because an infant in this age group is unlikely to be ambulating.[21,246–248] Recent studies demonstrate a varied incidence of inflicted femoral fractures in the infant population; however, many agree that these inflicted injuries are overrepresented in the younger than 1 year age group.[246,247,249] Different types of femur fractures can occur; however, no one type is predictive for abuse. Birth-associated femur fractures are extremely rare and are associated with difficult births (i.e., breech).[250]

Unexplained fractures pose more of a dilemma for the physician than does the dichotomous question of accidental or inflicted injuries. Variations of skeletal disorders can appear as injuries or accidental injuries and the disorder can make the child more at risk for certain pathology. It is important that physicians are aware of the possible disorders and the types of potential injuries resulting as they are of the signs and symptoms indicating abuse. A differential diagnosis of skeletal injury is presented in Table 18-4.

Osteogenesis imperfecta is perhaps one of the most common skeletal disorders considered when faced with a child with multiple fractures. It is an inherited connective tissue disorder, though spontaneous mutations can occur and thus genetic history may be negative. There is variable phenotypic expression regarding degrees of osteoporosis and bruisability that occurs with this condition regardless of the four different types with which the patient may be afflicted.[251] Of particular consideration are types I and IV because these are consistently missed at birth or in utero. In these types, there can be normal-appearing bones on X-ray and the presence of the visually diagnosed "blue sclera" is variable. The common metaphyseal fractures of inflicted injuries are not likely to be seen in osteogenesis imperfecta.[252] The diagnosis is often made clinically, but available testing can potentially confirm the diagnosis. The false-negative rate for these tests is considerable, so a negative test does not exclude the possibility of osteogenesis imperfect.[251,253] Common tests to confirm the diagnosis of OI include:

- Skin fibroblast biopsy
- Bone mineral density scanning is decreased
- Elevated plasma osteocalcin

Osteopenia may be the result of metabolic disorders not often seen currently in the United States, such as rickets (vitamin D deficiency), scurvy (vitamin C deficiency), and copper deficiency. Rickets is an uncommon vitamin D deficiency that is more common in exclusively breast-fed infants or in children not exposed to adequate sunlight. In infants with rickets, characteristic radiographic changes occur that are distinguishable from abusive injuries. Current American Academy of Pediatrics (AAP) guidelines include vitamin D supplementation for these infants. Scurvy is a rare condition in the United States in which subperiosteal bleeding occurs, causing large areas of subperiosteal calcification that can lead to misdiagnosis of abuse. Ascorbic acid levels must be obtained to make the diagnosis. Copper deficiency is primarily seen in preterm infants and presents commonly in the second 6 months of life. Characteristic radiographic bone changes and serologic findings tend to occur before the presentation of pathologic fractures. Additionally, osteopenia of prematurity may be seen, which presents between 6 and 12 weeks of age. Unfortunately, preterm infants are also at increased risk for abuse than are term infants.

Disuse osteoporosis potentially occurs in any child who has severe limitations on limb movements such as those with cerebral palsy or paralysis. Inflicted injuries in these children are particularly difficult to determine because not only are they at increased risk for abuse, but the fractures can occur with normal handling or physical therapy.

Hereditary multiple exostoses (HMEs)[254,255] is a rare autosomal dominant disorder characterized by painless bony protrusions (exostoses). The exostoses commonly involve the femur and tibia (70%), humerus (50%), radius and ulna (50%), and scapula (50%). The lesions can be mistaken for the classic metaphyseal lesions of nonaccidental trauma; however, exostoses occur more proximally in the metaphyses of long bones and point away from the epiphysis. Exostoses become more prominent with age—especially in childhood and adolescence. Thus, infants are rarely diagnosed because the

TABLE 18-4 **Differential Diagnosis of Skeletal Injury**

Skeletal dysplasia
- Osteogenesis imperfecta
- Infantile cortical hyperostosis = Caffey's disease
- Hereditary multiple exostoses

Nutritional/metabolic defects
- Rickets = vitamin D deficiency
- Scurvy = vitamin C deficiency
- Copper deficiency
- Menke's "kinky hair" disease
- Homocystinuria
- Hypophosphatasia

Osteopenia of prematurity

Neuromuscular
- Disuse osteoporosis
  - Cerebral palsy
  - Paralysis
  - Myelodysplasia
- Riley–Day syndrome = familial dysautonomia = congenital insensitivity to pain

Congenital syphilis

Toddler's fracture

Physiologic periosteal new bone

Neoplasm
- Leukemia
- Histiocytosis X
- Metastatic neuroblastoma

exostoses are small and not clinically detectable but may be seen on radiographs obtained for other purposes.

ABDOMINAL

Blunt abdominal trauma is not a common injury in child maltreatment (2–4%); however, it is the second most common cause of inflicted deaths (12%) with a mortality of greater than 50%.[75,256,257] Like inflicted head injuries, there is often no apparent external signs of trauma.[258,259] In asymptomatic children with a suspicion of abuse, liver serology may assist in determination of abdominal injury.[70] There is often a delay in seeking medical care for children with abdominal injuries, which may contribute to the mortality rate because the caretaker often acts once the child has obvious signs of illness (peritonitis, sepsis, hemodynamic instability).[258] Delay in seeking care, however, is not specific for inflicted injury.[260]

The mechanism is usually a direct blow to the abdomen with compression of the contents against a rigid spine. The injuries include rupture of the liver and/or spleen, ruptured viscous, duodenal hematoma, mesenteric vascular injury, pancreatic injury, and renal trauma.[108,258] The liver is the most common solid organ injury that occurs in inflicted abdominal trauma. Conversely, the spleen is rarely injured in physical child abuse.[261,262] Because of the retroperitoneal position of the duodenum, significant force needs to be applied to cause injury. A recent study found duodenal injury present in 0.5% to almost 3% of the children admitted for inflicted injury.[256,258,263] Pancreatic trauma is the most common cause of acute pancreatitis in childhood where 30% of all post-traumatic pancreatitis is the result of abuse.[109] More than 50% of pseudocysts are caused by trauma, and up to 30% of these patients have concurrent signs of abuse.[264] Other injuries associated with inflicted abdominal trauma are soft tissue (95%), head injury (45%), bony fractures (27%), and skull fractures (18%).[258]

SKIN

The skin is the most common organ injured in child abuse; however, the nature of children predisposes them to frequent falls and bruising. It is important to determine which areas are prone to bruising in differing pediatric populations and evaluate the pattern of bruising when evaluating for possible abuse. In nonambulatory children, bruises rarely occur (approximately 2%).[265,266] This differs from cruisers (about 17%) and walkers (about 50%).[266]

Generally, areas of isolated injuries suspicious for abuse are regions of the body usually protected: trunk, thigh, upper arms, cheeks, ears, neck, buttocks, genitalia. The face is the most frequently injured part of the body, and the cheek receives more trauma than any other facial area in inflicted injuries.[213] (See Figure 18-3.) The mechanism of injury has the utmost importance in determining inflicted versus accidental trauma in regard to bruising regions and patterns. (See Figures 18-4, 18-5, and 18-6.)

Previously, it was thought that age of cutaneous contusions could be estimated.[267] However, recent studies have refuted this assumption because the development of the bruise color varies depending on the location, injury, skin color, age of child, and chronic injury.[268] Bruising that occurs on the same person at the same time in different areas of the body has also shown to differ in terms of color changes and length of time of each color.[269] Currently, there is no method for

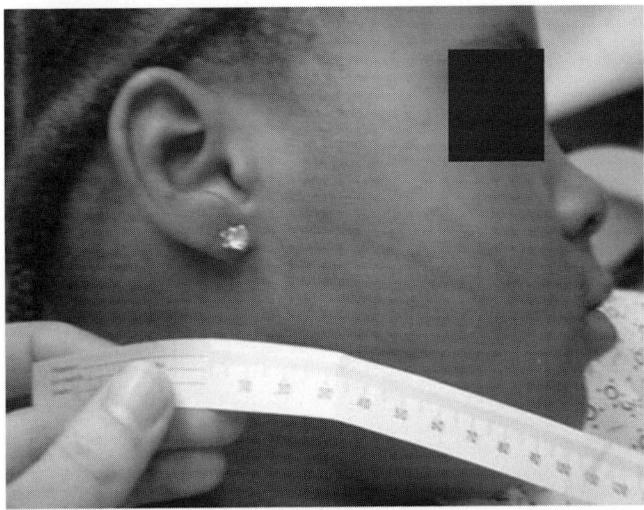

FIGURE 18-3 **Facial injury—child slapped in the face. Note the linear, parallel bruising representing the perpetrator's fingers.**

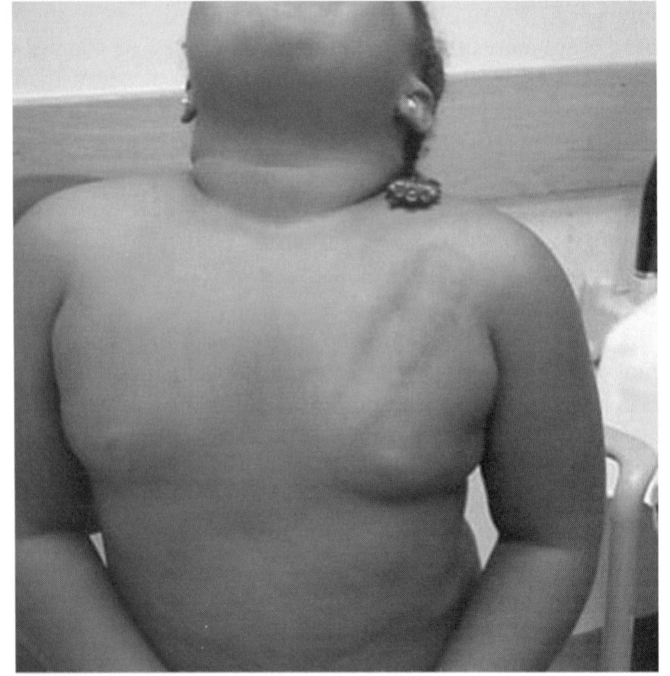

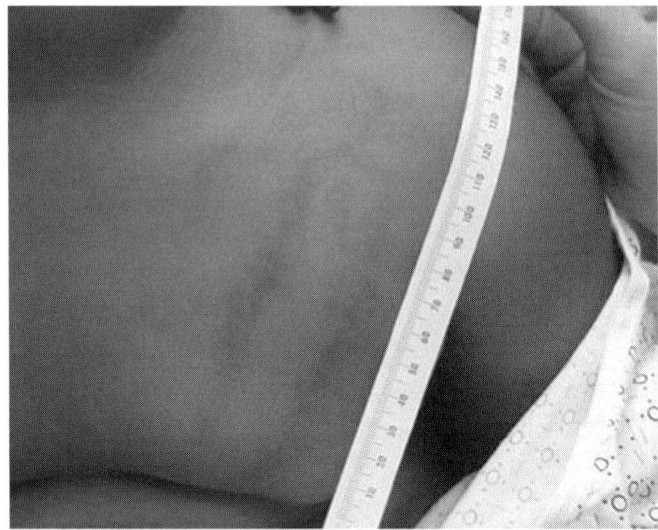

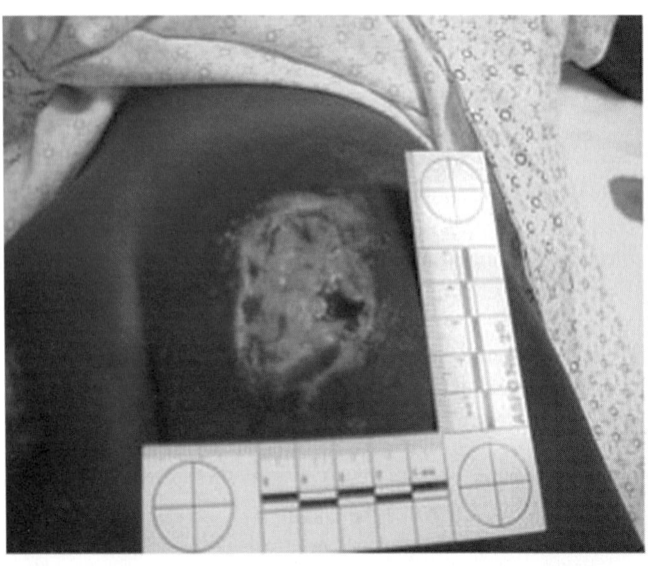

(a)

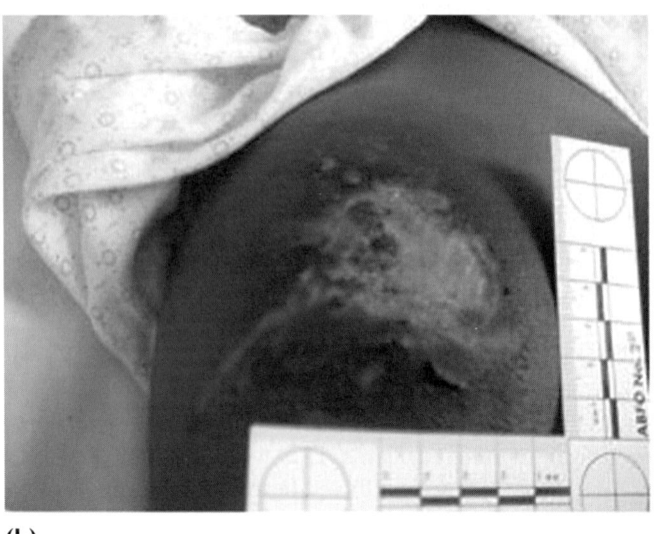

(b)

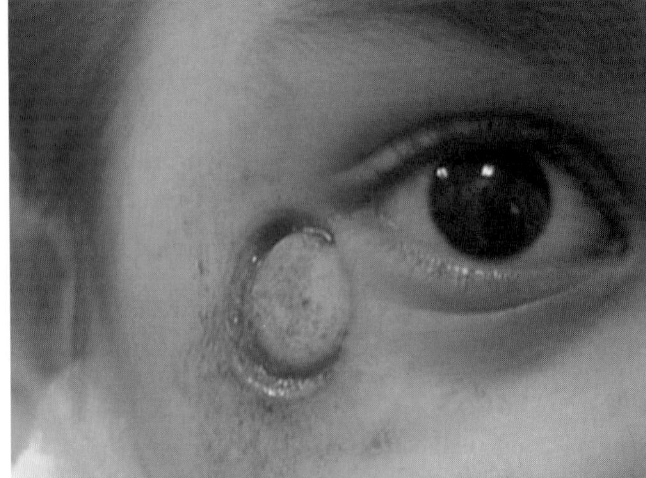

FIGURE 18-4 *(top row)* Pattern injury of the left upper chest. This injury was caused by a looped object being struck against the child.

FIGURE 18-5 *(middle row)* Repetitive injury in the right buttock (a) and left upper posterior thigh (b) in a child caused by a toilet plunger.

FIGURE 18-6 *(bottom left)* Pattern injury inflicted by the end of a curtain rod.

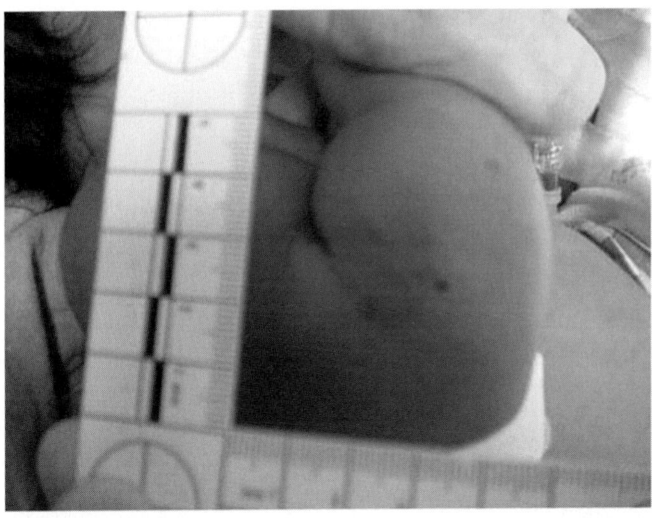

FIGURE 18-7 **Human bite to the forearm of a toddler.**

determining the timing of bruising. When a bruise occurs, the blood begins to deoxygenate and the sequence of color change is not always predicable (red to purple to blue to green to brown to yellow)—and neither is the time in which it takes for those changes to occur.[269-271]

Bites

Animal bites differ from human bites in that they tend to be deeper puncture wounds associated with soft tissue tearing. Human bites, on the other hand, are more elliptical in shape and superficial with more soft tissue bruising. If the intercanine diameter of the bite is greater than 3 cm, it is evidence of an adult bite; if the distance is less than 3 cm, the bite is likely from a child.[272] The most common sites for bite marks are the cheeks, back, sides, arms, buttocks, and genitalia.[273] (See Figure 18-7.)

In evaluation of bites, it is best to obtain photographs that can be reviewed at a later date by experts if required. It is important to position the camera directly above the bite mark to avoid any distortion of the lesion and to include a ruler in the photo. Additionally, if the bite is fresh, a saliva sample may be obtained using a sterile cotton applicator moistened with water, and then swabbed over the bite mark. The swab should be air dried, placed in a sterile vial or container, and then placed in a secured refrigerator until it can be retrieved by authorities. Table 18-5 lists other skin findings that can mimic child abuse.

Burns

Burns are uncommon in childhood; up to 25% of burns in children are inflicted.[281] Boys are more commonly inflicted with burn injuries than are girls, and the most common age for inflicted burns is 2–4 years.[282] There are different types of burns: scalds, dry contact, and microwave. Any of these can occur in maltreatment (though scalds are more common) and can produce recognizable patterns when inflicted.[108] Though burns may occur through accidental trauma (see Figure 18-8), they may also be classified as "inflicted" as a result of neglect or because a child was unsupervised and thus this becomes a variation of abuse causality.[283] (See Figure 18-9.)

TABLE 18-5 **Skin Findings That Mimic Child Abuse**

Normal variations
- Striae
- Mongolian spots

Congenital dermatologic manifestations
- Ehlers–Danlos syndrome type I (there are multiple known types)

Infections[274]
- Impetigo[275]
- Staph scalded skin syndrome (SSSS)
- Dermatitis
  - Fixed drug eruption
  - Severe diaper rash
- Henoch–Schonlein purpura[275,276]
- Purpura fulminans of meningococcemia
- Erythema multiforme[275,277]

Metabolic diseases
- Vitamin K deficiency from liver disease
- Cystic fibrosis[278]
- Salicylate toxicity can cause easy bruising

Bleeding disorders[274,279]
- Hemophilia
  - Inherited disorder that varies from mild to severe forms
  - PTT is not a sensitive screening test for mild forms and thus requires factor VIII and IX assays[280]
- Platelet disorders
  - ITP with petechiae
- Leukemia
- Neuroblastoma
- Vasculitis
  - Postinfectious vasculitis
  - Hypersensitivity of vasculitis can result in ecchymotic lesions

Homeopathic remedies
- Cao giao = coining
  - Vietnamese folk remedy that involves vigorously stroking oiled skin with a coin to remove harmful causes of fevers
- Cupping
  - A Latin American folk remedy in which a glass is heated and applied to the skin; a vacuum forms as the glass cools, leaving circular bruises or burns
  - Wet cupping: variation where the skin is abraded first
- Moxibustion
  - Asian folk remedy
  - Moxa herb (*Artemsia vulgaris*) is burned in an area of the body that needs healing
  - May cause full- or partial-thickness small, circular burns
- Maquas
  - Seen in Arabic, Bedouin, and Russian cultures
  - Deep burns with hot metal spits near the area of illness

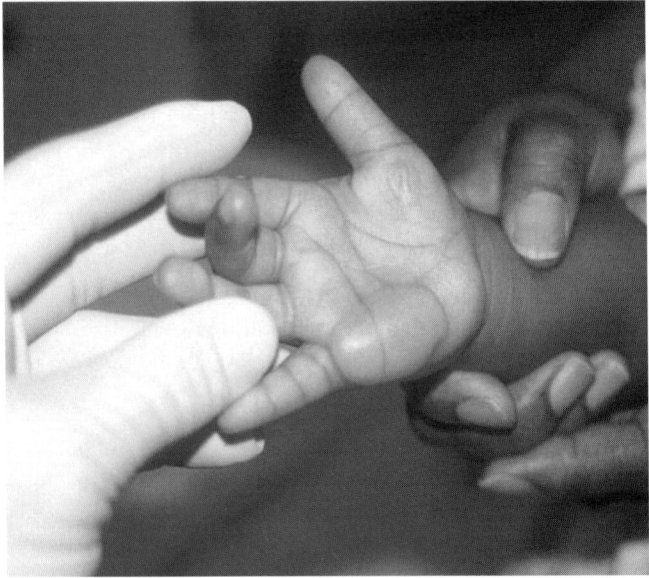

FIGURE 18-8 **Accidental burn to the palm of the right hand caused when the child contacted a hot surface.**

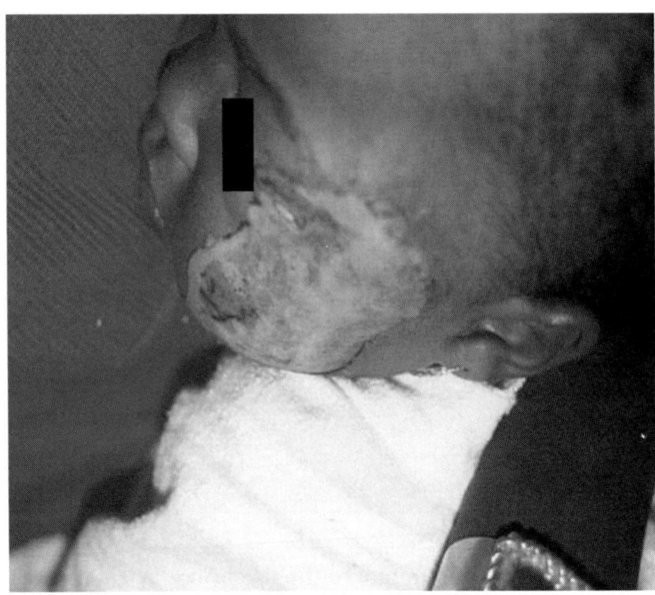

FIGURE 18-9 **Intentional burn injury to the left cheek.**

A delay in seeking medical attention is cited as an association with inflicted burns[284]; however, the family's role in the delay must be taken into account. Some burns do not initially appear impressive to caregivers, and caregivers may be more inclined to begin home remedies before an emergency department or doctor visit. Additionally, time, therapy, and physiology affect parts of the same burn differently and can alter the burn's appearance. Thus, it may be important to photograph the initial presentation of the burn and subsequent phases of healing.

Cumulative factors that cause concern for inflicted burn injury are as follows:

- Inconsistent history given by caretaker
- Delay in seeking medical help (without sound explanation)
- Lack of witnesses to event
- History of prior injuries of abuse, neglect
- Child is younger than 8 months or older than 2 years

Scald Burns

Accidental burns are typically caused by spills of hot liquid, which tend to produce a recognizable pattern that indicates a pouring or flowing of hot medium over the skin with splash and splatter marks.[285] The initial point of contact is typically the anterior chest and is the most severely burned area. As the hot liquid drips down, it cools, so the burns become less severe.

The developmental age of the child comes into question in burn injuries. Initially, it was thought that a nonambulatory child could not climb into a bathtub with the potential to sustain an immersion injury. Since then, a study was performed that evaluated the ability of a child to climb into a tub, and 35% of the children 10–18 months of age were able to climb into the tub, unassisted with stools or curtains—including a 10-month-old who was unable to walk independently.[286] Additionally, 25% of those who climbed in went in head first, and the rest climbed in sideways.

The following patterns are associated with inflicted scald burns:

- Deeper burn injury from forced submersion.
- Absence of splash marks.
- Immersion line (stocking or glove appearance); occurs in extremity immersion injuries.
- Symmetric/bilateral burns.
- "Zebra stripes" (sparing of the flexural areas as a result of the body's flexed position in hot liquid).
- Buttocks, perineal burns; the central aspect of the buttocks may be inadvertently spared resulting in a "donut" pattern in children who tend to be held down in the tub or sink.

The average temperature setting of a hot water heater is 140°F. A 3-second exposure to water this hot can cause first- or second-degree burns.[287] Thus, the depth of the burn is dependent on the time of exposure, the water temperature, the child's age, and the body region exposed. The relationship between hot water temperature and time to burn development is shown in Table 18-6.

Contact Burns

The patterns that emerge from dry contact burns tend to resemble the surface of the object involved.[285,288] Accidental injuries as a result of dry contact burns are commonly found on the palms because this is the mode used for tactile exploration by infants and children. Suspicious areas involve the dorsum of the hand or areas not easily contacted, such as the back or buttocks. When accidental, cigarette burns tend to be superficial because children brush against the lighted portion, and then immediately back away. If the wound is deep, well demarcated, and appears 7–10 mm round, it is less likely

TABLE 18-6 **Water Temperature and Length of Time Until Burn Development**

Water Temperature °C (°F)	Time of Exposure (sec) to Cause First- or Second-Degree Burns on Human Skin
52 (125.6)	70
54 (129.2)	30
56 (132.8)	14
58 (136.4)	6
60 (140.0)	3
62 (143.6)	1.6
64 (147.2)	1

Source: Adapted from Mortiz AR.[287]

accidental and more suspicious if there are multiple burns in the same area.

Microwave Oven Burns

Microwave ovens heat by a mechanism of molecular agitation that results in tissues with higher water content (such as muscle) heating to a greater extent than those with lower water content (such as fat).[289] This fact spares certain tissue levels in microwave oven burn injuries. Diagnosis is confirmed by a deep biopsy of the burned tissue down to and including the underlying muscle.

DROWNING AND NEAR DROWNING

Near drowning is rarely reported as a nonaccidental injury; however, there are cases reported in the literature. The typical scenario begins with the child in the bathtub. Some characteristics of accidental drowning and near drowning involve an unsupervised child who is younger than 15 months or who has developmental delay, or a child with a history of seizures. Nonaccidental submersions are associated with maternal mental illness, previous history of abuse, child outside the ages of 8–24 months, or the child is the youngest of the family.[290]

REPORTING CHILD MALTREATMENT

Child maltreatment requires a multifaceted intervention that includes medical specialists, social services, and law enforcement.

Though it may be difficult to inform the parents or caregivers of the decision to report the concern for maltreatment, it can be an opportune time to educate the parents about the proceedings and the possible services that can be offered to families with certain stressors. It is important to express to the caregivers that the main concern is child safety.

The literature proposes the following reasons for failure to report abuse:

- Inadequate training to diagnose the problem.
- Examiner does not want to get involved in perceived family situation or risk stigmatizing the family.
- Problem of defining child maltreatment.
- Fear of legal involvement.
- Disruption of doctor–patient relations.
- Fear of confrontation.
- Physician believes what is told in the history, and all decisions are based on that belief.
- When a severely injured child presents to the emergency department, staff members concentrate only on the medical issues at hand and not the overall etiology of maltreatment.

A listing of toll-free child abuse reporting numbers by state can be found at http://www.acf.dhhs.gov. Each state has its own system for reporting child maltreatment.

DISPOSITION AND FOLLOW-UP

Injuries suffered from abuse are more severe than are those of an accidental nature as noted by the higher hospitalization rates, longer hospital stays, and neurologic outcomes of the former.[16,175]

For those children who are discharged (whether in the custody of an agency or parent or other caregiver) without physical findings of injury, it is important that follow-up studies are conducted to reduce the likelihood of missed injury. Specifically, if initial skeletal survey is negative, it is recommended that the child have it repeated in 2 weeks.

CONCLUSION

The recognition of child maltreatment is important for all persons involved with children. The conditions that place children at risk for abuse are multifactorial and cumulative. Early detection of these risk factors is important in preventing the escalation of maltreatment that tends to occur as the exposure continues.[119,221,291-295] The presentation of child maltreatment can be on a number of scales from behavioral, to cognitive, and to medical, and possibly death.

Associated injuries of long bone and rib fractures of head-injured children are highly suggestive of abuse,[144,237] especially if differing stages of healing are noted for the fractures. This has been well described in the literature since 1962.[5,123] Since that time, additional associations have been made, including the relation of retinal hemorrhages[35,79,121,175] and a history of abuse within the family.[35,175] With this constellation of findings, the suspicion of abuse can be more confidently stated.[135,237] However, many children present with only one of the symptoms or a variation of this constellation of symptoms. With a suspicion of abuse, the diagnostic modalities chosen not only must evaluate for physical signs of injury, but also exclude other medical conditions that may mimic abusive conditions. Conditions that prompt suspicion of child maltreatment are presented in Table 18-7.

In a child who is younger than 2 years, the initial evaluation includes a skeletal survey with dilated retinal examination. Because of the minimal symptoms that many children with subdural hemorrhages have on presentation, a CT scan should be considered in any child younger than 2 years with retinal hemorrhages, suspicious bone fractures, unexplained neurologic findings, increasing head circumference,

TABLE 18-7 **Conditions That Prompt Suspicion of Child Maltreatment**

History[24]	Physical examination
• Conflicting/changing history • Delay in medical care with apparent injury • Denial of trauma with traumatic injuries • History inconsistent with mechanism, force required, or developmental capacity of child • Injury attributed to another child who lacks the force or development to inflict injury • Unexplained neurologic symptoms, respiratory distress, apnea, poor feeding without infectious, toxic, metabolic cause • Fatal or severe injuries related to short or household fall • Trauma caused by home resuscitation	• Multiple injuries • Multiple types of injuries (fractures, burns) • Multiple injuries at varied stages of healing • Patterned bruising • Injured sites other than those most injured in accidental injuries • Retinal hemorrhage without specific history of moderate to severe accidental trauma • Facial/scalp injuries in nonambulatory child, or involves the ear, or intraoral trauma **Documentation** • Describe and measure all traumatic skin lesions • Photograph if possible

Source: Adapted from Hymel KP, Hall CA.[296]

TABLE 18-8 **Diagnostic Studies for Suspected Maltreatment**

Infant or child younger than 2 years with any neurologic signs/findings	Infant or young child with bruising and/or bleeding
• Skeletal survey complete with skull radiographs • Noncontrast head CT scan with brain and bone windows **Initial studies negative** • Cranial MRI with T1 and T2 weighted windows • Ophthalmology consult for dilated retinal examination **Initial CT scan positive** • Cranial MRI with T1 and T2 weighted windows (more useful if 5–7 days post injury) • Ophthalmology consult for dilated retinal examination • Initial serology: PT, PTT, CBC with platelet count, thrombin time, fibrinogen level, fibrin split products, bleeding time, liver function tests • Consider studies for inherited metabolic disease	• If younger than 2 years, skeletal survey • PT, PTT, and CBC with platelet count • Inquire about family bleeding history **Initial coagulation tests or history abnormal** • Thrombin time, fibrinogen level, fibrin split products • Retinal hemorrhage without specific history of moderate to severe accidental trauma • Consider von Willebrand screening • Consider hematology consult **Suspicion of skeletal injury** • Age younger than 12 months – Skeletal survey – Head CT scan – Consider bone scan if initial skeletal survey negative • Age 12 months to 2 years – Skeletal survey – Consider head CT scan

nonaccidental bruising, or any child younger than 6 months old.[156] Laboratory studies are indicated based on the constellation of symptoms of the child. Table 18-8 lists the diagnostic studies that should be considered for a child with suspected maltreatment.

With the history, physical exam, and diagnostic workup, the clinician must determine whether the injuries and findings are supported by the mechanistic history provided and the level of safety being provided to the child. Although many abusers of children are caregivers, it is important that the appearance of the caregiver during the evaluation does not sway the physician in the determination of maltreatment because other persons can also be responsible for the safety of the child. It is the responsibility of social services and law enforcement to make the determination of maltreatment. It is the physician's role to report the suspicion and to better ensure the safety of the child.

REFERENCES

1. Jalongo MR. The story of Mary Ellen Wilson: tracing the origins of child protection in America. *Early Childhood Edu J.* 2006;34(1):1–4.
2. Caffey J. Multiple fractures in the long bones of infants suffering from chronic subdural hematoma. *Am J Roentgenol.* 1946;56(2):163–173.
3. Alexander RC. Education of the physician in child abuse. *Pediatr Clin N Am.* 1990;37(4):971–988.
4. Ewing-Cobbs L, et al. Acute neuroradiologic findings in young children with inflicted or noninflicted traumatic brain injury. *Child Nerv Sys.* 2000;16:25–34.
5. Kempe CH, et al. The battered child syndrome. *JAMA.* 1962;181(1):105–112.

6. Southall DP, et al. Apnoeic episodes induced by smothering: two cases identified by covert video surveillance. *BMJ.* 1987;294:1637–1641.
7. Southall DP, et al. Covert video recordings of life threatening child abuse: lessons for child protection. *Pediatrics.* 1997;100(5):735–760.
8. Chang DC, et al. The multi-institutional validation of the new screening index for physical child abuse. *J Pediatr Surg.* 2005;40:114–119.
9. US Department of Health and Human Services. *Child Maltreatment 2002.* Washington, DC: US Department of Health and Human Services; 2002.
10. American Academy of Pediatrics, Committee on Child Abuse and Neglect, and Committee on Community Health Services. Investigation and review of unexpected infant and child deaths. *Pediatrics.* 1999;104(5):1158–1160.
11. Agran PF, et al. Rates of pediatric injuries by 3 month intervals for children 0 to 3 years of age. *Pediatrics.* 2003;111(6):e683.
12. DiScala C, et al. Child abuse and unintentional injuries. *Arch Pediatr Adolesc Med.* 2000;154:16–22.
13. Overpeck MD, et al. Risk factors for infant homicide in the United States. *N Engl J Med.* 1998;339(17):1211–1216.
14. Zenel J, Goldstein B. Child abuse in the pediatric intensive care unit. *Crit Care Med.* 2002;30(11 suppl):s515–s523.
15. Chang D, et al. The tip of the iceberg for child abuse: the critical roles of pediatric trauma service and its registry. *J Trauma.* 2004;57:1189–1198.
16. Stewart G, Meert K, Rosenberg N. Trauma in infants less than three months of age. *Pediatr Emerg Care.* 1993;9(4):199–201.
17. Thomas DE, Leventhal JM, Friedlaender E. Referrals to a hospital-based child abuse committee: a comparison of the 1960s and 1990s. *Child Abuse Negl.* 2001;25:203–213.
18. Giardino AP, Hudson KM, Marsh J. Providing medical evaluations for possible child maltreatment to children with special health care needs. *Child Abuse Negl.* 2003;27:1179–1186.
19. Hobbs GF, Hobbs CJ. Abuse of children in foster and residential care. *Child Abuse Negl.* 1999;23(12):1239–1252.
20. Keenan HT, et al. Increased incidence of inflicted traumatic brain injury in children after a natural disaster. *Am J Prevent Med.* 2004;26(3):189–193.
21. Leventhal JM, et al. Fractures in young children: distinguishing child abuse from unintentional injuries. *Am J Dis Child.* 1993;147:87–92.
22. Duhaime AC, et al. The shaken baby syndrome. *J Neurosurg.* 1987;66:409–415.
23. Alexander R, et al. Incidence of impact trauma with cranial injuries ascribed to shaking. *Am J Dis Child.* 1990;144:724–726.
24. Hettler J, Greenes DS. Can the initial history predict whether a child with head injury has been abused? *Pediatrics.* 2003;111(3):602–607.
25. Willman KY, Bank DE, Chadwick DL. Restricting the time of injury in fatal inflicted head injuries. *Child Abuse Negl.* 1997;21(10):929–940.
26. Starling SP, et al. Analysis of perpetrator admissions to inflicted traumatic brain injury in children. *Arch Pediatr Adolesc Med.* 2004;158:454–458.
27. Case ME, et al. Position paper on fatal abusive head injuries in infants and young children. *Am J Forensic Med Pathol.* 2001;22(2):112–122.
28. Adams JH, et al. Diffuse brain damage of immediate impact type. *Brain.* 1977;100:489–502.
29. Hymel KP, et al. Abusive head trauma? A biomechanics-based approach. *Child Maltreatment.* 1998;3:116–128.
30. Helfer RE, Slovis TL, Black M. Injuries resulting when small children fall out of bed. *Pediatrics.* 1977;60(4):533–535.
31. Lyons TJ, Oates RK. Falling out of bed: a relatively benign occurrence. *Pediatrics.* 1993;92:125–127.
32. Wickham T, Abrahamson E. Head injuries in infants: the risks of bouncy chairs and car seats. *Arch Dis Child.* 2002;86:168–169.
33. Warrington SA, Wright CM, ALSPAC Study Team. Accidents and resulting injuries in premobile infants: data from the ALSPAC study. *Arch Dis Child.* 2001;85:104–107.
34. Williams RA. Injuries in infants and small children resulting from witnessed and corroborated free falls. *J Trauma.* 1991;31(10):1350–1352.
35. Johnson K, et al. Accidental head injuries in children under 5 years of age. *Clin Radiol.* 2005;60:464–468.
36. MacGregor DM. Injuries associated with falls from beds. *Inj Prev.* 2000;6:291–292.
37. Tarantino CA, Dowd MD, Murdock TC. Short vertical falls in infants. *Pediatr Emerg Care.* 1999;15(1):5–8.
38. Smith MD, Burrington JD, Woolf AD. Injuries in children sustained in free falls: an analysis of 66 cases. *J Trauma.* 1975;15(11):986–991.
39. Nimityongskul P, Anderson LD. The likelihood of injuries when children fall out of bed. *J Pediatr Orthoped.* 1987;7:184–186.
40. Wheeler DS, Shope TR. Depressed skull fracture in a 7 month old who fell from bed. *Pediatrics.* 1997;100(6):1033–1031.
41. Gruskin KD, Schutzman SA. Head trauma in children younger than 2 years: are there predictors for complications? *Arch Pediatr Adolesc Med.* 1999;153(1):15–20.
42. Greenes DS, Schutzman SA. Infants with isolated skull fracture: what are their clinical characteristics, and do they require hospitalization? *Ann Emerg Med.* 1997;30(3):253–259.
43. Reece RM, Sege R. Childhood head injuries: accidental or inflicted? *Arch Pediatr Adolesc Med.* 2000;154:11–15.
44. Ros SP, Cetta F. Are skull radiographs useful in the evaluation of asymptomatic infants following minor head injury? *Pediatr Emerg Care.* 1992;8(6):328–330.
45. Greenes DS, Schutzman SA. Clinical indicators of intracranial injury in head-injured infants. *Pediatrics.* 1999;104(4):861–867.
46. Hall JR, et al. The mortality of childhood falls. *J Trauma.* 1989;29(9):1273–1275.
47. Kim KA, et al. Analysis of pediatric head injury from falls. *Neurosurg Focus.* 2000;8(1):273–280.
48. Chadwick DL, et al. Deaths from falls in children: how far is fatal? *J Trauma.* 1991;31(10):1353–1355.
49. Joffe M, Ludwig S. Stairway injuries in children. *Pediatrics.* 1988;82:457–461.
50. Chiaviello CT, Christoph RA, Bond GR. Stairway-related injuries in children. *Pediatrics.* 1994;94:679–681.
51. Alario A, et al. Do retinal hemorrhages occur with accidental head trauma in young children? [abstract]. *Am J Dis Child.* 1990;144:445.
52. Peclet MH, Newman KD, et al. Patterns of injury in children. *J Pediatr Surg.* 1990;25:85–91.
53. Smith GA, et al. Babywalker-related injuries continue despite warning labels and public education. *Pediatrics.* 1997;100(2):e 1.
54. Chiaviello CT, Christoph RA, Bond GR. Infant walker-related injuries: a prospective study of severity and incidence. *Pediatrics.* 1994;93(6):974–976.
55. Selbst SM, Baker D, Shames M. Bunk bed injuries. *Am J Dis Child.* 1990;144:721–723.
56. Plunkett J. Fatal pediatric head injuries caused by short-distance falls. *Am J Forensic Med Pathol.* 2001;22(1):1–12.
57. Barlow B, et al. Ten years of experience with falls from a height in children. *J Pediatr Surg.* 1983;18(4):509–511.
58. Lehman D, Schonfeld N. Falls from heights: a problem not just in the Northeast. *Pediatrics.* 1993;92(1):121–124.
59. Musemeche CA, et al. Pediatric falls from heights. *J Trauma.* 1991;31(10):1347–1349.
60. Pitetti RD, et al. Prevalence of retinal hemorrhages and child abuse in children who present with an apparent life-threatening event. *Pediatrics.* 2002;110(3):557–562.
61. Meadow R. Suffocation, recurrent apnea, and sudden infant death. *J Pediatrics.* 1990;117(3):351–357.
62. Altman RL, et al. Abusive head injury as a cause of apparent life threatening events in infancy. *Arch Pediatr Adolesc Med.* 2003;157:1011–1015.
63. Peterson DR. Clinical implications of sudden infant death syndrome epidemiology. *Pediatrician.* 1988;15:198–203.
64. Bass M, Kravath RE, Glass L. Death scene investigation in sudden infant death. *N Engl J Med.* 1986;315(2):100–105.
65. McClain PW, et al. Estimates of fatal child abuse and neglect, United States, 1979 through 1988. *Pediatrics.* 1993;91(2):338–343.

66. Ewing-Cobbs L, et al. Neuroimaging, physical and developmental findings after inflicted and noninflicted traumatic brain injury in young children. *Pediatrics.* 1998;102(2):300–307.
67. Corathers SD. The alkaline phosphatase level: nuances of a familiar test. *Pediatr Rev.* 2006;27(10):382–384.
68. Hymel KP, et al. Coagulopathy in pediatric abusive head trauma. *Pediatrics.* 1997;99(3):371–375.
69. Makoroff KL, et al. Elevated lactate as an early marker of brain injury in inflicted traumatic brain injury. *Pediatr Radiol.* 2005;35:668–676.
70. Coant PN, et al. Markers for occult liver injury in cases of physical abuse in children. *Pediatrics.* 1992;89:274–278.
71. Cameron CM, Lazoritz S, Calhoun AD. Blunt abdominal injury: simultaneously occurring liver and pancreatic injury in child abuse. *Pediatr Emerg Care.* 1997;13(4):334–336.
72. Isaacman DJ, et al. Utility of routine laboratory testing for detecting intra-abdominal injury in the pediatric trauma patient. *Pediatrics.* 1993;92:691–694.
73. Brown T. Radiography's role in detecting child abuse. *Radiol Technol.* 1995;66:389–390.
74. Ablin DS, et al. Differentiation of child abuse from osteogenesis imperfecta. *Am J Roentgenol.* 1990;154:1035–1046.
75. Merten DF, Radkowski MA, Leonidas JC. The abused child: a radiological reappraisal. *Radiology.* 1983;146:377–381.
76. American College of Radiology. *Suspected physical abuse—child.* American College of Radiology; 1995. Available at: http://www.acr.org/SecondaryMainMenuCategories/quality_safety/app_criteria/pdf/ExpertPanelonPediatricImaging/SuspectedPhysicalAbuseChildDoc9.aspx. Accessed August 13, 2008.
77. McClelland CQ, Heiple KG. Fractures in the first year of life. *Am J Dis Child.* 1982;136:26–29.
78. Dos Santos LM, et al. Soft tissue swelling with fractures: abuse versus nonintentional. *Pediatr Emerg Care.* 1995;11(4):215–216.
79. Duhaime AC, et al. Head injury in very young children: mechanisms, injury types, and ophthalmologic findings in 100 hospitalized patients younger than 2 years of age. *Pediatrics.* 1992;90:179–185.
80. Ablin DS, Greenspan A, Reinhart MA. Pelvic injuries in child abuse. *Pediatr Radiol.* 1992;22: 454–457.
81. Nimkin K, Kleinman PK. Imaging of child abuse. *Pediatr Clin N Am.* 1997;44(3):615–633.
82. Belfer RA, Klein BL, Orr L. Use of the skeletal survey in the evaluation of child maltreatment. *Am J Emerg Med.* 2001;19:122–124.
83. Smith FW, et al. Unsuspected costo-vertebral fractures demonstrated by bone scanning in the child abuse syndrome. *Pediatr Radiol.* 1980;10:103–106.
84. Merten DF, Kirks DR, Ruderman RJ. Occult humeral epiphyseal fracture in battered infants. *Pediatr Radiol.* 1981;10:151–154.
85. Frye TR, et al. Radiological case of the month: child abuse. *Am J Dis Child.* 1984;138:323.
86. Cadzow SP, Armstrong KL. Rib fractures in infants: red alert! The clinical features, investigations and child protection outcomes. *J Paediatr Child Health.* 2000;36:322–326.
87. Ellerstein NS, Norris KJ. Value of radiologic skeletal survey in assessment of abused children. *Pediatrics.* 1984;74:1075–1078.
88. American Academy of Pediatrics and Section on Radiology. Diagnostic imaging of child abuse. *Pediatrics.* 2000;105(6):1345–1348.
89. Kleinman PK, et al. Follow up skeletal surveys in suspected child abuse. *Am J Roentgenol.* 1996;167:893–896.
90. Zimmerman S, et al. Utility of follow-up skeletal surveys in suspected child physical abuse evaluations. *Child Abuse Negl.* 2005;29:1075–1083.
91. Prosser I, et al. How old is this fracture? Radiologic dating of fractures in children: a systematic review. *Am J Roentgenol.* 2005;184:1282–1286.
92. Sty JR, Starshak RJ. The role of bone scintigraphy in the evaluation of the suspected abused child. *Radiology.* 1983;146:369–375.
93. Mandelstam SA, et al. Complementary use of radiological skeletal survey and bone scintigraphy in detection of bony injuries in suspected child abuse. *Arch Dis Child.* 2003;88:387–390.
94. Pickett WJ, et al. Comparison of radiographic and radionuclide skeletal surveys in battered children. *Southern Med J.* 1983;76(2):207–212.
95. Conway JJ, et al. The role of bone scintigraphy in detecting child abuse. *Semin Nucl Med.* 1993;23(4):321–333.
96. Jaudes PK. Comparison of radiography and radionuclide bone scanning in the detection of child abuse. *Pediatrics.* 1984;73:166–168.
97. Section on Radiology, et al. Diagnostic imaging of child abuse. *Pediatrics.* 1991;87(2):262–264.
98. Rosenthal L, Hill RO, Chuang S. Observation on the use of 99mTC–phosphate imaging in peripheral bone trauma. *Radiology.* 1976;119:637–641.
99. Dietrich AM, et al. Pediatric head injuries: can clinical factors reliably predict an abnormality on computed tomography? *Ann Emerg Med.* 1993;22(10):1535–1540.
100. Schunk JE, Rodgerson JF, Woodward GA. The utility of head computed tomographic scanning in pediatric patients with normal neurologic examination in the emergency department. *Pediatr Emerg Care.* 1996;12(3):160–165.
101. Shane SA, Fuchs SM. Skull fractures in infants and predictors of associated intracranial injury. *Pediatr Emerg Care.* 1997;13(3):198–203.
102. Hahn YS, et al. Head injuries in children under 36 months of age. *Child Nerv Sys.* 1988;4:340.
103. Rivara FP, et al. Poor prediction of positive computed tomographic scans by clinical criteria in symptomatic pediatric head trauma. *Pediatrics.* 1987;80:579–584.
104. Davis RL, et al. Cranial computed tomography scans in children after minimal head injury with loss of consciousness. *Ann Emerg Med.* 1994;24(4):640–645.
105. Greenes DS, Schutzman SA. Occult intracranial injury in infants. *Ann Emerg Med.* 1998;32(6):680–686.
106. Rubin DM, et al. Occult head injury in high risk abused children. *Pediatrics.* 2003;111(6):1382–1386.
107. Dias MS, et al. Serial radiography in the infant shaken impact syndrome. *Pediatr Neurosurg.* 1998;29(2):77–85.
108. Hyden PW, Gallagher TA. Child abuse intervention in the emergency room. *Pediatr Clin North Am.* 1992;39(5):1053–1081.
109. Lonergan GF,Baker AM, Morey MK, Boos SC. From the AFIP Archives: Child abuse: radiologic-pathologic correlation. *Radiographics.* 2003;23(4):811–845.
110. Alexander RC, Schor DP, Smith WL. Magnetic resonance imaging of intracranial injuries from child abuse. *J Pediatr.* 1986;109:975–979.
111. Zimmerman RA, et al. Head injury: early results of comparing CT and high-field MRI. *Am J Roentgenol.* 1986;147(6):1215–1222.
112. Harwood-Nash DC. Abuse to the pediatric central nervous system. *Am J Neuroradiol.* 1992;13:569–575.
113. Chabrol B, Decarie JC, Fortin G. The role of cranial MRI in identifying patients suffering from child abuse and presenting with unexplained neurological findings. *Child Abuse Negl.* 1999;23(3):217–228.
114. Packer RJ, et al. Magnetic resonance imaging of lesions of the posterior fossa and upper cervical cord in childhood. *Pediatrics.* 1985;76:84–90.
115. Scherl SA. Orthopaedic injuries in child abuse. *Curr Paediatr.* 2006;16:199–204.
116. Morris MW, et al. Evaluation of infants with subdural hematoma who lack external evidence of abuse. *Pediatrics.* 2000;105(3):549–553.
117. Laskey AL, et al. Occult head trauma in young suspected victims of physical abuse. *J Pediatr.* 2004;144:719–722.
118. Jenny C, et al. Analysis of missed cases of abusive head trauma. *JAMA.* 1999;281:621–626.
119. Benzel EC, Hadden TA. Neurologic manifestations of child abuse. *South Med J.* 1989;82(11):1347–1351.
120. Sirotnak AP, Grigsby T, Krugman RD. Physical abuse of children. *Pediatr Rev.* 2004;25(8):264–276.
121. Jayawant S, et al. Subdural haemorrhages in infants: population based study. *BMJ.* 1998;317(7172):1558–1561.
122. Duhaime AC, et al. Nonaccidental head injury in infants–the "shaken-baby syndrome." *N Engl J Med.* 1998;338:1822–1829.

123. Caffey J. On the theory and practice of shaking infants. *Am J Dis Child.* 1972;124(2):161–169.
124. Morad Y, et al. Normal computerized tomography of brain in children with shaken baby syndrome. *J AAPOS.* 2004;8:445–450.
125. Cox LA. The shaken baby syndrome: diagnosis using CT and MRI. *Radiol Technol.* 1996;67(6):513–520.
126. Morad Y, et al. Correlation between retinal abnormalities and intracranial abnormalities in the shaken baby syndrome. *Am J Ophthalmol.* 2002;134:354–359.
127. Kivlin JD, et al. Shaken baby syndrome. *Ophthalmology.* 2000;107:1246–1254.
128. Gilliland MGF, Folberg R. Shaken babies—some have no impact injuries. *J Forensic Sci.* 1996;41(1):114–116.
129. Billmire ME, Myers PA. Serious head injury in infants: accident or abuse? *Pediatrics.* 1985;75(2):340–342.
130. Alexander R, et al. Serial abuse in children who are shaken. *Am J Dis Child.* 1990;144:58–60.
131. Barnes PD, Robson CD. CT findings in hyperacute nonaccidental brain injury. *Pediatr Radiol.* 2000;30:74–81.
132. Zimmerman RA, Bilaniuk LT. Pediatric head trauma. *Pediatr Neuroradiol.* 1994;4(2):349–366.
133. Pierce MC, et al. Injury biomechanics for aiding in the diagnosis of abusive head trauma. *Neurosurg Clin North Am.* 2002;13:155–168.
134. Zimmerman RA, et al. Computed tomography of craniocerebral injury in the abused child. *Radiology.* 1979;130:687–690.
135. Hymel KP, et al. Comparison of intracranial computed tomographic findings in pediatric abusive and accidental head trauma. *Pediatr Radiol.* 1997;27:743–747.
136. Zimmerman RA, et al. Interhemispheric acute subdural hematoma: a computed tomographic manifestation of child abuse by shaking. *Neuroradiology.* 1978;16:39–40.
137. Smith C. Intracranial haemorrhage in infants. *Curr Diag Pathol.* 2006;12:184–190.
138. Heyman R, et al. Intracranial epidural hematoma in newborn infants: clinical study of 15 cases. *Neurosurgery.* 2005;57(5):924–929.
139. Mealey J. Acute extradural hematomas without demonstrable skull fractures. *J Neurosurg.* 1960;17:27–34.
140. Shurgerman RP, et al. Epidural hemorrhage: is it abuse? *Pediatrics.* 1996;97(5):664–669.
141. Arbogast KB, Marguiles SS, Christian CW. Initial neurologic presentation in young children sustaining inflicted and unintentional fatal head injuries. *Pediatrics.* 2005;116(1):180.
142. Denton S, Mileusnic D. Delayed sudden death in an infant following an accidental fall. *Am J Forensic Med Pathol.* 2003;24(4):371–376.
143. Merten DF, Carpenter BLM. Radiologic imaging of inflicted injury in the child abuse syndrome. *Pediatr Clin North Am.* 1990;37(4):815–837.
144. Tzioumi D, Oates RK. Subdural hematomas in children under 2 years. Accidental or inflicted? A 10 year experience. *Child Abuse Negl.* 1998;22(11):1105–1112.
145. Vinchon M, et al. Accidental and nonaccidental head injuries in infants: a prospective study. *J Neurosurg Pediatr.* 2005;102(4):380–384.
146. Rustamzadeh E, Truwit CL, Lam CH. Radiology of nonaccidental trauma. *Neurosurg Clin North Am.* 2002;13:183–199.
147. Feldman KW, et al. The cause of infant and toddler subdural hemorrhage: a prospective study. *Pediatrics.* 2001;108(3):636–645.
148. Whitby EH, et al. Frequency and natural history of subdural haemorrhages in babies and relation to obstetric factors. *Lancet.* 2004;362:846–851.
149. Piatt JH. A pitfall in the diagnosis of child abuse: external hydrocephalus, subdural hematoma, and retinal hemorrhages. *Neurosurg Focus.* 1999;7(4).
150. Papasian NC, Frim DM. A theoretical model of benign external hydrocephalus that predicts a predisposition towards extra-axial hemorrhage after minor head trauma. *Pediatr Neurosurg.* 2000;33(4):188–193.
151. Pittman T. Significance of a subdural hematoma in a child with external hydrocephalus. *Pediatr Neurosurg.* 2003;39(2):57–59.
152. Ravid S, Maytal J. External hydrocephalus: a probable cause for subdural hematoma in infancy. *Pediatr Neurol.* 2003;28:139–141.
153. Haworth JC, et al. Phenotypic variability in glutaric aciduria type 1: report of fourteen cases in five Canadian Indian kindreds. *J Pediatrics.* 1991;118:52–58.
154. Per H, et al. Intracranial hemorrhage due to late hemorrhagic disease in two siblings. *J Emerg Med.* 2006;31(1):49–52.
155. Clemetson CAB. Child abuse or Barlow's disease. *Pediatr Int.* 2003;45:758.
156. Kemp AM. Investigating subdural haemorrhage in infants. *Arch Dis Child.* 2002;86(2):98–102.
157. Wilkins B, Sunderland R. Head injury—abuse or accident? *Arch Dis Child.* 1997;76:393–397.
158. Green PM, et al. Idiopathic intracranial haemorrhage in the fetus. *Fetal Diagn Ther.* 1999;14(5):275–278.
159. Tokoro K, Nakajima F, Yamataki A. Infantile chronic subdural hematoma with local protrusion of the skull in a case of osteogenesis imperfecta. *Neurosurgery.* 1988;22(3):595–598.
160. Meyer FB, et al. Cerebral aneurysms in childhood and adolescence. *J Neurosurg.* 1989;70:420–425.
161. Donaldson JW, Edwards-Brown M, Luerssen TG. Arachnoid cyst rupture with concurrent subdural hygroma. *Pediatr Neurosurg.* 2000;32(3):137–139.
162. Grode ML, Saunders M, Carton CA. Subarachnoid hemorrhage secondary to ruptured aneurysms in infants. *J Neurosurg.* 1978;49:898–902.
163. Chadwick D, et al. Shaken baby syndrome—a forensic pediatric response. *Pediatrics.* 1998;101(2):321–323.
164. Kendall N, Woloshin H. Cephalohematoma associated fracture of the skull. *J Pediatrics.* 1952;41(2):125–132.
165. Sargent S, Kennedy JG, Kaplan JA. Hyperacute subdural hematoma: CT mimic of recurrent episodes of bleeding in the setting of child abuse. *J Forensic Sci.* 1996;41(2):314–316.
166. Greenberg J, Cohen WA, Cooper PR. The "hyperacute" extraaxial intracranial hematoma: computed tomographic findings and clinical significance. *Neurosurgery.* 1985;17(1):48–56.
167. Plunkett J. Shaken baby syndrome and the death of Matthew Eappen: a forensic pathologist's response. *Am J Forensic Med Pathol.* 1999;20(1):17–21.
168. Duhaime AC, et al. Disappearing subdural hematomas in children. *Pediatr Neurosurg.* 1996;25:116–122.
169. Lee KS, et al. Origin of chronic subdural hematomas and relation to traumatic subdural lesions: review. *Brain Injury.* 1998;12:901–910.
170. Tung GA, et al. Comparison of accidental and nonaccidental traumatic head injury on noncontrast computed tomography. *Pediatrics.* 2006;118(2):626.
171. Hamlin H. Subgleal hematomas caused by hair pull. *JAMA.* 1968;205:314.
172. Santucci KA, Hsiao AL. Advances in clinical forensic medicine. *Curr Opin Pediatr.* 2003;15:304–308.
173. Bechtel K, et al. Characteristics that distinguish accidental from abusive head injury in hospitalized young children with head trauma. *Pediatrics.* 2004;114 (1):165–168.
174. Dashti SR, et al. Current patterns of inflicted head injury in children. *Pediatr Neurosurg.* 1999;31(6):302–306.
175. Goldstein B, et al. Inflicted versus accidental head injury in critically injured children. *Crit Care Med.* 1993;21(9):1328–1332.
176. Morad Y, et al. Nonophthalmologist accuracy in diagnosing retinal hemorrhages in the shaken baby syndrome. *J Pediatrics.* 2003;142:431–434.
177. Gayle MO, et al. Retinal hemorrhage in the young child: a review of etiology, predisposed conditions, and clinical implications. *J Emerg Med.* 1995;13(2):233–239.
178. Greenwald MJ, et al. Traumatic reinoschisis in battered babies. *Ophthalmology.* 1986;93:618–625.
179. Tsao K, Kazlas M, Weiter JJ. Ocular injuries in shaken baby syndrome. *Int Ophthalmol Clin.* 2002;42:145–155.
180. Green MA, et al. Ocular and cerebral trauma in non-accidental injury in infancy: underlying mechanisms and implications for paediatric practice. *Br J Ophthalmol.* 1996;80:282–287.

181. Gilliland MGF, Luckenback MW, Chenier TC. Systemic and ocular findings in 169 prospectively studied child deaths: retinal hemorrhages usually mean abuse. *Forensic Sci Int.* 1994;68:117–132.
182. Pierre-Kahn V, et al. Ophthalmologic findings in suspected child abuse victims with subdural hematomas. *Ophthalmology.* 2003;110:1718–1723.
183. Curcoy Barcenilla AI, et al. When a fundoscopic examination is the clue of maltreatment diagnostic. *Pediatr Emerg Care.* 2006;22(7):495–496.
184. Levin AV. Ophthalmology of shaken baby syndrome. *Neurosurg Clin North Am.* 2002;13:201–211.
185. Aryan HE, et al. Retinal hemorrhage and pediatric brain injury: etiology and review of the literature. *J Clin Neurosci.* 2005;12(6):624–631.
186. Tyagi AK, Willshaw HE, Ainsworth JR. Unilateral retinal hemorrhages in non-accidental injury. *Lancet.* 1997; 349:1224.
187. Paviglianiti J, Donahue SP. Unilateral retinal hemorrhages and ipsilateral intracranial bleeds in nonaccidental trauma. *J AAPOS.* 1999;3(6):383–384.
188. Drack AV, Petronio J, Capone A. Unilateral retinal hemorrhages in documented cases of child abuse. *Am J Ophthalmol.* 1999;128:340–344.
189. Lantz PE. The evidence base for shaken baby syndrome: response to Reece et al from 41 physicians and scientists. *BMJ.* 2004;329:741–742.
190. Levin AV. Ocular manifestations of child abuse. *Ophthalmol Clin North Am.* 1990;3:249.
191. Lantz PE, et al. Perimacular retinal folds from childhood head trauma. *BMJ.* 2004;328:754–756.
192. Mills M. Fundoscopic lesions associated with mortality in shaken baby syndrome. *J AAPOS.* 1998;2:67–71.
193. Ou JI. Macular hole in the shaken baby syndrome. *Arch Ophthalmol.* 2006;124:913–915.
194. Schloff S, et al. Retinal findings in children with intracranial hemorrhage. *Ophthalmology.* 2002;109:1472–1476.
195. Johnson DL, Braun D, Friendly D. Accidental head trauma and retinal hemorrhage. *Neurosurgery.* 1993;33(2):231–235.
196. Christian CW, et al. Retinal hemorrhages caused by accidental household trauma. *J Pediatrics.* 1999;135:125–127.
197. Emerson MV, et al. Incidence and rate of disappearance of retinal hemorrhages in newborns. *Ophthalmology.* 2001;108:36–39.
198. Levin S, et al. Diagnostic and prognostic value of retinal hemorrhages in the neonate. *Obstet Gynecol.* 1980;55(3):309–314.
199. Hughes LA, et al. Incidence, distribution, and duration of birth-related retinal hemorrhages: a prospective study. *J AAPOS.* 2006;10(2):102–106.
200. Smith WL, et al. Magnetic resonance imaging evaluation of neonates with retinal hemorrhage. *Pediatrics.* 1992;89:332–333.
201. Kanter RK. Retinal hemorrhage after cardiopulmonary resuscitation or child abuse. *J Pediatrics.* 1986;108(3):430–432.
202. Odom A, et al. Prevalence of retinal hemorrhages in pediatrics patients after in-hospital cardiopulmonary resuscitation: a prospective study. *Pediatrics.* 1997;99(6):e3.
203. Fackler JC, Berkowitz ID, Green WR. Retinal hemorrhages in newborn piglets following cardiopulmonary resuscitation. *Am J Dis Child.* 1992;146:1294–1296.
204. Goetting MG, Sowa B. Retinal hemorrhage after cardiopulmonary resuscitation in children: an etiologic re-evaluation. *Pediatrics.* 1990;85:585–588.
205. Geddes JF, Talbert DG. Paroxysmal coughing, subdural and retinal bleeding: a computer modeling approach. *Neuropathol Appl Neurobiol.* 2006;32:625–634.
206. Ganesh A, et al. Retinal hemorrhages in type 1 osteogenesis imperfecta after minor trauma. *Ophthalmology.* 2004;111:1428–1431.
207. Tyagi AK, et al. Can convulsions alone cause retinal hemorrhages in infants? *Br J Ophthalmol.* 1998;82:659–660.
208. Goldman M, et al. Severe cough and retinal hemorrhage in infants and young children. *J Pediatrics.* 2006;148:835–836.
209. Herr S, et al. Does Valsalva retinopathy occur in infants? An initial investigation in infants with vomiting caused by pyloris stenosis. *Pediatrics.* 2004;113(6):1658–1661.
210. Clark RSB, et al. Retinal hemorrhages associated with spinal cord ateriorvenous malformation. *Clin Pediatr.* 1995;34:281–283.
211. Feldman KW. Patterned abusive bruises of the buttocks and pinnae. *Pediatrics.* 1992;90:633–636.
212. Hanigan WC, Peterson RA, Njus G. Tin ear syndrome: rotational acceleration in pediatric head injuries. *Pediatrics.* 1987;80:618–622.
213. Naidoo S. A profile of the oro-facial injuries in child physical abuse at a children's hospital. *Child Abuse Negl.* 2000;24(4):521–534.
214. Maguire S, et al. Torn labial frenulum—evidence of child abuse? A systemic review abstract. *Arch Dis Child.* 2005;90(suppl II):A41–A 43.
215. Chadwick D. The diagnosis of inflicted injury in infants and young children. *Pediatr Ann.* 1992;21(8):477–483.
216. Chan L, Hodes D. When is an abnormal frenulum a sign of child abuse? *Arch Dis Child.* 2004;89:277.
217. Jessee SA. Orofacial manifestations of child abuse and neglect. *Am Fam Physician.* 1995;52(6):1829–1834.
218. Pramuk LA, Sirotnak AP, Friedman NR. Esophageal perforation preceding fatal closed head injury in child abuse case. *Int J Pediatr Otorhinolaryngol.* 2004;68:831–835.
219. Lloyd DA, et al. Predictive value of skull radiography for intracranial injury in children with blunt head injury. *Lancet.* 1997;349:821–824.
220. Kleinman PK, Spevak MR. Soft tissue swelling and acute skull fractures. *J Pediatr.* 1992;121:737–739.
221. O'Neill JA, et al. Patterns of injury in the battered child syndrome. *J Trauma.* 1973;13(4):332–339.
222. Merten DF, et al. Craniocerebral trauma in the child abuse syndrome: radiological observations. *Pediatr Radiol.* 1984;14:272–277 .
223. Cohen RA, et al. Cranial computed tomography in the abused child with head injury. *Am J Roentgenol.* 1986;146:97–102.
224. Tsai FY, et al. Computed tomography in child abuse head trauma. *J Comput Assist Tomogr.* 1980;4:277–286.
225. Chasler CN. The newborn skull: the diagnosis of fracture. *Am J Roentgenol.* 1967;100:92–99.
226. Meservy CJ, et al. Radiographic characteristics of skull fractures resulting from child abuse. *Am J Roentgenol.* 1987;149:173–175.
227. Hiss J, Tzipi K. The medicolegal implications of bilateral cranial fractures in infants. *J Trauma.* 1995;38(1):32–34.
228. Hobbs CJ. Skull fracture and the diagnosis of abuse. *Arch Dis Child.* 1984;59:246–252.
229. Pierce MC, et al. Evaluating long bone fractures in children: a biomechanical approach with illustrative cases. *Child Abuse Negl.* 2004;28:505–524.
230. King J, et al. Analysis of 429 fractures in 189 battered children. *J Pediatr Orthoped.* 1988;8(5):585–589.
231. Kleinman PK, et al. Inflicted skeletal injury: a postmortem radiologic-histopathologic study in 31 infants. *Am J Roentgenol.* 1995;165:647–650.
232. Kahana T, Hiss J. Forensic radiology. *Br J Radiol.* 1999;72:129–133.
233. Bulloch B, et al. Cause and clinical characteristics of rib fractures in infants. *Pediatrics.* 2000;105(4):e48.
234. Barsness KA, et al. The positive predictive value of rib fractures as an indicator of nonaccidental trauma in children. *J Trauma.* 2003;54(6):1107–1110.
235. Kleinman PK, et al. Factors affecting visualization of posterior rib fractures in abused infants. *Am J Roentgenol.* 1988;150:635–638.
236. Zumwalt RE, Fanizza-Orphanos AM. Dating of healing rib fractures in fatal child abuse. *Adv Pathol.* 1990;3:193–205.
237. Kleinman PK. Diagnostic imaging in infant abuse. *Am J Roentgenol.* 1990;155:703–712.
238. Sewell RD, Steinberg MA. Chest compressions in an infant with osteogenesis imperfecta type II: no new rib fractures. *Pediatrics.* 2000;106(5):1130.
239. Feldman KW, Brewer DK. Child abuse, cardiopulmonary resuscitation and rib fractures. *Pediatrics.* 1984;73:339–342.
240. Spevak MR, et al. CPR and rib fractures in infants. *JAMA.* 1994;272:617–618.
241. Betz P, Liebhardt E. Rib fractures in children—resuscitation or child abuse? *Int J Legal Med.* 1994;106:215–218.

242. Caffey J. Some traumatic lesions in growing bones other than fractures and dislocations: clinical and radiological features. *Br J Radiol.* 1957;30(353):225–238.
243. Longergan GF, et al. Child abuse: radiologic-pathologic correlation. *AFIP Arch.* 2003;23(4):811–845.
244. Grayev AM, et al. Metaphyseal fractures mimicking abuse during treatment for clubfoot. *Pediatr Radiol.* 2001;31(8):559–563.
245. Worlock P, Stower M, Barbor P. Patterns of fractures in accidental and non-accidental injury in children: a comparative study. *BMJ.* 1986;293:100–102.
246. Anderson WA. The significance of femoral fractures in children. *Ann Emerg Med.* 1982;11(4):174–177.
247. Blakemore LC, Loder R, Hensinger RN. Role of intentional abuse in children 1 to 5 years old with isolated femur shaft fractures. *J Pediatr Orthopaed.* 1996;16(5):585–588.
248. Dalton HJ, et al. Undiagnosed abuse in children younger than 3 years with femoral fracture. *Am J Dis Child.* 1990;144:875–878.
249. Loder RT, O'Donnell PW, Feinberg JR. Epidemiology and mechanisms of femur fractures in children. *J Pediatr Orthoped.* 2006;26(5):561–566.
250. Morris S, et al. Birth-associated femoral fractures: incidence and outcome. *J Pediatr Orthoped.* 2002;22:27–30.
251. Cole WG. Advances in osteogenesis imperfecta. *Clin Orthopaed.* 2002;401:6–16.
252. Astley R. Metaphyseal fractures in osteogenesis imperfect. *Br J Radiol.* 1979;52:441–443.
253. Jenny C. Evaluating infants and young children with multiple fractures. *Pediatrics.* 2006;118(3):1299–1303.
254. Tay ET, Levin TL. Suspected abuse. *Clin Pediatrics.* 2004;43:583–585.
255. Schmale GA, Chansky HA, Raskind WH. Hereditary multiple exostoses. Gene Reviews. Original posting 2000, Updated 2005. Available at: http://www.ncbi.nlm.nih.gov/bookshelf/br.fcgi?book=gene&part=ext, Accessed August 26, 2008.
256. Kirks DR. Radiological evaluation of visceral injuries in the battered child syndrome. *Pediatr Ann.* 1983;12(12):888–893.
257. Ng CS, Hall CM, Shaw DG. The range of visceral manifestations of non-accidental injury. *Arch Dis Child.* 1997;77:167–174.
258. Cooper A, et al. Major blunt abdominal trauma due to child abuse. *J Trauma.* 1988;28(10):1483–1487.
259. Barnes PM, et al. Abdominal injury due to child abuse. *Lancet.* 2005;366:234–235.
260. Wood J, et al. Distinguishing inflicted versus accidental abdominal injuries in young children. *J Trauma.* 2005;59(5):1203–1208.
261. Gornall P, Ahmed S, Jolleys A, et al. Intra-abdominal injuries in the battered baby syndrome. *Arch Dis Child.* 1972; 47:211-244.
262. Ledbetter DJ, Hatch EI, Feldman KW, Fligner CL, Tapper D. Diagnostic and surgical implications of child abuse. *Arch Surg.* 1988;123(9):1101-1105.
263. Gaines BA, et al. Duodenal injuries in children: beware of child abuse. *J Pediatr Surg.* 2004;39(4):600–602.
264. Pena SD, Medovey H. Child abuse and traumatic pseudocyst of the pancreas. *J Pediatr.* 1973;83(6):1026-1028.
265. Sugar NF, et al. Bruises in infants and toddlers: those who don't cruise rarely bruise. *Arch Pediatr Adolesc Med.* 1999;153:399–403.
266. Labbe J, Caouette G. Recent skin injuries in normal children. *Pediatrics.* 2001;108(2):271–276.
267. Wilson EF. Estimation of the age of cutaneous contusions in child abuse. *Pediatrics.* 1977;60(5):750–752.
268. Stephenson T. Ageing of bruising in children. *J Royal Soc Med.* 1997;90:312–314.
269. Stephenson T, Bialas Y. Estimation of the age of bruising. *Arch Dis Child.* 1996;74:53–55.
270. Bariciak ED, et al. Dating of bruises in children: an assessment of physician accuracy. *Pediatrics.* 2003;112(4):804–807.
271. Langlios NE, Gresham GA. The aging of bruises: a review and study of the colour changes with time. *Forensic Sci Int.* 1991;50:227–238.
272. Lee LY, Ilan J, MulveyT. Human biting of children and oral manifestations of abuse: case report and literature review. *J Dent Child.* 2002;5:92–95.
273. Levine LJ. Bite mark evidence. *Dent Clin North Am.* 1977;21(1):145–158.
274. Wheeler DM, Hobbs CJ. Mistakes in diagnosing non-accidental injury: 10 years experience. *BMJ.* 1988;296:1233–1236.
275. Mudd SS, Findlay JS. The cutaneous manifestations and common mimickers of physical child abuse. *J Pediatr Health Care.* 2004;18(3):123–129.
276. Brown J, Melinkovich P. Schonlein-Henoch purpura misdiagnosed as suspected child abuse. *JAMA.* 1986;256(5):617–618.
277. Adler R, Kane-Nussen B. Erythema multiforme: confusion with child battering syndrome. *Pediatrics.* 1983;72(5):718–720.
278. Carpentieri U, Gustavson LP, Haggard ME. Misdiagnosis of neglect in a child with bleeding disorder and cystic fibrosis. *South Med J.* 1978;71(7):854–855.
279. O'Hare AE, Eden OB. Bleeding disorders and non-accidental injury. *Arch Dis Child.* 1984;59:860–864.
280. Hathaway WE, et al. Activated partial thromboplastin time and minor coagulopathies. *Am J of Clin Pathol.* 1979;71(1):22–25.
281. Dietch EA, Staats M. Child abuse through burning. *J Burn Care Rehab.* 1982;3:89–94.
282. Greenbaum AR, et al. Intentional burn injury: an evidence–based, clinical and forensic review. *Burns.* 2004;30:628–642.
283. Kharasch S, Vinci R, Reece R. Esophagitis, epiglottitis, and cocaine alkaloid ("crack"): "accidental" poisoning or child abuse? *Pediatrics.* 1990;86(1):117–119.
284. Hobbs CJ. When are burns not accidental? *Arch Dis Child.* 1986;61:357–361.
285. Peck MD, Priolo-Kapel D. Child abuse by burning: a review of the literature and an algorithm for medical investigations. *J Trauma.* 2002; 53(5):1013–1022.
286. Allasio D, Fischer H. Immersion scald burns and the ability of young children to climb into a bathtub. *Pediatrics.* 2005;115(5):1419–1421.
287. Moritz AR. Studies of thermal injury: pathology and pathogenesis of cutaneous burns: an experimental study. *Am J Pathol.* 1947;23(6):915–934.
288. Kibayashi K, Shojo H. Patterned injuries in children who have suffered repeated physical abuse. *Pediatr Int.* 2003;45:193–195.
289. Alexander RC, Surrell JA, Cohle SD. Microwave oven burns to children: an unusual manifestation of child abuse. *Pediatrics.* 1987;79:255–260.
290. Kemp AM, Mott AM, Sibert JR. Accidents and child abuse in bathtub submersions. *Arch Dis Child.* 1994;70:435–438.
291. Friedman SB, Morse CW. Child abuse: a five-year follow-up of early case finding in the emergency department. *Pediatrics.* 1974;54(4):404–410.
292. Fischer H, Allasio D. Permanently damaged: long term follow-up of shaken babies. *Clin Pediatr.* 1994;33(11):696–697.
293. McRae KN, Ferguson CA, Lederman RS. The battered child syndrome. *CMAJ.* 1973;108:859–866.
294. Johnson CF, Showers J. Injury variables in child abuse. *Child Abuse Negl.* 1985;9:207–215.
295. Handy TC, Nichols GR, Smock WS. Repeat visitors to a pediatric forensic medicine program. *J Forensic Sci.* 1996;41(5):841–844.
296. Hymel KP, Hall CA. Diagnosing pediatric head trauma. *Pediatr Ann.* 2005;34(5):358–370.

19 | Pediatric Sexual Abuse: Evaluation in the Emergency Department

Amita Sudhir, MD, Sarah Anderson, PhD, RN, CEN, SANE-A, and William J. Brady, MD, FACEP, FAAEM

INTRODUCTION

Sexual abuse affects children irrespective of age, sex, socioeconomic class, or geographic location. Annually, more than 1 million substantiated cases of child mistreatment occur in the United States—of these cases of child maltreatment, approximately 10% involve sexual abuse. Most often, the abuser is an adult male; yet female abuse of children, particularly adolescent males, is increasing. Most often, the sexually abused child has a favorable medical outcome—it is quite rare for a child to die from such abuse. Yet the psychological outcome can be severe, with higher rates of mental illness later in life as well as interpersonal difficulties in adulthood.

Certainly, the emergency department (ED) evaluation of the potentially abused child is difficult for all involved, including the patient, the family, and the ED staff. The consequences of misdiagnosis of sexual abuse can be damaging from two perspectives: overdiagnosis with defamation of character and altered trust issues, and failure to diagnose with ongoing danger to the patient. As a result, a basic awareness of the behavioral and physical manifestations of sexual abuse is critical to the detection of sexual abuse in the ED.

When a child presents to a healthcare setting with a report of sexual abuse or concerns of sexual abuse, several important pieces of information are needed prior to evaluation and evidence collection. The information collected prior to evidence collection has several purposes: to obtain details of the event and disclosure; establish a rapport with the child; assess the developmental stage and emotional status of the child in terms of the sexual abuse; and assess how cooperative the child might be with the examination.[1,2]

CLINICAL PRESENTATION

The caregiver and the child should be interviewed separately to avoid contamination (influence or distraction) of the information. When interviewed with a caregiver, the child may not disclose all information, especially if the child believes the information will upset the caregiver further, or the child may add information if he or she believes that is what the caregiver wants to hear. During the interview with the parent or caregiver, the following information should be obtained: past medical history including sexual and/or physical abuse; developmental information about the child's terminology for body parts; and who has access to the child and details about the current living arrangements. Additional information must be collected, including how the abuse was identified; the disclosure of events; who disclosed the events; if no disclosure, what lead to the suspicions of abuse; if the child disclosed, exactly what was said and the context of the disclosure; and how the caregiver reacted to the statements along with subsequent conversations with the child.[3] Clarification of information obtained is essential.

The Patient Interview

When the child is interviewed, the environment should be quiet to avoid distractions and interruptions, and if possible, only the child and the interviewer should be present. Because some information obtained as part of a medical examination may be admissible in court, medical practitioners must remember several important points. The interviewer needs to remain neutral throughout the interview and avoid asking leading questions, including yes/no questions.

Initially, interviewers need to establish a rapport with the child by introducing themselves and talking with the child about themselves. During this part of the interview, information about the child's verbal and cognitive skills can be assessed. At some point during the interview, it is important to establish the "rules" (that is, if you don't know the answer, it is okay to say so), and in this way establish the child's ability to tell about a past event. For example, ask the child about an old injury such as a scar on the knee. It is important for the interviewer to let the child know up front that he or she will explain each action in the interview and examination and that it should not hurt.

When the child feels comfortable, interviewers can introduce the reason why the child is present, which is usually done by asking the child, "So, do you know why we are meeting and talking today?" The child should be allowed to speak freely; ask open-ended questions after the child stops speaking. Avoid rewarding the child for information given.

The Physical Examination

There are two types of evidence collection examinations. One is the acute examination, within 72 hours of the event, and the nonacute examination, which is performed if the event occurred more than 72 hours ago. Based on recommendations, it is suggested that if the event is more distant than 72 hours, once child protective services has been involved, the child should be referred to a regional child sexual abuse specialist for evaluation.[4,5] The parent or caregiver, especially for younger children, may provide support and assistance during the examination as long as the caregiver is not the suspected perpetrator.

The purpose of the acute examination is to provide emergency medical assessment to identify injuries, detect sexually transmitted diseases, collect and preserve physical evidence from the child, and assess the child's safety.[6] Because only 14.3% of the children reporting sexual abuse have suspicious genital or anal injuries,[4] any evidence of sexual assault collected may be the only evidence present.[6]

The physical examination of the sexually abused child may reveal entirely normal findings. The absence of physical findings rarely confirms the absence of sexual abuse; for example, approximately 50% of female children with a documented history of vaginal penetration have a normal genital examination,[7,8] and only a small percentage of children evaluated for suspected sexual abuse have any physical findings. In fact, a substantial number of victimized children are not *physically* injured because the abuse act often involves only touching, fondling, or orogenital contact without vaginal or anal penetration with a finger or the penis,[9] or the injury has healed. The ultimate diagnosis of pediatric sexual abuse is made by an analysis of the history, examination findings, and subsequent investigation, which at times is supported by evidence from the physical examination. It must be stressed, however, that a normal physical examination is common in cases of documented child sexual abuse.

If the alleged sexual abuse occurred less than 72 hours prior to presentation, the examination should be performed in the emergency department because of the time sensitivity of possible forensic evidence. For patients who present more than 72 hours after the event, the clinician should consider deferring the examination to someone who specializes in the evaluation of sexual abuse.[10] If the child refuses the examination, it is up to the clinician to decide how important it is to proceed. If there is reasonable suspicion of injury that needs to be identified, it is appropriate to conduct the examination under sedation or general anesthesia.[3]

The goals of the physical examination are as follows:

- To identify and manage genital trauma
- To identify and manage other signs of physical abuse
- To diagnose medical conditions such as pregnancy or sexually transmitted disease
- To collect forensic evidence
- To address the concerns of both parent and child regarding what, if any, harm has been done

The general physical examination should be performed prior to examination of the genitalia, the perineum, and the anus. Evidence of traumatic injury including ecchymoses, abrasions, and lacerations to the head, neck, trunk, extremities, and—in particular—the breasts and buttocks must be sought (Figures 19-1 and 19-2). The oropharynx must be closely examined for signs of traumatic injury as well as for signs of sexually transmitted infections (STIs) such as exudate, erythema, chancre, vesicle, or ulcer. Additionally,

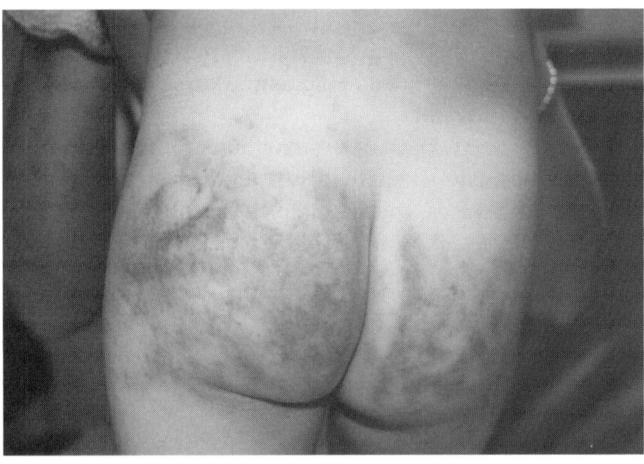

FIGURE 19-1 **Three-year-old male with ecchymosis to buttocks (medium-range photograph). Note patterned injury to left buttocks from "strap" used to discipline the child. See Color Plate 15.**

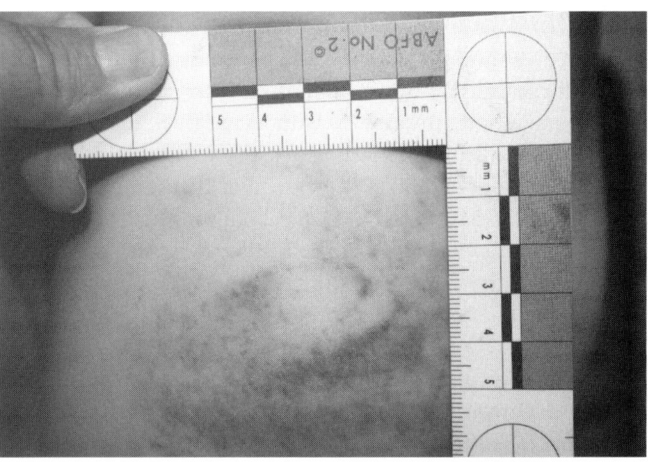

FIGURE 19-2 **Close-up photograph of patterned injury with a scale. See Color Plate 16.**

intra-abdominal injury must be ruled out in the standard fashion using the physical examination, laboratory testing, and radiographic imaging. Such findings consistent with either trauma or STI, however, are not specific for physical or sexual abuse in most cases; these findings must be incorporated into the overall picture of the medicolegal investigation.

After a general physical examination has been performed, the evaluation of the perineum and related areas obviously differs based upon the gender of the patient. In the female child, the external genitalia should be examined first. Visual inspection should be followed by gentle labial separation, and then labial traction while the child is in frog-leg position and knee–chest position (Figures 19-3 and 19-4). The presence or absences of injuries to the labia majora, labia minora,

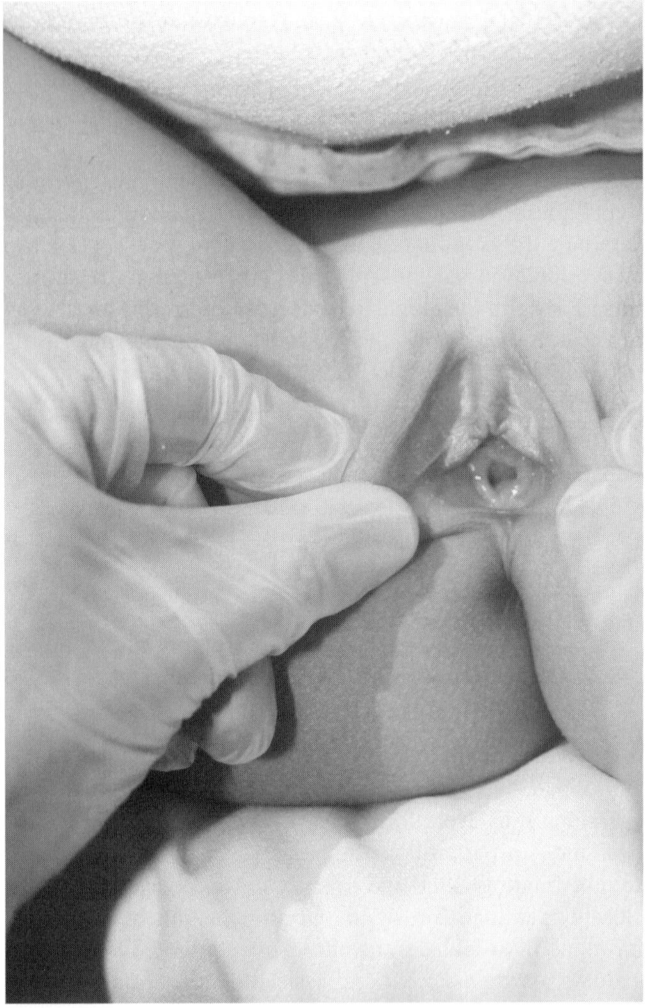

FIGURE 19-3 ***(left)*** **Ten-year-old female examined using labial traction in the frog-leg position. A "bump" is noted at the 4 to 6 o'clock position. See Color Plate 17.**

FIGURE 19-4 ***(bottom)*** **Ten-year-old female examined using labial separation in the knee–chest position to confirm finding in the frog-leg position. See Color Plate 18.**

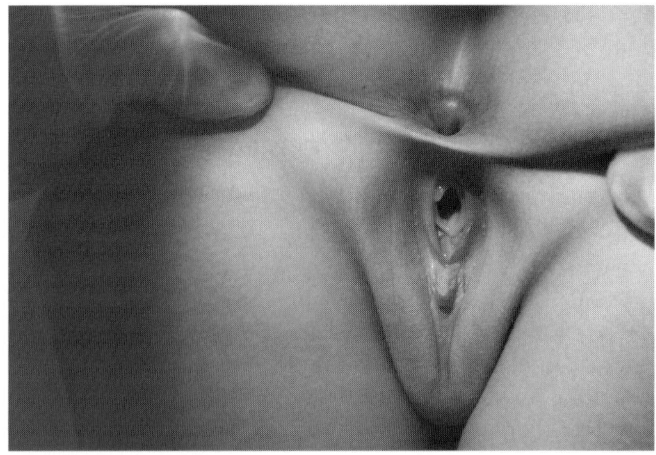

clitoris, urethra, hymen, vestibule, posterior fourchette, medial thighs, and perineum should be included in the documentation and a schematic diagram.

The term *intact* should be avoided in describing the hymen. If the tissue of the hymen appears folded in on itself, the tissue can be gently moved with a cotton swab dipped in saline.[3] Because the hymen in a prepubescent child is extremely sensitive, touching the hymen should be avoided until the exam is almost complete. An internal vaginal examination (the speculum is only used in adolescent girls who have started their menstrual cycle) should be conducted only if there is serious and persistent vaginal bleeding or other concern for internal injury. Strong consideration should be given to having this examination conducted by a gynecologist with the child under general anesthesia. The anus can be examined with the child in the supine position. The gluteal folds should be spread and anal area inspected for tears, abrasions, ecchymosis, and swelling. If anal dilatation occurs with gentle traction, note whether or not there is stool in the vault. As with the vaginal examination, digital or endoscopic examination should be performed only if there is bleeding or concern for serious internal injury.[3] Findings on anal examination should also be documented on a diagram.

A male child should be placed in lateral decubitus position with the child holding his knees. The prone knee–chest position, again, may create anxiety, especially because with male children, this may simulate the position of abuse.[10] The penis, scrotum, anus, and surrounding areas should all be examined with notation of any trauma or other physical findings; further, as with the female patient, the gluteal folds should be spread and the anal area inspected. As with the vaginal examination, digital or endoscopic examination should be performed only if there is bleeding or concern for serious internal injury.[3]

Physical examination findings of the genitalia that are associated with sexual abuse include evidence of acute trauma to the external genital/anal area, healing injuries, injuries associated with blunt force penetrating trauma, presence of STIs, pregnancy, or the presence of sperm found on the child. Findings of acute trauma healing injuries or blunt force penetrating trauma can also be caused by accidental trauma to the genital area. In addition to physical findings associated with sexual abuse, there may be other findings commonly referred to as "indeterminate" that may or may not be a result of sexual abuse or trauma. See Table 19-1 for a list of normal, variant, and indeterminate findings diagnostic of sexual abuse that is taken from the "Guidelines for Care of Children Who May Have Been Abused."[11]

The hymen is a small organ that surrounds the opening of the vaginal introitus with considerable normal anatomic variation. A number of descriptive terms have been suggested for these variations, including fimbriated, circumferential, and posterior rim[12] or crescent and concentric.[13] In general, the fimbriated and/or concentric hymen is most often encountered in infants less than 12 months of age while the crescentic hymen is usually found in children 2 years of age and older.[13,14] The hymenal appearance changes when estrogen is present (postnatal and with the onset of puberty). Estrogen causes the hymenal tissue to thicken and at times be redundant. The vast majority of female infants are born with hymens; the estimated frequency of congenital absence of the hymen is 0.01%. Disruption to the hymenal tissue occurs as a result of both accidental (nonabuse) and intentional (abuse) situations. Accidental injury, however, is rare and should be assumed only after a full investigation has been completed.[15,16] Injury to the hymen when noted in the emergency department must be assumed to have resulted from sexual abuse and should prompt the clinician to initiate a thorough investigation.

Manifestations of intentional injury to the hymen include transections, lacerations, notches, bumps, scarring, and attenuation.[17–20] Acute injuries to the hymen are manifested by lacerations and attenuation, whereas past injuries with varying degrees of healing are signified by notches or concavities, bumps with thickening of the mucosa, and scarring. The location of the hymenal abnormality is important in the determination of potential sexual injury as the etiology. Using the clock positioning method, abnormalities of the hymen in the 4 to 8 o'clock region are highly suggestive of sexual abuse.[7,14,21] Blurring the picture, hymenal bumps and notches have been noted during normal examinations where abuse had not occurred. Bumps have been found in 7–18% of normal examinations (i.e., no history of abuse), and notches have been documented in 7–8% of a similar group.[14] Hymenal scarring, lacerations, and attenuation of the tissue most often represent abuse.

Labial fusion is another physical finding associated with sexual abuse, though with much less sensitivity than hymenal injury. *Labial fusion*, also known as vulvar fusion, synechiae of the vulva, and agglutination of the labia minora, is defined as either partial or complete adherence of the labia minora. This entity results from a combination of poor hygiene, vulvovaginitis, and/or mechanical irritation in the setting of hypoestrogenism.[22–24] Labial fusion has been reported in victims of child abuse,[25,26] as well as in normal children without history of sexual injury at frequencies of approximately 20–40%.[13,27] At times, these fusions are only noted on colposcopic examination. Adhesions likely to have resulted from sexual abuse may appear thickened and irregular in texture, similar to typical scar tissue.[13]

Injuries to the posterior fourchette or commisure, the posterior union of the labia minora, can arise from a number of causes including gymnastic maneuvers, "doing the splits," and riding horseback, as well as sexual abuse. The tissue in this region is both thin and fragile; it is easily disrupted with direct pressure. Such injuries range from minor increases in vascularity to deep lacerations extending into the anus.[25,28] Careful attention must be applied to distinguish the naturally occurring midline perineal raphe, which extends from the posterior fourchette to the anus, from scar tissue representing past posterior injury.

TABLE 19-1 **Symptoms and Signs Associated with Sexual Abuse**[11]

Findings Documented in Nonabused Children	**Normal variants:** • Periurithral or vestibular bands • Intravaginal ridges or columns • Hymenal bumps or mounds • Hymenal tags or septal remnants • Linea vestibularis • Hymenal notch/cleft above the 3 to 9 o'clock line • Superficial/shallow hymenal notch below the 3 to 9 o'clock line • External hymenal ridge	• Congenital variants in appearance of hymen • Diastasis ani • Perianal skin tags • Hyperpigmentation of labia minora or perianal tissue • Dilation of the urethral opening with application of labial traction • Thickened hymenal tissue
Indeterminant Findings	**Findings commonly caused by other medical conditions:** • Redness of the vestibule, penis, scrotum, or perianal areas • Increased vascularity • Labial adhesions • Vaginal discharge • Friability of the posterior fourchette or commisure • Excoriations/bleeding/vascular lesions	• Perineal groove partial or complete • Anal fissures • Venous congestions or pooling in the perianal area with traction • Flattened anal folds • Partial or complete anal dilation to less than 2 cm with or without stool
	Physical findings: • Deep notches or clefts in the hymen between 4 and 8 o'clock • Deep notches or complete clefts in the hymen at 3 or 9 o'clock • Smooth, uninterrupted rim of the hymen between 4 and 8 o'clock that appears to be less than 1 mm wide	• Wart-like lesions in the genital or anal area • Vesicular lesions or ulcers in the genital or anal area • Marked, immediate anal dilation to 2 cm or more in the absence of predisposing factors
	Lesions with etiology confirmed: • Genital or anal condyloma in child in the absence of other indicators of abuse	• Herpes Type 1 or 2 in the genital or anal area with no indicators of sexual abuse
Findings Diagnostic of Trauma and/or Sexual Abuse	**Acute trauma to external genitalia/anal area:** • Lacerations or bruising to labia, scrotum, perianal tissue, or perineum (accidental trauma or sexual abuse)	• Acute lacerations to posterior fourchette
	Healing injuries: • Perianal scarring (accidental injury, disease process [Crohn's], previous medical procedures or sexual abuse)*	• Posterior fourchette or fossa scarring*
	Injuries associated with blunt force trauma: • Acute lacerations or transactions to the hymen • Ecchymosis to the hymen • Missing segment of hymen	• Healed transaction of the hymen (confirmed in both frog-leg and knee–chest position) between 4 and 8 o'clock
Findings Diagnostic of Sexual Contact	**Presence of infection most likely to have been sexual abuse:** • Positive confirmed culture of gonorrhea, from genital area, outside of the neonatal period • Confirmed diagnosis of syphilis, if perinatal transmission is ruled out • *Trichomonas vaginalis* in a child older than 1 year identified by culture or wet mount by an experienced clinician	• Positive culture from genital or anal area for chlamydia, if child is older than 3 at time of diagnosis and specimen was tested using cell culture or CDC-approved method • Positive HIV if perinatal transmission, transmission from blood products, and needle contamination has been ruled out
	Other evidence of sexual contact: • Pregnancy	• Detection of sperm taken directly from the child's body

*Pale areas to the midline may be due to labial adhesions or linea vestibularis.

Source: Adam JA, Kaplan RA, Starling SP, Mefta NH, Finkel MA, Botash AS, Kellogg ND. Guidelines for medical care of children who may have been sexually abused. *J Pediatr Adolesc Gynecol.* 2007;20:163–172.

LABORATORY INVESTIGATIONS

The clinical laboratory may aid the physician in the evaluation of patients suspected of sexual abuse, providing evidence of an STI and other signs of sexual contact such as sperm, saliva, or pregnancy. Clinical evidence confirming the presence of an STI—with an incidence of less than 4% in documented cases of abuse—is a specific finding consistent with sexual abuse.[29,30] The Centers for Disease Control and Prevention (CDC) states in its treatment guidelines that a pediatric STD infection, particularly in a prepubertal child, should be considered as evidence of sexual abuse until fully investigated and proven otherwise. Current basic knowledge of disease transmission, however, forces practitioners to place such infectious findings into categories of clinical suspicion for sexual abuse, including definite, probable, and possible.[31] The "definite" grouping includes *Treponema pallidum* (syphilis) and *Neisseria gonorrhea*, STI organisms that are virtually always transmitted through sexual contact. Members of the "probable" category, infections that are usually but not always transmitted through sexual contact, include *Trichomonas vaginalis*, Herpes simplex, *Condylma acuminata*, and *Chlamydia trachomatis*. It must be stressed that infections caused by members of the previous two categories must be considered highly suspect of abuse because nonsexual transmission is unlikely.[32,33]

Sexually transmitted diseases classified as "possible" are *Gardnerella vaginalis*, pediculosis, scabies, and human immunodeficiency virus (HIV). These STDs may be transmitted in a nonsexual manner and, therefore, are only possible indicators of sexual abuse. Additionally, certain members of these three categories (*T. pallidum*, *N. gonorrhoeae*, herpes simplex, *C. trachomatis*, and HIV) may undergo perinatal transmission; such a mechanism of disease contagion must be considered in appropriately aged patients. A standard urinalysis demonstrating pyuria and/or microscopic hematuria in the absence of bacteria may, in fact, represent lower genital tract infection from an STI organism and not urinary tract infection acquired in a nonsexual manner. Such an STI is confirmed by appropriate studies including positive genital tract and negative urinary cultures.

The presence of sperm or saliva is another laboratory finding diagnostic of sexual abuse. Any body surface area or cavity that may have been contaminated, particularly the anus, the vagina, and the oropharynx, must be sampled with saline-moistened swabs. Importantly, approximately one-third of positive findings are collected from areas distant from the orogenital tracts such as the back or internal aspects of the thighs.[34] Motile and nonmotile sperm may be found in the vagina as late as 3 to 12 hours and 2 to 10 days after the sexual assault, respectively.[35] The enzyme acid phosphatase, which is present in high concentrations in seminal fluid, is another indicator of the recent presence of semen.

And last, a positive test for pregnancy whether using urine or blood is confirmatory evidence that sexual intercourse has taken place. Such sexual contact must then be investigated to determine whether abuse has occurred.

EVIDENCE COLLECTION

The evidence collection process for a child is based on the information collected during the interview with the child and the caregiver along with a careful systematic head-to-toe physical examination. Most jurisdictions have a prepackaged evidence collection kit specific to sexual assaults. These kits contain the materials and directions to collect and preserve physical evidence after a sexual assault.

For evidence to be used in court, the chain of custody must be maintained. For purposes of litigation, for the evidence to be used in the court proceedings, the prosecutor must be able to prove the legal integrity of all samples and data introduced as evidence. There must be an accurate written record to track all samples from the time of collection until the evidence is presented. Verification of who has possessed the samples and where the samples have been is easier if medical practitioners follow chain-of-custody procedures.

During the medical and forensic examinations, potential evidentiary items are collected in a systematic fashion. The clothing worn at the time of the assault or immediately afterward should be collected. Clothing and linens are more likely to contain evidence longer than areas on the body, especially after 24 hours.[36] Other items collected during the examination include trace evidence or debris that is found on the child. Trace evidence can be found using visual inspection, magnification of an area, and combing through hair.

Each individual item is carefully packaged in its own separate paper—not plastic—envelope/container. If the item is damp or wet, exam table paper should be placed in between the layers prior to packaging. The evidence technician who takes the items needs to be notified that items are wet so that they can be dried prior to storage. The envelope/container is sealed using a piece of tape wide and long enough to cover the opening of the container. The evidence collector then initials across the edges of the tape in several locations. The container is labeled with the following information: name of the victim; date; time of collection; the item in the container; and the initials or signature of the evidence collector. This process of packaging is used for each item that is collected.

Other types of evidence that may be collected include body fluids such as saliva, semen, blood, urine, or gastric contents. There are several ways to decide where to collect possible body fluids. Based on information collected during the interview about contact with a body fluid along with the use of a Wood's lamp, swabs can be taken to try to collect foreign DNA. The Wood's lamp is used to look for areas that fluoresce and should be used as an adjunct to the investigative process.[37] It is important to understand that there are other substances that fluoresce such as detergents that contain bleach, certain bacterial or fungal skin infections, topical medications, lint, and soap residues.

To use the Wood's lamp correctly, the lamp should ideally be allowed to warm up for about 1 minute. The examination room should be perfectly dark, preferably a windowless room or a room with black occlusive shades. The examiner should become dark adapted to see the contrast clearly. The light source should be 4 to 5 inches from the area.[38]

To increase the chance of collecting evidence with swabbing the skin, the best method is referred to as the double-swab technique in which a wet cotton swab is used followed by a dry cotton swab.[39] All areas identified with the Wood's lamp should be swabbed with the double-swab technique and looked at again with the Wood's lamp to ensure a specimen was collected. Any area of suspected body fluid exposure (i.e., urine, saliva, seminal fluid, blood) should be swabbed using this method.

Photography should be utilized to document any injuries or findings during the head-to-toe examination. Photographs taken should include an overall, medium-range, and close-up picture with and without a scale. In addition to the photographs, written documentation with actual measurements and schematic drawings should be included in documentation.

Colposcopy should be utilized to document the genital examination even if no injuries are found. Standard photographs with the colposcope should include an overall picture of the genital area with close-up views that show the edges of the hymen, the posterior fourchette, labia minora, labia majora, clitoral hood, and the anal area. This can be extremely important when expert consultation is needed at a later time.

CONDITIONS MIMICKING SEXUAL ABUSE

The diagnosis of pediatric sexual abuse is difficult for a number of reasons, including a lack of physician awareness of age-adjusted genital anatomy and also a host of nonabuse conditions that mimic or that are confused with intentional genital trauma. There is evidence to suggest that many physicians are unable to recognize both normal and abnormal female prepubertal anatomy. A survey of 129 medical practitioners—including 77% in pediatrics or family medicine—revealed lack of a solid knowledge base concerning prepubertal female anatomy.[40] When asked to label genital structures in a photograph of a 6-year-old female, only 59% correctly identified the hymen, 78% the urethral opening, and 89% the clitoris. Further, an inability to firmly establish a diagnosis of sexual abuse was one justification given by physicians for not referring patients to child protective services for abuse investigation.[41]

A variety of dermatologic, traumatic, infectious (non-STI), gastrointestinal, urologic, and congenital conditions can mimic or be mistaken for physical findings caused by sexual abuse. The most common dermatologic syndrome mistaken for sexual abuse is lichen sclerosis. Lichen sclerosis manifests as subepidermal hemorrhage of the genital tissues—usually caused by minimal trauma to the area such as wiping after using the toilet—occasionally accompanied by vesicular, blistering, or bullous lesions. The characteristic hourglass configuration of atrophic and hypopigmented skin around the genitalia and/or anus is consistent with the diagnosis, which is confirmed by biopsy.[42–44] Other abnormal skin and mucous membrane findings of the genitalia including erythema, edema, and excoriations may be caused by such nonabuse conditions as diaper dermatitis, irritation from bath soap, poor hygiene, pinworms, or *Candida albicans* infection.[45,46]

Unintentional injury to the genital, anal, or perineal tissues may be mistaken for sexual abuse. In general, such injuries result from straddle mechanisms, producing damage to external structures in a unilateral distribution that are anterior or lateral to the hymen. Vaginal lacerations have been noted in young females falling astride sharp objects. The hymen and other internal genital tissues are rarely involved; hymenal damage should alert the clinician to an increased risk of sexual abuse.[15,47,48] Trauma occurring in motor vehicle crashes has been reported to cause genital injury. For example, an improperly placed lap belt was responsible for perineal tears and labial abrasions sustained in an automobile accident; the hymen was without evidence of injury.[49] Additionally, intentional, surgical trauma—manifested by adhesions and scarring—to the genitals of young African or Middle Eastern females may represent circumcision.[48]

Infectious disorders from non-STD organisms may also produce findings similar to child abuse. Pinworms and *Candida albicans* both cause erythema, edema, and excoriations. Perineal streptococcal cellulitis presents with bleeding, anal fissures, painful bowel movements, and profuse Erythema.[42,50] Acute varicella (chickenpox) infection may initially appear in the genital area, prompting the physician to make the diagnosis of herpes simplex infection. Only after the typical exanthem pattern is noted and/or viral culture results are available is the correct diagnosis made.[51]

Gastrointestinal and urologic maladies have also been incorrectly diagnosed as sexual abuse. Crohn's disease presents with a tendency for fistulization, rectal tumors, chronic constipation with anal fissuring, rectal prolapse, and megacolon.[52–56] A word of warning concerning rectal prolapse is warranted: such a physical finding has been reported as being caused by sexual abuse.[53] Urologic conditions mistaken for abuse including urethral prolapse, urethral caruncle, and urethral hemangiomas may come to the attention of concerned parents, presenting with pain and vaginal bleeding.[42,57,58] Again, caution is advised; as with rectal prolapse, urethral prolapse has been reported as a result of sexual abuse. In both situations, a number of other etiologies other than abuse have been reported. A thorough investigation of the history will aid in making the diagnosis.[59]

Last, a number of congenital anomalies masquerade as sexual abuse. A general guideline suggests that abnormalities of midline structures in the genital, perianal, and anal areas may represent congenital abnormality rather than intentional, malicious injury. Failure of midline fusion across the posterior fourchette, a congenital cleft superior to the urethra, and anomalies of the anal sphincter have all been wrongly diagnosed as the sequelae of past sexual abuse.[42,60] Hemangiomas of the hymen, the vaginal wall, and the vulva have all been incorrectly identified as signs of sexual abuse.[42,61]

THE TEAM APPROACH

To adequately investigate allegations of or concerns about child sexual abuse, a multidisciplinary team approach is necessary because 85–95% of the reported cases of child sexual abuse have no physical findings. Without physical findings, a complete investigation of the circumstances of the event, the living situation, adults who have access to the child, and past history of prior sexual abuse (founded or unfounded) needs to be performed.

Many communities have established child advocacy teams. The team members may vary, but most include child protective services, law enforcement, medical personnel, and mental health services. Communities, depending on services available and financial means, may have a child advocacy center where all members of the team can evaluate the child and services are provided. Even if there is not a formal center or team established, the agencies identified should have informal agreements.

Members and Roles of the Child Advocacy Team

Child protective service agencies are responsible for receiving and investigating reports of child abuse and neglect. In addition to sexual abuse services, child protective service agencies provide services for child physical abuse and child neglect along with coordinating services for children and families when the situation involves a child's caregiver. If the case does not involve a caregiver or someone who is acting in that position, child protective services will involve the local prosecutor's office and law enforcement. These agencies may be involved even if the situation involves a caregiver.

Medical professionals, such as physicians, nurses, emergency medical services personnel, and social workers, are required to report all cases of suspected child sexual abuse to child protective services. Because healthcare providers are more likely to come in contact with children, they provide a large number of the reports made to child protective services.

Even with mandatory reporting requirements, there are barriers to reporting suspected child sexual abuse.[62–65] To decrease these barriers, certain provisions are in place: immunity for good faith reporting; standards to guide reasonable suspicion; rules regarding anonymity; relaxation of privileged communication rights; procedures for reporting and how information is processed; guidelines regarding protective custody; and penalties for not reporting.

Some physicians and nurses (usually pediatric sexual assault nurse examiners) have additional training in evaluating child sexual abuse patients. The child sexual abuse examination can involve evidence collection, injury documentation, interpretation of findings, detection of sexually transmitted diseases, and expert testimony in court proceedings. Law enforcement agencies are responsible for investigations where criminal activity may be involved because they are tasked and trained to conduct interviews, collect evidence at the crime scene, and interrogate suspects. Many times law enforcement and child protective services work concurrently, especially in cases of child sexual abuse.

Mental health professionals provide assessments and treatment to deal with the short- and long-term impact of child sexual abuse. It is not uncommon for a mental health professional to work with a child if there are concerns of sexual abuse but there has been no disclosure of an event.

CONCLUSION

Pediatric sexual abuse is a common problem and one that requires a multidisciplinary approach. Acute forensic evidence collection is often not needed, but a pelvic examination may reveal previous trauma. Physicians and SANEs should be familiar with the approach to the pediatric survivor. There may be long lasting psychological trauma to the child, and any system that treats children should have counseling and social services readily available.

REFERENCES

1. Lahoti SL, Mclain N, Girardet R, McNeese M, Cheung K. Evaluating the child for sexual abuse. *Am Fam Phys.* 2001;63(5):883–892.
2. Kellog N, Committee on Child Abuse and Neglect. The evaluation of sexual abuse in children. *Pediatrics.* 2005;116(2): 506-512.
3. Sugarman J. Evaluation of child sexual abuse. In: Giardino A., Datner EM, Asher JB, eds. *Sexual Assault Victimization Across the Life Span: A Clinical Guide.* St. Louis, Mo: GW Medical Publishing; 2003.
4. Adams JA. Medical evaluation of suspected child abuse: it's time for standardized training, referral centers, and routine peer review [comment]. *Arch Pediatr Adolesc Med.* 1999;153(11):1121–1122.
5. Arnold DH, Spiro DM, Nichols MH, King WD. Availability and perceived competence of pediatricians to serve as child protection team medical consultants: a survey of practicing pediatricians. *South Med J.* 2005;98:423–428.
6. Palusci VJ, Cox EO, Shatz EM, Schultze JM. Urgent medical assessment after child sexual abuse. *Child Abuse Negl.* 2006;30(4):367–380.
7. Muram D. Child sexual abuse: relationship between sexual acts and genital findings. *Child Abuse Negl.* 1989;13:211–216.
8. Marshall WN. New child abuse spectrum in an era of increasing awareness. *Am J Dis Child.* 1988;142:668–673.
9. Rimsza ME, Niggemann EH. Medical evaluation of sexually abused children: a review of 311 cases. *Pediatrics.* 1982;8:69–76.
10. Kini N, Brady WJ, Lazoritz S. Evaluating child sexual abuse in the emergency department: clinical and behavioral indicators. *Acad Emerg Med.* 1996;3:966–976.
11. Adam JA, Kaplan RA, Starling SP, Mefta NH, Finkel MA, Botash AS, Kellogg ND. Guidelines for medical care of children who may have been sexually abused. *J Pediatr Adolesc Gynecol.* 2007;20:163–172.
12. Pokorny SF. Configuration of the prepubertal hymen. *Am J Obstet Gynecol.* 1987;157:950–956.
13. McCann J, Wells R, Simon M, et al. Genital findings in prepubertal girls selected for nonabuse: a descriptive study. *Pediatrics.* 1990;86:428–439.
14. Berenson AB, Heger AH, Hayes JM, et al. Appearance of the hymen in prepubertal girls. *Pediatrics.* 1992;89:387–394.
15. Bond GR, Dowd MD, Landsman I, Rimsza M. Unintentional perianal injury in prepubescent girls: a multicenter, prospective report of 56 girls. *Pediatrics.* 1995;95:628–631.
16. Pokorny SF, Kozinetz CA. Configuration and other anatomical details of the prepubertal hymen. *Adolesc Pediatr Gynecol.* 1988;1:97–103.
17. Herman-Giddens ME, Frothingham TE. Prepubertal female genitalia: examination for evidence of sexual abuse. *Pediatrics.* 1987;80(22):203–208.
18. Muram D. Child sexual abuse: genital tract findings in prepubertal girls. *Am J Obstet Gynecol.* 1989;160:328–333.
19. Claytor RN, Barth KL, Shubin CI. Evaluating child sexual abuse: observations regarding ano-genital injury. *Clin Pediatr.* 1989;28:419–422.
20. Emans SJ, Woods ER, Flagg NT, et al. Genital findings in sexually abused, symptomatic and asymptomatic, girls. *Pediatrics.* 1987;79:778–785.
21. Berenson AB, Heger AH, Andrew S. Appearance of the hymen in newborns. *Pediatrics.* 1991;87:458–465.
22. Teton JR, Treadwell NC. The management of nonspecific vulvitis in children. *Am J Obstet Gynecol.* 1956;72:674–676.

23. Bowles HE, Childs LS. Synechiae of vulva in small children. *Am J Dis Child.* 1953;66:258–263.
24. Finlay HVL. Adhesions of the labia minora in childhood. *Proc R Soc Med.* 1965;58:929–931.
25. McCann J, Voris J, Simon M. Labial adhesions and posterior fourchette injuries in childhood sexual abuse. *Am J Dis Child.* 1988;142:659–663.
26. Berkowitz CD, Elvik SL, Logan MK. Labial fusion in prepubescent girls: a marker for sexual abuse? *Am J Obstet Gynecol.* 1987;156:16–20.
27. Emans SJ, Woods ER, Flagg NT, et al. Genital findings in sexually abused, symptomatic and asymptomatic, girls. *Pediatrics.* 1987;79:778–785.
28. Teixeira WRG. Hymenal colposcopic examination in sexual offenses. *Am J Forensic Med Pathol.* 1980;2:209–215.
29. De Jong AR. Sexually transmitted disease in sexually abused children. *Sex Transm Dis.* 1986;13:123–126.
30. Dattel BJ, Landers DV, Coulter K, et al. Isolation of *Chlamydia trachomatis* and *Neisseria gonorrhea* from the genital tract of sexually abused prepubertal females. *Adolesc Pediatr Gynecol.* 1989;2:217–220.
31. Ludwig S. Child abuse. In: Fleisher GR, Ludwig S, eds. *Textbook of Pediatric Emergency Medicine.* Baltimore, Md: Williams and Wilkins; 1993:1429–1463.
32. Neinstein LS, Goldenring J, Carpenter S. Nonsexual transmission of sexually transmitted disease: an infrequent occurrence. *Pediatrics.* 1984;74:67–76.
33. Kaplan KM, Fleisher GR, Paradise JE, et al. Social relevance of genital Herpes simplex in children. *Am J Dis Child.* 1984;138:872–876.
34. Enos WF. Forensic evaluation of the sexually abused child. *Pediatrics.* 1986;77:433–440.
35. Ricci LR. Child abuse: the emergency department response. *Ann Emerg Med.* 1986;6:711–716.
36. Christian CW, Lavelle JM, De Jong AR, Loiselle J, Brenner L, Joffe M. Forensic evidence findings in prepubertal victims of sexual assault. *Pediatrics.* 2000;106:100–104.
37. Santucci KA, Nelson DG, McQuillen KK, Duffy SJ, Linakis JG. Wood's lamp utility in the identification of semen. *Pediatrics.* 1999;104:1342–1344.
38. Gupta LK, Singhi MK. Wood's lamp. *Indian J Dermatol Venereol Leprol.* 2004;70:131–135.
39. Sweet D, Lorente JA, Lorente M, Valenzuela A, Villanueva E. An improved method to recover saliva from human skin: the double swab technique. *J Forensic Sci.* 1997;42:320–322.
40. Ladson S, Johnson CF, Doty RE. Do physicians recognize sexual abuse? *Am J Dis Child.* 1987;141:411–415.
41. Morris JL, Johnson CF, Clasen M. To report or not report: physician's attitudes toward discipline and child abuse. *Am J Dis Child.* 1985;139:194–197.
42. Bays J, Jenny C. Genital and anal conditions confused with child sexual abuse trauma. *Am J Dis Child.* 1990;144:1319–1322.
43. Handfield-Jones SE, Hinde FRJ, Kennedy CTC. Lichen sclerosus et atrophicus in children misdiagnosed as sexual abuse. *BMJ.* 1987;294:1404–1405.
44. Jenny C, Kirby P, Fuquay D. Genital lichen sclerosus mistaken for child sexual abuse. *Pediatrics.* 1989;83:597–599.
45. Paul DM. The medical examination in sexual offenses against children. *Med Sci Law.* 1977;17:251–258.
46. McCann J, Voris J, Simon M, et al. Perianal findings in prepubertal children selected for non-abuse: a descriptive study. *Child Abuse Negl.* 1989;13:179–193.
47. Muram D. Genital tract injuries in the prepubertal child. *Pediatr Ann.* 1986;15:616–620.
48. Unuighe JA, Giwa-Osagie AW. Pediatric and gynecological disorders in Benin City, Nigeria. *Adolesc Pediatr Gynecol.* 1988;1:257–261.
49. Baker R. Seat belt injury masquerading as sexual abuse. *Pediatrics.* 1986;77:435.
50. Spear RM, Rothbaum RJ, Keating JP, et al. Perianal streptococcal cellulitis. *J Pediatr.* 1985;107:557–559.
51. Boyd M, Jordan SW. Unusual presentation of varicella suggestive of child abuse. *Am J Dis Child.* 1987;141:940.
52. Hey F, Buchan PC, Littlewood JM, et al. Differential diagnosis in child sexual abuse. *Lancet.* 1987;1:283.
53. Hobbs CJ, Wynne JM. Sexual abuse of English boys and girls: the importance of the anal examination. *Child Abuse Negl.* 1989;13:195–210.
54. Lazar LF, Muram D. The prevalence of perianal and anal abnormalities in a pediatric population referred for gastrointestinal complaints. *Adolesc Pediatr Gynecol.* 1989;2:37–39.
55. Clayden GS. Reflex anal dilation associated with severe constipation in children. *Am J Dis Child.* 1988;63:832–836.
56. Zempsky WT, Rosenstein BJ. The cause of rectal prolapse in children. *Am J Dis Child.* 1988;142:338–339.
57. Johnson CF. Prolapse of the urethra: confusion of clinical and anatomic characteristics with sexual abuse. *Pediatrics.* 1991;87:722–723.
58. Roberts JW, Devine CJ. Urethral hemangioma: treatment by total excision and grafting. *J Urol.* 1983;129:1053–1054.
59. Lowe FC, Hill GS, Jeffs RD, et al. Urethral prolapse in children: insights into etiology and management. *J Urol.* 1986;135:100–103.
60. Adams JA, Horton M. Is it sexual abuse? *Clin Pediatr.* 1986;28:146–148.
61. Levin AV, Selbst SM. Vulvar hemangioma simulating child abuse. *Clin Pediatr.* 1988;27:213–215.
62. Delaronde S, King G, Bendel R, Reece R. Opinions among mandated reporters toward child maltreatment reporting policies. *Child Abuse Negl.* 2000;24(7):901–910.
63. Ladson S, Johnson CF, Doty RE. Do physicians recognize sexual abuse? *AJDC.* 1987;141:411–415.
64. Lentsch KA, Johnson CF. Do physicians have adequate knowledge of child sexual abuse? Results of surveys of practicing physicians. *Child Maltreat.* 2000;5:72–78.
65. Savell S. Childhood sexual abuse: are health care providers looking the other way? *J Foren Nurs.* 2005;1(2):78–81,85.

20 Elder Abuse and Neglect

Matthew R. Bartholomew, MD, FAAEM, Jean Cheek, RN, FNE, and Jennifer Hoyt, MD

INTRODUCTION

Why should we worry about elder abuse? Elder abuse is a growing health and social problem in the United States and the world. The sheer numbers alone should startle most people, and healthcare providers should be especially concerned. As of July 2003, 35.9 million people in the United States were aged 65 years or older, about 12% of the population. This number is expected to double by the year 2030 and represent about 20% of the US population. Worldwide the elderly population is on a similar tract. In 2000, 420 million people in the world were aged 65 years or older, and that number is expected to rise to 974 million by 2030.[1]

Each year somewhere between 1 and 2 million elderly Americans experience some form of abuse.[2] But only about 10% of cases are reported. In 1996, only 293,000 cases of elder abuse were reported.[3] In one study, it was found that only 1 out of every 14 cases of elder abuse or neglect is reported to authorities.[4] Why are the numbers of reported cases so small? There are many factors involved that may lead to underreporting or, more likely, misdiagnosis of elder abuse: denial by both victim and perpetrator, reluctance to report victims by clinicians, disbelief by healthcare providers, and lack of awareness of the warning signs.[5]

Hospital protocols have been recommended by the American Medical Association and the American College of Emergency Physicians to aid in the detection and management of elder abuse and neglect.[6,7] Many emergency departments lack protocols for elder abuse, and many physicians are unaware that they exist, even if present.[8] These protocols should be developed at your institution and, if already present, should be updated on a regular basis. Elder abuse and neglect may be detected by screening protocols in the emergency department.[9]

The goals of this chapter are for you to obtain a better understanding of the many different types of elder abuse and neglect, and to be more prepared to recognize elder abuse and neglect and to identify who is at risk of becoming a victim or a perpetrator. Also, this chapter can give you an idea of what you should do if you suspect elder abuse or neglect and a few ideas on how to help this group of patients. Not only can you help the patient you have under your care, but your early intervention may help prevent a caretaker at risk from becoming an abuser and the damage to both that follows.

DEFINING ELDER ABUSE

There are six types of elder abuse: physical abuse, emotional abuse, sexual abuse, financial exploitation, neglect, and abandonment (see Table 20-1). Extreme and heinous cases can be easily identified, such as gunshot wounds, knife wounds, bite marks, and rope burns; however, other cases are not as clear-cut and the signs may be subtle in nature.[10] The ability to identify signs of abuse may help indicate cases of elder abuse. There is no gold standard test for elder abuse or neglect; you must rely on history and forensic markers.[11](Refer to Table 20-2.) This is difficult because some markers of natural disease processes overlap those of abuse and neglect. Signs and symptoms of abuse or neglect may include abrasions, lacerations, bruising, fractures, restraints, decubitus ulcers, weight loss, dehydration, burns, cognitive and mental health problems, hygiene issues, burns, and sexual abuse.[11] The identification of injuries associated with elder abuse is vital to the medical and legal determination of whether elder abuse or neglect has occurred.[10]

TABLE 20-1 **Types of Elder Abuse**

Physical Abuse
Emotional Abuse
Sexual Abuse
Financial Exploitation
Neglect and Self-Neglect
Abandonment

TABLE 20-2 **Questions to Screen for Elder Abuse**

Physical abuse
- Are you afraid of anyone at home?
- Have you been struck, slapped, or kicked?
- Have you been tied down or locked in a room?
- Has anyone touched you without your permission?

Emotional abuse
- Do you ever feel alone?
- Have you been threatened with punishment, deprivation, or institutionalization?
- Have you received the "silent treatment"?
- Have you been force-fed?
- What happens when you and your caregiver disagree?

Neglect
- Do you lack aids such as eyeglasses, hearing aids, or false teeth?
- Have you been left alone for long periods?
- If you need assistance, how do you obtain it?
- How do you get help?

Financial abuse
- Does your caregiver depend on you for shelter or financial support?
- Has money been stolen from you?

Source: Used with permission from Carney et al. Elder abuse: is every bruise a sign of abuse? *Mt Sinai J Med.* 2003;70(2):69–74.

Physical abuse is the intentional use of physical force that may result in bodily injury and pain or impairment. This is the most easily identified type of abuse.[12,13] Signs of physical abuse are bruises, lacerations, ligature marks, and there may also be skull or other fractures. Fractures of the head, spine, and trunk are found to be more indicative of assault injuries than are limb fractures, sprains, or other musculoskeletal injuries. Fractures with a rotational component and spiral fractures of a large bone without a history of gross injury may be indicative of abuse.[10,11] Another sign is untreated injuries at various stages of healing. A National Institutes of Health (NIH)–funded study to explore injuries of physical abuse found that accidental bruises occur in a predictable pattern in older adults, and most large bruises that are accidentally inflicted occur on the extremities.[14] In the elderly, bruises occur more frequently and resolve more slowly than in a younger person and can last for months rather than 1 to 2 weeks.[11] Elder skin becomes thin, loose, and transparent with a decreased vascularity and atrophy that makes it fragile. Elders bruise under less force or pressure than younger individuals do.[15] The elder may report that he or she is being hit, slapped, or kicked.

Emotional abuse is the psychological abuse of the elder by inflicting emotional anguish and pain through verbal and nonverbal actions. Psychological or emotional abuse commonly includes verbal or nonverbal insults, humiliation, and is often defined as an act carried out with the intent of causing emotional pain or injury.[10,16] The caretaker may make threats of harm and blame the elder for the increased responsibility and financial strain on the caretaker. Signs of emotional abuse may present as the elder being withdrawn, noncommunicative, or refusing to respond to questioning. Elders may also report being intentionally kept isolated from others.

Sexual abuse is nonconsensual sexual contact with an elderly person, and this may include elders who are mentally incapacitated. The contact may include inappropriate sexual touching or fondling, nonconsensual sexual intercourse, and other forms of sexual assault. Signs of sexual abuse can include bruising around the breasts or genital areas; however, the signs are often subtle and may manifest as behavioral changes, withdrawal, fear of male caregivers, and health decline. Again, as individuals age, skin becomes thin, loose, and transparent.[15] As such, an elder sexual assault victim will exhibit more skin and mucous membrane injury than a younger victim would.[10] There may also be signs of sexually transmitted disease and unexplained vaginal and/or rectal bleeding. Bruising to the inner thighs is a common finding in elder sexual assault victims.[15] Clinicians should be alert to signs of difficulty sitting or walking; a bloody or stained undergarment; and a reddened, ecchymosed, pruritic, or painful genital area because these findings may be indicators of elder sexual abuse.[10,17] It is important to preserve potential evidence should the alleged perpetrator be prosecuted. The victim should not be bathed, the physical environment should be left as intact as possible, and the victim will need to be escorted to a trained professional for a postassault examination.[10,18]

Financial exploitation is the illegal or improper use of the elder's funds, property, or assets. There may be a sudden change in the elder's bank account with missing funds or additional names added to the account. Forgery of the elder's signature, changes in the will, or transfer of assets to family members or others can occur. This is most likely to be noticed by bank personnel and dealt with by law enforcement agencies.

Neglect is the most common form of elder abuse. Neglect is the refusal of the caretaker or family member to provide the elder with adequate necessities such as food, water, clothing, or personal hygiene. Neglect may be further divided into intentional neglect, as when there is deliberate failure in caregiving responsibilities with the intent to harm or punish an elderly person; or unintentional neglect, which may be the result of ignorance or an inability to provide care.[10,16] Malnutrition could be attributed to multiple causes, including neglect of oneself or the caretaker's refusal or inability to provide the adequate time to assist with feeding, ill-fitting dentures, medications, or medical problems. Bowden and colleagues examined the relationship of adult abuse and neglect to burns and found that 70% of the cases were due to neglect and abuse.[19] In another study, it was determined that 40% of burn cases in patients older than age 60 were a result of abuse or neglect and 36% of the cases were a result of negligence.[20] Data suggest burns may be a forensic marker for self-neglect, caregiver neglect, or abuse.[10,11] Signs of neglect are dehydration, weight loss, dirty and stained clothing, malodor, and lack of eye glasses or dentures.

Another form of neglect is self-neglect. This is the most common case reported to adult protective services. Self-neglect is the behavior of the elder that adversely affects his or her own health and safety. The elder may deny him- or herself adequate food, water, clothing, shelter, and personal hygiene. This may be an individual who has difficulty performing activities of daily living skills and refuses assistance despite resulting problems.[21] This presents the ethical dilemma of patient autonomy versus beneficence, and in some cases, the belief is that this reflects more a failure of society than an issue of elder abuse.[10,21] The capacity for self-care decreases as dependence on others grows, which increases the risk for abuse and neglect by caregivers who may be unable or unwilling to provide assistance.[10]

Abandonment is the desertion of an elderly person by a caretaker or family member who has physical custody of the elder. Elders may be deserted at hospitals, nursing homes, shopping centers, or other public locations. One survey reported that a median of 24 elderly patients were abandoned annually per emergency department, with 41% being left in the emergency department by a family member or a caregiver.[12]

When assessing a patient for signs of elder abuse, a practitioner should also be aware of the risk factors that make elders more susceptible to elder abuse. The risk factors include a history of mental illness or substance abuse, history of family violence, and isolation of the elder. (See Table 20-3.) Evaluation of stressful events in the life of the elder or caregiver can also predict abuse. Numerous factors could contribute to the possibility of an elder becoming a victim of abuse. The practitioner needs to be aware that all factors are difficult to define and the possibility of abuse should be considered for all elderly patients.[12] Table 20-4 lists pertinent history and physical exam findings in elder abuse. The presence of any of the items listed in the table does not necessarily indicate abuse but can be used by clinicians to heighten awareness to the possibility of abuse or neglect.

THE LEGAL ASPECT

All 50 states and the District of Columbia have adult protective services (APS) laws to establish a system for the reporting and investigation of elder abuse and for the provision of social services to help the victim and ameliorate the abuse.[22,23] Individual states vary in the way the laws are written and who is covered. In some states, the laws cover only disabled adults, and in others, the laws cover all elderly persons. Some other differences between the laws in states include the age at which or circumstances in which a victim is eligible; the definitions of abuse; types of abuse, neglect, and exploitation that are covered; classifying the abuse as criminal or civil; reporting (mandatory or voluntary); investigation responsibility and procedures; and remedies for abuse.[22] States with mandatory reporting requirements may vary on the definition of a mandatory reporter. Penalties for failing to report can include fines and jail sentences.[24] At this time, there are no known cases of healthcare providers being convicted for failure to report elder abuse. All states and Washington, DC, have laws authorizing the Long-Term Care Ombudsman

TABLE 20-3 **Risk Factors for Elder Abuse**

Advanced age of the elder (greater than 80 years)
Impairment of the dependent elder (physical or mental)
Dementia
Incontinence
Alcoholism or drug abuse in the elder and/or caregiver
Transgenerational history of abuse
Poor premorbid relationship between elder and younger perpetrator
Mental illness of caregiver
Financial problems of the caregiver
Lack of family or community resources and support for caregiver
Lack of knowledge related to the elderly person's condition and needs

TABLE 20-4 **History and Physical Exam Clues to Elder Abuse**

Physical Abuse and Neglect
- Patterned injuries: ligature marks, slap marks, fingertip pressure bruises, objects
- Bruises especially on areas of body not over bony prominence
- Multiple bruises in various healing stages
- Wounds including decubiti and those in multiple stages of healing
- Burns, including cigarette burns, immersion burns, lack of splash burns
- Sprial/oblique fractures without plausible explanation
- Delay in seeking treatment
- Doctor/hospital/ED hopping
- Subdural hematoma from violent shaking
- Dehydration, cachexia, electrolyte disturbances
- Subtherapeutic or toxic drug levels
- Drugs not prescribed for patient or illegal drug presence
- Poor hygiene
- Lack of assistive devices, canes, walkers, dentures, glasses, shoes, hearing aids, etc.
- Poor living conditions: fire hazard, infestation, lack of heat, lack of plumbing

Sexual Abuse
- Breast and genitalia wounds
- Inner thigh bruising
- Sexually transmitted infections
- Unexplained vaginal or rectal bleeding
- Pain/tenderness on pelvic/rectal examination
- Behavioral changes: withdrawal, fear, depression
- Fear of people who are same sex as perpetrator

Psychological Abuse and Neglect
- Poor eye contact
- Ambivalence and/or withdrawal
- Cowering
- Noncommunication
- Paranoia
- Fear and apprehension
- Involuntary movement, rocking, sucking, trembling
- Decreased or poor appetite
- Altered sleep patterns
- Post-traumatic stress disorder
- Elder fear of the caregiver
- Caregiver insists on being with elder at all times

Program (LTCOP) to advocate on behalf of long-term care facility residents who experience abuse.

Physicians and other healthcare workers have many misconceptions about mandatory reporting. Some believe that they can be held liable for breaching confidentiality with their patient. All APS laws provide immunity to those who report in good faith.[6] In most states, healthcare workers are required by law to report all cases of suspected abuse to adult protective services. Some believe that only substantiated cases should be reported.[25] Others believe that the law requires the provider to obtain consent from a competent patient prior to contacting APS.[26] In contrast, a mandatory reporting law does not exempt a physician from reporting simply because a competent elderly patient insists that the physician not do so.[24] It is the provider's job to recognize situations of abuse and report. It is APS's job to investigate the claim once filed. Once a report has been filed and services are offered to the patient, a competent elderly adult will have the right to refuse assistance from APS.[24]

Providers continue not to report cases of suspected abuse, despite mandatory reporting laws, for numerous reasons. One of the most common concerns is expressed by a physician: "I think you really hurt the relationship of the family as a family, as well as with you, if you report prematurely or inadequately.... They're subjective decisions you make, unless there is obvious evidence of injury... you don't want to hurt the family or the relationship you have, so you want the strongest evidence that there is."[27] Physicians are concerned that they will exacerbate an already unsafe situation the elderly patient is in by reporting.[27] Others fear reporting will interfere with the provider–patient relationship.[28,29] Some physicians recognize that the patient may be taken out of the environment in which he or she lives and placed in a worse situation.[27] In this case, a social worker with experience with the elderly population would be a vital part of a team geared to helping those at risk.

Emergency medicine providers are in a unique position in detecting and reporting suspected abuse, whether it is elderly, child, or incompetent adult abuse. The emergency providers often do not have the relationship with a patient that the patient has with the primary care doctor, so they are not risking damaging the provider–patient relationship. Patients are also seen in the emergency room in their most acute state, when the suspicion of abuse should be acknowledged.

It is recommended that all providers become familiar with the laws regarding elder abuse and the reporting requirements in the state in which they practice. Some resources include the Administration on Aging (www.aoa.gov), Long-Term Care Ombudsman Resource Center (www.ltcombudsman.org), American Bar Association Commission on Law and Aging (www.abanet.org/aging), and the National Center on Elder Abuse (www.elderabusecenter.org).

PREVENTION AND INTERVENTION

Healthcare providers have many options to prevent and protect elders from abuse. All elderly patients and their caregivers, whether or not suspicion of abuse exists, should be educated on the different types of abuse and how to recognize it. Visits to the primary care doctor or the emergency room are often the only contact, besides family, that the elderly have with others.[6] It is important to take this opportunity to inform them of the availability of resources. It has been found that higher rates of reporting to APS directly correlate with increased public awareness of elder abuse.[30]

Victims often deny abuse is occurring or rationalize the behavior, especially if the suspected perpetrator is a family member. The National Center on Elder Abuse found that more than two-thirds of the perpetrators of elder abuse were relatives, with adult children followed by spouses being the most likely. Victims may fear being placed in a worse situation or putting the abuser whom they love in a bad situation such as being homeless or in jail. Many victims will tolerate the abuse over disrupting their relationship with their loved one who is abusing them and the rest of the family.[31] If the person denies abuse, the person's right not to disclose to the provider should be respected. If suspicion of immediate danger is present, the provider should call 9-1-1, or if in the emergency room, the patient may be admitted to the hospital until the situation is investigated by APS and safety is ensured.[25]

Documenting the details of suspected abuse is critical to the legal aspects of a case and is a means of communicating with other providers regarding a particular patient. Verbatim descriptions of events, relevant medical and social history, drawings or photographs of injuries, pertinent laboratory and imaging results, and physician's assessment should all be documented in the chart.[25]

Utilizing a multidisciplinary team including a primary care doctor, nurses, home health agencies, social workers, forensic team members, and psychiatrists is recommended for managing abuse.[25] Initiating a 24-hour response team, such as the forensic nurse examiners at Virginia Commonwealth University Health System, can help facilitate reporting, documentation, and treatment. Readily available social workers can help to determine a safe place for a victim of abuse to go while APS is conducting an investigation. Social workers can be of assistance by ensuring the patient has follow-up, notifying the primary care provider of a visit to an emergency room, and sharing records. They can also facilitate the call to APS and arrange resources in the community including services like meals on wheels and recruitment and placement of community volunteers. Helping to facilitate follow-up with a practitioner who is from the same cultural background and speaks the same language as the patient can be invaluable.[32]

According to the National Center on Elder Abuse, APS caseworkers are the first responders to reports of abuse, neglect, and exploitation of adults. The job of the caseworker includes receiving reports, investigating, gauging the patient's risk, and assessing the patient's capacity to understand the risk and ability to give informed consent. The caseworker will then, based on the investigation, develop a case plan and arrange emergency shelter, medical care, legal assistance, and supportive services.[33]

Interventions from APS may include shelter, home repair, meals, transportation, and assistance with financial management, home health services, and medical and mental health services. Victims who have the capacity to understand their circumstances have the right to refuse services, regardless of level of risk. The goal of APS is to use the least restrictive services first; this may include community-based rather than institutionally based resources and utilizing family and informal support systems in the best interest of the adult. APS strongly believes in "do no harm" and that inadequate or inappropriate intervention may be worse than no intervention.[33]

CONCLUSION

Elder abuse and neglect will become an increasing problem in the coming years. It is important for all providers to become familiar with how to recognize the at-risk patient and caretaker alike. Each provider should have at least a basic understanding of his or her responsibilities regarding mandatory reporting, as per individual state's laws. Providers should also familiarize themselves with any hospital protocols and the resources available in their area. The best way to begin to fix any problem is to first recognize that it exists. Then, we can all work toward developing multidisciplinary plans to combat it.

REFERENCES

1. Wan H, Sengupta M, Velkoff VA, DeBarros KA. *65+ in the United States: 2005.* Washington, DC: US Government Printing Office; 2005. US Census Bureau Current Population Reports, P23-209.
2. Shields LB, Hunsaker DM, Hunsaker JC, III. Abuse and neglect: a ten-year review of mortality and morbidity in our elders in a large metropolitan area. *J Forensic Sci.* January 2004;49(1):122–127.
3. Pillemer K, Finkelhor D. The prevalence of elder abuse: a random sample survey. *Gerontologist.* February 1988;28(1):51–57.
4. Jones JS, Veenstra TR, Seamon JP, et al. Elder mistreatment: national survey of emergency physicians. *Ann Emerg Med.* October 1997;30(4):473–479.
5. Levine JM. Elder neglect and abuse. A primer for primary care physicians. *Geriatrics.* October 2003;58(10):37–40, 42–43.
6. American Medical Association. *Diagnostic and Treatment Guidelines on Elder Abuse and Neglect.* Chicago, Ill: American Medical Association; 1992.
7. American College of Emergency Physicians. Management of elder abuse and neglect. *Ann Emerg Med.* January 1998;31(1):149–150.
8. Cammer Paris BE. Violence against elderly people. *Mount Sinai J Med* (New York). March 1996;63(2):97–100.
9. Fulmer T, Paveza G, Abraham I, et al. Elder neglect assessment in the emergency department. *J Emerg Nurs.* October 2000;26(5):436–443.
10. Pearsall C. Forensic biomarkers of elder abuse: what clinicians need to know. *J Forensic Nurs.* Winter 2005;1(4):182–186.
11. National Research Council (US), Panel to Review Risk and Prevalence of Elder Abuse and Neglect, Bonnie RJ, Wallace RB. *Elder mistreatment: abuse, neglect, and exploitation in an aging America.* Washington, DC: National Academies Press; 2003.
12. Anglin D, Schneider DC. Elder abuse and neglect. In: Marx JA, Rosen AP, Hockberger RS, Walls RM, eds. *Rosen's Emergency Medicine: Concepts and Clinical Practice.* 6th ed. Philadelphia: Mosby; 2006:1008-1016.
13. Schneider DC, Li X. Sexual abuse of vulnerable adults: the medical director's response. *J Am Med Direct Assoc.* September 2006;7(7):442–445.
14. Schofield RB. Office of Justice Programs focuses on studying and preventing elder abuse. *J Forensic Nurs.* Fall 2006;2(3):150–153.
15. Brown K, Streubert GE, Burgess AW. Effectively detect and manage elder abuse. *Nurse Pract.* August 2004;29(8):22–27, 31–33.
16. Lachs MS, Pillemer K. Abuse and neglect of elderly persons. *N Engl J Med.* February 16 1995;332(7):437–443.
17. Wieland D. Abuse of older persons: an overview. *Holistic Nurs Prac.* July 2000;14(4):40–50.
18. Carney MT, Kahan FS, Paris BB. Elder abuse: is every bruise a sign of abuse? *Mount Sinai J Med* (New York). March 2003;70(2):69–74.
19. Bowden ML, Grant ST, Vogel B, et al. The elderly, disabled and handicapped adult burned through abuse and neglect. *Burns.* December 1988;14(6):447–450.
20. Bird PE, Harrington DT, Barillo DJ, et al. Elder abuse: a call to action. *J Burn Care Rehab.* November–December 1998;19(6):522–527.
21. Kleinschmidt KC. Elder abuse: a review. *Ann Emerg Med.* October 1997;30(4):463–472.

22. Irizarry A. Pilot study of the differences among the Puerto Rican aged by gender in opinion, attitude and exposure to abuse, mistreatment and neglect. *Puerto Rico Health Sci J.* December 2005;24(4):303–311.
23. National Center on Elder Abuse. *Information about Laws Related to Elder Abuse.* American Bar Association Commission on Law and Aging. 2005. Available at: http://www.ncea.aoa.gov/ncearoot/Main_Site/pdf/publication/InformationAboutLawsRelatedtoElderAbuse.pdf. Accessed September 5, 2008.
24. Welfel EF, Danzinger PR, Santoro S. Mandated reporting of abuse/maltreatment of older adults: a primer for counselors. *J Couns Dev.* 2000(78):284–292.
25. Wei GS, Herbers JE, Jr. Reporting elder abuse: a medical, legal, and ethical overview. *J Am Med Womens Assoc.* Fall 2004;59(4):248–254.
26. Daniels RS, Baumhover LA, Clark-Daniels CL. Physicians' mandatory reporting of elder abuse. *Gerontologist.* June 1989;29(3):321–327.
27. Rodriguez MA, Wallace SP, Woolf NH, et al. Mandatory reporting of elder abuse: between a rock and a hard place. *Ann Family Med.* September–October 2006;4(5):403–409.
28. Clark-Daniels CL, Baumhover LA. Physicians' and nurses' responses to abuse of the elderly: a comparative study of two surveys in Alabama. *J Elder Abuse Neglect.* 1989(1):57–72.
29. Williams G. Elder abuse reporting and ethical dilemmas. *Iowa Med.* January 1996;86(1):20–22.
30. Jogerst GJ, Daly JM, Brinig MF, et al. Domestic elder abuse and the law. *Am J Public Health.* December 2003;93(12):2131–2136.
31. Kahan FS, Paris BB. Why elder abuse continues to elude the health care system. *Mount Sinai J Med* (New York). January 2003;70(1):62–68.
32. Montoya V. Understanding and combating elder abuse in Hispanic communities. *J Elder Abuse Neglect.* 1997;9(2):5–17.
33. Kenney JP. Domestic violence: a complex health care issue for dentistry today. *Forensic Sci Int.* May 15 2006;159(suppl 1):S121–125.

21 | Sudden Infant Death Syndrome (SIDS)

Jennifer Sellakumar Tom, MD, Ron V. Hall Jr, MD, and Neil Gandhi, MD

A startling commotion interrupts a busy emergency room. Coming toward the nurse are obviously upset parents with a listless infant in the mother's arms. The nurse and the physician quickly attend to the infant only to discover that the infant is dead. The entire emergency department staff is in shock with questions remaining as to what happened to the infant.

INTRODUCTION

Sudden infant death syndrome (SIDS), formally defined in 1969, continues to be a phenomenon of unknown cause and, despite marked reductions in rates over the past decade, still is responsible for more infant deaths in the United States than any other cause of death during infancy beyond the neonatal period.[1] Most SIDS deaths occur when babies are between 2 months and 4 months of age. Although there is ongoing discussion about changing the definition,[2] the current generally accepted definition of SIDS is the sudden death of an infant under 1 year of age, which remains unexplained after a thorough case investigation, including performance of a complete autopsy, death scene investigation, and review of the clinical history.[3]

Each year between 1983 and 1992, the average number of reported SIDS deaths ranged from 5,000 to 6,000. Over the past few years, especially since the mid-1990s, the number of SIDS deaths has declined significantly. According to the National Center for Health Statistics, the infant mortality rate for 2004 was 6.79 infant deaths per 1,000 live births. (See Table 21-1.) Sudden infant death syndrome is listed in 10 leading causes of infant mortality for 2004; a total of 2,246 SIDS death occurred in 2004.[4] Still, when considering the number of live births each year, SIDS remains the leading cause of death in the United States among infants between 1 month and 1 year of age and the third leading cause of death overall among infants less than 1 year of age.[5]

TABLE 21-1 **SIDS Deaths and Mortality Rates per 1,000 Live Births for 1990 to 2004**

Year	Infant Mortality Total	Infant Mortality Rate	SIDS Total	SIDS Rate
1990	38,351	9.2	5,417	1.30
1991	36,766	8.9	5,349	1.30
1992	34,628	8.5	4,890	1.20
1993	33,466	8.4	4,669	1.17
1994	31,710	8.0	4,073	1.03
1995	29,505	7.6	3,397	0.87
1996	28,419	7.3	3,050	0.78
1997	27,968	7.2	2,991	0.77
1998	28,325	7.2	2,822	0.71
1999	27,864	7.0	2,648	0.66
2000	27,960	6.9	2,523	0.62
2001	27,523	6.8	2,234	0.55
2002	28,034	7.0	2,295	0.57
2003	28,025	6.8	2,162	0.52
2004	27,936	6.7	2,246	0.55

Source: For 1979–2004 data: National Vital Statistics Reports, National Center for Health Statistics (NCHS). Available at: http://www.cdc.gov/nchs/deaths.htm.

Although the overall SIDS rates have declined in all populations throughout the United States, disparities in SIDS rates and prevalence of risk factors remain in certain groups. SIDS rates are highest among African Americans and American Indians and are lowest among Asians and Hispanics.[6] (See Table 21-2.)

The following have been consistently identified across studies as independent risk factors for SIDS: prone sleep position, sleeping on a soft surface, maternal smoking during pregnancy, overheating, late or no prenatal care, young maternal age, prematurity and/or low birth weight, co-sleeping, and male gender.[7–10]

Although the exact cause of SIDS is unknown, researchers have discovered trends in SIDS deaths that may help them understand this mysterious fatal problem:

- SIDS is the leading cause of death in babies older than 1 month of age.
- Most SIDS deaths occur in babies younger than 6 months old.
- Babies placed to sleep on their backs are less likely to die from SIDS than are those who are placed on their stomachs to sleep.
- Babies are more likely to die from SIDS when they are placed on or covered by soft bedding.
- African American babies are twice as likely to die from SIDS than are white babies.
- American Indian babies are nearly three times more likely to die of SIDS than are white babies.

TABLE 21-2 **SIDS Deaths by Race and Hispanic Origin of Mother, 2003**

Race	Number	Rate*
All races	2,162	52.9
White	1,173	50.5
African American	627	108.8
American Indian	53	124
Asian/Pacific Islander	61	27.7
Hispanic/Latino	234	25.6

*Per 100,000 live births by group.

Source: National Vital Statistics Reports: Infant mortality statistics from the 2003 period linked birth/infant death data set.[5]

HISTORY

SIDS was formally defined in 1969 with little insight as to what the cause of death was. At one point, SIDS was first thought to be the act of parents murdering their newborn infants. This theory was proposed by Dr. Roy Meadows, a former British pediatrician, who postulated that most of these deaths occurred as a result of child abuse by Munchausen's syndrome by proxy. As a result, many parents were convicted of infanticide despite little evidence to support the claim.[11] However, many people who were convicted of infanticide soon had their ruling overturned as a result of better forensic investigations and SIDS research.

Finally, the SIDS Act of 1974 stated that SIDS was a public health concern and attempted to reduce the number of SIDS deaths in the United States. During the last 40 years, a dramatic decrease has occurred in the number of SIDS cases in the United States and globally. The decrease in prevalence is attributed to worldwide research mostly conducted in Australia, the United Kingdom, and Scandinavia. Researchers reviewed thousands of clinical presentations as well as forensic evidence collected from the cases. They discovered several relationships common to SIDS. The most notable relationship was the sleeping position. Infants who were placed in the prone position for sleep had a greater risk of SIDS or experiencing an acute life-threatening event (ALTE). As result of these findings, the National Institutes of Child Health and Human Development (NICHD) created a campaign and easy slogan to help decrease the number of SIDS. The NICHD promoted the "Back to Sleep" campaign, established in 1994.[10,12]

PRESENTATION

SIDS is unexpected, usually occurring in healthy-appearing infants younger than 1 year of age. A SIDS death occurs quickly and usually during sleep. SIDS is rare during the first month of life. Although SIDS can occur in older infants, most SIDS deaths occur by the end of the sixth month, with the greatest number occurring in infants between 2 and 4 months of age.[13] More SIDS cases are reported in the fall and winter than in spring or summer. SIDS occurs more often in boys than in girls (approximately a 60% to 40% male-to-female ratio).

In the United States, SIDS occurs in all racial and ethnic groups. Consistently higher SIDS rates are found in African Americans and American Indian/Alaska Native children—2 to 3 times the national average.[6,13] Several government agencies are intensifying efforts to reach these populations with the latest information about SIDS. Racial makeup appears to be an independent risk factor related to SIDS. Several studies conducted by state departments of health have attempted to explain this racial disparity. The goal was to identify these differences to decrease SIDS disparities. For example, Minnesota demonstrated that 31% of African American families were placing their infants in the supine sleeping position as compared to 47% of whites. Overall, 43% of families in the state were placing their infants in the supine position. The state also discovered that the primary source of medical advice for African Americans came from family members as compared with whites, whose primary source of medical advice came from physicians.[14]

Other factors that increased the risk of SIDS were low birth weight, cigarette smoking, bedding materials, young mother, multiparity, and male sex. The male:female ratio was 3:2. In terms of health disparities, African Americans and Native Americans are more prone to have low birth weight babies and smoke cigarettes.[8,10]

Historically, infants who died from SIDS have been regarded as being normal, healthy babies. This idea originated primarily from the inability to find anything abnormal during autopsy. Later, Dr. Hannah Kinney argued that SIDS infants were not born as healthy individuals and that SIDS infants possessed an abnormality in brainstem function leading to loss of homeostatic controls. She later postulated that rapid growth periods and exogenous stressors challenge these abnormalities in homeostatic controls.[15] These factors are also known as the Triple Risk Model for SIDS.[15] Kinney and Filiano also postulated that SIDS babies have abnormal brainstems that make it difficult for them to maintain homeostasis. The three risks of abnormal brainstem, critical growth periods, and inability to handle exogenous stressors combined—not individually—have been implicated as the cause of SIDS.

Autopsies done by neuropathophysiologists have implicated abnormal brainstem function in SIDS deaths. Developmental pathology in these infants was thought to be abnormal in neurotransmitter activity and structural development of the arcuate nucleus, as well as a few other structures. There are three mechanisms by which neurotransmitters are felt to play a role in SIDS. One is in the central nervous system (CNS) where dopamine beta-hydroxylase and tyrosine hydroxylase have demonstrable differences in neurotransmitter activity.[16] Another mechanism is the development of abnormal adrenergic pathways in the pons and medulla. The third is deficient serotonin binding.[17]

The critical development period seems to be universal to all infants who die from SIDS. This period is from the ages of 1 to 6 months. During this period, it is postulated that there is some subtle change that occurs in behavioral development that predisposes infants to SIDS. Early in infancy, protective mechanisms possibly keep infants from becoming apneic. One of these protective reflexes is infant gasping.[18] Gasping is thought to occur when an infant becomes hypoxic and needs to reset the respiratory rate. SIDS researchers have noticed this mechanism begins to fade after the first month of life. Therefore, when infants become hypoxic, they no longer may have this mechanism to compensate.[19]

The third risk in the triad is the inability to handle environmental stressors or precipitating events. The most notable stressors are carbon monoxide, secondhand smoke, overheating, and upper respiratory tract infections.

Management of SIDS in the Emergency Department

When a previously healthy infant, usually younger than 6 months, apparently dies while sleeping, SIDS is suspected. The infant may be declared dead by the emergency medical service (EMS) workers, or cardiopulmonary resuscitation may be started at the home and continued en route to the hospital where the infant is declared dead. Often the decision to begin resuscitation and transport of an infant with signs of death in the field is a difficult one. The home is usually chaotic with distressed family members asking, sometimes begging EMS to initiate care. One of the benefits of initiating transport to the ED is the presence of additional personnel to provide care for the family and the infant, including physician, clergy, and social services.

In most cases cardiopulmonary resuscitation is unsuccessful, and the emergency physician must provide supportive care to the grieving family, including information about SIDS and referral to a local SIDS support group.[20] A thorough clinical history from the family should be respectfully obtained as soon as they are emotionally ready in the emergency department. Appropriate samples must be obtained (i.e., urine, blood), and an autopsy should be performed in all SIDS deaths. If local protocols, statutes, and the medical examiner permit, the family may be given the opportunity to see and hold the infant with an unrelated observer present following the pronouncement of death.

Clinical History

Classically, the presentation of SIDS involves an infant put to bed, usually after being breast or bottle fed. Despite checks on the infant made by the caregiver, the infant is found dead in the position he or she was originally placed in. Most SIDS victims are healthy, but many parents state that their infants "were not themselves" hours before they were found dead. There is no outcry heard by the infant during death. Thirty percent to 50% of SIDS victims have an infection, usually an upper respiratory infection, at the time of the event. Once the family is calmed down, it is important to obtain a detailed history including the occurrence of apnea, trauma, ingestion, foreign body, or ALTE. Usually, in the case of a SIDS death, the infant was apparently healthy, had a silent death, and was found lifeless.

A sudden unexplained infant death is suspicious for child abuse when the history is atypical for SIDS or is unclear, discrepant, or the time interval between bedtime and death is prolonged. It is estimated that between 1% and 5% of all SIDS deaths are related to infanticide.[21] Any previous unexpected deaths of siblings or unrelated infants under the care of the suspected individual should create a strong suspicion of child abuse. Caregivers involved with multiple deaths also need to be investigated for Munchausen's syndrome by proxy. This term describes when parents or caregivers intentionally fabricate symptoms in their children that result in their child being subjected to unwarranted medical exams and procedures. This syndrome constitutes child abuse. The evaluating parties should always keep child abuse in the differential when evaluating a SIDS case because abusers may go on to hurt other children. Age at death of 6 months or older is suspicious for child abuse, whereas age at death of between 2 and 4 months is consistent with SIDS.

Prenatal care in SIDS cases ranges from maximal to minimal. However, there is frequently a history of cigarette usage in the mother and premature delivery or low birth weight of the SIDS infant. Other factors that sometimes present in the history of SIDS infants are gastroesophageal reflux (GER), decreased postnatal height and weight gain, twins, triplets, thrush, pneumonia, tachypnea, tachycardia, and cyanosis. There may be defects in feeding, crying, and neurological status (including lethargy, hypotonia, irritability).

Alternately, factors that raise suspicion for child abuse include unwanted pregnancy, scant or no prenatal care, no well-baby care visits, and lack of immunizations. Other suspicious factors include deviant feeding routines, history of unexplained medical disorders (e.g., seizures), and previous apnea in the presence of the same person. The occurrence of previous infant deaths in the same family remains an area of controversy. The Committee on Child Abuse and Neglect finds suspicious the previous unexplained death of one or more siblings while under the care of the same person. However, some studies have supported that siblings of SIDS victims are at higher risk of SIDS. The history of previously unexplained infant death does raise the possibility of inborn errors of metabolism or child abuse. Typically, a SIDS victim is the first unexplained infant death in the household. Also, the history of previous law enforcement or child protective services involvement two or more times raises the suspicion of child abuse.[22]

Physical Exam

The clinical examination of the SIDS infant should be carefully documented, including the cardiopulmonary resuscitation, because it contributes to the death investigation and autopsy. Upon examination of the body, there may be found serosanguineous, watery, blood-tinged, frothy, or mucoid discharge from the mouth or nose. There may also be evidence of terminal motor activity such as clenched fists. Postmortem lividity in the dependent parts of the infant's body or infant's face and skin mottling are commonly found. The SIDS infant usually has no evidence of skin trauma and appears well cared for. Pressure points may have some marks present.

Findings suspicious for child abuse include signs of neglect, malnutrition, skin injuries, or abnormalities of the body and head. Suspicions are also raised when there is presence of pressure ischemia over the nose and mouth of the infant or when the distribution of hypostasis suggests the infant was in a different position than was stated. It is important to look for the presence of truncal bruising and contusions in the soft sites (e.g., cheeks), which suggest abuse. Pinch marks, bite marks, wounds at varying stages of healing, burns, fractures, and oronasal hemorrhage suggest child abuse. Retinal hemorrhages are strongly associated with shaken baby syndrome but can also be seen in other conditions such as accidental trauma, sepsis, and vaginally delivered newborns. It is very important to note that the absence of physical signs of child abuse still may not indicate that the infant death was natural. "Gentle battering" leaves no physical mark (e.g., when a hand or pillow is placed over the face). EMS providers and emergency medical personnel must be trained in recognizing normal findings such as postmortem anal dilatation and lividity from trauma secondary to abuse.[23]

Death Scene Investigation

It is very important that in a SIDS case, the pre-hospital providers report the death scene details, including the location and position of the infant. Other important details from the death scene investigation include the marks on the body, temperature of the body and room, type of crib/bed/bedding material and any defects, presence of soft toys and pillows, amount and position of clothing, type of ventilation and heating, reaction of caregivers, and general condition of the house.

In 1996, the Centers for Disease Control and Prevention (CDC) put out guidelines for death scene investigation, including a Sudden Unexplained Infant Death Investigation Report Form (SUIDIRF), in a short and a more comprehensive model. The SUIDIRF and the guidelines put forth by the CDC provide a standardized method of collecting and recording information on a sudden, unexplained infant death, which in turn provides further information to the pathologist.[24] (See Figure 21-1, which begins on page 177.)

Postmortem Imaging and Pathology

The skeletal survey is performed prior to autopsy in all potential SIDS cases to look for trauma or skeletal abnormalities related to a naturally occurring illness. It is then reviewed by a radiologist who is experienced in child abuse. The National Association of Medical Examiners and the American Academy of Pediatrics both recommend autopsy on infants who die suddenly and unexpectedly by forensic pathologists who are experienced in SIDS. Although there are no pathognomonic findings for SIDS victims on autopsy, there are some commonalities. Petechial hemorrhages occur in 68–95% of cases[24] and are more extensive than those found in explained infant deaths. Pulmonary congestion is found in 89% of SIDS cases, and pulmonary edema is present in 63% of SIDS cases. In autopsies performed based upon a research protocol, SIDS infants had several changes in the lungs, brainstem, and other organs.[25] Two-thirds had tissue markers of chronic low-grade asphyxia.

One of the leading hypotheses of SIDS is that it may be secondary to a deficient or delayed arousal response. Supporting this theory, hypoplasia of the arcuate nucleus in up to 60% of SIDS cases has been seen on autopsy.[25] The arcuate nucleus is a region in the brainstem involved in the hypercapneic ventilatory response, chemosensitivity, and blood pressure response. In some SIDS cases, neurotransmitter studies have shown receptor abnormalities involved with autonomic control. The deficits in binding were to kainite, muscarinic cholinergic, and 5-HT receptors. There were persistent increases in dendritic spines (signaling neuronal maturational delay), delayed maturation of synapses in the medullary respiratory center, and decreased tyrosine hydroxylase immunoreactivity in catecholaminergic neurons.[25–27]

In cases of fatal child abuse, the most common postmortem findings are cranial injuries, abdominal trauma (e.g., liver laceration), burns, or drowning. There have been a small percentage of sudden unexplained deaths in infants with autopsy findings that are consistent with SIDS that were implicated with inborn errors of metabolism. Blood and bile are analyzed for these errors in metabolism, especially in cases involving SIDS within siblings. On autopsy, it is very difficult (some suggest impossible) to distinguish between SIDS and accidental or intentional suffocation with a soft object.[22] Certain circumstances suggest the possibility of deliberate suffocation, including the following:

- Repeated episodes of cyanosis, apnea, or ALTEs while under the care of the same individual
- Previously unexplained or unexpected deaths of one or more siblings or previous death of infants under the care of the same person
- Age at death greater than 6 months
- Simultaneous or nearly simultaneous death of twins
- Evidence of previous pulmonary hemorrhage

SIDS is a diagnosis of exclusion requiring complete autopsy, investigation of circumstances of death, and review of case records that fail to reveal another cause of death. Without these three entities, there can be failure to identify fatal child abuse or other preventable hazards that can cause sudden infant death. For example, without the thorough investigation of SIDS cases, potential hazards of water beds, defective infant furniture, and bean bag mattresses would not have been identified as risks for SIDS deaths.[22,28,29] Infant deaths that do not have a comprehensive death investigation or infant deaths that reveal uncertainty regarding the manner of death are designated "undetermined." Undetermined cases of infant death include suspected (but unproven) death resulting from infection, metabolic disease, asphyxiation, and child abuse.

A diagnosis of SIDS can be made when the following conditions are met:

- A complete autopsy, including cranium and cranial contents, is performed and autopsy findings are consistent with SIDS.
- There is no evidence of trauma or significant bone disease seen on skeletal radiologic survey, postmortem examination, and reliable clinical history.
- Other causes of death are sufficiently excluded, including meningitis, sepsis, aspiration pneumonia, myocarditis, trauma, dehydration, fluid and electrolyte imbalance, significant congenital defects, inborn metabolic disorders, asphyxia, drowning, burns, and poisoning.
- There is no evidence for toxic exposure to alcohol, drugs, or other substances.
- Thorough death and incident scene investigation and review of the clinical history reveal no other cause of death.

Apparent Life-Threatening Events

An apparent life-threatening event (ALTE) is defined as "an episode that is frightening to the observer and that is characterized by some combination of apnea (central or occasionally obstructive), color change (usually cyanotic or pallid but occasionally erythematous or plethoric), marked change in muscle tone (usually marked limpness), choking, or gagging. In some cases, the observer fears that the infant has died."[1] The term *ALTE* denotes a complaint from parents and caregivers who have noticed an abnormality in their infant. ALTE is not a diagnosis. The occurrence of ALTE ranges from 0.05% to 3% of all infants under the age of 1 year in several studies done in multiple countries.[30] Infants who present to the emergency department with prolonged resuscitation including CPR or who experience ALTEs during sleep tend to have significantly worse outcomes than do infants with "uncomplicated" ALTEs or who experience ALTEs where the infant is easily revived after minor stimulation, including lifting up the child or gently patting them.

ALTE infants represent a diverse group of patients with no particular pathology that links them together. ALTE itself has not been proven to be an independent risk factor for SIDS, but between 1% and 5% of all SIDS cases have had an ALTE. The problem with correlating ALTEs and SIDS lies in the fact that there is a significantly higher number of reported ALTEs when compared to the total number of documented SIDS cases. Numerous risk factors are associated with ALTEs, including gastrointestinal, neurologic, cardiac, and respiratory abnormalities. Roughly 50% of infants evaluated for ALTE are found to have one or more of the following diagnoses: gastroesophageal reflux disease (GERD), respiratory syncytial virus (RSV), and seizure.[30] This fact also means that 50% of infants have their ALTE designated as unsolved.

After a child has an ALTE and presents to a physician, a detailed history and physical must be performed. During the evaluation of ALTE, a possible diagnosis of child abuse or infanticide must be considered. Because the evaluation of ALTE often occurs in the setting of an emergency department, further care must be taken when obtaining history information from the parents and caregivers because a lack of familiarity with the history may lead to important information being missed. Once this initial information has been gathered, further testing aids in the evaluation of the infant. The most common tests ordered include CBC, SMA7, RSV, urinalysis, toxicology screen, EKG, and chest radiograph. If the history or physical is suspicious for a particular etiology causing the ALTE, head CT, EEG, radiographs, toxicology screen, and dilated fundoscopic exam should be considered. If an inborn error of metabolism is suspected, then liver enzymes, ammonia level, and lactate should be checked. Nearly all infants presenting with ALTE should be admitted to the hospital for observation in a monitored environment (neonatal or pediatric intensive care unit) and further workup.

An EKG provides particularly useful information when screening infants for ALTE. The EKG can allow the physician to detect heart arrhythmias, structural abnormalities, and prolonged QT, all with a relatively benign and inexpensive test. *Prolonged QT* refers to a QT interval greater than 440 ms. Infants with long QT are predisposed to electrical instability in their heart, which can cause fatal ventricular arrhythmias leading to sudden death. All siblings of patients with long QT should be screened for similar pathologies because oftentimes this is an inherited condition.

Metabolic abnormalities have been shown to play a role in ALTE and SIDS.[31] The most common abnormalities are defects in the metabolism of fatty acids.[30] Numerous different etiologies for metabolic disease have been uncovered as culprits for SIDS, including medium-chain acyl-CoA dehydrogenase deficiency, urea cycle disorders, and propionic and methylmalonic acidemias, to name a few. Fatty acid oxidation disorders can cause fatty livers, which have been discovered on autopsy of SIDS cases. Thorough evaluation for metabolic disorders given a likely history (ALTE with any one of the following: neonatal hypoglycemia, muscular hypotonia, or vomiting) can lead to the particular metabolic error being identified and in some cases corrected before infant death occurs.

Prevention of SIDS

The devastating impact that SIDS has on families and communities has led to much research on areas of prevention. In 1994, the "Back to Sleep" campaign was introduced from the NICHD. This campaign simply states that healthy babies should be placed on their back while sleeping during the first year of life. This simple slogan has been embraced by pediatricians, health professionals, child care providers, and parents. The end result has been a nearly 50% reduction in SIDS since 1994.

Other evidence-based recommendations include using firm bedding, avoiding cigarette smoke exposure, and using a pacifier. Parents should be informed of these recommendations during periodic well-check pediatric exams. Several studies have questioned the safety of cobedding. Many pediatricians have recommended the avoidance of sharing a bed with infants. Further research is still needed in this area to determine whether this recommendation will lead to reduction in death similar to the "Back to Sleep" campaign.

CONCLUSION

With public education and the "Back to Sleep" Campaign, the number of SIDS cases has dramatically decreased. However, emergency physicians still need to be prepared to care for these infants and their families. It truly is a multi-disciplinary team approach involving the family, the hospital staff, social services, child services, law enforcement, and the medical examiner's office.

(References for Chapter 21 appear on page 185.)

Sudden Unexplained Infant Death Investigation

SUIDI Reporting Form

INVESTIGATION DATA

Infant's Information: Last ______ First ______ M. ______ Case # ______

Sex: ☐ Male ☐ Female Date of Birth ____/____/____ (Month Day Year) Age ____ Months SS# ______

Race: ☐ White ☐ Black/African Am. ☐ Asian/Pacific Islander ☐ Am. Indian/Alaskan Native ☐ Hispanic/Latino ☐ Other

Infant's Primary Residence Address:

Address ______ City ______ County ______ State ____ Zip ______

Incident Address:

Address ______ City ______ County ______ State ____ Zip ______

Contact Information for Witness:

Relationship to the deceased: ☐ Birth Mother ☐ Birth Father ☐ Grandmother ☐ Grandfather
☐ Adoptive or Foster Parent ☐ Physician ☐ Health Records ☐ Other: ______

Last ______ First ______ M. ______ SS # ______

Home Address ______ City ______ State ____ Zip ______

Place of Work ______ City ______ State ____ Zip ______

Phone (H) ______ Phone (W) ______ Date of Birth ____/____/____ (Month Day Year)

WITNESS INTERVIEW

1 Are you the usual caregiver? ☐ Yes ☐ No

2 Tell me what happened: ______

3 Did you notice anything unusual or different about the infant in the last 24 hrs? ☐ No ☐ Yes ⇨ Describe: ______

4 Did the infant experience any falls or injury within the last 72 hrs? ☐ No ☐ Yes ⇨ Describe: ______

5 When was the infant *LAST PLACED*? .... ____/____/____ (Month Day Year) ____:____ (Military Time) ______ Location (room)

6 When was the infant *LAST KNOWN ALIVE(LKA)*? ____/____/____ (Month Day Year) ____:____ (Military Time) ______ Location (room)

7 When was the infant *FOUND*? .... ____/____/____ (Month Day Year) ____:____ (Military Time) ______ Location (room)

8 Explain how you knew the infant was still alive. ______

9 Where was the infant - (P)laced, (L)ast known alive, (F)ound (circle P, L, or F in front of appropriate response)?

P L F Bassinet	**P L F** Bedside co-sleeper	**P L F** Car seat	**P L F** Chair
P L F Cradle	**P L F** Crib	**P L F** Floor	**P L F** In a person's arms
P L F Mattress/box spring	**P L F** Mattress on floor	**P L F** Playpen	**P L F** Portable crib
P L F Sofa/couch	**P L F** Stroller/carriage	**P L F** Swing	**P L F** Waterbed

P L F Other ______

Page 1

FIGURE 21-1 **SUIDIRF, the Sudden Unexplained Infant Death Investigation Reporting Form.**

WITNESS INTERVIEW (cont.)

10 **In what position was the infant *LAST PLACED*?** ☐ Sitting ☐ On back ☐ On side ☐ On stomach ☐ Unknown
Was this the infant's usual position? ☐ Yes ☐ No ⇨ What was the infant's usual position? ______

11 **In what position was the infant *LKA*?** ☐ Sitting ☐ On back ☐ On side ☐ On stomach ☐ Unknown
Was this the infant's usual position? ☐ Yes ☐ No ⇨ What was the infant's usual position? ______

12 **In what position was the infant *FOUND*?** .... ☐ Sitting ☐ On back ☐ On side ☐ On stomach ☐ Unknown
Was this the infant's usual position? ☐ Yes ☐ No ⇨ What was the infant's usual position? ______

13 **FACE position when *LAST PLACED*?** ..... ☐ Face down on surface ☐ Face up ☐ Face right ☐ Face left

14 **NECK position when *LAST PLACED*?** ..... ☐ Hyperextended *(head back)* ☐ Flexed *(chin to chest)* ☐ Neutral ☐ Turned

15 **FACE position when *LKA*?** .... ☐ Face down on surface ☐ Face up ☐ Face right ☐ Face left

16 **NECK position when *LKA*?** .... ☐ Hyperextended *(head back)* ☐ Flexed *(chin to chest)* ☐ Neutral ☐ Turned

17 **FACE position when *FOUND*?** .... ☐ Face down on surface ☐ Face up ☐ Face right ☐ Face left

18 **NECK position when *FOUND*?** .... ☐ Hyperextended *(head back)* ☐ Flexed *(chin to chest)* ☐ Neutral ☐ Turned

19 **What was the infant wearing?** *(ex. t-shirt, disposable diaper)* ______

20 **Was the infant tightly wrapped or swaddled?** ☐ No ☐ Yes ⇨ Describe: ______

21 **Please indicate the types and numbers of layers of bedding both over and under infant (not including wrapping blanket):**

Bedding UNDER Infant	None	Number	Bedding OVER Infant	None	Number
Receiving blankets	☐	____	Receiving blankets	☐	____
Infant/child blankets	☐	____	Infant/child blankets	☐	____
Infant/child comforters *(thick)*	☐	____	Infant/child comforters *(thick)*	☐	____
Adult comforters/duvets	☐	____	Adult comforters/duvets	☐	____
Adult blankets	☐	____	Adult blankets	☐	____
Sheets	☐	____	Sheets	☐	____
Sheepskin	☐	____	Pillows	☐	____
Pillows	☐	____	Other, specify: ______		
Rubber or plastic sheet	☐	____			
Other, specify: ______					

22 **Which of the following devices were operating in the infant's room?**
☐ None ☐ Apnea monitor ☐ Humidifier ☐ Vaporizer ☐ Air purifier ☐ Other ______

23 **What was the temperature of the infant's room?** ☐ Hot ☐ Cold ☐ Normal ☐ Other ______

24 **Which of the following items were near the infant's face, nose, or mouth?**
☐ Bumper pads ☐ Infant pillows ☐ Positional supports ☐ Stuffed animals ☐ Toys ☐ Other ______

25 **Which of the following items were within the infant's reach?** ☐ Blankets ☐ Toys ☐ Pillows
☐ Pacifier ☐ Nothing ☐ Other ______

26 **Was anyone sleeping with the infant?** ☐ No ☐ Yes ⇨ Name these people.

Name	Age	Height	Weight	Location in Relation to Infant	Impaired *(intoxicated, tired)*

27 **Was there evidence of wedging?** ☐ No ☐ Yes ⇨ Describe: ______

28 **When the infant was found, was s/he:** ☐ Breathing ☐ Not breathing
If not breathing, did you witness the infant stop breathing? ☐ No ☐ Yes

Page 2

FIGURE 21-1 **SUIDIRF, the Sudden Unexplained Infant Death Investigation Reporting Form.** *(continued)*

WITNESS INTERVIEW (cont.)

29 What had led you to check on the infant? ______

30 Describe infant's appearance when found.

	Unknown	No	Yes	Describe and specify location:
a) Discoloration around face/nose/mouth	☐	☐	☐	⇨ ______
b) Secretions *(foam, froth)*	☐	☐	☐	⇨ ______
c) Skin discoloration *(livor mortis)*	☐	☐	☐	⇨ ______
d) Pressure marks *(pale areas, blanching)*	☐	☐	☐	⇨ ______
e) Rash or petechiae *(small, red blood spots on skin, membranes, or eyes)*	☐	☐	☐	⇨ ______
f) Marks on body *(scratches or bruises)*	☐	☐	☐	⇨ ______
g) Other	☐	☐	☐	⇨ ______

31 What did the infant feel like when found? *(Check all that apply.)*

☐ Sweaty ☐ Warm to touch ☐ Cool to touch
☐ Limp, flexible ☐ Rigid, stiff ☐ Unknown
☐ Other ⇨ Specify: ______

32 Did anyone else other than EMS try to resuscitate the infant? ☐ No ☐ Yes ⇨ Who and when?

Who ______ ___/___/___ (Month Day Year) ___:___ (Military Time)

33 Please describe what was done as part of resuscitation:

______

______

34 Has the parent/caregiver ever had a child die suddenly and unexpectedly? ☐ No ☐ Yes ⇨ Explain

______

INFANT MEDICAL HISTORY

1 Source of medical information: ☐ Doctor ☐ Other healthcare provider ☐ Medical record
☐ Mother/primary caregiver ☐ Family ☐ Other: ______

2 In the 72 hours prior to death, did the infant have:

	Unknown	No	Yes
a) Fever	☐	☐	☐
b) Excessive sweating	☐	☐	☐
c) Lethargy or sleeping more than usual	☐	☐	☐
d) Fussiness or excessive crying	☐	☐	☐
e) Decrease in appetite	☐	☐	☐
f) Vomiting	☐	☐	☐
g) Choking	☐	☐	☐
h) Diarrhea	☐	☐	☐
i) Stool changes	☐	☐	☐
j) Difficulty breathing	☐	☐	☐
k) Apnea *(stopped breathing)*	☐	☐	☐
l) Cyanosis *(turned blue/gray)*	☐	☐	☐
m) Seizures or convulsions	☐	☐	☐
n) Other, specify ______			

3 In the 72 hours prior to death, was the infant injured or did s/he have any other condition(s) not mentioned?

☐ No ☐ Yes ⇨ Describe: ______

4 In the 72 hours prior to the infants death, was the infant given any vaccinations or medications?
(Please include any home remedies, herbal medications, prescription medicines, over-the-counter medications.)

☐ No ☐ Yes ⇨ List below:

Name of vaccination or medication	Dose last given	Date given (Month / Day / Year)	Approx. time (Military Time)	Reasons given/ comments:
1. ______	______	___/___/___	___:___	______
2. ______	______	___/___/___	___:___	______
3. ______	______	___/___/___	___:___	______
4. ______	______	___/___/___	___:___	______

Page 3

FIGURE 21-1 **SUIDIRF, the Sudden Unexplained Infant Death Investigation Reporting Form.** *(continued)*

INFANT MEDICAL HISTORY (cont.)

5 At any time in the infant's life, did s/he have a history of?

	Unknown	No	Yes	Describe:
a) Allergies *(food, medication, or other)*	☐	☐	☐	⇨ ______
b) Abnormal growth or weight gain/loss	☐	☐	☐	⇨ ______
c) Apnea *(stopped breathing)*	☐	☐	☐	⇨ ______
d) Cyanosis *(turned blue/gray)*	☐	☐	☐	⇨ ______
e) Seizures or convulsions	☐	☐	☐	⇨ ______
f) Cardiac *(heart)* abnormalities	☐	☐	☐	⇨ ______
g) Metabolic disorders	☐	☐	☐	⇨ ______
h) Other	☐	☐	☐	⇨ ______

6 Did the infant have any birth defects(s)? ☐ No ☐ Yes

Describe: ______

7 Describe the two most recent times that the infant was seen by a physician or health care provider:
(Include emergency department visits, clinic visits, hospital admissions, observational stays, and telephone calls)

	First most recent visit	Second most recent visit
a) Date	___/___/___ Month Day Year	___/___/___ Month Day Year
b) Reason for visit	______	______
c) Action taken	______	______
d) Physician's name	______	______
e) Hospital/clinic	______	______
f) Address	______	______
g) City	______	______
h) State, ZIP	______ ______	______ ______
i) Phone number	(___)___-______	(___)___-______

8 Birth hospital name: ______

Street ______

City ______ State ______ Zip ______

Date of discharge ___/___/___ Month Day Year

9 What was the infant's length at birth? ______ inches **or** ______ centimeters

10 What was the infant's weight at birth? ______ pounds ______ ounces **or** ______ grams

11 Compared to the delivery date, was the infant born on time, early, or late?

☐ On time ☐ Early—How many weeks early?______ ☐ Late—How many weeks late?______

12 Was the infant a singleton, twin, triplet, or higher gestation?

☐ Singleton ☐ Twin ☐ Triplet ☐ Quadruplet or higher gestation

13 Were there any complications during delivery or at birth? *(emergency c-section, child needed oxygen)*

☐ No ☐ Yes ⇨ Describe the complications: ______

14 Are there any alerts to pathologist? *(previous infant deaths in family, newborn screen results)*

☐ No ☐ Yes ⇨ Specify: ______

Page 4

FIGURE 21-1 **SUIDIRF, the Sudden Unexplained Infant Death Investigation Reporting Form.** *(continued)*

INFANT DIETARY HISTORY

1 On what day and at what approximate time was the infant last fed?

_____/_____/_________ _____:_____
Month Day Year Military Time

2 What is the name of the person who last fed the infant? ____________________

3 What is his/her relationship to the infant? ____________________

4 What foods and liquids was the infant fed in the last 24 hours (include last fed)**?**

	Unknown	No	Yes		Quantity	Specify: *(type and brand if applicable)*
a) Breast milk *(one/both sides, length of time)*	☐	☐	☐	⇨	_____ ounces	____________
b) Formula (*brand, water source - ex. Similac, tap water*)	☐	☐	☐	⇨	_____ ounces	____________
c) Cow's milk	☐	☐	☐	⇨	_____ ounces	____________
d) Water *(brand, bottled, tap, well)*	☐	☐	☐	⇨	_____ ounces	____________
e) Other liquids *(teas, juices)*	☐	☐	☐	⇨	_____ ounces	____________
f) Solids	☐	☐	☐	⇨	____________	
g) Other	☐	☐	☐	⇨	____________	

5 Was a new food introduced in the 24 hours prior to his/her death?
☐ No ☐ Yes ⇨ Describe *(ex. content, amount, change in formula, introduction of solids)*

____
____
____

6 Was the infant last placed to sleep with a bottle?
☐ Yes ☐ No ⇨ Skip to question **9** below

7 Was the bottle propped? (i.e., object used to hold bottle while infant feeds)
☐ No ☐ Yes ⇨ What object was used to prop the bottle? ____________________

8 What was the quantity of liquid (in ounces) in the bottle? ____________________

9 Did death occur during? ☐ Breast-feeding ☐ Bottle-feeding ☐ Eating solid foods ☐ Not during feeding

10 Are there any factors, circumstances, or environmental concerns that may have impacted the infant that have not yet been identified? *(ex. exposed to cigarette smoke or fumes at someone else's home, infant unusually heavy, placed with positional supports or wedges)*
☐ No ☐ Yes ⇨ Describe concerns: ____________________

____
____
____

PREGNANCY HISTORY

1 Information about the infant's birth mother:

First name ____________________ Middle name ____________________

Last name ____________________ Maiden name ____________________

Date of Birth: _____/_____/_________ SS # _______-______-_______
Month Day Year

Current Address: ____________________ City __________ ______ ______
State Zip

How long has the birth mother been a resident at this address? _____ and _____ Previous Address __________ ______
Years Months City State

2 At how many weeks or months did the birth mother begin prenatal care?
_____ Weeks _____ Months ☐ No prenatal care ☐ Unknown

3 Where did the birth mother receive prenatal care? *(Please specify physician or other health care provider name and address.)*

Physician/provider ____________________ Hospital/clinic ____________________ Phone (____) __________

Street ____________________ City ____________________ ______ ______
State Zip

Page 5

FIGURE 21-1 **SUIDIRF, the Sudden Unexplained Infant Death Investigation Reporting Form.** *(continued)*

PREGNANCY HISTORY (cont.)

4 During her pregnancy with the infant, did the birth mother have any complications?
(ex. high blood pressure, bleeding, gestational diabetes)

☐ No ☐ Yes ⇨ Specify: ____________

5 Was the birth mother injured during her pregnancy with the infant? *(ex. auto accident, falls)*

☐ No ☐ Yes ⇨ Specify: ____________

6 During her pregnancy, did she use any of the following?

	Unknown	No	Yes	Daily consumption
a) Over the counter medications	☐	☐	☐	________
b) Prescription medications	☐	☐	☐	________
c) Herbal remedies	☐	☐	☐	________
d) Cigarettes	☐	☐	☐	________
e) Alcohol	☐	☐	☐	________
f) Other	☐	☐	☐	________

7 Currently, does any caregiver use any of the following?

	Unknown	No	Yes	Daily consumption
a) Over the counter medications	☐	☐	☐	________
b) Prescription medications	☐	☐	☐	________
c) Herbal remedies	☐	☐	☐	________
d) Cigarettes	☐	☐	☐	________
e) Alcohol	☐	☐	☐	________
f) Other	☐	☐	☐	________

INCIDENT SCENE INVESTIGATION

1 Where did the incident or death occur? ____________

2 Was this the primary residence? ☐ Yes ☐ No

3 Is the site of the incident or death scene a daycare or other childcare setting?

☐ Yes ☐ No ⇨ Skip to question 8 below.

4 How many children were under the care of the provider at the time of the incident or death? ______ *(under 18 years old)*

5 How many adults were supervising the child(ren)? ______ *(18 years or older)*

6 What is the license number and licensing agency for the daycare?

License number: ____________ Agency: ____________

7 How long has the daycare been open for business? ____________

8 How many people live at the site of the incident or death scene?

______ Number of adults *(18 years or older)* ______ Number of children *(under 18 years old)*

9 Which of the following heating or cooling sources were being used? *(Check all that apply.)*

☐ Central air
☐ A/C window unit
☐ Ceiling fan
☐ Floor/table fan
☐ Window fan
☐ Gas furnace or boiler
☐ Electric furnace or boiler
☐ Electric space heater
☐ Electric baseboard heat
☐ Electric (*radiant*) ceiling heat
☐ Wood burning fireplace
☐ Coal burning furnace
☐ Kerosene space heater
☐ Other ⇨ Specify: ____________
☐ Unknown
☐ Open window(s)
☐ Wood burning stove

10 Indicate the temperature of the room where the infant was found unresponsive:

______ Thermostat setting ______ Thermostat reading ______ Actual room temp. ______ Outside temp.

11 What was the source of drinking water at the site of the incident or death scene? *(Check all that apply.)*

☐ Public/municipal water source
☐ Well
☐ Bottled water
☐ Unknown
☐ Other ⇨ Specify: ____________

12 The site of the incident or death scene has: *(check all that apply)*

☐ Insects
☐ Smoky smell *(like cigarettes)*
☐ Dampness
☐ Visible standing water
☐ Mold growth
☐ Pets
☐ Peeling paint
☐ Rodents or vermin
☐ Odors or fumes ⇨ Describe: ____________
☐ Presence of alcohol containers
☐ Presence of drug paraphenalia
☐ Other ⇨ Specify: ____________

13 Describe the general appearance of incident scene: *(ex. cleanliness, hazards, overcrowding, etc.)*

____
____
____

Page 6

FIGURE 21-1 **SUIDIRF, the Sudden Unexplained Infant Death Investigation Reporting Form.** *(continued)*

INVESTIGATION SUMMARY

1 Are there any factors, circumstances, or environmental concerns about the incident scene investigation that may have impacted the infant that have not yet been identified?

____

____

2 Arrival times: Law enforcement at scene: ______:______ Military Time DSI at scene: ______:______ Military Time Infant at hospital: ______:______ Military Time

Investigator's Notes

Indicate the task(s) performed.

- ☐ Additional scene(s)? (forms attached)
- ☐ Materials collected/evidence logged
- ☐ Notify next of kin or verify notification
- ☐ Doll reenactment/scene re-creation
- ☐ Referral for counseling
- ☐ 911 tape
- ☐ Photos or video taken and noted
- ☐ EMS run sheet/report

If more than one person was interviewed, does the information differ?

☐ No ☐ Yes ⇨ Detail any differences, inconsistencies of relevant information: *(ex. placed on sofa, last known alive on chair.)*

____

____

____

____

INVESTIGATION DIAGRAMS

1 Scene Diagram:

2 Body Diagram:

FIGURE 21-1 **SUIDIRF, the Sudden Unexplained Infant Death Investigation Reporting Form.** *(continued)*

SUMMARY FOR PATHOLOGIST

Case Information

Investigator Information: Name ____________ Agency ____________ Phone ____________

Investigated: ____/____/____ (Month Day Year) ____:____ (Military Time) Pronounced Dead: ____/____/____ (Month Day Year) ____:____ (Military Time)

Infant's Information: Last ____________ First ____________ M. ____________ Case # ____________

Sex: ☐ Male ☐ Female Date of Birth ____/____/____ (Month Day Year) Age ____ Months

Race: ☐ White ☐ Black/African Am. ☐ Asian/Pacific Islander ☐ Am. Indian/Alaskan Native ☐ Hispanic/Latino ☐ Other ____

1 Indicate whether preliminary investigation suggests any of the following:

Yes No

Sleeping Environment

☐ ☐ Asphyxia *(ex. overlying, wedging, choking, nose/mouth obstruction, re-breathing, neck compression, immersion in water)*
☐ ☐ Sharing of sleep surface with adults, children, or pets
☐ ☐ Change in sleep condition *(ex. unaccustomed stomach sleep position, location, or sleep surface)*
☐ ☐ Hyperthermia/Hypothermia *(ex. excessive wrapping, blankets, clothing, or hot or cold environments)*
☐ ☐ Environmental hazards *(ex. carbon monoxide, noxious gases, chemicals, drugs, devices)*
☐ ☐ Unsafe sleep condition *(ex. couch/sofa, waterbed, stuffed toys, pillows, soft bedding)*

Infant History

☐ ☐ Diet *(e.g., solids introduced, etc.)*
☐ ☐ Recent hospitalization
☐ ☐ Previous medical diagnosis
☐ ☐ History of acute life-threatening events *(ex. apnea, seizures, difficulty breathing)*
☐ ☐ History of medical care without diagnosis
☐ ☐ Recent fall or other injury
☐ ☐ History of religious, cultural, or ethnic remedies
☐ ☐ Cause of death due to natural causes other than SIDS *(ex. birth defects, complications of preterm birth)*

Family Info

☐ ☐ Prior sibling deaths
☐ ☐ Previous encounters with police or social service agencies
☐ ☐ Request for tissue or organ donation
☐ ☐ Objection to autopsy

Exam

☐ ☐ Pre-terminal resuscitative treatment
☐ ☐ Death due to trauma (injury), poisoning, or intoxication

Investigator Insight

☐ ☐ Suspicious circumstances
☐ ☐ Other alerts for pathologist's attention

Any "Yes" answers should be explained and detailed.

Brief description of circumstances: ____________

Pathologist

2 Pathologist Information:

Name ____________ Agency ____________

Phone (____)____-____________ Fax (____)____-____________

Page 8

FIGURE 21-1 **SUIDIRF, the Sudden Unexplained Infant Death Investigation Reporting Form.** *(continued)*

REFERENCES

1. Arias E, MacDorman MF, Strobino DM, Guyer B. Annual summary of vital statistics—2002. *Pediatrics.* 2003;112:1215–1230.
2. American Academy of Pediatrics, Task Force on Infant Sleep Position and Sudden Infant Death Syndrome. The changing concept of sudden infant death syndrome: diagnostic coding shifts, controversies regarding the sleeping environment, and new variables to consider in reducing risk. *Pediatrics.* 2005;1169(5):1245–1255.
3. Willinger M, James LS, Cotz C. Defining the sudden infant death syndrome (SIDS): deliberations of an expert panel convened by the National Institute of Child Health and Human Development. *Pediatr Pathol.* 1991;11(5): 677–684.
4. National Vital Statistics Reports, National Center for Health Statistics (NCHS). Available at: http://www.cdc.gov/nchs/deaths.htm. Accessed January 15, 2008.
5. Mathews TJ, MacDorman MF. National Vital Statistics Reports: Infant mortality statistics from the 2003 period linked birth/infant death data set. 2006:54(16). Available at: http://www.cdc.gov/nchs/data/nvsr/nvsr54/nvsr54_16.pdf Accessed: September 28, 2008.
6. National Institute of Child Health and Human Development, National Institutes of Health. *From Cells to Selves. Targeting Sudden Infant Death Syndrome (SIDS): A Strategic Plan.* Bethesda, Md: National Institute of Child Health and Human Development; 2001.
7. Committee on Child Abuse and Neglect, 1999–2000. American Academy of Pediatrics. Investigation and review of unexpected infant and child deaths. *Pediatrics.* 1999;104(5): 1158–1159.
8. Cote A, Russo P, Michaud J. Sudden unexpected deaths in infancy: what are causes? *J Pediatr.* 1999;135(4).
9. Martin RJ, Miller MJ, Redline S. Screening for SIDS: a neonatal perspective. *Pediatrics.* 1999;103(4):812–813.
10. Mitchell E, Tuohy P, Brunt J, et al. Risk factors for sudden infant death syndrome following the prevention campaign in New Zealand: a prospective study. *Pediatrics.* 1997;100(5): 835–840.
11. Dyer O. Meadows faces GMC over evidence given in child deaths. *BMJ.* 2004;328.
12. Oyen N, Markestad T, Skjaerven R, et al. Combined effects of sleeping position and prenatal risk factors in sudden infant death syndrome. The Nordic Epidemiological SIDS study. *Pediatrics.* 1997;100:613–621.
13. American Academy of Pediatrics, Task Force on Infant Sleep Position and Sudden Infant Death Syndrome. Changing concepts of sudden infant death syndrome: implications for infant sleeping environment and sleep position. *Pediatrics.* March 2000; 105(3):650–656.
14. Minnesota Department of Health. *Eliminating Health Disparities: Infant Mortality—Sudden Infant Death Syndrome (SIDS).* Fact sheet. Available at: http://www.health.state.mn.us. Accessed March 2001.
15. Filiano JJ, Kinney HC. A perspective on neuropathologic findings in victims of the sudden infant death syndrome: the triple risk model. *Biol Neonate.* 1994;65:194–197.
16. Kinney HC, Filiano JJ, Harper RM. The neuropathology of the sudden infant death syndrome. *J Neuropath Exp Neurol.* 1992;51:115–126.
17. Kinney HC, Filiano JJ, White WF. Medullary serotonergic network deficiency in the sudden infant death syndrome: review of a 15-year study of a single database. *J Neuropath Exp Neurol.* 2001;60:228–247.
18. Guntheroth WG, Kawabori I. Hypoxic apnea and gasping. *J Clin Invest.* 1975;56:1371–1377.
19. Waggener TB, Southall DP, Scott LA. Analysis of breathing patterns in a prospective population of term infants does not predict susceptibility to SIDS. *Pediatric Res.* 1990;27:113–117.
20. Gausche-Hill M. Sudden infant death and apparent life threatening events. In: Marx J, Hockberger R, Walls R, eds. *Rosen's Emergency Medicine: Concepts and Clinical Practices.* 6th ed. Philadelphia: Mosby; 2006:2713–2717.
21. Reece RM. Fatal child abuse and sudden infant death syndrome: a critical diagnostic decision. *Pediatrics.* February 1993; 91(2):423–429.
22. Barkley Burnett L, Adler J. Pediatrics, Sudden Infant Death Syndrome. eMedicine 2006. Available at: http://www.emedicine.com/EMERG/topic407.htm. Accessed December 10, 2007.
23. American Academy of Pediatrics, Hymel K, et al. Distinguishing sudden infant death syndrome from child abuse fatalities. *Pediatrics.* 2006;118:421–427.
24. Centers for Disease Control and Prevention. Guidelines for death scene investigation of sudden, unexplained infant deaths: recommendations of the Interagency Panel on Sudden Infant Death Syndrome. *MMWR.* 1996:45(RR-10):1–23.
25. Hunt CE, Hauck FR. Sudden infant death syndrome. *CMAJ.* 2006;174(13):1861–1869.
26. Thompson MW, Hunt CE. Control of breathing: development, apnea of prematurity, apparent life-threatening events, SIDS. In: Macdonald MG, Mullett MD, Seshia MMK, eds. *Avery's Neonatology: Pathophysiology and Management of the Newborn.* 6th ed. Philadelphia: Lippincott Williams & Wilkins; 2005:535–552.
27. Hunt CE, Hauck FR. Sudden infant death syndrome. In: Behrman RE, Kliegman RM, Jenson HB, eds. *Nelson Textbook of Pediatrics.* 17th ed. Saunders Elsevier, Philadelphia; 2004:1380–1385.
28. Kemp JS, Thach BT. Sudden death in infants sleeping on polystyrene-filled cushions. *N Eng J Med.* 1991;324:1858–1864.
29. Ramanathan R, Chandra S, et al. Sudden infant death syndrome and water beds [letter]. *N Eng J Med.*1988;318:1700.
30. Corwin MJ. Suddent infant dealth syndrome. UpToDate Version 16.3. Available at: www.uptodate.com. Accessed: December 10, 2007.
31. Bonham JR, Downing M. Metabolic deficiencies and SIDS. *J Clin Pathol.* November 1992;45(11 suppl):33–38.

22 Youth and Gang Violence: Identification and Prevention Strategies

S. Ivan Riley Jr, MD, and Jayne Batts, MD, FACEP
Special Thanks to Mitchell J. Goldman, DO

INTRODUCTION

Gang culture is evolutionary with dynamic changes occurring over time. Therefore, this chapter focuses on the more consistent characteristics of gangs and gang violence. The scope of information incorporates current trends associated with most major gang categories such as street, prison, motorcycle, and hate gangs.

Defining the parameters of a gang or a gang member continues to be an issue of debate because the spectrum of involvement can be quite diverse. However, most authorities generally agree on the definition of a gang as an ongoing organization, association, or group of three or more people with a common interest, bond, or activity. The behavior of the members, either individually or collectively, may be disruptive or antisocial, involving a pattern of criminal or delinquent behavior.[1] Estimating the scope of gang activity is convoluted by the complexity of gang hierarchy. Members range from the "wannabe" to the "hard-core" and vary in degrees of criminal activity. Many sources of gang-related statistics are unreliable, secondary to the inherent furtive nature of gangs. Thus, survey and population studies performed can be easily misinterpreted or distort gang epidemiology.[1]

Despite these challenges, longitudinal studies such as by the National Youth Gang Center estimate 760,000 youth gang members nationwide with 24,000 active gangs not including motorcycle, hate, prison, and adult gang affiliates.[2] These trends have remained relatively stable since 1995. Youth gang activity is present in 80% of US cities with populations greater than 50,000 people and is present in approximately 10–30% of rural jurisdictions. Fifty-two percent of US law enforcement agencies have reported an increase in the number of documented gang members in more recent survey studies.[2] Statistics also indicate the number of female gang members, currently accounting for 6–10% of the gang population, is rising.[3,4] Thus, gangs remain a substantial problem nationwide, affecting millions of Americans.

ECONOMIC IMPACT

The fiscal impact of gang violence is devastating. The average cost of criminal acts in the United States is estimated to be more than $655 billion each year.[5] Each adolescent involved in 10 or more years of criminal activities costs taxpayers approximately $1.7 million to $2.3 million.[5,6] Gang members are accountable for a disproportionate share of these violent and nonviolent offenses. Seattle gang members were 3 times more likely to report involvement in larceny and assaults, 4 times more likely to commit felony theft, 8 times more likely to be involved in robberies, 3 times more likely to be arrested, and 5 times more likely to have sold drugs compared to nongang members.[7]

The medical cost of gang violence is just as crippling. Los Angeles County estimates nearly a $1 billion budget for gang-associated violence.[8] One trauma center study estimated $5 million spent on 856 gunshot wound injures—one-fourth of the victims being gang-related.[8,9] Most of this fiscal burden is absorbed by the hospital or taxpayers because more than 50% of the patients have no third-party reimbursement.[9] These estimates still may not fully include additional costs of rehabilitation, long-term facility care, psychological support, family counseling, and other medical assistance.

FIREARM MORBIDITY AND MORTALITY

Unfortunately, the United States firearm death rate is one of the highest and far exceeds most industrialized nations in comparison.[10] Firearm-related injuries are the second leading cause of death among adolescents and the primary cause for African American boys.[11] For each death, four additional children will sustain a firearm-related injury.[11]

In general, gang members are 60 times more likely than nonmembers to be involved in a homicide.[12] Nearly half of all homicides in densely populated cities such as Los Angeles and one-fourth of the homicides in medium to large cities are associated with gang violence.[12,13] These gang-related homicides have increased more than 30% in recent years.[14] Firearms are used in 95% of the cases.[8] The gunshot wounds are located in proportion to the body surface area with the head, chest, and abdomen each accounting for 20% of the wounds while the extremities account for approximately one-third. Nearly half of these injuries require emergent surgery, including the following: laparotomy, craniotomy, laparoscopy, vascular, orthopedic, endoscopic, and thoracostomies.[10]

Gang members maim or kill for numerous reasons. Youth gang-bangers cite revenge, retaliation, disrespect, put in work (gang repayment) for the hood, wearing the wrong color, mad-dogging (staring), self-defense, graffiti warfare, drugs, and money as some of the more common reasons. However, other answers for killing have included boredom and peer pressure.[15]

DRIVE-BY SHOOTINGS

Drive-by shooting is one of the more common forms of homicidal killings in gang organizations. The police define this crime as a gang-motivated incident in which the suspect discharges a firearm from a vehicle and causes a homicide, attempted murder, or felonious assault or shoots into an inhabited dwelling.[16] The reasons behind such acts are many and can include retaliation, drug trade, gang warfare, initiation ceremonies, or even recreational purposes. The primary goal usually involves provoking terror and fear by a rival gang, with secondary intentions of killing and maiming the victims.[9]

One LA-based study retrospectively reviewed 677 adolescent drive-by shooting cases. Findings suggest approximately two-thirds of the victims sustained a gunshot wound with half the injuries involving the extremities. Only 5% of the victims died from associated injuries. Two-thirds of the victims were rival gang members. The majority of injuries occurred openly on city streets with less than 15% involving gangs shooting into a car or into a home. Most commonly handguns are used, with a third of these involving semiautomatic capabilities. Occasionally, shotguns, rifles, and rarely assault weapons are used.[17] However, some of the more violent gangs such as MS-13 are paramilitary trained and can access more elaborate weaponry.

These drive-by shootings are well documented in gang mass media writing and video production. The most publicized drive-by shootings involve rapper Tupac Shakur who was killed in a Las Vegas drive-by in 1996 and rival gang member Notorious B.I.G. during a drive-by shooting in 1997.[18] Multiple popular video games now incorporate drive-by shootings as a strategic means of killing opponents. *Grand Theft Auto: San Andreas* requires the player to recruit various gang members to shoot police and opposing gangs.[19] Rockstar Games, the publisher of the Grand Theft Auto franchise, grossed more than $1 billion in US sales alone and sold more than 6.6 million copies of the game.[20,21]

Furthermore, dozens of gang documentaries, including video media usually codirected by current or ex-gang members, romanticize urban warfare or glorify gang lifestyle. Significant mass media exposure from the hip-hop culture and lucrative multimedia software programs are but a few negative influences desensitizing our current youth population. The overall impact of publicized drive-by shootings remains controversial. Yet, increasing drive-by shooting trends support Thrasher's 1927 analysis that hypermasculine violent imagery promulgates the contagious copycat phenomenon where youth imitate and simulate visual media.[22]

RISK FACTORS FOR YOUTH GANG INVOLVEMENT

Multiple risk factors have been postulated as reasons why certain youths are more vulnerable to gang involvement. These risk factors, listed in Table 22-1, can be subdivided into groups including individual, family, school, peer, and community-based factors. General risk factors for an individual may encompass younger age, male gender, poor self-esteem, early delinquency, dating, sexual promiscuity, antisocial behaviorism, or other biopsychosocial attributes.[23–25]

Family factors may include a poor nurturing infrastructure with single parent involvement or foster care, drugs and alcoholism, abuse, negligence, poverty, poor parental discipline, family gang members, or even wealth.[24,26] School factors may involve poor individual performance, low achievement, truancy, lack of a safety network, or being mislabeled by surrounding role models. The most influential risk factor is peer pressure with one survey study suggesting approximately half of all gang members follow friends or family members as the main reason for gang involvement.[7,27] Community factors vary depending on the locality, but most communities lack safe recreational activities and jobs while adulterated with poverty, drugs, preexisting gangs, and racial or cultural conflicts.[28,29] Financial factors include the pecuniary need to obtain food, shelter, drugs, materialistic items, or to impress peers or a significant other.[25]

Female gang members have similar risk factors; however, they are more commonly subject to abuse. Nine out of 10 incarcerated female offenders in one LA study were victims of "some form of emotional, physical, and/or sexual abuse" at the median age of 13 years.[21,22] Minority females are often further alienated by the consequences of teenage pregnancy, sexual discrimination, and unemployment.[32]

The combination of these risk factors kindles gang involvement. Children 10–12 years of age with 3 risk factors are 3 times more likely to join a gang, whereas 7 or more risk factors increase the likelihood of gang involvement 13-fold compared to youth with 1 or fewer risk factors.[7,33,34]

At-risk youth may be further captivated by the overglamorization of gang lifestyle. Such attractive features include a sense of belonging or attachment, respect, adventure, a surrogate family, recognition, protection, sex, shelter, and monetary gain. Obviously, more factors contribute to the equation, and identifying these influences can aid in further research, profiling at-risk youth, gang prevention strategies, and forensic data gathering.

RECRUITMENT AND INITIATION (LOC'ING-IN)

Gang initiation is an urban rite of passage for at-risk youth to be formally inducted as a gang member. Prior to initiation, the inductee often memorizes basic gang principles,

TABLE 22-1 **Common Youth Risk Factors for Gang Involvement**

Financial Factors:
Lack of food
Unsuitable shelter
Drug addiction
Materialistic needs

Family Factors:
Single parent
Foster care
Poor parenting
Drugs and alcoholism
Abuse and negligence
Poverty
Lack of discipline
Family gang members

Individual Factors:
Young age
Male gender
Poor self-esteem
Early delinquency
Sexual promiscuity
Antisocial behaviorism
Aggressiveness
Pregnancy

Community Factors:
Lack of recreation
Lack of jobs
Poverty
Drugs
Gang activity
Racial segregation

School Factors:
Truancy
Poor performance
Low achievement
Unsafe environment
Mislabeled
Lack of role models
Peer pressure

codes of conduct, hand signals, and symbols often referred to as "knowledge."[35] The most common initiation strategies utilized by nationally based gangs are subdivided into the following categories: assault, homicide, sexual relations, larceny, and nonviolent methods as listed in Table 22-2.[36–38] Hybrid or occult gangs may perform more unusual or bizarre hazing tactics. Generally, the inductee must endure a limited but severe beating by one or more assailants. Women can usually forfeit the beating for a sexual act.[39]

During this hazing process, the new inductee can suffer multiple injuries both physically and sexually. According to one survey study, 5% of female gang members listed sex with gang leaders as their primary role.[40] Homicidal acts are rarely performed for gang membership and are generally reserved for prison or aggressive gangs. Some gang family members or friends, as well as highly educated public figures, can bypass the initiation process altogether through nonviolent means. Familiarization with these practices is important in identifying gang or associated gang injuries. In fact, a new gang member may present to the hospital with injuries afflicted from gang initiation.

STREET GANGS

A majority of street gangs are generally composed of urban-dwelling adolescents. However, older members are found in prison gangs, gang affiliates, and multigenerational Hispanic gangs from South America. These older gangsters continue to influence younger populations through various media including music, television, and the Internet, thus kindling further recruitment and involvement.

Modern-day street gangs are more organized, widespread, and violent with advancements in weaponry, warfare tactics, drug trading, and monetary stature. Most street gangs are structured with a majority of gang members being associates or "wannabes" generally 10 to 15 years. They attempt to advance by involvement in petty crimes, graffiti, drug trafficking, or dressing and acting as a gang member. Survey studies suggest that approximately 1–2% of youths in this age range are active gang members.[7] New recruits undergo one or more various induction rituals as mentioned earlier usually around the age of 15 to 17 with peak gang affiliation between 15 and 21 years of age.[41] Incarcerated members join the ranks as hard-core members. Membership is set for life with older members becoming habitual felons. Migrating out of a gang can be difficult and potentially fatal. The most notorious street gangs include the following LA-, Chicago-, and Hispanic-based gangs. Most sets or local street gangs have conglomerated into larger "nations" and are listed in Table 22-3.[42–45]

LA-BASED GANGS

The two most commonly known Los Angeles–based street gangs include the Bloods and the Crips. Prior to these two factions, Mexican American *pachuco* gangs and smaller black social clubs predominated in Los Angeles and conjugated for camaraderie and protection.[46] In the late 1960s,

TABLE 22-2 **Initiation Strategies for Gang Members**

Assault	
Jumped in/Beaten in/Rolled in	Multiple gang members assaulting the inductee over a period of time
Lined in/walk the line/gauntlet	Multiple gang members assaulting the inductee who walks through two gang lines
Punched in	Inductee is punched in the chest one or more times
Circled in	Gang members surround and assault the inductee who must try to escape the gang circle
Freein Hoover	Assaulting the inductee who attempts to pick up coins off the ground
Assault	Assault to an innocent bystander or rival gang member by the inductee
Homicide	
Cop killing	Rare phenomenon, however significant reputation is achieved
Russian roulette	Inductee risks death by a semi-loaded weapon
Blood in/blood out	Common prison initiation tactic where the inductee kills someone or dies for initiation and retirement from a gang
Larceny	
Jacked in	Committing an armed robbery or theft by the inductee
Non-Violent	
Courted in/Deeded in	Gang membership granted secondary to inductee's special talents, credentials, or education (e.g., drug dealer, wealthy benefactor, lawyer, police, judge, doctor)
Blessed in/Born in	Gang membership granted secondary to inductee's family ties
Sexual	
Rape	Sexual abuse usually involving the inductee and an innocent victim
Sexed in	Forced or voluntary sexual intercourse usually involving a female inductee with one or more gang-bangers; sometimes, this tactic is in lieu of a beat in and the gang members are potentially known to have HIV/AIDS

Source: Courtesy of Michael Carlie, PhD. Missouri State University. *Into the Abyss: A Personal Journey into the World of Street Gangs*. 2002.

TABLE 22-3 **Gang Nations and Associated Sets**

Blood Nation	135 Piru, Avenue Piru, Campenella Park Piru, Center Park Blood, Cedar Block Piru, 706 Blood, 92 Bishops, Be-Bopp Watts Bishops, Athens Park Boys, Black P Stones, Bounty Hunters, Fruit Town Brims, Leuders Park Piru, Mad Swan Blood, Rollin 20s Neighborhood Blood, Tree Top Piru, West Side Piru, Crenshaw Mafia Gang, Mob Piru, Rollin 50s Brims
Crip Nation	Acacia Block Compton Crip, Avalon 40's Crip, Compton Avenue Crip, East Coast Crip, East Side Players, Gangster Crip, Hard Time Hustler Crip, Hoover, Insane Crip, Kitchen Crip Gang, Mafia Crip, Neighbor Hood Crip, Original Blocc Crip, Original Blocc Crip, Rollin 40s, West Side Mafia
Folk Nation	Black Gangster Disciples, Gangster Disciples, Imperial Gangsters, La Raza, Spanish Cobras, Latin Eagles, Latin Disciples, Simon City Royals, Two Sixers, Spanish Gangsters
People Nation	Latin Kings, Latin Counts, Kents, Spanish Lords, Vice Lords, Gaylords, Insane Duces, Black P. Stones, Insane Unknowns, El Rukns, Bishops
La Gran Raza	Mexican Boys, Crazy Homies, Chidos Picudos, Cachandos, Wild Chicanos, Santaneros, Los Primos, Necios, Santiago Muchacan, Reyes Locos (Affiliations: La Eme)
La Gran Familia	Ninos Malos, Southside, Traviesos, Cacos, 18th Street, Sureno Trece, LA 13, Brown Pride, Vagabondos, Compadres, La Tremendas, Escandolosos, Barrio Kings, La Cien, Cueristos (Affiliations: Nuestra Familia)

adolescent gang sets began congregating in local neighborhoods taking on street names along Compton.[43] By the early 1970s, dozens of youth sets including the Hoovers, the Rollin Street Set, and East Coast Boys incorporated into the Crip Nation to become the largest gang faction in Los Angeles. The Bloods (also known as Black Liberation Organization of Defense) thus developed as a means of retaliation through a similar pact of sets such as the Pirus, Brims, Athens Park Boys, and the Pueblos.[42,43]

The Crips and Bloods adopted the blue and red, respectively, railroad-manufactured bandannas (a.k.a. flags) for gang identification purposes.[15] Hand signing or "flaggin'" became popular as an encrypted method for communication. Graffiti symbolism littered the street becoming the ghetto's newspaper declaring rivalry gang concentrations and gang feud warfare. LA gangs grew in a race to control territory and the drug trade, particularly crack cocaine. Weapons advanced from common household items like bats and knives to hand guns and high-caliber assault firearms as drug money paved the way to further territorial domination.

By the end of the Los Angeles riots of 1992, some sets established truces, although significant violence continues. The strong media coverage of the riots, gangs, and the hip-hop culture helped to spread the seed to the current international infestation. Current census studies estimate 39,000 gang members reside in Los Angeles County alone, with nearly half involved in black gangs.[47] These members belong to more than 250 Crip and 300 Blood sets, although Crips outnumber Bloods by about 2 to 1.[47]

Bloods commonly call themselves CKs (Crip-killers), MOBs (member of bloods), dawgs, or "ballers" (drug dealers), while referring to Crips as "crabs."[43] Crips address themselves as "cuz," BKs, or "high rollers" (drug dealers), while calling Bloods "slobs" or "snoops."[15,48]

CHICAGO-BASED GANGS

The two major Chicago-based gangs include the People and the Folk Nation, which formed in similar fashion to the LA-based gangs. Initially, local youth social cliques spawned along particular streets giving rise to set names such as 2-7s or 1-9s, meaning 27th and 19th Streets, respectively. As street violence increased, sets merged into larger "camps" such as the Black Gangster Disciples, Gangster Disciples, Imperial Gangsters, La Raza, Spanish Cobras, Latin Eagles, and Latin Disciples to eventually form the Folk Nation. To combat this alignment in the late 1970s, sets including the El Rukns (a.k.a. Black P. Stones), Vice Lords, and Latin Kings formed an alliance known as People Nation. Additional recruitment into the People Nation included the Mickey Cobras, Latin Counts, Norteños, Bishops, Insane Unknowns, and the Spanish Lords.[46] As a means for stronger alliances, gang support, and drug trading, the Bloods and People Nation are allies combating the cohesive forces of the Crips and Folk Nation.[15]

Unlike the LA-based gangs, Chicago gangs embrace more religious Islamic and Christian doctrines. These influences are exemplified by their rules of conduct and symbolism. The People Nation uses Islamic symbols such as the five-pointed star and the crescent moon. They adopted moral codes of "street conduct" such as "All is all" and "All is well."[43] They identify to the left, hats tilted or "broke" to the left, left pants leg up, earring in left ear, fading clothes to the left, and so forth. Folk Nation adopted some Christian symbolism such as the six-pointed Star of David in honor of deceased leader "King" David Barksdale and the upright devil's pitchfork. Folk Nation's code of conduct includes "I will not let my brother fall to a knee" or "All is One." Folk Nation members identify to the right in an opposite fashion as the People Nation.[49,50]

Some argue that these gangs are more structured in comparison to their LA counterparts. The structure involves numerous ranks and positions emulating a military ranking system. For example, People Nation's structure incorporates associate members as foot soldiers or "pee-wees" that advance 10 to 15 ranks to the El Rukn level. The infrastructure provides strength, protection, and an authoritarian structure for commanding officers. Such features are attractive for terrorist organizations seeking aide from US-based anti-governmental factions. In fact, the El Rukn Jeff Fort was arrested in the 1990s for his involvement in drafting a multi-million-dollar contract with Libyan foreigners for a proposed covert terrorist plot. A Latin Disciple member was arrested more recently in 2002 training as an al-Qaida terrorist.[51,52]

LATIN GANGS

For more than a century, the United States has been home to multiple Latin gangs. However, their strength and presence have grown exponentially over the last decade. Experts believe the North American Free Trade Agreement, enacted in 1993 in efforts to increase South American and Mexican employment, along with the 1990s Mexican economic crash known as the Peso Crisis significantly affected the influx of illegal aliens. Often, immigrants crossing illegally together form cliques known as Border Brothers or "Hermanos de la Frontera."[53] This strong bonding intermixed with social protection morphs into gang formation similar to the formation of LA- and Chicago-based gangs. Mexican street gangs also formed major alliances known as the *La Gran Raza,* or "The Great Race," and *La Gran Familia,* or "The Great Family." These gang nations combine more than a dozen sets, forming an incredible force to counteract rival gangs. These gangs are affiliated with popular Hispanic prison gangs such as *La Eme,* or "The Mexican Mafia," and the *Nuestra Familia.* Other non-aligned Mexican-based gangs include *La Raza, Vatos Locos,* Sons of Mexico, and Chicano Nation to name a few.[53] Many of these Mexican-based gangs share common symbols and tattoos such as the Lady of Guadalupe, praying hands, cholo, and the dog paw or *Mi Vida Loco* hand tattoo (see Figure 22-1).

The MS-13s, or *Mara Salvatrucha,* now identified by the FBI as one of the most dangerous gangs in the country, consists mostly of El Salvadoran illegal aliens. The organization was initially founded in the 1980s in Los Angeles as a source of protection for Salvadoran immigrants.[54] However, these *cholos,* or Hispanic gangsters, were raised in a country with severe economic turmoil and corruption, with broken families commonly integrated with multiple generations of gang members. The youth are often trained in paramilitary tactics and weaponry, are extremely violent, are minimally educated, and view law enforcement as enemies of the state. These gangsters are heavily tattooed (Figure 22-2) all across the body and face, proclaiming their lifelong MS-13 loyalty. They are renowned for vicious assaults on rival gang members by dismembering limbs with machete knifes or brutally killing police officers. Some population studies estimate more than 10,000 members in the United States, while more than 40,000 remain in El Salvador. Local authorities in Washington, DC, which contains a significant population of Salvadoran immigrants, estimate approximately 6,000 MS-13 members.[54,55] The abundance of drugs in their mother country and the surplus of guns manufactured in the United States led to a symbiotic bartering system involving MS-13s using border labor to ship the goods. Many of the gang members have been deported multiple times only to resurface in another injunction by police.[54] Gang members can also obtain immunity by fleeing the United States after committing crimes because present international agreements greatly interfere with the return of criminals.[55]

One of the most popular Hispanic street gangs is the Latin Kings. The gang formed nearly a half a century ago in Chicago similarly to other Chicago-based gangs, as a social organization that grew into corruption. Well known for their violent reputation and hostile attacks on rival gangs, this gang started cloning in every Hispanic neighborhood along the East Coast. The Almighty Latin Kings was later created as the prison counterpart in a New York City corrections center.[56] The males refer to one another as kings and wear gold and black jewelry and gang attire. Often, they are tattooed with elaborate kings, crowns, and lions to suggest strength and power. The Latin Queens, or the gang's female auxiliary unit, is one of the largest and most well respected units in

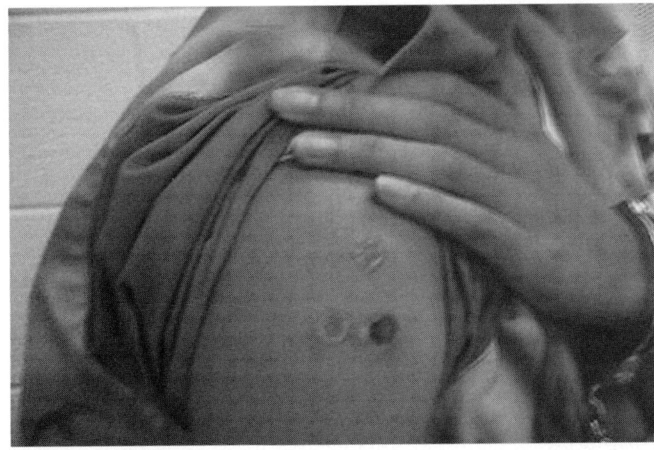

(a)

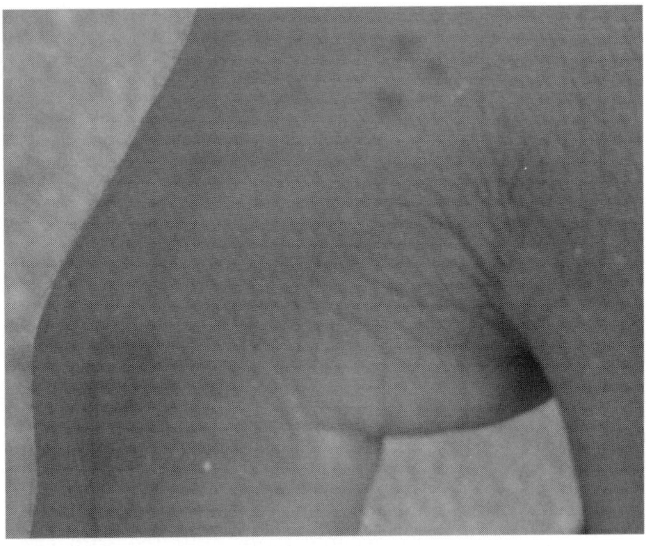

(b)

FIGURE 22-1 (a) and (b) **The dog paw or *Mi Vida Loco* hand tattoo.**

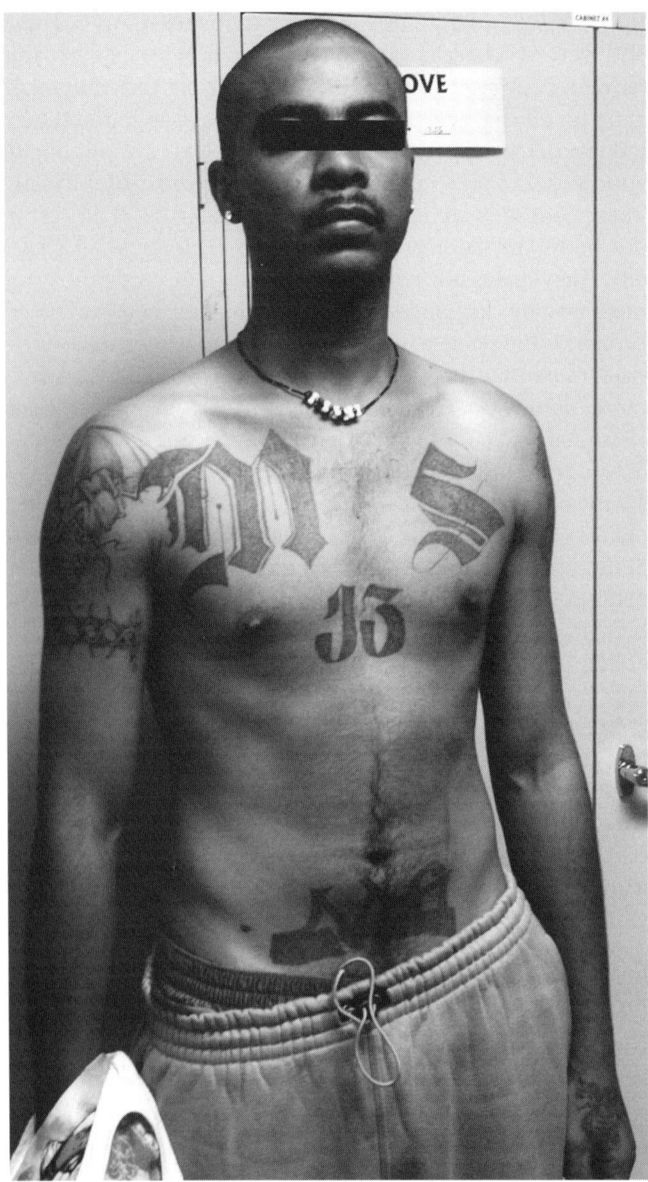

FIGURE 22-2 **MS-13 gang member with multiple tattoos.**

the country. Disrespecting a "sister" or "queen" could mean death.[57] The gang is deeply affiliated with the People Nation. And the Latin King name is an international icon with members in nearly every state, South America, and Europe, with operations continuing to expand abroad. The gang is the second largest in Chicago with estimates of nearly 20,000 members or more.[57]

PRISON GANGS

According to the 2003 prison census, nearly 2 million Americans are incarcerated, 4 million on probation, and nearly 1 million on parole. This total population is equivalent to 3% of the US adult population. More than 10% of these criminals are actively involved in gangs and the numbers are rising.[58] As prison populations become more saturated with gang members, officials will need to watch for emerging prison gangs such as the Consolidated Crip Organization (CCO), United Blood Nation (UBN), Almighty Latin Kings, Aryan Brotherhood, Mexican Mafia, La Nuestra Familia, Black Guerilla Family, and the Texas Syndicate. Law enforcement agents estimate nearly one-third of all violent incidents in prisons are prison gang related.[58] The white supremacy gang Aryan Brotherhood is responsible for nearly one-fifth of all prison-related murders.[59]

Gang leadership is well established in prison settings and the physical encapsulation prevents little disruption to the ongoing violence and drug trade. Larry Hoover, ex-leader of the Black Gangster Disciples, orchestrated a $100 million annual drug profit while incarcerated.[58] Although these gangs have only surfaced in isolated areas, there will be a natural growth inside the prisons as more members are sentenced.

MOTORCYCLE GANGS

For more than half a century, motorcycle gangs have been a growing faction, with an estimated 800 gangs worldwide.[60] The most notorious gangs in the United States include the Hells Angels, One Percenters, the Bandidos, Pagans, Outlaws, Warlocks, and the Avengers. These dangerous outlaw gangs are well versed in criminal activity including drug production and distribution, prostitution, money laundering, and extortion.[60] Their capricious and aggressive nature often leads to local bar brawls and gang fighting. However, these wars can escalate well beyond the use of firearms to include pipe bombs and explosives.

As motorcyclists, they have certain advantages over street gangs because their mobility aids in evading law enforcement. Most of the larger gangs have close ties and connections to some law enforcement through bribes and extortion. One US District Court judge was even convicted for accepting bribes from Hells Angels.[60] They network with smaller motorcycle or "puppet" gangs, street gangs, and organized crime including the Mafia and Aryan Brotherhood for drug trades and contract murders. Even police-based motorcycle gangs such as the Wild Pigs, Blood Brothers, and the Chosen Sons are suspected of socializing with these outlaw gangs.[60]

The gang "colors" or vest or jacket is essential to the gang's identity. Composed of a three-tier system, the back of the jacket incorporates the gang label along the top, a centrally located gang logo, and a bottom rocker with the gang chapter.[60] Most gang chapters have particular membership requirements regarding race, type of motorcycle, sex, and criminal history.

HATE GANGS

The most notorious hate crime organizations are white supremacist factions that are deeply rooted in anti-government, anti-black, and anti-Semitic beliefs. Common white supremacist groups include the Ku Klux Klan, Aryan Brotherhood, National Alliance, National Vanguard, the Nationalist Movement, World Church of the Creator, and the White Revolution. The groups generally accept a pan-Aryanism culture with a neo-Nazi fascist belief system misconstrued by falsely justified Christian doctrine.

The Aryan Brotherhood charters membership in every state and major federal prison with an estimated collective force of 15,000 members.[59] However, the skinhead recruitment soared more than 30% after the September 11 World Trade Center attack as a result of the resurgence of nationalism.[61] The organization is heavily tainted by criminal acts from armed robbery to murder—they justify their acts in the name of white supremacy.

SHARP (Skinheads Against Racial Prejudice) are the antithesis of most modern white supremacy groups with anti-fascist, anti-racist ideals while enjoying the skinhead lifestyle of razor-blade-shaven haircuts, punk clothing, and radical neo-hardcore music. As the American melting pot stirs, hate crime organizations are persecuting more minorities such as homosexuals and Hispanic populations.[62]

FEMALE GANGS

Female juvenile delinquents are one of the fastest growing populations in the correctional system. In 2001, females were responsible for 28% of aggravated assault charges.[63] Survey studies estimate 10% to 20% of gang members are female.[64] Most gangs are composed of an integrated or an auxiliary system, and rarely an autonomous system for female members.[26] Exclusive all-female gangs do exist but generally focus on street drug trading and prison domination.

Little is known regarding the role of female members. Surveys conducted show nearly half of the females are dating a gang member, a third are expected to carry a weapon for their male companions, and one-fourth have a specified role or designated duty in the gang.[65] Some experts believe female gang members are more violent in comparison to their male counterparts; however, this a relative point and no systematic research proves it.

HYBRID GANGS

Although the purpose of this chapter is to provide a sense of organization and structure to the field of gangology, true gang dynamics entail a bastardized process composed of new and old gangs converging and diverging with so-called hybrid gangs popping up across the United States. These gangs may adopt a combination of Chicago- and Los Angeles–based philosophies while proclaiming loyalty to multiple affiliations or displaying a combination of colors. For example, a small hybrid gang in Charlotte, North Carolina, known as the Grape Vine Crips is composed of Blood and Crip members, and thus represents the blue and red colors with purple attire (author's knowledge). Local gangs and gang members may "flip" or suddenly change gang affiliations, proclaim allegiance to multiple nationally based gangs, or label themselves independent. These nontraditional practices make gang tracking and recognition a difficult task for many local law enforcement agencies.[66]

GANG CLOTHING, ACCESSORIES, AND IDENTIFIERS

Gang fashion is evolutionary and incorporates current fashion trends into the daily attire. Typical gang bedizenment includes affiliated colors, loose-fitting apparel, particular brands with gang symbolism, embroidered gang names, beaded necklaces, belt buckles with initials, key chains, belts, and bandannas commonly called "rags."[26] Gang members embellish in dark shades of a single color nuance; the most common gang-affiliated colors are listed in Table 22-4. Loose-fitting apparel may include oversized T-shirts, plaid shirts, Starter jackets, "sagging" pants, long belts, and untied suede shoes or boots. Elephantine gold or silver jewelry (a.k.a. "bling-bling") may be worn as rings, watches, earrings, necklaces, or even "grills" (dental decoration). Multicolored beaded necklaces, popular with Chicago-based gangs, often signify rank and stature through the use of recognized patterns.[67]

Gang branding is another key component of gang fashion where commercial brands and associated symbols are integrated into gang style. Table 22-5 highlights common gang branding, oftentimes overlooked by the untrained eye.[68,69] The brand's logo or symbol may be displayed on hats, shirts, pants, or shoes. Some members may embroider clothing with gang names, symbols, or associated artwork. Others may simply draw graffiti on clothing, book bags, notebooks, weapons, wallets, belts, or accessories with permanent markers (Figure 22-3). Bandanas, belts, and beaded key chains are important components for members to display, "throw," or "flash" their colors (Figure 22-4). These appurtenances may also serve multiple purposes (i.e., bandanas to cover the face, wipe down weapons, or store drugs).

TABLE 22-4A **Gang Colors**

Blue	Folk Nation, Crips, Surenos, Gaylords, Black Disciples, Gangster Disciples, Latin Disciples, Spanish Gangster Disciples, Two-Two Boys, Latin Disciples, Saints
Copper	Bishops
Gold	Latin Kings, Vice Lords, Four Corner Hustlers
Grey	Latin Eagles
Maroon	Spanish Vice Lords
Green	King Cobras, Mickey Cobras, Spanish Cobras, Insane Deuces
Purple	Grape Vine Crips, Get Down Boys
Red	People Nation, Bloods, Nortenos, La Gran Familia, Latin Counts, Black P. Stones, Vice Lords, Hell's Angels
Yellow	Gangster Satan Disciples
White/Black	Vice Lords, Latin Dragons, Neo-Nazi groups, Aryan Brotherhood, Gothic groups

TABLE 22-4B **Gang Flag Colors**

White, Blue	MS-13s (El Salvador)
Red, White, Blue, Yellow	Vargas Gang (Philippines)
Red, White, and Blue	Neto (Puerto Rico)
Red, White, Green	La Raza Nation (Mexico)

TABLE 22-5 **Gang-Affiliated Brands**

4 Corner Hustlers	Cincinnati Reds (color)
Black Disciples	Denver Broncos (initials)
Black Peace Stone Nation	Chicago Bulls (color); Phoenix Suns (initials)
Bloods	Charlotte Knights (Crip Killer); Pittsburgh Pirates (P = Piru)
Crips	British Knights (Blood Killer); Burger King (Blood Killer)
Folk	Duke (color, devil symbol); Georgetown (initials); Georgia Tech (G = Gangster); Kansas City Royals (color); Los Angeles Raiders; North Carolina Tar Heels (color); Orlando Magic (symbol, color); Nike (color)
Gangster Disciples	Detroit Lions (color); Detroit Tigers (blue/black color, initials); Georgetown Hoyas (Hoyas = [Larry] Hoover's on your a**); LA Dodgers (D symbol); NY Yankees (color)
Imperial Gangsters	Indiana University (pitchfork symbol)
Latin Counts	Chicago Bulls (color); Chicago Cubs (initials)
Latin Kings	LA Kings (crown symbol, initials)
Maniac Latin Disciples	Michigan State (initials); Minnosota Twins (initials)
People Nation	Atlanta Braves (initial "A" for Almighty); Chicago Bulls (color); Converse All Star shoe (star symbol); Dallas Cowboys (star symbol); LA Kings (crown symbol); Miami Hurricanes (color); Philadelphia Phillies (initials); Texas Rangers (pitchfork T symbol); Starter apparel (star symbol)
Simon City Royals	Colorado Rockies (initials); Kansas City Royals (initials)
Spanish Cobras	Oakland A's (green/black color)
Vice Lords	Chicago Bulls (color); Louis Vitton (initials); St. Louis Cardinals (color); University of Nevada at Las Vegas (color, initials UNLV = Vice Lord Nations United)

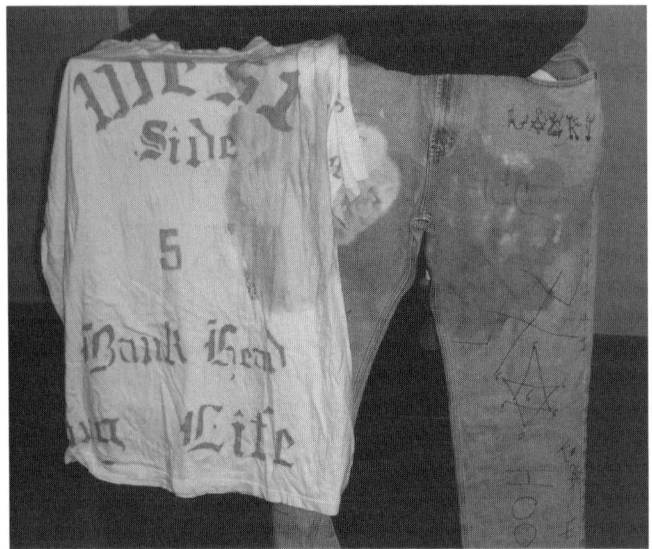

(a)

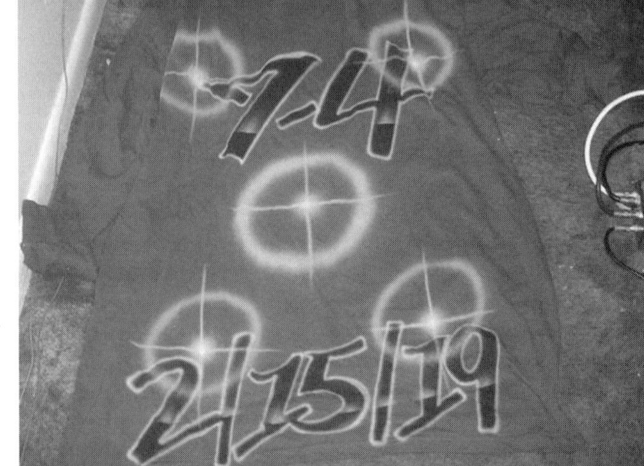

(b)

FIGURE 22-3 **Clothing with graffiti, embroidery, and airbrushing. (a) The shirt was worn by a West Side Blood gang member, and the pants by a Folk Nation gang member. Notice the pitchforks, six-pointed star, and the moniker "loc-ky" on the pants. (b) The shirt demonstrates the numeric code 7-4 for Gangster Disciples and 2-15-19, which represents the Brothers of Struggle. (c) The hats are embroidered with MS-13 and Sur (South) logos.**

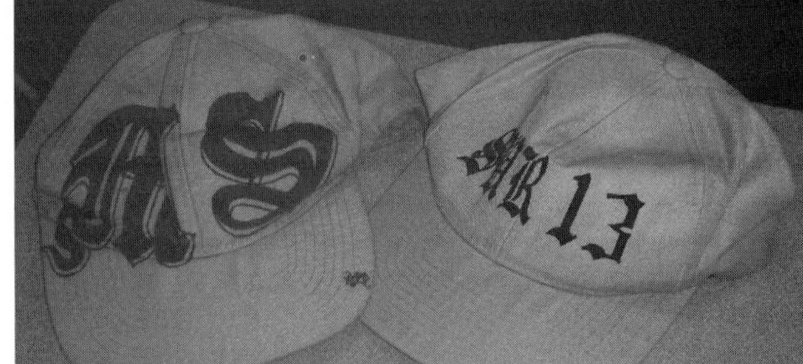

(c)

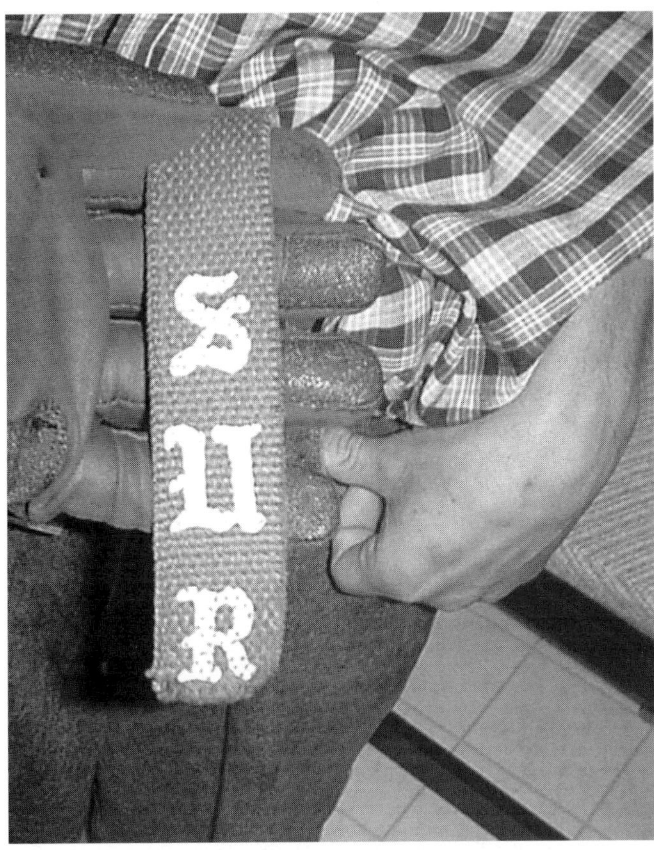

(a)

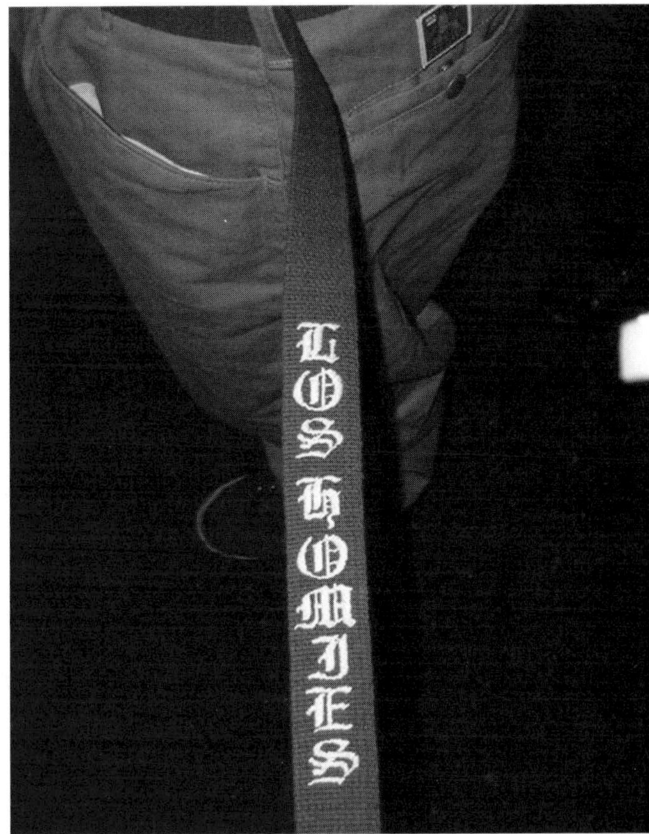

(b)

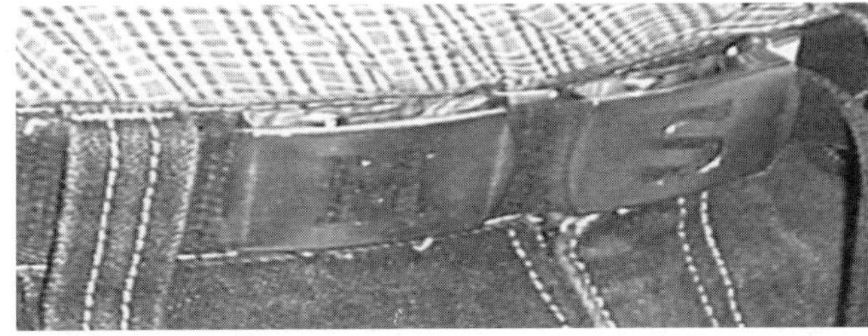

(c)

FIGURE 22-4 **Accessories demonstrating belts used to "flash" or "drop" gang-affiliated logos that are commonly used by Hispanic gangs such as (a) the Surenos, (b) Los Homies, and (c) MS-13.**

Excessive dark-colored makeup or facial paint is popular among female and occult gangsters. Some gangs such as the Juggalos, an emerging Insane Clown Posse horror-core rap cult, paint themselves in diabolic clown-like makeup.[70] This new breed is mainly devoted to public terrorizing, but also is responsible for multiple horrific machete assaults. The traditional dress of skinheads is a razor-shaved head, suspenders, and steel-toed boots. Realize that as local law enforcement agencies crack down on gang violence, some gangs are camouflaging their once conspicuous attire with minimal identifying features.[68]

Street gang fashion entails dress codes beyond color and style by encompassing elements of "fading." Gang members commonly will wear certain clothing placed strategically to one side as a means of further gang identification or gang status. Jackets or button-down shirts will be open or removed on side, as illustrated in Figure 22-5. Pant legs will be drawn up or rolled on one side. Hats, jewelry, belts, belt buckles, earrings, or embroideries may be angled or predominantly located on one side.[49]

Hair styles play a role in gang identification. Street gang members may shave elaborate designs or gang symbols into the hairline whereas white supremacy members have shaven

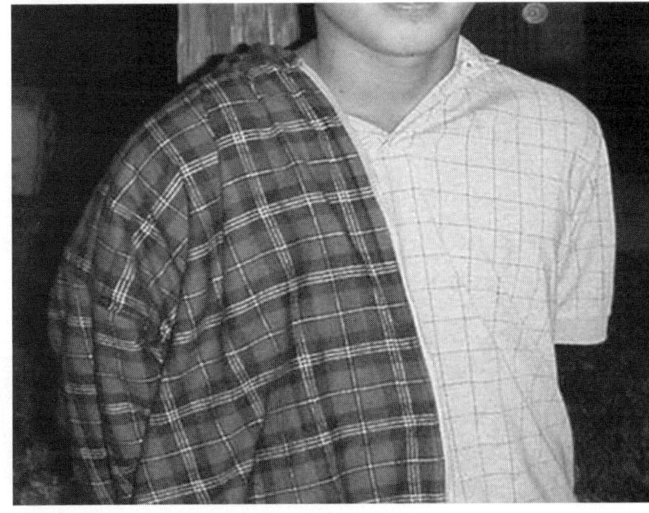

FIGURE 22-5 **Example of a Crip gang member "fading" his shirt.**

heads. Gothic or occult groups dye hair, eyebrows, and facial hair dark colors and occasionally incorporate bizarre colored highlights. Incarcerated gang members may tattoo or brand symbols onto the scalp.[71] Hair accents include beads, barrettes, rubber bands, or combs distinguishing members by color or location.[49]

GANG SYMBOLS AND CODING

Gangs communicate through various media such as artwork, tattoos, graffiti, e-mail, Web sites, and letters. The language is encrypted in symbols and numeric coding. Each symbol may represent one or more meanings.[49] Figure 22-6 shows some of the most common gang symbols.[42,69] Gangs disrespect

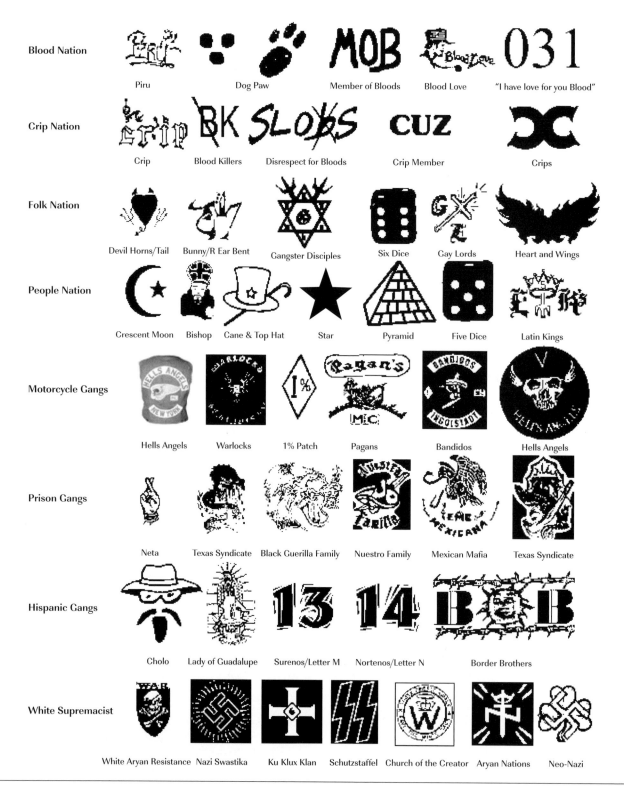

FIGURE 22-6 **Associated gang symbols.**

other gangs by slashing out or drawing a rival gang symbol upside down, as demonstrated in Figure 22-7.

Skinheads use acronyms including war (white Aryan resistance), AYM (Aryan youth movement), or AF (abraxas foundation) to show allegiance. Neo-Nazi symbols include the swastika or the double lighting bolt. Other white supremacy symbols include cloverleafs, coats of arms, and shields.[49,69] Occult or gothic gangs display demonic symbolism such as the inverted cross, pentagram, hexagram, or cross of Nero. Satanic symbols often depict the mark of the beast in the form of triple 6s, Fs, or circles.[49] The symbols may be found on religious documents, drawings, clothing, animal carcasses, or dead bodies. Prison gangs have more consistent and easily recognizable symbols. The Mexican Mafia use the "Mexican flag" symbol consisting of an eagle and serpent with the acronym "EME" translating to Mexican pride. Other prison gangs such as the Nuestra, Texas Syndicate, and Black Guerilla Family share similar dragon and sword type logos.[69] Outlaw motorcycle gangs strut with leather jackets placarded with the gang's colors or emblems on the back surrounded by patches, badges, or memorabilia.[49]

Covert alpha and numeric coding is also common in gang language. Telephone area codes, zip codes, streets, and addresses represent a gang territory or location.[72] Other codes may mimic federal, state, or penal criminal coding systems. For instance, the California criminal codes 211 and 187 mean armed robbery and homicide, respectively.[35] Simple codes substitute the alphabet with corresponding numbers with each code separated by a dash or period. For example, the 2.7.4 stands for B.G.D., or Black Gangster Disciple. The code of conduct "1-1-15" symbolizes the phrase "all as one."[49] Codes may be interjected in a gangster's alias name. The moniker "t-loc" represents the first initial of the gangster's name and the slang "loc," short for the Spanish term *loco* or crazy.[69,73] More complex codes such as "031" translate into "I have love for you, Blood" and may require a specialized gang cryptographist to decode.[48]

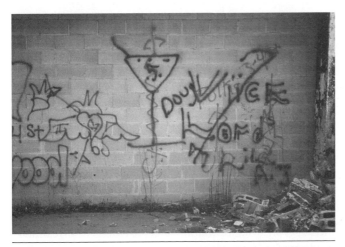

FIGURE 22-7 **Black graffiti representing the Vice Lords with blue Folk Nation graffiti scribbled over as a sign of disrespect.**

Body Language

Gangs have other active forms of nonverbal communication including body stance, hand signing, or specialized ceremonial dances. The body stance may incorporate the crossing of arms or legs to form a symbol and is often performed when addressing ally or rival gang members.[49]

"Throwing up" hand signs conveys messages or threats by "claiming" gang loyalty.[73] "Stacking" multiple hand signs in rapid sequence constitutes gang sign language. Gangs will disrespect or "challenge" gang opposition by imitating rival gang hand signs upside down. Figure 22-8 demonstrates the most common hand signs from various gangs.[35,37,49,50]

Certain gangs such as the Bloods and Crips have deeply rooted ceremonial dances known respectively as the "b-walk" and "c-walk." Members may be identified by "walking it out" or performing a "G-check." These dances involve repetitive heel-to-heel and toe-to-toe combinations, performed to insult or after killing rival gang members.[74,75] Although these dances have been around for 20 years, their popularity has reached national acclaim after live performances by rap artists Snoop Dogg (former Crip member) and Rapper WC. Now derivations of the dance like the Harlem Shake are gaining popularity.[74]

Tattoos

Gang tattoos vary depending on the gang and degree of association. They may display the gang name, acronym, symbol, or logo. Street gang members usually tattoo one or more gang symbols or logos (Figure 22-9).[35,37,49,50,69,76] In contrast, Hispanic gangs such as the Mexican Mafia, Surenos, and Netas may tattoo abstract artwork or elaborate pictorials of mystical landscapes and naked women. The Mara Salvatrucha are notorious for blanketing themselves in tattoos. Markings include "MS," "13," and "Devil Horns."[55] White supremacists share iconic neo-Nazi symbols of lightning bolts and swastikas or gang acronyms. Similarly, prison tattoos are generally composed of a symbolic gang logo. Native American gangs are notorious for branding or burning gang symbols into the skin and emulating aboriginal war chief tattooing ceremonies.[77] "Slashing" marks into the skin with a knife or "scarring" the skin with cigarette burns to produce symbols or dots is a common practice for Asian gangs, with less of an emphasis on tattooing.[78] Occult gang members may use a combination of the preceding techniques to produce demonic carvings in their skin or the skin of a victim.

HEALTHCARE PREVENTION STRATEGIES

It's 4:15 a.m. on a busy Saturday night and a victim of a drive-by shooting is found in the medic bay lying across the front seat of his car. Despite attempts at resuscitation, he is pronounced dead shortly after arrival. When his friends attempt to leave in the vehicle, they are stopped by hospital security and the police are notified. Over the next few hours, nearly 40 gang members arrive demanding entrance into the emergency department (ED) to retaliate against the security officers and to see their "dawg." Although security personnel and the police work to alleviate the situation, the ED is ultimately

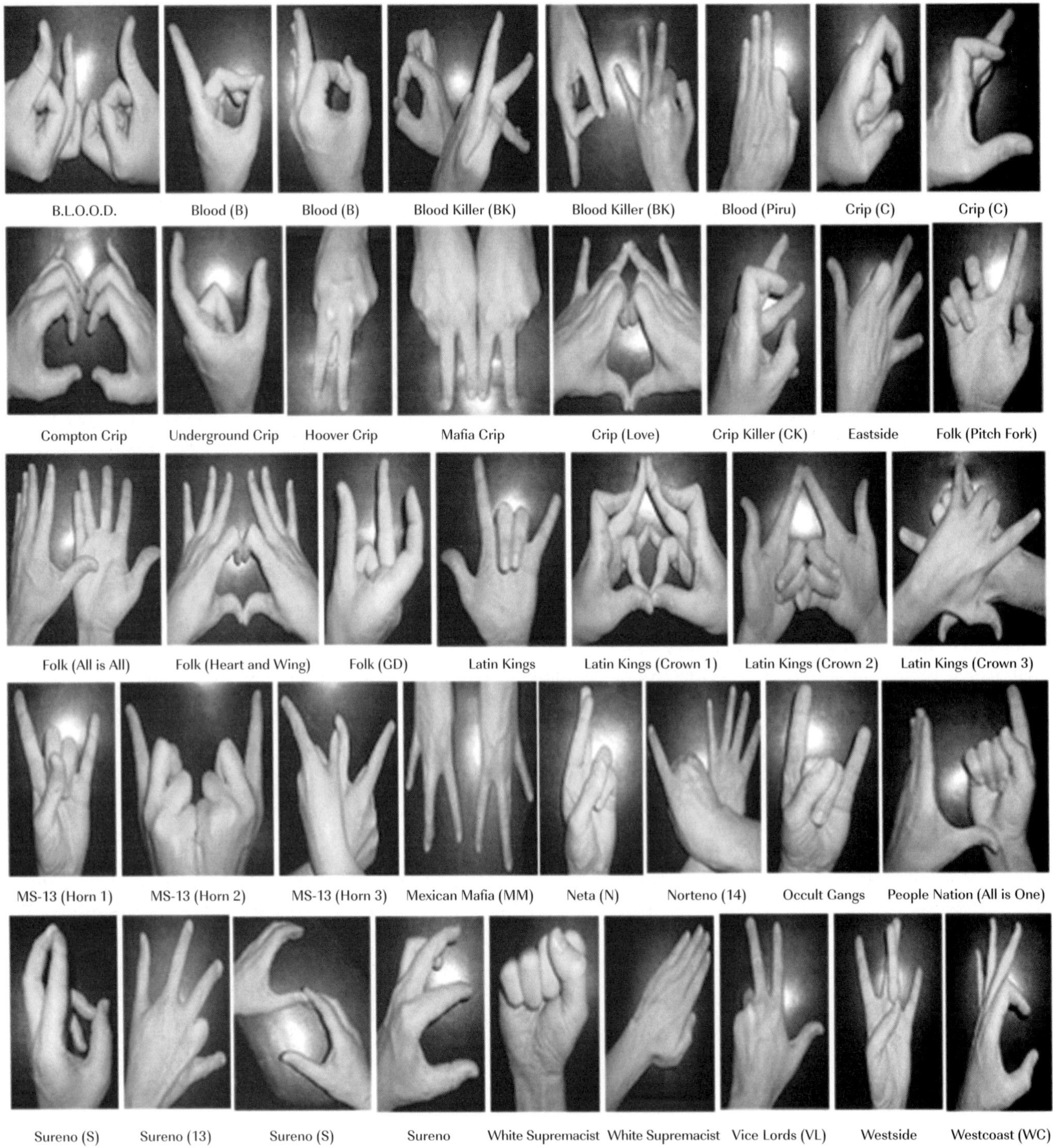

FIGURE 22-8 **Common gang hand signs.**

"locked down" for the rest of the night, resulting in the arrest of 14 armed gang members. Police later discover the victim's car was also loaded with multiple semiautomatic weapons planned for gang retaliation.

Hospitals, once thought of as "violence-free" areas, are becoming more common ground for gang warfare and retaliation, resulting in hospital staff injuries.[79] Studies on workplace violence found a third of ED physicians report being physically assaulted.[80] These events occasionally make the press but are down-played by public relations. Less than a handful of these clinical cases are documented in medical literature despite daily violent encounters by hospital staff. When gang members are seen for routine or acute emergency treatment, healthcare workers are at risk for injury or even death. Risk reduction strategies include staff education, security enforcement, and specific protocols when violence erupts in the ED.

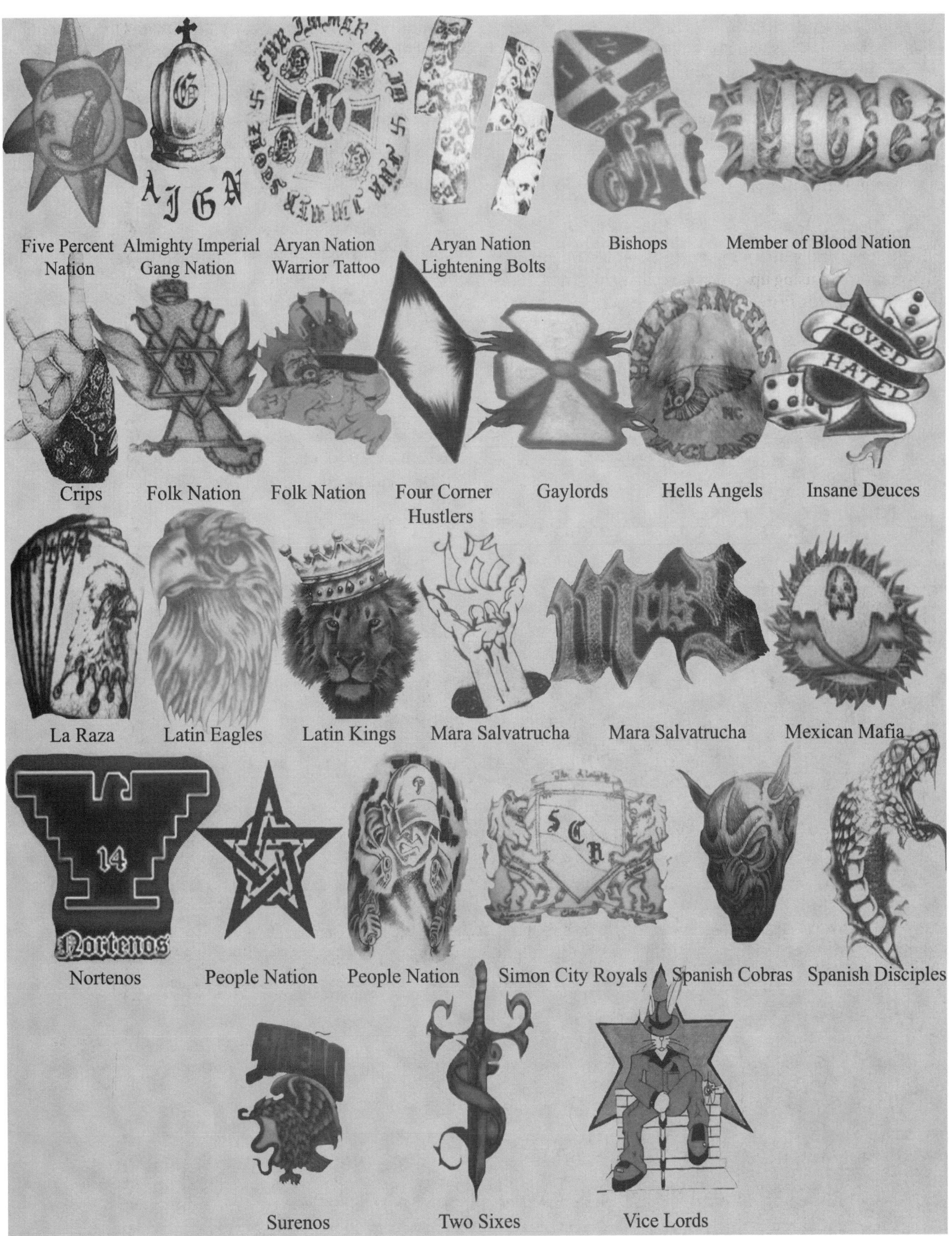

FIGURE 22-9 **Common gang tattoos and security threat group markings.**

Staff Education

Healthcare providers should be educated to recognize gang tattoos, numbers, clothing, colors, accessories, hand signals, and gang-associated trauma. Understanding gang formation, the effects of gang violence, and how to institute prevention strategies are equally important. Educational courses should focus on simple, common gang identifiers, as shown in Figure 22-10.

Security Protocols

All entrances and exits to the hospital should be continuously monitored using upgraded surveillance cameras. Special entry and exit systems such as card access readers or key punch locks can secure access to restricted areas. Studies demonstrate that metal detectors and bullet-resistant glass can ultimately decrease in-hospital weapon contamination and potential fatal assaults.[81] Panic alarms strategically placed throughout the department with easily assessable overhead paging violence protocols such as "code Armstrong" are mandatory to summon security staff efficiently.

Pre-hospital and Emergency Department Protocols

Hospital security should be notified prior to the arrival of any known or suspected gang members. Multiple injured gang members should be placed in separate treatment areas or transferred to different hospitals if possible—secondary to concerns of in-hospital retaliation by rival gang members. Access to the patient should be limited to primary family members with appropriate identification, and the patient should be given an alias to prevent rival gang members from tracking the person down. During the primary survey, the patient should be completely exposed and his or her belongings searched for weapons.

Always assume gang members are carrying a weapon. More than 50% of arrested gang members have a history of firearm use to commit crimes.[82] A general rule of thumb is any instrument that can cause harm can and will be used by gang members. Weapons include bats, razor blades, brass knuckles, maces, sharpened utensils, guns, and even heavy explosives. Figure 22-11 is an example of some of the weapons confiscated by police during a street gang war. Notice that weapons can be concealed in even seemingly benign items.

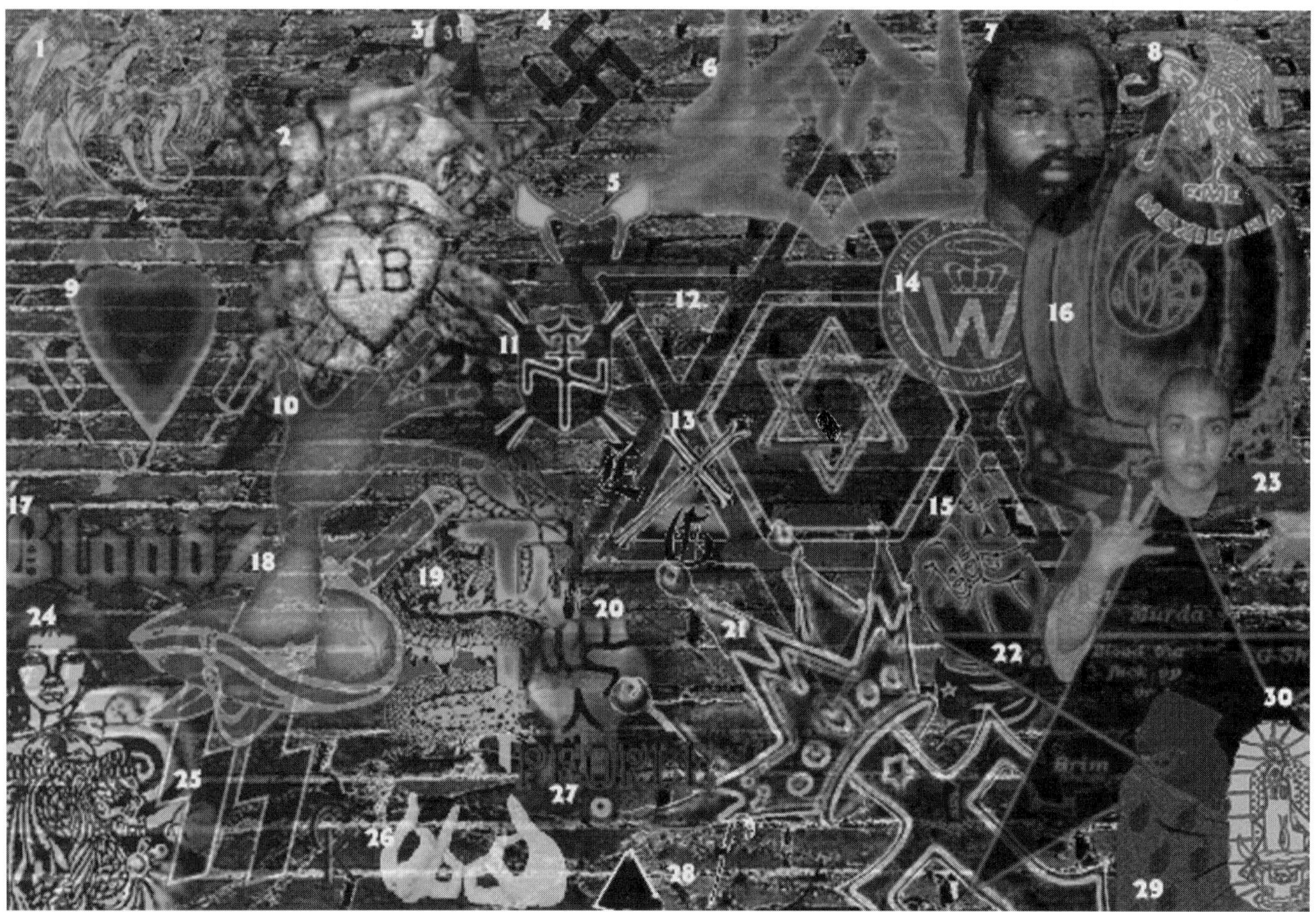

FIGURE 22-10 **Collage of gang colors, tattoos, graffiti, and hand signs.**

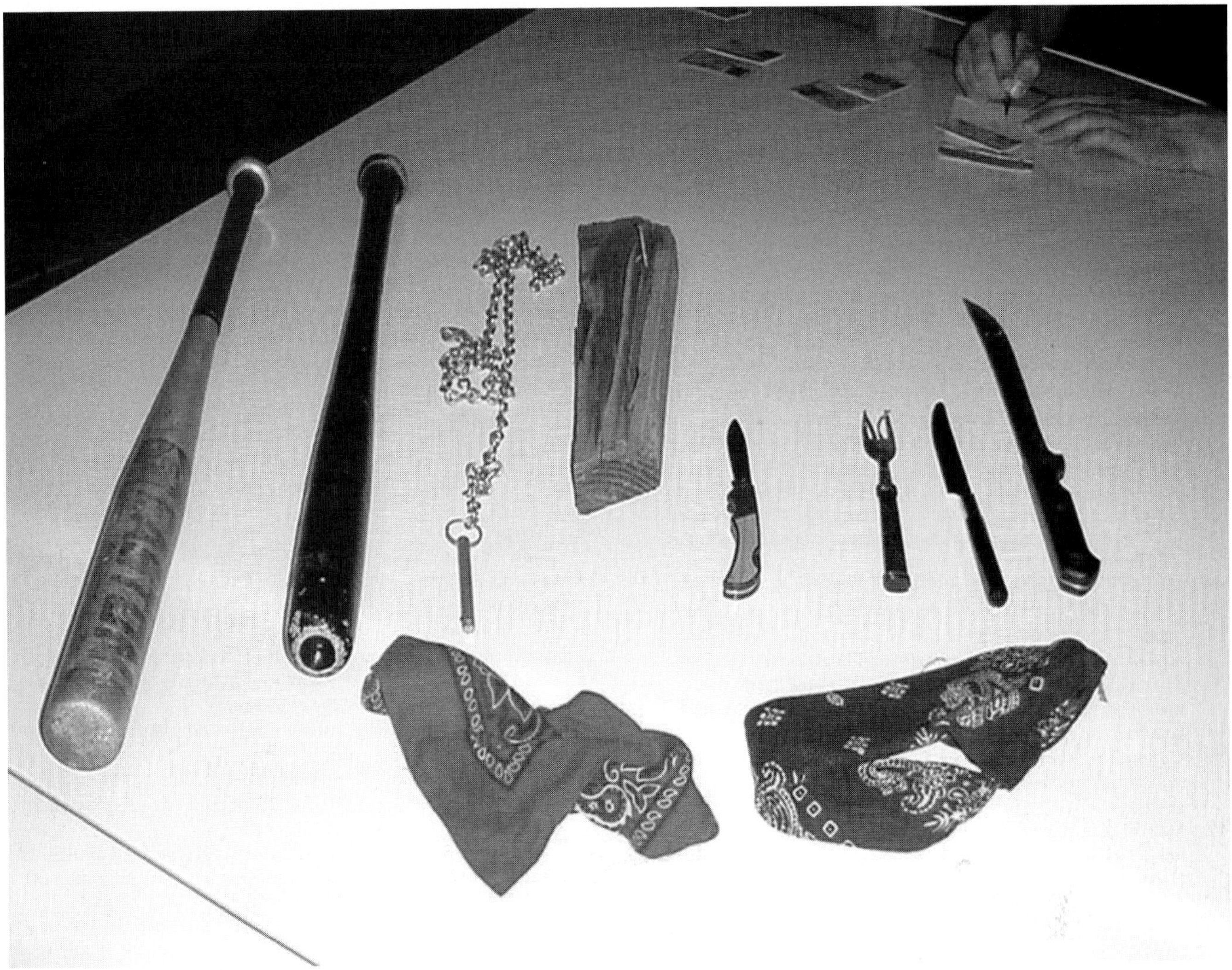

FIGURE 22-11 **Weapons confiscated by police during a feud between the rival Blood and Crip gangs.**

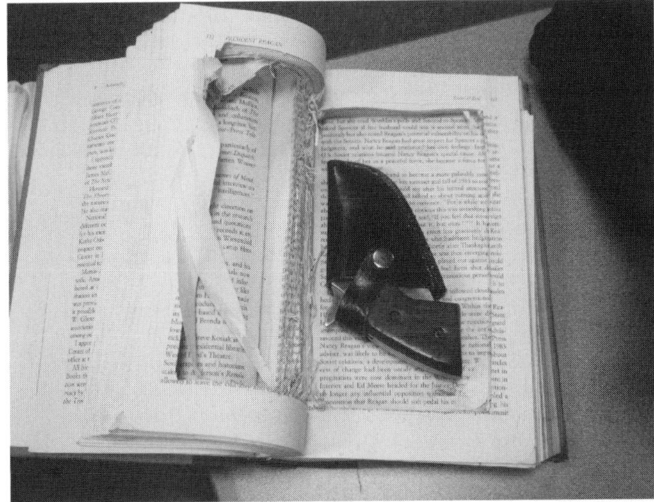

If a weapon is located, it should be placed in a clean storage vessel and given to the security staff for safe-keeping. This will prevent cross-contamination of the weapon and avoid possible injury to the staff. If violence erupts in the ED, there should be specific protocols in place to address it, including a procedure to lock down the ED, and if necessary, patients, visitors, and staff should be escorted to predetermined safe zones.

Psychosocial Support

Following any incident of gang-related violence, all hospital personnel involved should participate in a critical incidence stress debriefing. This allows the staff to discuss the event and their associated reactions in efforts to decrease the incidence of post-traumatic stress syndrome.

CONCLUSION

Gangs and gang violence are becoming increasing problems in the United States. Gang members are often victims of violence and seek care in the ED. Staff knowledge and recognition of gang violence and gang behaviors can help to protect the patient and staff from further injury and harm.

REFERENCES

1. Lyddane D. Understanding gangs and gang mentality: acquiring evidence of gang conspiracy. *United States Attorneys Bull.* 2006;54:1–14. Washington, DC: US Department of Justice Executive Office for United States Attorneys.
2. Egley A, Ritz CE. *Highlights of the 2004 National Youth Gang Survey.* Washington, DC: US Department of Justice, Office of Justice Programs, Office of Juvenile Justice and Delinquency Prevention; 2006.
3. Archer L, Grascia AM. Girls, gangs, and crime: profile of the young female offender. *J Gang Res.* 2006;13:37–48.
4. Chesney-Lind M, Sheldon, RG, Joe KA. Girls, delinquency, and gang membership. In: Huff CR, ed. *Gangs in America.* 2nd ed. Newbury Park, Calif: Sage; 1996:185–204.
5. Fight Crime: Invest in Kids. *Caught in the Crossfire: Arresting Gang Violence by Investing in Kids.* Washington, DC: Fight Crime: Invest in Kids; 2004.
6. Cohen M. The monetary value of saving a high-risk youth. *J Quant Criminol.* 1998;14:5–33.
7. Snyder HN, Sickmund M. 2006. *Juvenile Offenders and Victims: 2006 National Report.* Washington, DC: US Department of Justice, Office of Justice Programs, Office of Juvenile Justice and Delinquency Prevention.
8. Huston HR, Anglin D, Mallon W. Injuries and deaths from gang violence: they are preventable. *Ann Emerg Med.* 1992;21:1234–1236.
9. Song, DH, Naude GP, Gilmore KA, Mongard F. Gang warfare: the medical repercussions. *J Trauma.* 1996;40:(5);810–815.
10. Krug EG, Powell KE, Dahlberg LL. Firearm-related deaths in the United States and 35 other high- and upper-middle-income countries. *Int J Epidemiol.* 1998;27:214–221.
11. Centers for Disease Control and Prevention. Rates of homicide, suicide and firearm-related death among children—26 industrialized countries. *MMWR.* 1997;46:101–105.
12. Morales A. A clinical model for the prevention of gang violence and homicide. In: Cervantes RC, ed. *Substance Abuse and Gang Violence.* Newbury Park, Calif: Sage; 1992:105–118.
13. Egley A, Howell JC, Major AK. *Recent Patterns of Gang Problems in the United States: Results from the 1996–2002 National Youth Gang Survey.* Washington, DC: US Department of Justice, Office of Justice Programs, Office of Juvenile Justice and Delinquency Prevention; 2004.
14. Curry GD. *Youth Gang Homicide Trends in the National Youth Gang Survey.* Report to the National Youth Gang Center. Tallahassee, Fla: National Youth Gang Center; 2004.
15. Bing L. *Do or Die.* Los Angeles: Harper Perennial; 1991:115–127.
16. Los Angeles Police Department. Order no. 8, 1990.
17. Hutson HR, Anglin D, Pratts MJ. Adolescents and children injured or killed in drive-by shooting in Los Angeles. *New Engl J Med.* 1994;330:324–327.
18. Philips C. Who killed Tupac Shakur? *Los Angeles Times.* September 6, 2002.
19. Wikipedia. *Drive-by shooting.* 2007. Available at: http://en.wikipedia.org/wiki/Drive-by_shooting. Accessed September 5, 2008.
20. Vargas JA. Gamers' intersection: "Grand Theft Auto: San Andreas" plays to a generation from the streets to suburbia. *Washington Post.* September 27, 2005:C01.
21. Garrelts N. *The Meaning and Culture of Grand Theft Auto: Critical Essays.* Jefferson, NC: McFarland and Company, Inc; 2006.
22. Knox G. The promulgation of gang-banging through the mass media. *J Gang Res.* 1999;6:19–38.
23. Hawkins JD, Herrenkohl T, Farrington DP, Brewer D, Catalano RF, Harachi TW. A review of predictors of violence. In: R Loeber, DP Farrington, eds. *Serious and Violent Juvenile Offenders: Risk Factors and Successful Interventions.* Thousand Oaks, CA: Sage Publications; 1998.
24. Kosterman R, Hawkins JD, Hill KG, Abbott RD, Catalano RF, Guo J. The developmental dynamics of gang initiation: when and why young people join gangs. Paper presented at the annual meeting of the American Society of Criminology; November, 1996; Chicago, IL.
25. Hill KG, Howell JC, Hawkins JD, Battin SR. Childhood risk factors for adolescent gang membership: results from the Seattle Social Development Project. *J Res Crime Delinq.* 1999;36(3):300–322.
26. Spergel IA. *The Youth Gang Problem.* New York: Oxford University Press; 1995.
27. Curry GD, Spergel IA. Gang involvement and delinquency among Hispanic and African-American adolescent males. *J Res Crime Delinq.* 1992;29(3):273–291.
28. Moore JW. *Going Down to the Barrio: Homeboys and Homegirls in Change.* Philadelphia, PA: Temple University Press; 1991.
29. Sanchez-Jankowski MS. *Islands in the Street: Gangs and American Urban Society.* Berkeley, CA: University of California Press; 1991.
30. Acoca L, Austin J. *Investing in Girls: A 21st Century Strategy.* Washington, DC: US Department of Justice, Office of Justice Programs, Office of Juvenile Justice and Delinquency Prevention; 1999.
31. Acoca L, Dedel K. *No Place to Hide: Understanding and Meeting the Needs of Girls in the California Juvenile Justice System.* San Francisco, CA: National Council on Crime and Delinquency; 1998.
32. Harris MG. *Cholas: Latino Girls and Gangs.* New York: AMS Press; 1988.
33. Hawkins JD, Herrenkohl TI, Farrington DP, et al. *Predictors of Youth Violence.* Washington, DC: US Department of Justice, Office of Justice Programs, Office of Juvenile Justice and Delinquency Prevention; 2000.
34. Hill KG, Howell JC, Hawkins JD, Battin-Pearson SR. Childhood risk factors for adolescent gang membership: results from the Seattle social development project. *J Res Crime Delinquency.* 1999;36:300–302. Newbury Park, Calif: Sage Publications.
35. Nawojczyk S. *Street Gang Dynamics.* North Little Rock, Ark: Nawojczyk Group; 1997.
36. Walker R. *Initiations.* Robert Walker's Gangs OR Us. 2007. Available at: http://www.gangsorus.com/initiations.html. Accessed September 5, 2008.
37. Youth Crime Service Unit. *Gang Awareness: A Handbook for Parents, Teachers, and Concerned Citizens.* San Antonio, Tex: San Antonio Police Department; 2007.
38. Carlie M. 2002. *Into the Abyss: A Personal Journey into the World of Street Gangs.* Available at http://www.faculty.missouristate.edu/m/MichaelCarlie/what_I_learned_about/GANGS/gangs.htm. Accessed March 8, 2009.
39. Wiener V. *Winning the War Against Youth Gangs: A Guide for Teens, Families, and Communities.* Westport, CT: Greenwood Publishing Group; 1991.
40. Chang J. A comparative study of female gang and non-gang members in Chicago. *J Gang Res.* 1996;4:14.
41. Vigil JD. *Barrio Gangs: Street Life and Identity in Southern California.* Austin: University of Texas Press; 1988.
42. Kontos L, Brotherton D. *Encyclopedia of Gangs.* Westport, CT: Greenwood Publishing Group; 2008.
43. Phillips SA. *Wallbangin: Graffiti and Gangs in LA.* Chicago: University of Chicago Press; 1999.
44. *The Rap Dictionary.* Gangs. 2005. Available at: http://www.rapdict.org/Category:Gangs. Accessed March 8, 2009.
45. Walker R. Street Gang Pages. *Gangs or Us.* 2007. Available at http://www.gangsorus.com/crips.htm. Accessed March 8, 2009.
46. Hagedorn JM, Macon P. *People and Folks: Gangs, Crime and the Underclass in Rustbelt City.* Chicago: Lake View Press; 1998.
47. Garvey M, McGeevy P. Racial attacks by gangs rising, L.A. officials fear. *LA Times.* January 14, 2007.
48. *Bloods.* Gangsta411.com. 2003. Available at: http://gangsta411.com/Bloods.htm. Accessed September 5, 2008.
49. Dunston MS. *Street Signs: An Identification Guide of Symbols of Crime and Violence.* New York: Performance Dimensions; 1992.
50. Security Threat Intelligence Unit. *Street Gangs—Chicago Based or Influenced.* Gang and Security Threat Group Awareness. Tallahassee: Florida Department of Corrections; 1998. Available at: http://www.dc.state.fl.us/pub/gangs/chicago2.html. Accessed September 5, 2008.

51. Dart RW. The future is here today: street gang trends. *J Gang Res.* 1992;1:87–88.
52. Sadovi C. El Rukns had early terror ties. *Chicago Sun Times.* June 11, 2002.
53. Savelli L. *East Coast Gangs.* National Alliance of Gang Investigators' Association. 2000. Available at: http://www.nagia.org/Gang%20Articles/East%20Coast%20Gangs.htm. Accessed September 5, 2008.
54. Buchanan PJ. *State of Emergency: The Third World Invasion and Conquest of America.* New York: Macmillan; 2006.
55. Domash SF. America's most dangerous gang. *Police: Law Enforcement Magazine.* 2005;29:2.
56. Daily W. *Almighty Latin King Nation.* National Alliance of Gang Investigators' Association. 2000. Available at: http://www.nagia.org/Gang%20Articles/Almighty%20Latin%20Kings.htm. Accessed September 5, 2008.
57. Knox GW. *Gang Profile: The Latin Kings.* National Gang Crime Research Center. 2000. Available at: http://www.ngcrc.com/ngcrc/page15.htm. Accessed September 5, 2008.
58. National Alliance of Gang Investigators' Associations. *2005 National Gang Threat Assessment.* Washington, DC: Bureau of Justice Assistance, US Department of Justice; 2005. Available at: http://www.ojp.usdoj.gov/BJA/what/2005_threat_assesment.pdf. Accessed September 5, 2008.
59. Holthouse D. Smashing the shamrock. *SPLC Intelligence Report.* Fall 2005. Available at: http://www.splcenter.org/intel/intelreport/article.jsp?aid=569
60. Smith RC. Dangerous motorcycle gangs: a facet of organized crime in the mid Atlantic region. *J Gang Res.* 2002;9:33–44.
61. Washington Crime News Service. Hate groups recruit in wake of terrorism. *Organized Crime Digest.* 2001;22:2–4.
62. Herek GM, Berrill KT. *Hate Crimes: Confronting Violence Against Lesbians and Gay Men.* Newbury Park, CA: Sage Publications; 1992.
63. Synder HN. Juvenile arrests 2001. *Juvenile Justice Bulletin.* Washington, DC: US Department of Justice, Office of Justice Programs, Office of Juvenile Justice and Delinquency Prevention; 2001:1–11.
64. Moore J, Hagedorn J. Female gangs: a focus on research. *Juvenile Justice Bulletin.* Washington, DC: US Department of Justice, Office of Justice Programs, Office of Juvenile Justice and Delinquency Prevention; 2001:1–11.
65. Knox GW. *Female Gang Members and the Rights of Children.* National Gang Crime Research Center. 2008. Available at: http://www.ngcrc.com/ngcrc/page16.htm. Accessed September 5, 2008.
66. Starbuck D. 2000. *Breaking all the Rules: Hybrid Gangs.* National Alliance of Gang Investigators' Association. 2000. Available at: http://www.nagia.org/Gang%20Articles/Hybrid%20Gangs.htm. Accessed September 5, 2008.
67. Gutierrez R. *Gangs!* Parents in Crisis home page. 1998. Available at: http://www.geocities.com/Athens/4111/nogangs.html. Accessed September 5, 2008.
68. Walker R. *Clothing.* Robert Walker's Gangs OR Us. 2007. Available at: http://www.gangsorus.com/clothing.html. Accessed September 5, 2008.
69. Watkins D, Ashby R. *Gang Investigations: A Street Cop's Guide.* Sudbury, MA: Jones and Bartlett Publishers; 2006.
70. Sullivan J. Pierce County park visitors assaulted by gang of thugs. *Seattle Times.* July 12, 2006.
71. Orlando-Morningstar D. Prison gangs. *Special Needs Offenders BULL.* 1997;2:1–13.
72. *Area Codes.* Know Gangs. 2006. Available at: http://www.knowgangs.com/gang_resources/411/area_codes/area_codes.php. Accessed September 5, 2008
73. Niemann L, Heyer C. *Community Partners Crime Awareness Guide.* Austin: Texas Apartment Association Education Foundation; 2002.
74. Libaw O. *The New Forbidden Dance: Schools Ban Popular "Crip Walk" Because of Gang Ties.* ABC News. June 2002. Available at: http://www.streetgangs.com/topics/2002/061402dance.html. Accessed September 5, 2008.
75. Urban Dictionary. *B-walk.* 2003. Available at: http://www.urbandictionary.com/define.php?term=b+walk. Accessed September 5, 2008.
76. Valentine B. *Gangs and Their Tattoos: Identifying Gangbangers on the Street and in Prison.* Boulder, CO: Paladin Press; 2001.
77. Grant C. *Native Gangs.* Know Gangs. 2004. Available at: http://www.knowgangs.com/gang_resources/native/native_001.htm. Accessed September 5, 2008.
78. Walker R. Asian gang members: marks, scars, and tattoos. Robert Walker's Gangs OR Us. 2006. Available at: http://www.gangsorus.com/asianmrks.htm. Accessed September 5, 2008.
79. Robinson KS. Nurses caught in the crossfire: assisting patients outside. *J Emerg Nurs.* 1998;24:380–381.
80. Kowalendo T, Walters B, Khare R, Compton S, et al. Workplace violence: a survey of emergency physicians in the state of Michigan. *Ann Emerg Med.* 2005;46:142–147.
81. Mattox EA, Wright SW, Bracikowski AC. Metal detectors in the pediatric emergency department: patron attitudes and national prevalence. *Pediat Emerg Care.* 2000;16:163–165.
82. Decker SH, Pennel S, Caldwell A. *Illegal Firearms: Access and Use by Arrestees.* Washington, DC: US Department of Justice, Office of Justice Programs, National Institute of Justice; 1997.

23 | Suspect Evaluation and Evidence Collection

Bohdan (Dan) M. Minczak, MS, MD, PhD, FACEP, FAAEM

INTRODUCTION

Every patient presenting to a healthcare facility for a medical evaluation of a potential illness, physical or mental, has certain expectations and inalienable rights. The healthcare provider (physician, nurse, technician, etc.) who is involved in evaluating this patient has certain duties and responsibilities with respect to the patient and society. When a doctor–patient relationship is initiated between the physician and the patient, a specific set of parameters must be adhered to so that an appropriate patient encounter is executed. During this encounter, the patient often may provide the physician with personal, private information that must be protected and/or kept confidential; that is, the information exchanged is privileged.

Data gathered during the subsequent history and physical examination are also sensitive and must be kept confidential. There are certain circumstances when the data obtained during this medical evaluation can be released to other parties involved in the care of the patient, such as other physicians, nurses, technicians. Under these circumstances sharing of data does not violate any regulations or laws, either local, federal, or social (i.e., the Health Insurance Portability and Accountability Act, or HIPAA). If the data must be released for billing, insurance reasons, or medical consultation, then an appropriate release must be prepared in writing. However, when the patient in this encounter is either a victim of a crime or a known/alleged perpetrator of a crime, then a new set of responsibilities and obligations are superimposed onto this physician–patient encounter. Any data gathered may be used as evidence relevant to a crime. This data must be *appropriately collected* and *appropriately protected*, without biasing or altering the data. Failure to execute caution in this phase of evidence collection and transfer may introduce *confounders,* which may contaminate the data and compromise the chain of custody/evidence, rendering the evidence misleading, useless, and/or potentially inadmissible in court. This chapter addresses data and evidence collection from the patient.

EVIDENCE

Before proceeding any further, it is important to define the term *evidence.* Evidence is something submitted via the appropriate legal process to a qualified panel of judges for the purpose of ascertaining the truth regarding an alleged matter of fact presented for investigation. Evidence can be in the form of testimonial evidence, or statements made under oath from a witness or expert. This evidence is usually obtained when a witness undergoes questioning about an alleged crime. There is a deposition of an expert witness or cross-examination of an individual with potentially relevant information regarding the event in question. Evidence can also be physical evidence, that is, something that has an obvious physical existence; matter with shape, size, and dimension. Pieces or particles of evidence can be macroscopic such as a car or microscopic such as a spore or fiber removed from a specimen, victim, or suspect. Odors that are detected or stains that are present on clothing, shoes, and so forth may become evidence, depending on the context of the situation. This type of evidence is collected either at a crime scene or from a suspect and/or victim of a crime while in the emergency department (ED).

Recognizing, gathering, or procuring the evidence, preserving it, and presenting it appropriately for evaluation require training and knowledge. ("The eyes cannot see what the mind does not know.") Therefore, the individual charged with the duty of collecting evidence must be thoroughly familiar with the evidence collection process. In addition, the individual who will be evaluating a potential suspect or victim of a crime should be informed regarding the context of the given examination because this may facilitate and enhance the efficiency of the evaluation. This will further ensure that the data and information collected are appropriately gathered. Evidence collection with a focus will ensure that the information is valid and useful and that the evidence has relevance to a given case.[1]

In addition to being prepared to conduct an evaluation within the context of a forensic investigation, it is advisable that the healthcare provider be aware of the circumstances regarding the patient; that is, is this a suspect in a crime or a victim of an alleged crime? Also, the evidence collector should be familiar with the laws within a given region, county, state, and/or federal jurisdiction to ensure that proper protocol is followed in the legal sequestration of information/materials potentially destined to be used as evidence in a litigious process. An attempt to ascertain this information prior to initiating the evaluation and potential evidence collection process is advised to prevent loss of or inadvertent destruction of potential evidence (e.g., is this an alleged perpetrator of a violent crime who may have used a handgun and may have gunpowder residue on his hands? or is this the victim of an alleged rape where evidence of penetration, blood, or bodily fluids may be needed to establish the identity of the perpetrator?).

VALUE OF EVIDENCE

Usefulness of appropriately collected evidence is multifold.[2] Evidence can be used to prove that a crime has been committed (that there was forcible action taken with a victim, such as bruising, lacerations, defensive wounds). Furthermore, the information gathered can also help identify key elements of a crime (an accelerant detected at the scene of a suspicious fire may imply arson, or cut brake cables discovered in a car at a fatal accident scene may indicate that a potential homicide has occurred). Evidence can help establish that a suspect was indeed at the crime scene or that the suspect had contact with the victim. In addition, some evidence can even establish the identity of the person(s) associated with the crime (hair sample, blood, bodily fluids containing DNA, fingerprints, footprints, and palm prints).

On the other hand, physical evidence can be used to exonerate the innocent suspect, sometimes by the presence of a negative result; for example, a negative blood alcohol level in a driving while intoxicated case. Evidence can strengthen the case for the victim (the victim's blood stains are found on the perpetrator's clothing).

After the evidence is collected and appropriately processed, the presentation of evidence to a suspect can sometimes bring about an admission or confession of the circumstances and the crime. When evidence is presented to a jury, evidence often bears more weight than eyewitness testimony.[3]

Therefore, evidence must be recognized, gathered, and processed appropriately, and a complete, accurately documented chain of custody must be maintained.

PATIENT'S BILL OF RIGHTS

As mentioned earlier, every patient presenting for a medical evaluation, regardless of mitigating circumstances, is entitled to an unbiased, appropriately complete, and directed medical evaluation. Attention must also be given to privacy of the patient encounter, regardless of mitigating circumstances. Following is a summary of some key elements regarding the rights of a patient as presented in the "Patient's Bill of Rights" adopted by the US Advisory Commission on Consumer Protection and Quality in the Healthcare Industry in 1988.[4,5]

Each and every patient is entitled to appropriate, considerate, respectful, professional care. This evaluation and care should be provided in a timely fashion, appropriate for the nature of the chief complaint or illness that the patient proclaims or declares on presentation for a medical evaluation. If the patient's situation is deemed sufficiently emergent, then appropriate action should be taken, if applicable, to transfer the patient to the appropriate level of care (i.e., transfer by emergency medical services [EMS] to an ED, trauma center, obstetrical/gynecologic care in the case of a pregnant female or female of child-bearing age, psychiatric facility, etc.). If the services or anticipated diagnostics and interventions are available at the presenting facility, then the usual procedures for evaluation and indicated treatment should be followed.

If the presenting patient has difficulty communicating with the healthcare staff subsequent to a language barrier, then every attempt to facilitate communication with the patient should be made through a qualified, neutral interpreter.

The patient should be made aware of his or her rights as a patient. If the patient is an incarcerated or detained individual and/or a suspect in an alleged crime, these patients also have rights.[6,7] Patients should be informed of their right to appropriate access for medical evaluation and care, regardless of their circumstances as a detainee, suspect, prisoner, and so forth. At no time should there be any disrespect or discrimination introduced into the medical encounter with the patient.[8]

The patient has the right to know the identity and qualifications of the healthcare provider(s). The patient should be advised of the assessment made by the medical evaluator and the proposed diagnostics and therapeutics. Patients also have the right to question the provider regarding matters of their care that they may not fully understand. Every attempt should be made to explain the procedures and tests and so forth to the patient. This is especially important if informed consent will be needed for a given test or intervention. The patient also reserves the right to participate in the decision process regarding his or her care. If the patient chooses not to proceed for a further diagnostic test, treatment, or medication, the patient is entitled to refuse and an informed refusal or suspension of care under the conditions of "against medical advice/AMA" must be appropriately documented if applicable. This must be done with the patient's full understanding of the consequences of refusing care such as bad outcome, mortality/morbidity, and so forth.

The patient may also request transfer to a different facility if applicable. However, if there is a court order or other legal circumstances that necessitate the evaluation of a patient for legal purposes and with the intent of collecting evidence (e.g., DUI alcohol level determination), then the healthcare provider must proceed accordingly, in compliance with local legal directives.

Subsequent to the evaluation and/or treatment, the patient is entitled to appropriate continuity of care and follow-up as needed. Arrangements should be made for the appropriate follow-up, including appointment or provision of contact information and telephone numbers so that the patient can obtain the needed subsequent care. The patient should also have instructions for what to do if an emergency occurs. If any medication or prescriptions are indicated, these should be provided for the patient at the time of treatment. If the suspect is a detainee going to a facility such as a prison or jail, then arrangements and communication must be made with the facility and the local authorities to ensure compliance with aftercare and medications. The patient also has the right to review his or her medical record and question or appeal findings if appropriate. Also, these patients have the right to file a grievance if applicable.

INCARCERATED PATIENTS AND SUSPECT NEEDS

The emergency physician (EP) and healthcare providers rendering care to patients have many challenges and difficult circumstances to deal with. When dealing with a patient presenting to their facility while incarcerated or detained as a suspect in an alleged crime, the situation can become even more complex and convoluted.

Emergency department (ED) visits are increasing at alarming levels. The characteristic patient mix presenting is also increasing[9] in prisoners and detainees presenting to the ED.[10,11] Many of these patients have barriers to health care as a result of changing prison regulations and procedures. Oftentimes, these patients may experience a delay in receiving an evaluation and care. Sometimes, because of the lack of privacy in prisons, patients may not want to divulge information relevant to their health because they fear retaliation or ridicule for diseases such as HIV/AIDS, tuberculosis, and so forth. Some detainees may fear potential self-incrimination. These circumstances can lead the detainee to delay seeking care. Therefore, the healthcare provider must be sensitive to these issues when evaluating these patients. Hopefully, a comfortable atmosphere can be created to facilitate this encounter.

When these patients arrive at the healthcare facility, there may be a bias introduced into the evaluation and care of these individuals because they may arrive in handcuffs and shackles and be thought of as "undesirable criminals" or "social outcasts." In addition, they are usually brought directly back to the ED and not kept in the waiting area. This may cause disruption of the usual order of triage and compromise the evaluation of the patient because of time constraints, such as rushing through the evaluation and examination or compromising potential attention to detail. However, these patients do have rights. These rights must be respected, and an appropriate detailed evaluation must be performed. This standard must be adhered to so that if there is any need for evidence collection, the circumstances do not void the admissibility of the evidence.

THE EXAMINATION OF THE PATIENT: SUSPECT EVALUATION AND COLLECTION OF EVIDENCE

When a patient who is a potential suspect or victim of a crime, or who is incarcerated or a detainee, presents, the following approach should be utilized:

1. Record the mode of arrival: police department vehicle, or fire department/EMS vehicle.
2. Have the patient appropriately escorted to an available, cleaned, and, if possible, dedicated area for further evaluation.
3. Have the law enforcement officers and/or security personnel from your facility present and readily available during the examination, if warranted. Rely on your personal level of comfort and security when seeking assistance. Do not let bias or input from the accompanying police/sheriff/prison officials affect the nature, climate, and mood of the examination, and certainly do not let it affect the type or quality of care provided.
4. Have an egress route available for yourself at all times: Position yourself so that you can quickly leave the area if needed. Remember, *do not place the patient between you and the door.*
5. If both an alleged suspect and alleged victim are brought to the same facility for evaluation, make

every effort to ensure that the respective evaluations are conducted in distinctly separate areas to avoid the potential transfer or exchange of evidence between the two individuals. Failure to do so may cause contamination or compromise of the evidence and may lead to erroneous, inaccurate conclusions when the evidence is examined and scrutinized; that is, the evidence ultimately becomes useless or equivocal to the case at hand.

6. Attempt to verify whether this is a victim or suspect of a crime.
7. Initiate prompt documentation of the encounter from the moment of initial patient contact. Proper documentation should include date and time of each entry, and all paperwork should be sequentially numbered and labeled with at least two appropriate identifiers, such as date of birth (DOB) and name. Also a medical record number and or case number may be used if applicable. Do *not* use words such as *alleged* or *implied* when documenting the chief complaint or patient history. Just document the information in quotation marks as stated by the patient.
8. Obtain pertinent information regarding the nature of the chief complaint, presenting symptoms, and reason for the evaluation.
9. Record the vital signs. Record any abnormalities in gait, posture, or mental affect.
10. Document the patient's appearance in appropriate detail: type of clothing, missing buttons, stains, tears, type of shoes, and so forth.
11. Have the patient disrobe appropriately while positioned or standing over a paper drape on the floor. (This will help capture possible fibers, soil, hair, blood, bodily fluids, etc.)
12. *Be careful when handling the patient's personal effects.* Be aware of the possibility of sharp objects or needles even though the patient may have already been screened and cleared of potential weapons and contraband by police and security personnel. Exercise caution when handling clothing, and use universal precautions when dealing with bodily fluids. Use gloves when handling the patient's personal belongings to avoid contamination of the evidence or transfer of materials between the healthcare provider and the patient.
13. Place the suspect's shoes and each item of clothing into *separate* paper bags, *not* plastic, and appropriately label and seal them with the appropriate identifiers, such as name, date of birth, and time, and document who will be receiving and holding these materials, for example, a police officer or a security guard, so that an appropriate chain of custody of the evidence is documented. Note unusual clothing, buckles, and accessories, remove belts and objects that may cause possible injury, and appropriately secure them in the evidence bags.
14. Any stains present should be sampled and placed in the appropriate kit that is often provided by the investigating law enforcement team. Consider using a UV light source to identify unusual stains or bodily fluids if applicable.
15. If there is a question of gun powder or other chemical residue on the hands or other body parts of the suspect, protect these areas with a brown paper bag or use the materials that may be provided by the law enforcement personnel that will be taking custody of the evidence once it has been collected (for example, a paper bag wrapped around the limb may be useful to prevent loss of evidence). Usually the investigative team will have the appropriate kit for evidence collection.
16. Conduct a thorough directed history and physical (H&P) examination, which consists of the following:
    - Chief complaint
    - Vital signs: temperature, pulse, respirations, blood pressure, pulse oximetry
    - Review of systems (ROS)
    - Social history/family history
    - History of present illness (HPI)
    - Skin:
        - Document any lesions or wounds, and so forth.
        - *Do not make conclusions or speculate* on what caused a wound or whether it is an entrance or exit wound. Just note where wounds are, their size and length, characteristic shape, and any unique features.
        - Record the presence of any rash, tattoos, body art, body piercing, or jewelry.
        - Make notations of any obvious abnormalities, such as missing digits or limbs, or the presence of a prosthesis.
        - If applicable, describe the visual appearance of external genitalia, whether or not the person is circumcised, presence or absence of pubic hair, its distribution, and any other unique characteristics.
        - When appropriate, document any lesions, moles, birthmarks, and bite marks on the skin, noting the location, color, length, and any unique identifying features.
        - Look for and record any identifying impressions that may have been left on the skin or body from solid objects.
        - Take color photographs if possible and document the existence of this evidence appropriately.
        - Draw or use a body diagram, such as a scaled-down human silhouette, to indicate and further describe the location of any unique characteristics or injuries. As mentioned earlier, if possible take photos of injuries, scars, discolorations, birthmarks, and so forth because these may be of value in identifying and/or vindicating an individual if the need arises.

- Head, eyes, ears, nose, throat: Note lesions, hair color and type: curly, straight, and so forth. If applicable, note hair line pattern and/or any baldness. If requested to do so, collect several hair samples. This is usually done by pulling hair from the scalp to ensure that DNA is obtained. Place the hair in an evidence envelope and label it appropriately. Note the condition of the scalp, recording any unusual dermatologic conditions. Samples of cornified skin cells can be removed or scraped from the scalp and placed in a paper envelope for subsequent chemical or DNA processing if needed. There may be trace elements, pollen, insects, plant material, or dust from a crime scene present in this sample. Store accordingly as per kit instructions if applicable.
- Eyes: Note any abnormalities in extraocular muscle movement because this may be a factor in the visual acuity/depth perception of the individual.
    - » Note the color of iris, and document any abnormalities of the pupils (anisocoria, coloboma, prior eye surgery).
    - » Some cases may warrant the photographing of the retina and/or doing a retinogram via fluorescence. A retinal print can be used to identify a suspect or victim. Also, retinal examination can provide clues regarding other disease processes that may be important or relevant in an investigation.
    - » Perform a visual acuity examination and document accordingly. This may be important when describing the visual capabilities of either a suspect or a victim.
    - » If the patient wears corrective lenses or contacts, document this as well.
- Oral exam: Examine the oral cavity, noting the dentition and any surgical alteration of the posterior pharynx.
    - » An impression of the dentition can be extremely useful in suspect identification and linkage to a victim via a discovered bite mark. Dental impressions can be deferred to a forensic odontologist.
    - » A buccal swab for DNA analysis can be obtained.
    - » Patients/suspects can often hide evidence or contraband in their mouth; therefore, do an oral cavity search, especially under the tongue and in the cheek "pouch" areas.
- Neck:
    - » Look for any evidence of bruising, scarring, and discoloration.
    - » Look for a potentially recognizable pattern or impression from jewelry or from a possible struggle or choking.
    - » Look for and document old tracheostomy sites or surgical scars.
- Chest: Perform a cardiovascular and pulmonary exam. Note any abnormalities such as murmur and abnormal breath sounds. These may be useful in describing or determining the physical capabilities of an individual.
- Abdomen: Note the appearance, presence, and location of any scars. Consider radiographic imaging of the abdomen and pelvis if there is a suspicion of ingested contraband, such as drug packets or jewelry. Cathartics may be administered to recover items. This may require collection and examination of excrement and fecal material for evidence of these items.
- Rectal examination: A rectal examination should be performed to ensure that no contraband such as medications, drugs, or weapons are being hidden in this cavity. If there is a concern of a possible weapon or object that may injure the examiner, then radiographs can be obtained to confirm such an object's presence.
- Pelvis: Document the appearance of the genitalia.
    - » If there is concern or need to collect evidence from an alleged rape, collection should proceed following usual protocols.
    - » Use a UV light source to identify the presence of seminal fluid.
    - » Samples of pubic hair should be obtained via combing to detect the transfer of victim or perpetrator hair and serve for identification and/or implication of contact with a given individual. If required by protocol, pubic hair sampling may also include pulled samples.
    - » Evaluate the vagina for contraband.
- Extremities: Examine the extremities for abnormalities, prior trauma, current injuries, prior surgery, and so forth.
    - » Collect footprints, hand prints, palm prints, and fingerprints.
    - » Scrape any debris from underneath fingernails and toenails and package them in separate envelopes, labeled appropriately.
    - » Document any abrasions, lacerations, and bruises because these may indicate defensive posture.

17. Inform the patient regarding the findings of the H&P. Discuss the diagnostic and treatment plan with the patient and answer all pertinent questions so that the patient has a full understanding of the process involved. If informed consent is needed for diagnostic procedures or therapy, obtain it now.
18. Perform radiographs as needed and draw appropriate labs:
    - CBC
    - Serum chemistries and liver enzymes
    - PT/PTT/INR
    - Urine drug screen, alcohol level
    - Pregnancy test in females

19. All specimens collected for evidence should be inventoried and labeled. Any forms should be completed, and remember to document what was done with the evidence and to whom it was turned over.
20. Once the diagnostics and treatment have been completed and a disposition is made on the patient, communicate and establish the appropriate follow-up care and prescriptions, and inform the patient of what he or she must do to complete the care and follow-up. If the patient is to be incarcerated and will need medication or additional care, communicate this to the destination correctional facility and the officers who will be transporting the patient to or back to the prison/jail.

CONCLUSION

Emergency department personnel are often called upon to perform suspect evaluations on patients by law enforcement. A systematic head to toe approach with attention to details like physical characteristics, injury, and body art/modifications will greatly assist in this process. Standard forensic evidence collection policies and procedures should be followed.

REFERENCES

1. Nordby J. *Dead Reckoning: The Art of Forensic Detection*. Boca Raton, Fla: CRC Press; 2000.
2. Bergman RA. The impact of technological advancement on forensic science practice. *J Can Soc Forensic Sci*. 1988;21:169.
3. Fisher BAJ. *Techniques of Crime Scene Investigation: Introduction*. 7th ed. Boca Raton, Fla: CRC Press; 2004.
4. President's Advisory Commission on Consumer Protection and Quality in the Health Care Industry. *Patient's Rights and Responsibilities*. Available at: http://www.hcqualitycommission.gov/final/append_a.html. Accessed September 8, 2008.
5. US Office of Personnel Management. *Patients' Bill of Rights and the Federal Employees Health Benefits Program*. Available at: http://www.opm.gov/insure/health/billrights.asp#what. Accessed September 8, 2008.
6. National Commission on Correctional Health Care (NCCHC). Legal considerations in the delivery of healthcare services in prisons and jails. *Correctional Healthcare: Guidelines Management Adequate Delivery System*. 2001:43–65.
7. Sloan CDRM. Legal origins and issues behind correctional nursing. *Nurs Spectrum*. 2003;16 (71L).
8. American College of Emergency Physicians (ACEP). *Practice Resources: Recognizing the Needs of Incarcerated Patients in the Emergency Department*. Available at: http://www.acep.org/practres.aspx?id=30164. Accessed September 8, 2008.
9. Butterfield F. US "correctional population" hits record 6.9 million. *Chicago Tribune*. July 25, 2004.
10. Too many convicts. *Economist*. August 10, 2002.
11. Prison and beyond: a stigma that never fades. *Economist*. August 10, 2002:25–27.

24 | Forensics for EMS

James P. McCans, MS, NREMT-P

INTRODUCTION

A crime scene can be defined as "anyplace that a crime has occurred, a place where a perpetrator has been while preparing for a crime, anyplace where the perpetrator has been after the crime, and anyplace where a victim has been after the crime."

Emergency medical services (EMS) has its greatest impact in the third part of this definition, where the victim is located. Obviously, a victim's treatment takes priority over the preservation of evidence. This chapter explores methods, ideas, and suggestions that will provide the EMS provider with the tools to reduce the loss of evidence and possibly enhance the collection of some evidence.

Nothing in this chapter is to be construed as a suggestion that patient care should be altered, interrupted, or delayed to preserve evidence. We must, however, take into consideration that the recovery of evidence may lead to the conviction of those responsible and may prevent others from becoming victims. The recovery may also lead toward exonerating those who are innocent.

EMS is unique in that, by its nature, it creates a larger crime scene. Merely by transporting the victim of a crime, the ambulance becomes a crime scene, as does the receiving hospital. This chapter explores how EMS personnel can identify, secure, and report potential evidence that they may inadvertently spread to the ambulance and the receiving facility.

ON ARRIVAL

EMS personnel are taught very early in their training to assess the scene from a safe distance before taking any action. Whether the dispatch is for an overturned tanker truck, a structure fire, or a violent crime situation, as EMS we are taught to use our skills to evaluate the safety of the situation. It is during this phase that we start to form a working hypothesis as to what sort of incident we are dealing with on arrival. It is in this phase that we are, perhaps unknowingly, collecting evidence.

Consider a structure fire dispatch as an example. Upon arrival, we invariably look at the structure that is involved and immediately size it up for EMS potential; that is, a working elementary school fire during the school day will have an EMS potential different from a fire in the middle of the night.

During this initial sizing-up phase, we can make note of several important pieces of evidence. At the threshold, ask: *Where is the fire most intense?* The answer may give a clue as to where the fire started. Also ask: *What is the color of the fire and smoke?* A deep red fire and very black smoke can suggest the presence of a petroleum product; perhaps an accelerant of some sort was utilized. *Does there appear to be evidence of an explosion?* Perhaps there is debris in the form of windows, shingles, or doors displaced around the structure. *Is there a readily noticeable odor in the area?* Besides the smoke, is there a smell of natural gas? Is there a gunpowder-like odor? Is there a gasoline/flammable liquid-like odor?

Finally, ask: *Are there any obvious points of entry that are open and should not be?* An open window on a structure may be out of place certain times of the year and perfectly natural during other seasons; make note of this. An open door may have been the route of egress for an occupant or the perpetrator, so this is a noteworthy observation.

All of these points are potential evidence and will frequently change or be eliminated if the fire continues. The EMS provider may be on the scene early enough to take notice, not to collect or investigate, but to observe, make notes, and report to the investigating authority such as the fire marshal or police.

HAZ-MAT

Perhaps nowhere in EMS is the identification of evidence more important and relevant than during a Hazardous Materials ("Haz-Mat") incident.

I recall several occasions over my career where EMS personnel have died as a result of not properly assessing a Haz-Mat incident. Understanding and reading placards is only a portion of the proper response to a Haz-Mat incident. Proper protective equipment, available resources for containment, vehicle placement, public health/environmental threats, decontamination, and specific medical treatments are all concerns for EMS responders. Moreover, the responder must be proficient at identifying the product in question, have current resources to reference the material, and have knowledge of the geography and demographics of the threatened area.

The EMS responder must also evaluate the capabilities of the local medical facilities. Can the facility decontaminate? Can it handle caustic burns? Does it have enough personnel? How do they enact a disaster plan? Is the facility affected by the incident itself and therefore unable to accept patients?

The answers to these questions are readily available if you have preplanned how to handle the situation. I recommend proper Haz-Mat training for all EMS personnel.

THE CRIME SCENE

All scenes should be treated as a crime scene until shown to be otherwise. If the responding EMS crew assumes otherwise, they may destroy valuable evidence and their actions may disrupt or confuse the crime scene.

As many in the pre-hospital field have been taught in Pre-Hospital Trauma Life Suport (PHTLS) or Basic Trauma Life Suport (BTLS) or other classes, EMS should always be vigilant upon arrival at a scene for personal safety's sake. When responding to a known violent crime, the proper protocol for EMS is to have the scene controlled by law enforcement prior to EMS inclusion. If EMS arrives first, EMS should stage at a safe distance, in the vehicle, with several avenues of egress, to allow for rapid escape if the threat engages EMS and to permit the unit to move quickly to the area that has been secured. It is essential that EMS have direct communication with the responding police units so that care is not further delayed.

Once the scene is deemed safe and EMS has been requested into the scene, providers should take care to touch or move only that which must be touched. If an item is inadvertently moved, a mental note should be made but no effort should be made to return the item to the original state. Where the patient was located and a general impression of the scene are excellent points to be documented. While treating the patient, if it is necessary to remove clothing via cutting, the rescuer should not use the damaged areas of the material as a starting point. Bullet holes and knife holes should be bypassed by shears and left intact. No appreciable time will be saved by cutting through these zones, but crucial evidence will be destroyed.

The rescuer should note any dying declarations or statements by the injured. These words should be documented verbatim and be put in written form as soon as possible. Any removed clothing and medical waste (excluding sharps) should be left as is at the scene. Although EMS personnel are trained to be professional and not leave their trash behind, this is the exception. Cleaning up may remove evidence from the scene and further displace items that may be of evidentiary value. Let the investigating officers decide what is to stay and what is to be discarded. The presence of medical trash can note the general orientation of the body (airway equipment by the head, dressing wrappers near the wounds) and give an idea as to the position of the rescuers during the resuscitation. These points may seem trivial, but they may assist the investigators in putting together the entire story.

FORCIBLE ENTRY

Occasionally, EMS personnel are tasked with forcing entry into a dwelling to assist someone who is sick or injured inside the facility. A neighbor or concerned friend who is not able to reach someone at an assigned time may call for EMS, or perhaps the subject can be seen through a window or other vantage point and is deemed incapacitated.

In these situations, EMS may have to make entry via forcible means. Usually a Halligan tool or other form of pry bar is utilized, depending on the situation. If the situation is being treated as a crime scene, it is important that the rescuer note where and how entry was made and what tool was used.

It is not enough to state what type of tool but which exact tool. This is where unit-specific serial numbers are crucial to rescue equipment. Each and every piece of equipment should either be marked with the unit's designation name/number or the item's serial number should be noted in an equipment log that states when it was placed in or removed from that specific vehicle.

The reason for such accuracy lies in the advanced capabilities of investigators. Today's investigators take toolmark identification to a microscopic level, and if there is an unexplained toolmark at an entry site, this would obviously have an impact on the investigation. All tools should be logged in and logged out as repair and replacement dictate.

Once entry is made, the EMS personnel should not attempt to replace the forced access point to its predamaged state. More damage and disruption of the original simple toolmarks may result. The repairs should be left to the police after they have completed their investigation. When the run is completed, the documenting personnel should note which tool was used, where, and by whom.

Forcible entry is more often required in the vehicular accident scenario. High-powered hydraulic and pneumatic rescue tools allow rescuers to gain access and extricate victims more rapidly than ever before. With these rapid and powerful capabilities, it is important for EMS personnel to mentally note, and eventually document, patient position in the vehicle, to help identify the mechanism of injury, as well as who may have been operating the vehicle.

All removed portions of the vehicle should be kept together and not mingled with other vehicles from the same incident. This will prevent the mixing of paint and glass fragments that may be used to determine vehicle placement at the time of impact as well as other objects that the vehicle may have come in contact with during the impact phase.

Subject Versus Vehicle Scenario

The importance of potential evidence on the subject and the subject's clothing cannot be understated. Indeed, in cases of a hit-and-run event it is possible that the only evidence linking the vehicle to the victim will be on the victim.

Microscopic traces of paint, tire marks, and glass fragments are usually left on the patient's clothing, skin, and in wounds. While treating the victim, it is imperative to retain all clothing in a paper bag to promote drying, catch fragments that fall from the material, and prevent unrelated materials from contaminating the clothing. Obvious pattern marks, likely to be tire tracks, grille marks, vehicle emblems, and so forth, should be noted and documented.

If the situation, department policy, and human resources allow for the photographing of these marks, this would be beneficial for the investigation as well. These patterns are made up of dirt and tire compound, both of which may be washed off in a rapid prep for surgery. (Note on photography: A good quality digital camera, preferably with date and time stamping, is necessary. For a photograph to have good evidentiary value there must be an item in the photograph to note scale. For example, a 4 × 4 type bandage, an ECG electrode, or some other clean, readily available object can be useful to show scale.)

OBSERVATION

Pre-hospital personnel are trained observers; their talents of observation may be of great value to an investigation. EMS personnel are frequently the only people to see a crime scene before it is altered or destroyed.

For example, in cases of abuse we are summoned to the scene of the crime to care for the victim. Frequently, the initial report to dispatch will be deliberately inaccurate in an effort to cover up the crime of abuse. In the process of caring for the victim, we become witness to the injury but also to the surroundings as well. We must ask ourselves, "Does the injury fit the scene?"

Example 1

Assume that EMS is summoned to a home where it is reported that a 3-year-old has fallen down a flight of steps. The provider notices that the child has bruising on the cheeks, soft tissue of the lower back and buttocks. All appear to have various degrees of healing. Medical priorities allowing, the rescuer may note the steps in question. The steps were six carpeted, regular size steps, clear of debris, and they had a standard wooden rail.

What's the Call?

These areas are inconsistent with the expected bruising areas secondary to exploration such as the knees, shins, and forearms. The bruises in various stages of healing, although normal for a toddler, are not in typical toddler injury areas. A rescuer would expect the injuries on exposed skin to have an abrasion factor, hence the term *rug burn*.

The provider should quickly note whether the steps are carpeted, cluttered, the presence of safety devices, including gates and rails, and their general height. The EMS provider should evaluate by asking the question, *"Are the steps likely to have caused these injuries?"* but not the more widely inclusive question, *"Could these steps have possibly caused these injuries?"*

It must be stressed that it is not appropriate for the EMS provider to openly call attention to his or her suspicion at the scene, but to follow through and report the incident as soon as possible to the police and to the receiving staff. If the police are on location, a private and professional note should be made of the suspicion to the responding officer, as well as follow-up documentation.

Example 2

Assume EMS is called to a home where a child has reportedly been injured in a snowball fight. On arrival, the provider notes evidence of play in the snow and blood in the snow leading to the dispatched address. Inside the address, wet winter clothing is present in the child's immediate area. The patient is a 10-year-old child being attended to by his mother in the family's kitchen; the child has a significant facial swelling with underlying fracture of several teeth.

What's the Call?

This incident is of low suspicion. The scene fits the reported events thus far, and they are consistent with the injury. The rescuer should hear the child's version of events to make any further judgment.

CONCLUSION

EMS providers come in contact with forensic evidence. Rescuers should note what they have done to alter the scene in the act of providing care and note it to the investigating entity. Providers must also realize that as patient advocates they are *mandated* to report cases of abuse and assault.

It is in the role of good witnesses that EMS providers have their greatest impact on justice. The job of investigating and collecting evidence belongs to the police and is not an EMS function, but securing of evidence that would otherwise be altered or destroyed in the process of medical care and transport is within the realm of EMS providers. This realm does not include judgment or accusation, but does include reporting and recording that which was seen, heard, found, and changed.

SUGGESTED READING

Rovere R. Role of EMS prehospital care providers. In Giardino AP, Datner EM, Asher JP, eds. *Sexual Assault: Victimization Across the Life Span, A Clinical Guide.* St. Louis, Mo: GW Medical Publishing; 2003:487–493.

Rooms RR, Shapiro PD. Approach for emergency medical personnel. In Lynch VA, ed. *Forensic Nursing.* St. Louis, Mo: Elsevier Mosby; 2006:341–350.

25 | In-Custody Death

Kenneth G. Lavelle, MD, NREMT-P, and Theodore Corbin, MD, MPP

INTRODUCTION

Death of subjects in police custody is a significant public concern and frequently results in litigation.[1] Many of the issues and concerns can be seen in other situations in which patients are restrained as well, such as mental institutions or hospital emergency departments. These deaths can be divided into two primary situations: death of an individual during or shortly after restraint and arrest, and death of an individual who has been in custody for a period of time. Although we discuss the latter briefly, the primary emphasis of this chapter is on the arrest-related death, which is more likely to result in public attention and litigation and where there is opportunity for prevention by emergency medical service (EMS) staff and medical directors.

MEDICAL DEATHS AND DEATHS AFTER A PERIOD OF ARREST

Just as death occurs in any environment, it can occur while a subject is in custody as well. However, there is evidence that the death rate is higher for those in custody. Wobeser and associates reviewed this death rate in Ontario and found that the death rate in both federal and provincial prisons (420 and 212 per 100,000, respectively) was higher than that of similar-aged Canadian men (188 per 100,000). During the 10-year period from 1990 to 1999, there were 308 inmates who died, and information was available on 291. Eight of these were women, 5 died from suicide, and 3 from natural causes. Among the 283 men, the mean age was 40.9 years, and half died from violent causes. Two of the most significant causes of death included overdose and suicide by strangulation. The rate of cardiovascular death was also higher, 3.5 times in federal prisons and 1.7 times as high in provincial prisons. The reason for the difference in the type of prison is unclear because it was expected that the preventative medicine efforts should have been better in the federal prison system.[2]

Deaths of those in custody at the local level have also been reported several hours after arrest. The reasons certainly are varied, but the scenario can be imagined. An individual under arrest may have a physical complaint that may be ignored or may receive only a cursory medical examination. Law enforcement officers may not be aware of the seriousness of the type of complaint or may believe that the suspect is feigning the complaint to avoid jail or diminish the likelihood of successful prosecution. Thus, the position in which law enforcement is placed is difficult. If every suspect with any complaint is taken to the hospital for a full evaluation, this adversely affects staffing and can increase the risk of escape. However, if the complaint is ignored, the liability of the law enforcement agency is significant.

Some communities may have a hospital with a jail ward, which could make the transfer and assessment more secure, but this is a rare luxury. All arrested individuals should receive a medical screening exam by a medical professional familiar with the unique risks of those in custody. A system should be in place to obtain appropriate routine medications for suspects that may not have brought their prescriptions with them. Attempts to determine and confirm medical history may also benefit the agency. Protocols for the prompt but secure transfer of suspects with serious medical complaints should be established.

GUNSHOT WOUNDS AND SUICIDE BY COP

Suicide by cop is a phenomenon in which an individual intentionally engages in life-threatening behavior toward the public or the police with a lethal weapon. The individual does so with the intent of committing suicide by provoking the law enforcement officer to shoot the individual. This phenomenon was reviewed by Hudson and associates in 1998.[3] They found that in the 11-year period between 1987 and 1997, the Los Angeles Sheriff's Office investigated 437 officer-involved shootings. These were fatal in 45.8% (200) of the cases. Overall, 10.5% (46) of the 437 shootings were determined to be suicide by cop. These incidents progress rapidly, with 70% of the shootings occurring within 30 minutes of law enforcement officer arrival, rather than being a protracted event.

This is an actual form of suicide, and the numbers may be increasing. In 1997, suicide by cop may have accounted for 25% of officer-involved shootings. This phenomenon lends to reasons that perpetrators and victims of violence do not trust the police.[4] Domestic violence was involved in 39% of cases, and stress in a relationship is a recognized risk factor for suicide.

It is important that the medical provider be familiar with this form of suicide or suicide attempt so that appropriate psychological evaluation may be provided to an individual who survives the incident.[3]

LESS-LETHAL WEAPONS

The need for "less-lethal" weapons results from the desire for a level of force in between physical confrontation and the deadly force of a firearm. The intent is to provide an alternative to deadly force. Two of the more common less-lethal weapons include the conducted electrical weapon and pepper spray.

Conducted Electrical Weapons

The TASER (Thomas A. Swift Electrical Rifle, TASER International) is a conducted electrical weapon (CEW) that is used throughout the country. The TASER has two electrode-tipped, fishhook barbs (#8, 9.5 mm) that are ejected from the weapon by compressed nitrogen up to 35 feet. These are expelled at a speed of 170 feet per second, slightly less fast than recreational paintball guns. The device delivers about 1.76 joules or 26 watts per pulse. The device can deliver up to 50,000 volts in rapid pulses during 5-second periods.

The latest generation and most popular version is the X26. The average current of this weapon is 2.1 mAmps. The threshold for ventricular fibrillation is thought to be around 50–100 mAmps. The current that is sent through the barbs can cross up to 2 inches of clothing, so it can be used on individuals wearing coats or similar thick apparel. Skin penetration is not necessary for transmission. Once deployed, the current results in involuntary contraction of skeletal muscle that makes the individual incapable of voluntary movement. This permits the law enforcement officers to approach suspects and render them safe so as to pose less risk to them and the public.[5]

A relationship between the use of CEW such as the TASER and subject death has been suggested. However, there are several studies that seem to indicate that it is not solely the use of the TASER that is a risk factor for in-custody death, but rather the full set of circumstances involving its deployment.

It has been postulated that the TASER causes an arrhythmia such as ventricular fibrillation. The fact that death, if it occurs, occurs 15 or more minutes after the application would seem to discount this mechanism.[6] Also, the TASER has been used on tens of thousands of individuals during training without ill effect.

An animal study found that an experimental device similar to the TASER failed to cause ventricular fibrillation in pigs unless a minimum of 15 times the charge of the TASER device was used.[7] In two manufacturer-sponsored studies, the TASER failed to cause ventricular fibrillation when directly applied to dog hearts.[8,9] Ho and Associates studied the cardiovascular and physiologic effects of the TASER on resting adults.[5] All individuals that undergo a TASER training course are required to receive a shock from the weapon. This study was accomplished during one of these training classes. Adult volunteers received a 5-second application of the weapon with support personnel in place to assist them to the ground. The volunteers were 65 men and 1 woman between the ages of 29 and 55 years. Six had a history of hypertension, 6 had hyperlipidemia, and 1 had a history of myocardial infarction with coronary artery bypass graft (CABG). Labs (electrolytes, cardiac enzymes, lactate, and creatinine kinase levels) were drawn 0, 16, and 24 hours after application, and a 12-lead EKG was done at this time. In one individual, a troponin I level of 0.6 ng/mL (reference level 0–0.4 mg/mL) was noted at the 24-hour mark. This individual was transported to a hospital where he received a full evaluation by a cardiologist that included a treadmill stress test and a rest/adenosine-augmented perfusion study, which were normal.

This level returned to normal within 8 hours and occurred in a very physically fit individual. No cause for the elevation was found.[5]

Although this and other studies suggest that there is no significant cardiac damage as a result of TASER application, it should be noted that most of these studies involve law enforcement officers who are generally in excellent physical condition. A TASER is generally not applied solely to this type of individual. Suspects in which the TASER is applied may be in excellent condition or may have significant medical problems.

It is more reasonable to be concerned not only because a suspect has had a TASER applied, but because of the specific circumstances involved or reason for its deployment. It is therefore becoming more common in many jurisdictions that the deployment of the TASER requires the medical evaluation of the individual at the hospital. Some districts require only an evaluation by EMS staff. However, most EMS providers are not trained or familiar with the specific risks involved with this type of situation, and relying on them to provide medical reassurance may be imprudent.

Most likely, the emergency physician will be confronted with the patient who is alive following TASER application. These patients require a thorough head-to-toe physical examination looking for signs of injury. The involuntary muscle contraction induced by the device usually leads to a fall. Patients should be evaluated and worked up like any other fall from standing patient. The patient should be screened for the presence of excited delirium. Routine electrocardiogram is not indicated unless signs or symptoms of excited delirium or other reasons to obtain it exist.[10]

Emergency physicians may be faced with the patient who has a TASER barb embedded. Because of its relatively small size, the barb poses no significant risk to the lungs, heart, or bowel. At-risk structures may include the eye, neck vasculature, and genitalia, but there has been no reported cases of significant injury. If a barb is embedded near major vascular structures, consultation with a trauma or vascular surgeon is warranted. Barbs embedded elsewhere can be removed at the bedside. One hand is placed on the skin around the barb to pull it taut, and the other hand grasps the barb and applies steady inline traction. Unlike with other fishhooks, there is no need to advance the end of the barb through the skin to cut off the tip. Local anesthetic can be used at the site of the wound for patient comfort. A small scalpel can be used to cut down to the base of the barb tip.[10]

Oleoresin Capsicum

Pepper spray, or oleoresin capsicum (OC), is an extract of the pepper plant of the genus Capsicum. Its use is designed to cause pain and decrease the ability of the individual to continue to resist because of this pain and the inability to see because of tearing of the eyes and other mucous membranes. There has been speculation that pepper spray may have a role in the death of victims who are resisting. However, there is not a significant risk that has been identified in victims who are not showing signs of excited delirium.

Most exposures to pepper spray produce irritation of the skin and mucous membranes. Treatment required is often only supportive and involves irrigation of affected regions with water.

EXCITED DELIRIUM

Excited delirium is a state of severe agitation, delirium, hypertension, and hyperthermia and was described in the mid-1980s.[11] In the hospital, this had been seen in psychiatric patients, particularly those on phenothiazines. Other names for this state include exhaustive mania, Bell's mania, lethal catatonia, and acute exhaustive psychosis.[1] This state, if it occurs in public, can result in a response by both law enforcement and EMS because of violence, recklessness, or removal of clothes. The individual is unlikely to become calm when confronted by law enforcement so that some degree of force is required to restrain the individual to protect him or her and others.[12] Individuals in a state of excited delirium can be quite strong and require significant resources to control them. Stimulant drugs are often involved.

SUDDEN IN-CUSTODY DEATH SYNDROME

Sudden in-custody death syndrome (SICDS) can be defined as the unexpected death of a subject while in custody restraint, following an episode of excited delirium, where the autopsy fails to find a diagnosis or cause of death.[6] SICDS was first described in 1982 in Seattle and involved acute psychiatric agitation, increased activity, and restraint by law enforcement.[13,14] These individuals are usually showing signs of excited delirium, and then are restrained. Several factors involved in the syndrome increase the risk that excited delirium will progress to death (see Table 25-1).

Restraint and Positional Asphyxia

The role of the position of the restraint has been considered to be a significant factor in the syndrome. Positional asphyxia is related to the position of the individual; restraint asphyxia is a subset of this, where the restraint prevents the individual from changing position or otherwise improving the conditions that place them at risk.[1] A common restraint position that has been used is the hog-tie or hobble restraint. In this method, the individual is prone, with the wrists handcuffed behind the back and the ankles tied together.[1] The knees can be flexed and the ankles brought up toward the hands. This

TABLE 25-1 **Characteristics of SICDS**

- Acute onset
- Delirium
- Combativeness
- Physical restraint
- Sudden cardiac death
- No response to CPR
- History of stimulant abuse or mental illness

Source: DiMaio TG, DiMaio VJM. *Excited Delirium Syndrome.* Boca Raton, Fla: CRC Press; 2006.

position has been hypothesized to adversely affect breathing and limit chest and abdominal movement.[15] Weight on the back, such as an individual holding the subject down, can further impair ventilation.[16]

Chan and associates studied the role of restraint position in 1997. They studied 15 healthy men in various positions and administered pulmonary function tests and monitored arterial blood gases and vital signs. They found that there was a decline in forced vital capacity (FVC) and forced expiratory ventilation in 1 minute (FEV1), but there was no hypoxia or difference in heart rate recovery. They concluded that the hog-tie restraint itself does not cause hypoventilation and asphyxia. They acknowledge that a combination of factors that were not present in these healthy subjects, such as intoxication, agitation, and others, may together cause respiratory compromise.[17]

Preexisting Medical Conditions

Obesity can be a risk factor for death. Increased weight can limit diaphragmatic motion, and increased body mass can predispose persons to hyperthermia.[1] The large abdomen, particularly when the victim is prone, can force abdominal contents toward the diaphragm and restrict diaphragmatic excursion and movement. Other medical conditions that affect breathing can place the victim at higher risk of death also.[18]

Intoxicants

Rhabdomyolysis associated with intoxicants, particularly cocaine, has been reported since the mid-1980s.[19] The characteristics of cocaine-associated excited delirium are similar to the characteristics of excited delirium, including hyperthermia, but also include bizarre, psychotic behavior and hyperactivity, leading to the consideration that these two processes may be different stages of the same syndrome.

Ruttenber and associates studied the various hypotheses for the cause of cocaine-associated rhabdomyolysis. They considered that chronic cocaine use alters dopamine receptors, and that victims of excited delirium may have difficulty clearing dopamine, which predisposes the victim to fatal arrhythmias.[20] The level of cocaine in these subjects is usually not exceedingly high, indicating that a massive overdose is not alone the cause of mortality.[19]

In addition to precipitating the behavior that places the victim at risk, the stress of the delirium or the arrest and restraint may increase the toxicity of certain substances.[21] Other intoxicants, such as methamphetamines or PCP, can also increase the risk for the syndrome.[13] Chronic users may also be at higher risk because they are more susceptible to coronary vasoconstriction when exposed to increased levels of catecholamines such as norepinephrine, which are present in higher levels after the use of stimulants. This coronary vasoconstriction, right at a time when there is increased myocardial demand as a result of the struggle and increased heart rate, predisposes the individual to myocardial ischemia. Additionally, the cardiotoxic effects such as myocarditis and myocardial necrosis may play a role.[6]

Sudden Death

Often during restraint or transport, the individual will suddenly stop resisting, suffer respiratory arrest, coma, and death.[12] Even if the death is witnessed by EMS, resuscitation is unlikely.[15] Stratton and associates[15] studied the syndrome in 2001 in Los Angeles. They reviewed 216 subjects that were restrained and appeared to have signs of excited delirium between 1992 and 1998. There were 20 deaths, 2 of which were excluded from the study; 1 because of a pulmonary embolism found on autopsy and 1 because of ligature marks noted on the victim. Stimulant drug use was noted in 78% of these deaths, and 45% had a history of chronic cocaine use. The TASER was deployed in 28% and capsicum in 33%. Obesity was noted in 56%; however, it is noted that more than 60% of Americans are overweight or obese; therefore, it is unclear how much of a risk it is. It is also noted that all 20 of these deaths occurred with EMS in attendance, but resuscitation was unsuccessful.

It seems that several factors are often present for sudden in-custody death syndrome:

- Agitation or excited delirium
- Stimulant ingestion or mental illness
- Physical confrontation or restraint

These factors place the victim at high risk. Restraint position may be one of the final factors involved.

IMPLICATIONS FOR THE EMERGENCY PHYSICIAN

Pre-hospital Medical Direction

Physicians who are medical directors of law enforcement agencies should ensure that the officers have some understanding of this condition and the risks associated. The officer should be able to recognize respiratory distress and monitor the suspect while calling for emergency medical services. Once restrained, victims should be placed on their side (left lateral decubitus position) as soon as it is safe to do so, rather than be left prone.[18] Placing the victim on the side will prevent aspiration of vomitus.

Emergency Department Care

It is important that the emergency provider immediately evaluate any patient that arrives in restraints and attempt to determine any organic cause for the agitation that required restraint use.[11] The emergency department staff should consider the possibility of drug and/or alcohol intoxication and place the victim on a cardiac monitor and pulse oximeter. A subject in the prone position is difficult to monitor, and an alternative method of restraint is indicated.[14] Medical personnel have the benefit of chemical restraint, which should be used liberally to minimize the need for physical restraint.

Laboratory and radiologic studies should be obtained based on history and physical exam findings. Patients should be monitored for the development of metabolic acidosis and rhabdomyolysis and treatment for them initiated. Be prepared to treat cardiac arrest, especially if the victim becomes unexpectedly docile.[18]

CONCLUSION

The death of subjects who are in custody certainly involves multiple factors. Suspects in custody who have signs and symptoms of excited delirium and are restrained are at high risk for a fatal outcome. Bloom in her practice notes how the trauma of physical restraints of acute psychotic patients demonstrates negative outcomes.[22] It is important that all emergency responders, from the law enforcement officer to the emergency physician, are aware of the risks and provide immediate medical attention and evaluation.[13] Training should be provided to all responders regarding the risks involved and methods to prevent these deaths.

REFERENCES

1. O'Halloran RL, Frank JG. Asphyxial death during prone restraint revisited: a report of 21 cases. *Am J Forensic Med Pathol.* March 2000; 21(1):39–52.
2. Wobeser WL, Datema J, Ford P, Bechard B. Causes of death among people in custody in Ontario, 1990–9. *CMAJ.* November 12, 2002;167(10).
3. Hudson HR, Anglin D, Yarbrough J, et al. Suicide by cop. *Ann Emerg Med.* December 1998;32(6).
4. Rich JA, Grey CM. Pathways to recurrent trauma among young Black men: traumatic stress, substance use, and the "code of the street." *Am J Public Health.* May 2005;95(5):816–824.
5. Ho JD, Miner JR, Lakireddy DR, Bultman LL, Heegaard WG. Cardiovascular and physiologic effects of conducted electrical weapon discharge in resting adults. *Acad Emerg Med.* 2006;13(6):589–595.
6. DiMaio TG, DiMaio VJM. *Excited Delirium Syndrome.* Boca Raton, Fla: CRC Press; 2006.
7. McDaniel WC, Stratbucker RA, Nerheim M, et al. Cardiac safety of neuromuscular incapacitating defensive devices. *PACE.* 2005;28:S284–7.
8. Anonymous. Advanced TASER M26 Less-Lethal EMD weapon. Medical Safety Information. TASER International, 2000. Available at: www.taser.com.
9. Bleetman A, Steyn R. The advanced TASER: a medical review. Available at www.Taser.com. Accessed October 1, 2007.
10. Lutes M. Focus on: management of TASER injuries. *ACEP News.* May 2006. Available at: http://www.acep.org/publications.aspx?id=24740. Accessed on March 2, 2007.
11. McCarron M, Challoner K. Emergency department treatment of patients in police custody. *Top Emerg Med.* September 1999;21(3)39–48.
12. Parent R. Deaths during police intervention. *FBI Law Enforcement Bull.* April 2006;75(4). Available at: http://www.fbi.gov/publications/leb/2006/april2006/april06leb.htm#page18. Accessed September 22, 2007.
13. Robinson D, Hunt S. Sudden in-custody death syndrome. *Top Emerg Med.* 2005;27(1):26–45.
14. O'Halloran RL. Reenactment of circumstances in deaths related to restraint. *Am J Forensic Med Pathol.* 2004;25:190–193.
15. Stratton SJ, Rogers C, Green K. Sudden death in individuals in hobble restraint during paramedic transport. *Ann Emerg Med.* May 1995;25:710–712.
16. O'Halloran RL, Lewman LV. Restraint asphyxia in excited delirium. *Am J Forensic Med Pathol.* 1993;14:289–295.
17. Chan TC, Vilke GM, Neuman T, Clausen JL. Restraint position and positional asphyxia. *Ann Emerg Med.* November 1997;30:578–586.
18. Reay DT. Death in custody. *Clin Lab Med.* 1998;28(1):1–22.
19. Wetli C, Mash D, Karch S. Cocaine associated agitated delirium and the NMS. *Am J Emerg Med.* July 1996;14(4).
20. Ruttenber AJ, McAnally HB, Wetli CV. Cocaine associated rhabdomyolysis and excited delirium: different stages of the same syndrome. *Am J Forensic Med Pathol.* June 1999;20(2):120–127.
21. Park KS, Korn CS, Henderson SO. Agitated delirium and sudden death: two case reports. *Prehospital Emerg Care.* April/June 2001;5(2):214–216.
22. Bloom S. *Creating Sanctuary.* New York, NY: Routledge; 1997.

APPENDIX I Adult Forms

A. California Sexual Assault Form—OCJP 923 220

B. Philadelphia Sexual Assault Form 229

C. California Domestic Abuse Form—OES 502 239

D. California Elder Abuse Form—OES 602 247

E. California Sexual Assault Suspect Examination Form—OCJP 950 . . 257

State of California
Governor's Office of Criminal Justice Planning

FORENSIC MEDICAL REPORT: ACUTE (<72 HOURS) ADULT/ADOLESCENT SEXUAL ASSAULT EXAMINATION

OCJP 923

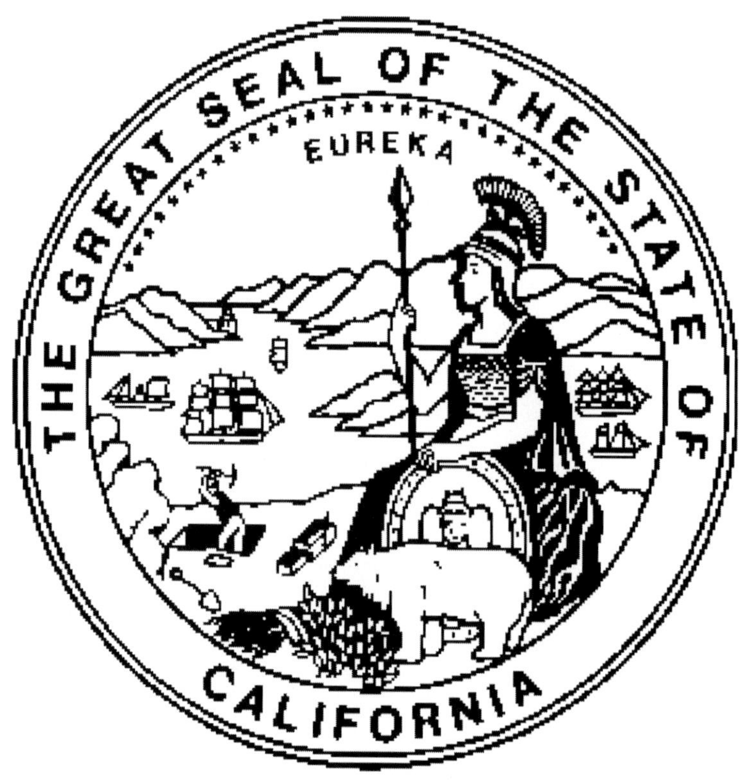

For more information or assistance in completing the OCJP 923 please contact University of California, Davis California Medical Training Center at:
(916) 734-4141

This form is available on the following Web site:
www.ocjp.ca.gov

FORENSIC MEDICAL REPORT: ACUTE (<72 HOURS)
ADULT/ADOLESCENT SEXUAL ASSAULT EXAMINATION

STATE OF CALIFORNIA
OFFICE OF CRIMINAL JUSTICE PLANNING

OCJP 923

Confidential Document

Patient Identification

A. GENERAL INFORMATION (print or type)

Name of Medical Facility:

1. Name of patient				Patient ID number			
2. Address		City		County	State	Telephone (W) (H)	
3. Age	DOB	Gender M F	Ethnicity	Arrival Date	Arrival Time	Discharge Date	Discharge Time

B. REPORTING AND AUTHORIZATION

Jurisdiction (☐city ☐county ☐other):

1. Telephone report made to law enforcement agency Name of Officer	Agency	ID Number	Telephone	Reported by: Name	Date	Time
2. Responding Officer	Agency	ID Number	Telephone			

3. I request a forensic medical examination for suspected sexual assault at public expense.

Law enforcement officer	ID number	Agency	
Telephone	Date	Time	Case Number

Telephone Authorization
Agency:
Authorizing party:
ID number:
Date/time:

C. PATIENT INFORMATION

- I understand that hospitals and health care professionals are required by Penal Code Sections 11160-11161 to report to law enforcement authorities cases in which medical care is sought when injuries have been inflicted upon any person in violation of any state penal law. The report must state the name of the injured person, current whereabouts, and the type and extent of injuries. ________ (Initial)
- I have been informed that victims of crime are eligible to submit crime victim compensation claims to the State Victims of Crime (VOC) Restitution Fund for out-of-pocket medical expenses, psychological counseling, loss of wages, and job retraining and rehabilitation. ________ (Initial)

D. PATIENT CONSENT

Minors: Family Code Section 6927 permits minors (12 to 17 years of age) to consent to medical examination, treatment, and evidence collection for sexual assault without parental consent. See instructions for parental notification requirements for minors.

- I understand that a forensic medical examination for evidence of sexual assault at public expense can, with my consent, be conducted by a health care professional to discover and preserve evidence of the assault. If conducted, the report of the examination and any evidence obtained will be released to law enforcement authorities. I understand that the examination may include the collection of reference specimens at the time of the examination or at a later date. I understand that I may withdraw consent at any time for any portion of the examination. ________ (Initial)
- I understand that collection of evidence may include photographing injuries and that these photographs may include the genital area. ________ (Initial)
- I hereby consent to a forensic medical examination for evidence of sexual assault. ________ (Initial)
- I understand that data without patient identity may be collected from this report for health and forensic purposes and provided to health authorities and other qualified persons with a valid educational or scientific interest for demographic and/or epidemiological studies. ________ (Initial)

Signature ______________________________ ☐ Patient ☐ Parent ☐ Guardian

DISTRIBUTION OF OCJP 923

☐ Original - Law Enforcement ☐ Copy within evidence kit - Crime Lab ☐ Copy - Child Protective Services (if patient is a minor) ☐ Copy - Medical Facility Records

OCJP 923 (Rev 7/02) 1

E. PATIENT HISTORY

1. Name of person providing history:	Relationship to patient:	Date	Time

2. Pertinent medical history:

- Last menstrual period

- Any recent (60 days) anal-genital injuries, surgeries, diagnostic procedures, or medical treatment that may affect the interpretation of current physical findings? ☐ No ☐ Yes
  If yes, describe:

- Any other pertinent medical condition(s) that may affect the interpretation of current physical findings? ☐ No ☐ Yes
  If yes, describe:

- Any pre-existing physical injuries? ☐ No ☐ Yes
  If yes, describe:

3. Pertinent pre- and post-assault related history:

	No	Yes	Unsure
• Other intercourse within past 5 days?	☐	☐	
If yes,			
anal (within past 5 days)? When ______	☐	☐	
vaginal (within past 5 days)? When ______	☐	☐	
oral (within past 24 hours)? When ______	☐	☐	
If yes, did ejaculation occur?	☐	☐	☐
If yes, where? ______			
If yes, was a condom used?	☐	☐	☐
• Any voluntary alcohol use within 12 hours prior to assault?	☐	☐*	
• Any voluntary drug use within 96 hours prior to assault ?	☐	☐*	
• Any voluntary drug or alcohol use between the time of the assault and the forensic exam?	☐	☐*	

* If yes, collection of toxicology samples is recommended according to local policy. ☐ Blood ☐ Urine

4. Post-assault hygiene/activity: ☐ **Not applicable if over 72 hours**

	No	Yes
Urinated	☐	☐
Defecated	☐	☐
Genital or body wipes	☐	☐
If yes, describe: ______		
Douched	☐	☐
If yes, with what ______		
Removed/inserted tampon☐ diaphragm☐	☐	☐
Oral gargle/rinse	☐	☐
Bath/shower/wash	☐	☐
Brushed teeth	☐	☐
Ate or drank	☐	☐
Changed clothing	☐	☐
If yes, describe: ______		

5. Assault-related history:

	No	Yes
Loss of memory? If yes, describe:	☐	☐*
Lapse of consciousness? If yes, describe:	☐	☐*

*If yes, collection of toxicology samples is recommended according to local policy. ☐Blood ☐Urine

	No	Yes
Vomited? If yes, describe:	☐	☐
Non-genital injury, pain and/or bleeding? If yes, describe:	☐	☐
Anal-genital injury, pain, and/or bleeding? If yes, describe:	☐	☐

Patient Identification

F. ASSAULT HISTORY

1. Date of assault(s):	Time of assault(s):

2. Pertinent physical surroundings of assault(s):

3. Alleged assailant(s) name(s)	Age	Gender	Ethnicity	Relationship to patient: Known	Unknown
#1.		M F			
#2.		M F			
#3.		M F			
#4.		M F			

4. Methods employed by assailant(s):

	No	Yes	If yes, describe:
Weapons	☐	☐	
Threatened?	☐	☐	
Injuries inflicted?	☐	☐	
Type(s) of weapons?	☐	☐	
Physical blows	☐	☐	
Grabbing/holding/pinching	☐	☐	
Physical restraints	☐	☐	
Choking/strangulation	☐	☐	
Burns (thermal and/or chemical)	☐	☐	
Threat(s) of harm	☐	☐	
Target(s) of threat(s)	☐	☐	
Other methods	☐	☐	

Involuntary ingestion of alcohol/drugs ☐No ☐Yes ☐ Unsure

If yes, ☐ Alcohol ☐ Drugs

If yes, ☐ Forced ☐ Coerced ☐ Suspected

If yes, toxicology samples collected: ☐ Blood ☐ Urine ☐ None

5. Injuries inflicted upon the assailant(s) during assault? ☐ No ☐Yes
If yes, describe injuries, possible locations on the body, and how they were inflicted.

G. ACTS DESCRIBED BY PATIENT

- **Any penetration of the genital or anal opening, however slight, constitutes the act.**
- **Oral copulation requires only contact**
- **If more than one assailant, identify by number.**

Patient Identification

1. Penetration of vagina by:

	No	Yes	Attempted	Unsure
Penis	☐	☐	☐	☐
Finger	☐	☐	☐	☐
Object	☐	☐	☐	☐

If yes, describe the object:

Describe: ______

2. Penetration of anus by:

	No	Yes	Attempted	Unsure
Penis	☐	☐	☐	☐
Finger	☐	☐	☐	☐
Object	☐	☐	☐	☐

If yes, describe the object:

Describe: ______

3. Oral copulation of genitals:

	No	Yes	Attempted	Unsure
Of patient by assailant	☐	☐	☐	☐
Of assailant by patient	☐	☐	☐	☐

Describe: ______

4. Oral copulation of anus:

	No	Yes	Attempted	Unsure
Of patient by assailant	☐	☐	☐	☐
Of assailant by patient	☐	☐	☐	☐

Describe: ______

5. Non-genital act(s):

	No	Yes	Attempted	Unsure
Licking	☐	☐	☐	☐
Kissing	☐	☐	☐	☐
Suction injury	☐	☐	☐	☐
Biting	☐	☐	☐	☐

Describe: ______

6. Other act(s):

No	Yes	Attempted	Unsure
☐	☐	☐	☐

Describe: ______

7. Did ejaculation occur?

No	Yes	Unsure
☐	☐	☐

If yes, note location(s):

- ☐ Mouth
- ☐ Vagina
- ☐ Anus/Rectum
- ☐ Body surface
- ☐ On clothing
- ☐ On bedding
- ☐ Other

Describe: ______

8. Contraceptive or lubricant products:

	No	Yes	Unsure
Foam used?	☐	☐	☐
Jelly used?	☐	☐	☐
Lubricant used?	☐	☐	☐
Condom used?	☐	☐	☐

Describe Type/Brand, if known: ______

H. GENERAL PHYSICAL EXAMINATION

Record all findings using diagrams, legend, and a consecutive numbering system.

1. Blood Pressure	Pulse	Resp	Temp	2. Exam Started		Exam Completed	
				Date	Time	Date	Time

3. Describe general physical appearance	4. Describe general demeanor

Patient Identification

5. Describe condition of clothing upon arrival.

6. Collect outer and underclothing if indicated. ☐ Not indicated

7. Conduct a physical examination. ☐ Findings ☐ No Findings

8. Collect dried and moist secretions, stains, and foreign materials from the body. Scan the entire body with a Wood's Lamp.
☐ Findings ☐ No Findings

9. Collect fingernail scrapings or cuttings according to local policy.

Diagram A

Diagram B

LEGEND: Types of Findings

AB	Abrasion	**DF**	Deformity	**FB**	Foreign Body	**MS**	Moist Secretion	**PE**	Petechiae	**TB**	Toluidine Blue ⊕
BI	Bite	**DS**	Dry Secretion	**IN**	Induration	**OF**	Other Foreign Materials (describe)	**PS**	Potential Saliva	**TE**	Tenderness
BU	Burn	**EC**	Ecchymosis (bruise)	**IW**	Incised Wound			**SHX**	Sample Per History	**V/S**	Vegetation/Soil
CS	Control Swab	**ER**	Erythema (redness)	**LA**	Laceration	**OI**	Other Injury (describe)	**SI**	Suction Injury	**WL**	Wood's Lamp ⊕
DE	Debris	**F/H**	Fiber/Hair					**SW**	Swelling		

Locator #	Type	Description	Locator #	Type	Description

RECORD ALL CLOTHING AND SPECIMENS COLLECTED ON PAGE 8

I. HEAD, NECK, AND ORAL EXAMINATION

Record all findings using diagrams, legend, and a consecutive numbering system.

1. **Examine the face, head, hair, scalp, and neck for injury and foreign materials** ☐ Findings ☐ No Findings
2. **Collect dried and moist secretions, stains, and foreign materials from the face, head, hair, scalp, and neck.** ☐ Findings ☐ No Findings
3. **Examine the oral cavity for injury and foreign materials (if indicated by assault history). Collect foreign materials.** **Exam done:** ☐ Not applicable ☐ Yes ☐ Findings ☐ No Findings
4. **Collect 2 swabs from the oral cavity up to 12 hours post assault and prepare one dry mount slide from one of the swabs.**
5. **Collect head hair reference samples according to local policy.**

Patient Identification

Diagram C

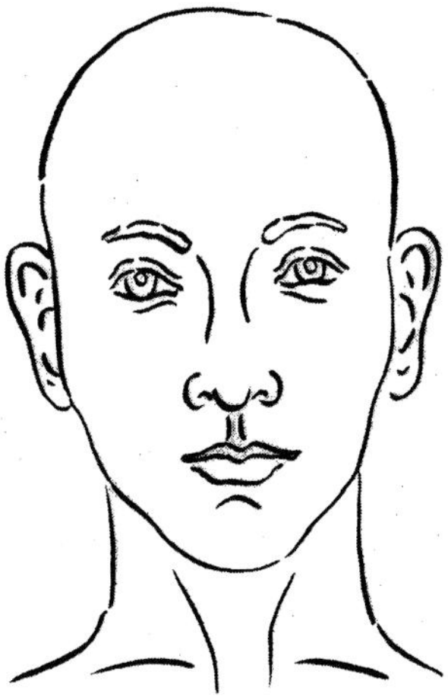

Diagram D

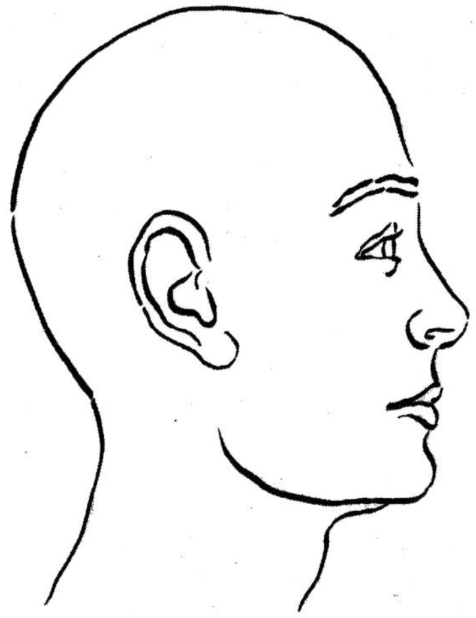

Diagram E

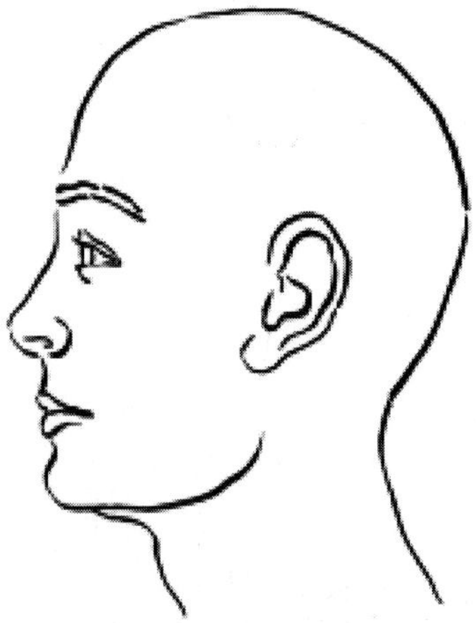

Diagram F

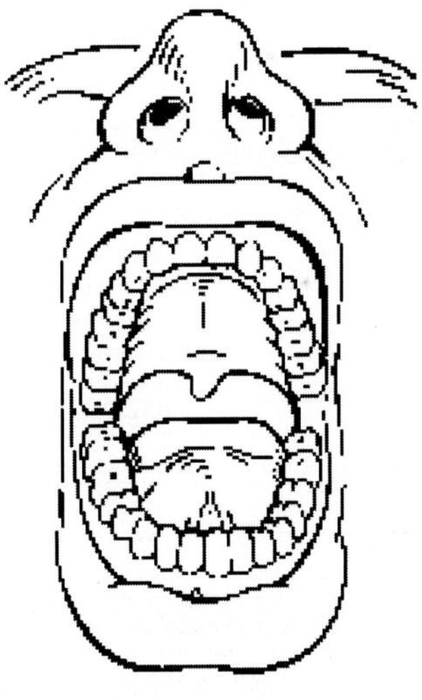

LEGEND: Types of Findings

AB	Abrasion	**DF**	Deformity	**FB**	Foreign Body	**MS**	Moist Secretion	**PE**	Petechiae	**TB**	Toluidine Blue ⊕
BI	Bite	**DS**	Dry Secretion	**IN**	Induration	**OF**	Other Foreign Materials (describe)	PS	Potential Saliva	**TE**	Tenderness
BU	Burn	**EC**	Ecchymosis (bruise)	**IW**	Incised Wound			**SHX**	Sample Per History	**V/S**	Vegetation/Soil
CS	Control Swab	**ER**	Erythema (redness)	**LA**	Laceration	**OI**	Other Injury (describe)	**SI**	Suction Injury	**WL**	Wood's Lamp ⊕
DE	Debris	**F/H**	Fiber/Hair					**SW**	Swelling		

Locator #	Type	Description	Locator #	Type	Description

RECORD ALL SPECIMENS COLLECTED ON PAGE 8

J. GENITAL EXAMINATION - FEMALES

Record all findings using diagrams, legend, and a consecutive numbering system.

1. **Examine the inner thighs, external genitalia, and perineal area. Check the box(es) if there are assault related findings:**
   - ☐ No Findings
   - ☐ Inner thighs ☐ Periurethral tissue/urethral meatus
   - ☐ Perineum ☐ Perihymenal tissue (vestibule)
   - ☐ Labia majora ☐ Hymen
   - ☐ Labia minora ☐ Fossa navicularis
   - ☐ Clitoris/surrounding area ☐ Posterior fourchette
2. **Collect dried and moist secretions, stains, and foreign materials. Scan the area with a Wood's Lamp.** ☐ Findings ☐ No Findings
3. **Collect pubic hair combing or brushing.**
4. **Collect pubic hair reference samples according to local policy.**
5. **Examine the vagina and cervix. Check the box(es) if there are assault related findings.**
   ☐ No Findings ☐ Vagina ☐ Cervix
6. **Collect 4 swabs from the vaginal pool. Prepare one wet mount slide and one dry mount slide.**
7. **Collect 2 cervical swabs (if over 48 hours post assault).**
8. **Examine the buttocks, anus, and rectum (if indicated by history).**
   Exam done: ☐ **Yes** ☐ **Not applicable**
   Check the box(es) if there are assault related findings:
   - ☐ No Findings
   - ☐ Buttocks ☐ Anal verge/folds/rugae
   - ☐ Perianal skin ☐ Rectum
9. **Collect dried and moist secretions, stains, and foreign materials.**
   ☐ Findings ☐ No Findings
10. **Collect 2 anal and/or rectal swabs and prepare one dry mount slide.**
11. **Conduct an anoscopic exam if rectal injury is suspected or if there is any sign of rectal bleeding.**
    Rectal bleeding ☐ No ☐ Yes
    If yes, describe:__________
12. **Exam position used:**
    ☐ Supine ☐ Other Describe:

LEGEND: Types of Findings

AB Abrasion	**EC** Ecchymosis (bruise)	**MS** Moist Secretion	**SI** Suction Injury
BI Bite	**ER** Erythema (redness)	**OF** Other Foreign Materials (describe)	**SW** Swelling
BU Burn	**F/H** Fiber/Hair		**TB** ToluidineBlue⊕
CS Control Swab	**FB** Foreign Body	**OI** Other Injury (describe)	**TE** Tenderness
DE Debris	**IN** Induration	**PE** Petechiae	**V/S** Vegetation/Soil
DF Deformity	**IW** Incised Wound	**PS** Potential Saliva	**WL** Wood's Lamp⊕
DS Dry Secretion	**LA** Laceration	**SHX** Sample Per History	

Locator #	Type	Description

Patient Identification

Diagram G

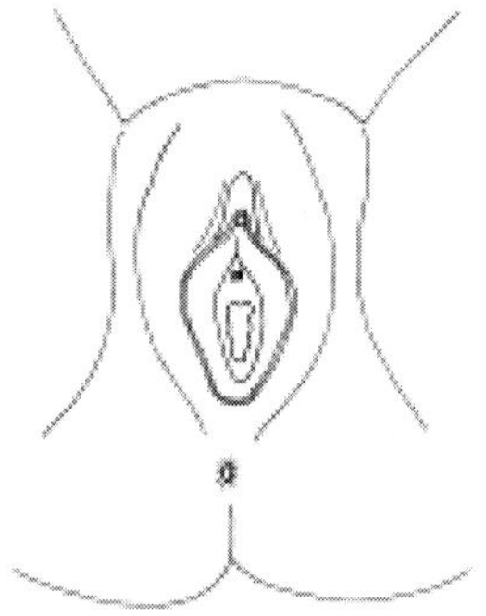

Diagram H

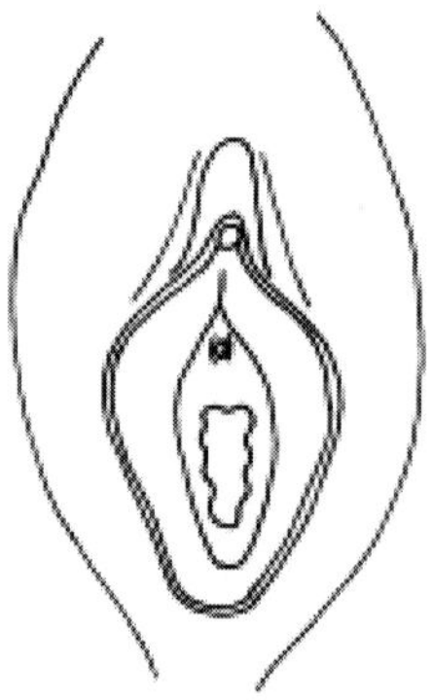

Diagram I

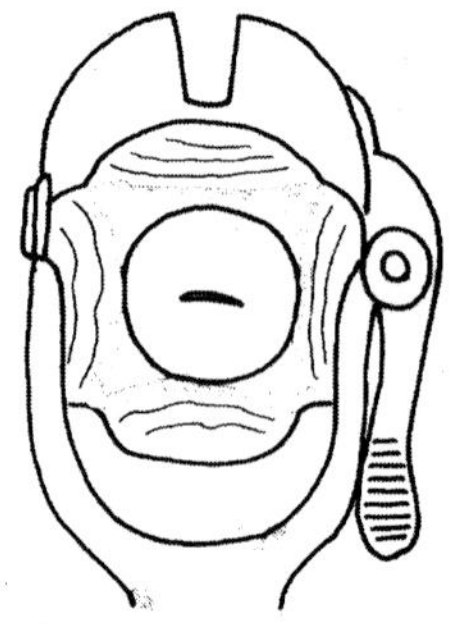

Diagram J

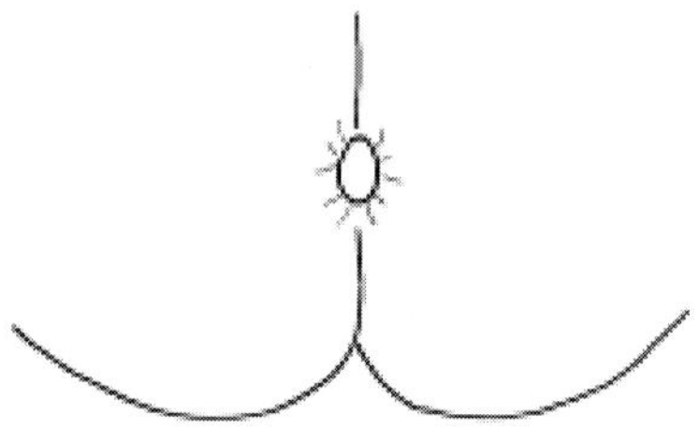

RECORD ALL SPECIMENS COLLECTED ON PAGE 8

K. GENITAL EXAMINATION – MALES

Record all findings using diagrams, legend, and a consecutive numbering system.

1. **Examine the inner thighs, external genitalia, and perineal area. Check the box(es) if there are assault related findings:**
   ☐ No Findings

   ☐ Inner thighs ☐ Glans penis ☐ Scrotum
   ☐ Perineum ☐ Penile shaft ☐ Testes
   ☐ Foreskin ☐ Urethral meatus
2. **Circumcised:** ☐ No ☐ Yes
3. **Collect dried and moist secretions, stains, and foreign materials. Scan the area with a Wood's Lamp.** ☐ Findings ☐ No Findings
4. **Collect pubic hair combing or brushing.**
5. **Collect pubic hair reference samples according to local policy.**
6. **Collect 2 penile swabs, if indicated by assault history.** ☐ N/A
7. **Collect 2 scrotal swabs, if indicated by assault history.** ☐ N/A
8. **Examine the buttocks, anus, and rectum (if indicated by history)**
   Exam done: ☐ **Yes** ☐ **Not applicable**
   Check the box(es) if there are assault related findings:
   ☐ No Findings

   ☐ Buttocks ☐ Anal verge/folds/rugae
   ☐ Perianal skin ☐ Rectum
9. **Collect dried and moist secretions, stains, and foreign materials.**
   ☐ Findings ☐ No Findings
10. **Collect 2 anal and/or rectal swabs and prepare one dry mount slide.**
11. **Conduct an anoscopic exam if rectal injury is suspected or if there is any sign of rectal bleeding.**
    Rectal bleeding: ☐ No ☐ Yes
    If yes, describe: ______
12. **Exam position used:**
    ☐ Supine ☐ Other Describe:

LEGEND: Types of Findings

AB	Abrasion	**EC**	Ecchymosis (bruise)	**MS**	Moist Secretion	**SI**	Suction Injury
BI	Bite	**ER**	Erythema (redness)	**OF**	Other Foreign Materials (describe)	**SW**	Swelling
BU	Burn	**F/H**	Fiber/Hair			**TB**	ToluidineBlue⊕
CS	Control Swab	**FB**	Foreign Body	**OI**	Other Injury (describe)	**TE**	Tenderness
DE	Debris	**IN**	Induration	**PE**	Petechiae	**V/S**	Vegetation/Soil
DF	Deformity	**IW**	Incised Wound	**PS**	Potential Saliva	**WL**	Wood's Lamp⊕
DS	Dry Secretion	**LA**	Laceration	**SHX**	Sample Per History		

Locator #	Type	Description

Patient Identification

Diagram K

Diagram L

Diagram M

Diagram N

RECORD ALL SPECIMENS COLLECTED ON PAGE 8

L. EVIDENCE COLLECTED AND SUBMITTED TO CRIME LAB

1. Clothing placed in evidence kit	Other clothing placed in bags

2. Foreign materials collected

	No	Yes	Collected by:
Swabs/suspected blood	☐	☐	______
Dried secretions	☐	☐	______
Fiber/loose hairs	☐	☐	______
Vegetation	☐	☐	______
Soil/debris	☐	☐	______
Swabs/suspected semen	☐	☐	______
Swabs/suspected saliva	☐	☐	______
Swabs/Wood's Lamp⊕ area(s)	☐	☐	______
Control swabs	☐	☐	______
Fingernail scrapings/cuttings	☐	☐	______
Matted hair cuttings	☐	☐	______
Pubic hair combings/brushings	☐	☐	______
Intravaginal foreign body	☐	☐	______
If yes, describe: ______			
Other types	☐	☐	______
If yes, describe:			

3. Oral/genital/anal/rectal samples

	# Swabs	# Slides	Time collected	Collected by:
Oral				
Vaginal				
Cervical				
Anal				
Rectal				
Penile				
Scrotal				

Aspirate/washings (optional) ☐ No ☐ Yes

4. Vaginal wet mount slide

	No	Yes	Time	Examiner:
Slide prepared				
Motile sperm observed				
Non-motile sperm observed				

M. TOXICOLOGY SAMPLES

	No	Yes	Time	Collected by:
Blood alcohol/toxicology (gray top tube)				
Urine toxicology				

N. REFERENCE SAMPLES

	No	Yes	Collected by:
Blood (lavender top tube)			
Blood (yellow top tube)			
Blood Card (optional)			
Buccal swabs (optional)			
Saliva swabs			
Head hair			
Pubic hair			

O. PHOTO DOCUMENTATION METHODS

	No	Yes	Colposcope/ 35mm	Macrolens/ 35mm	Colposcope/ Videocamera	Other Optics
Body	☐	☐	☐	☐	☐	☐ ______
Genitals	☐	☐	☐	☐	☐	☐ ______

Photographed by:

Patient Identification

P. RECORD EXAM METHODS

	No	Yes		No	Yes
Direct visualization only	☐	☐	Toluidine Blue Dye	☐	☐
Colposcopy	☐	☐	Anoscopic exam	☐	☐
Other magnifier	☐	☐	Anal speculum exam	☐	☐
Other	☐	☐			

If yes, describe: ______

Q. RECORD EXAM FINDINGS

☐ **Physical Findings** ☐ **No Physical Findings**

R. RECORD ASSESSMENT OF FINDINGS

☐ Exam consistent with history
☐ Exam inconsistent with history

S. SUMMARIZE FINDINGS

T. PRINT NAMES OF PERSONNEL INVOLVED

History taken by:	Telephone:
Exam performed by:	
Specimens labeled and sealed by:	
Assisted by: ☐ N/A	
Signature of examiner	License No.

U. EVIDENCE DISTRIBUTION

U. EVIDENCE DISTRIBUTION	GIVEN TO:
Clothing (item(s) not placed in evidence kit)	
Evidence Kit	
Reference blood samples	
Toxicology samples	

V. SIGNATURE OF OFFICER RECEIVING EVIDENCE

Signature: ______

Print name and ID #: ______

Agency: ______

Date: Phone:

City of Philadelphia
Department of Public Health
Medical Report—Sexual Assault Complaint

PATIENT INFORMATION:

Last Name:______________________________ First Name:_________________________

Date:_______________ Age:__________ DOB:___________ Female Male

Race:_______________ Language Spoken:____________________________________

Interpreter:____________________________ Relationship to Patient___________________

Police Vehicle #_______________________ Arrival Time:_____________

SAFE / MD Name:____

WOAR Representative:____

TIME / LOCATION OF ASSAULT

Information Provided by:____________________________________

Date/Time of Assault:_______________________________________

Place of Occurrence:____

Narrative:____

OFFENDER INFORMATION

Number of Offenders:_______________ Gender of Offender(s):_____________________

Race of Offender(s):____

Offender(s) Relationship to Victim:____

Offender is Partner / Acquaintance, history of previous violence:________________________

Examiner's Initials:________

Attending's Initials:________

PATIENT HISTORY FORM

DATE / TIME of Arrival at Hospital:______/_______/_______ @ ____________am pm

DATE / TIME of Examination:______/_______/_______ @ ____________am pm

Past Medical History:____

Past Surgical History:____

Past Psychiatric History:______________________________________

Tetanus Status:____________________ Hepatitis Status:______________________

Medications:____

Allergies:____

Social History:
Tobacco____________ Alcohol_____________ Drug Abuse___________

Review of Systems:____

□ All other ROS negative

GYN: LMP:_______________

Last Consensual Intercourse:_______________ with____________________
Condom: Yes No
Areas of Penetration:____

Tampon in place during assault Y N Removed? Y N
Location:____

Gravida__________ Para__________

Birth Control Used:___________________________________

Previous STD History:_________________________________

Examiner's Initials:_______

Attending's Initials:_______

ACTS OF ASSAULT

Key: Yes = Y
No = N
Unsure = U

Kissing, Licking, Biting of Victim	N	Y	U	Location____________________
Fondling of Victim	N	Y	U	Location____________________
Vaginal Penetration with:				
Penis	N	Y	U	
Offender's Fingers	N	Y	U	
Offender's Tongue	N	Y	U	
Foreign Object	N	Y	U	Describe:____________________
Other	N	Y	U	Describe:____________________
Anal Penetration with:				
Penis	N	Y	U	
Offender's Fingers	N	Y	U	
Offender's Tongue	N	Y	U	
Foreign Object	N	Y	U	Describe:____________________
Other	N	Y	U	Describe:____________________
Oral Penetration with:				
Penis	N	Y	U	
Offender's Fingers	N	Y	U	
Offender's Tongue	N	Y	U	
Foreign Object	N	Y	U	Describe:____________________
Other	N	Y	U	Describe:____________________
Other Oral Acts:				
Victim Mouth to Offender Genitals	N	Y	U	
Victim Mouth to Offender Anus	N	Y	U	
Offender Mouth to Victim Genitals	N	Y	U	
Offender Mouth to Victim Anus	N	Y	U	
Did offender ejaculate?	N	Y	U	
Vagina	N	Y	U	
Anus	N	Y	U	
Mouth	N	Y	U	
Other	N	Y	U	Describe:____________________

Examiner's Initials:________

3

Attending's Initials:________

ACTS OF ASSAULT Cont'd

Did offender use a condom?	N	Y	U	
Was it left at site?	N	Y	U	
Did offender use lubricant?	N	Y	U	
Was it left at site?	N	Y	U	
Type:____				
Verbal Threat	N	Y	U	Describe:__________________
Knife	N	Y	U	Describe:__________________
Gun	N	Y	U	Describe:__________________
Choking	N	Y	U	
Hitting	N	Y	U	Describe:__________________
Pushing	N	Y	U	Describe:__________________
Gag	N	Y	U	
Blindfold	N	Y	U	

Other Acts:____

____

Examiner's Initials:________

Attending's Initials:________

HISTORY SINCE ATTACK

Since the Attack have you....

Bathed or Showered?	No	Yes
Washed your Hair?	No	Yes
Changed clothes?	No	Yes
Washed clothes?	No	Yes
Urinated?	No	Yes
Defecated?	No	Yes
Douched?	No	Yes
Vomited?	No	Yes
Used any contraceptives?	No	Yes
Drank or ate?	No	Yes
Drank any alcohol?	No	Yes
Brushed your teeth?	No	Yes
Used mouthwash?	No	Yes
Used dental floss?	No	Yes

Used tissue / towel / paper / clothing to wipe off any fluid?	No	Yes
Used tissue / towel / paper / clothing to wipe off genitals?	No	Yes
Used / discarded any tampon or pad since assault?	No	Yes

Examiner's Initials:________

Attending's Initials:________

PHYSICAL EXAM

Temp________ Pulse_________ Resp_______ BP___________

General:____

Mental Status:___________________________________
Orientation:_____________________________________
Cognition:______________________________________
Affect/Mood:____________________________________

	NL	ABN	Comments
HEENT	[]	[]	________________________________
Neck	[]	[]	________________________________
Lungs	[]	[]	________________________________
Chest/Heart	[]	[]	________________________________
Breasts	[]	[]	________________________________
Abdomen	[]	[]	________________________________
Upper Ext.	[]	[]	________________________________
Lower Ext.	[]	[]	________________________________
Buttocks	[]	[]	________________________________
Neuro	[]	[]	________________________________

LEFT RIGHT LEFT RIGHT RIGHT LEFT

LEFT

Examiner's Initials:________

Attending's Initials:________

6

PHYSICAL EXAM

Tanner Stage:_______________

Female:

	NL	ABN	Comments
Ext. Genitalia	[]	[]	______
Labia Majora	[]	[]	______
Labia Minora	[]	[]	______
Fossa Navicularis	[]	[]	______
Posterior fourchette	[]	[]	______
Vagina	[]	[]	______
Cervix	[]	[]	______
Perineum	[]	[]	______
Bimanual Exam	[]	[]	______
Anus	[]	[]	______

Male:

	NL	ABN	Comments
Penis	[]	[]	______
Scrotum	[]	[]	______
Testes	[]	[]	______
Perineum	[]	[]	______
Anus	[]	[]	______

UV Light Reaction [] No []Yes [] Not indicated
If Yes, describe_______________

Toluidine Dye Uptake [] Negative uptake [] Yes (+) [] Not indicated
If uptake (+), describe_______________

Colposcopy Used [] No [] Yes [] Not indicated

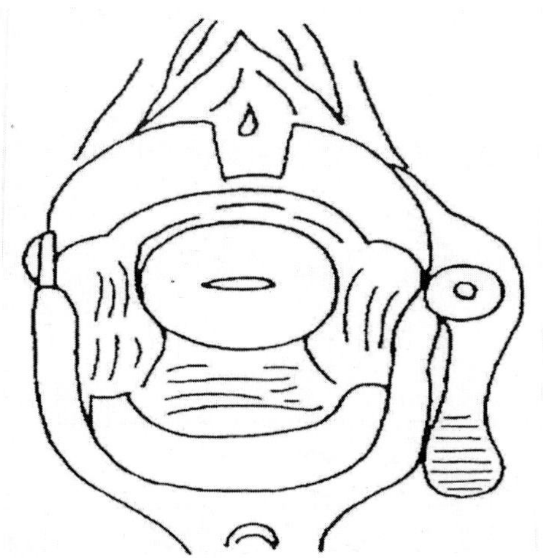

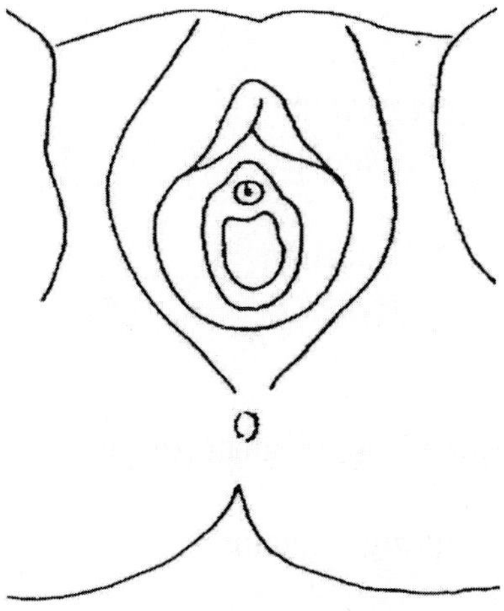

Examiner's Initials:_______

Attending's Initials:_______

DISPOSITION

Laboratory Studies:

Urine hCG	[] Yes [] Not indicated		Result: [] Pos [] Neg
RPR	[] Yes [] Not indicated		
STD Probe	[] Vaginal	[] Anal	[] Oral

Other:____

□ Pregnancy Prophylaxis
- □ Plan B: Levonogesterol 1 pill now and 1 in 12 hours
- □ Ovral: 2 pills now and 2 in 12 hours

□ Gonorrhea Prophylaxis
- □ Rocephin 250mg IM
- □ Ciprofloxacin 500mg po x 1
- □ Cefixime 400mg po x 1

□ Chlamydia Prophylaxis
- □ Azithromycin 1gram po x 1
- □ Doxycycline 100mg po now, then 1 po BID x 7 days

□ Trichomonas Prophylaxis
- □ Flagyl 500mg 4 pills po x 1

□ Tetanus Prophylaxis
- □ dT 0.5cc IM x1

□ Hepatitis B Prophylaxis
- □ Heptavax 1cc IM now then again in 1 month and 6 months

FOLLOW-UP

Date:____________________ at ______:______ am/pm

Location______________________________________

Examiner(s) Signature:____

Attending Signature:____

Examiner's Initials:______ 8

Attending's Initials:______

PATIENT CONSENT

Authorization to Evaluate Patient for Possible Abuse

A. Conditions

1. I understand that the examination for evidence of physical/sexual assault can, with my consent, be conducted by an examiner to discover and preserve evidence of the assault. I understand that I may withdraw my consent at any time for any portion of the evidential examination.

2. Photographs and video prints may be taken as evidence. Like all evidence collected in this evaluation, these records are to be used for medical treatment and legal purposes.

B. Authorization

I give permission for ____ to evaluate me or ________________________________. I certify that I have read, understand, and agree to the conditions described in section A.

________________________ ________________ ____________
Signature Witness Date

I understand that the collection of evidence may include photographing injuries and in cases of sexual assault, may include the genital area. Knowing this, I consent to having photographs taken.

________________________ ________________ ____________
Signature Witness Date

I understand that any photographs taken may be used for educational purposes and if used for such purposes, my identity will be kept confidential.

- ☐ I consent to the use of photography for educational purposes
- ☐ I refuse to consent to the use of photography for educational purposes

________________________ ________________ ____________
Signature Witness Date

C. Release of Information

I hereby authorize______________________________Hospital to release medical information and reports regarding any examination and treatment for sexual assault to the Philadelphia Police and to the Philadelphia District Attorney's Office.

Date:______________ Patient Signature:________________________________

Date:______________ Parent/Guardian Signature______________________________
Relationship______________________________

Witness:________________________ Address:______________________________

Examiner's Initials:________

Attending's Initials:________

City of Philadelphia
Department of Public Health
Medical Report—Sexual Assault Complaint

EVIDENCE COLLECTED

CLOTHING

□ None
□ Panties/Underpants-Describe____________________
□ Shirt/Blouse-Describe____________________
□ Pants/Slacks-Describe____________________
□ Skirt/Dress-Describe____________________
□ Bra/Undershirt-Describe____________________
□ Jacket/Coat-Describe____________________
□ Nightgown/PJ's-Describe____________________
□ Other:____________________
□ Other:____________________

RAPE KIT

□ None
□ Changing sheet
□ Oral Swab
□ Vulvar Swab
□ Vaginal Swab
□ Cervix Swab
□ Rectal Swab
□ Perineum Swab
□ Debris-Source________________
Description________________
□ Secretions-Source____________
Description________________
□ Bite Mark Size________________
□ Hair Combings-Source
□ Blood / Purple Top

PHOTOGRAPHS

Taken: YES NO

Type: Camera Colposcope

\# of photos:_______
Photographer:__________________________

CHAIN OF CUSTODY

□ All items listed are labeled, sealed, and locked in evidence refrigerator.

□ All items listed received from:

Name:________________________ by:____________________ Badge:__________

Date:__________________ Time:____________________

Signature____

Signature____

Examiner's Initials:_______

Attending's Initials:_______

State of California
Governor's Office of Emergency Services

FORENSIC MEDICAL REPORT: DOMESTIC VIOLENCE EXAMINATION

OES 502

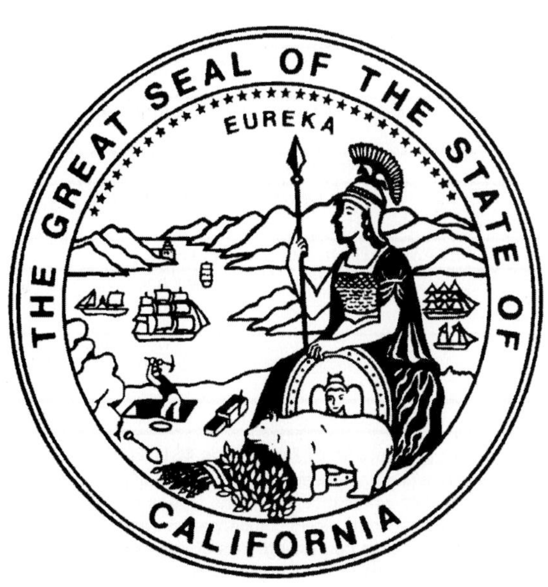

For more information or assistance in completing the OES 502, please contact University of California, Davis California Medical Training Center at: (888) 705-4141or **www.calmtc.org**

This form is available on the following website:
http://www.oes.ca.gov
Criminal Justice Programs Division
Publications and Brochures

FORENSIC MEDICAL REPORT: DOMESTIC VIOLENCE EXAMINATION
State of California
Governor's Office of Emergency Services
OES 502

Confidential Document: Restricted Release

Patient Identification: Date:

A. GENERAL INFORMATION

1. Patient's Last Name First Name M.I.

2. Street Address (optional) | City | County | State | Zip Code | Telephone (optional) (Home) (Work) (Safe)

3. Age | DOB | Gender F M MTF FTM | Ethnicity (check all that apply)
☐ White ☐ Black / African American ☐ Hispanic / Latino ☐ Asian ☐ American Indian / Alaskan Native ☐ Native Hawaiian / Other Pacific Islander ☐ Other_____

4. Name of Facility Where Forensic Exam Performed | Address of Facility

5. Patient Arrival		Patient Discharge		6. Exam Started		Exam Completed	
Date	Time	Date	Time	Date	Time	Date	Time

7. Interpreter Used ☐ No ☐ Yes Language Used:_____

Name of Interpreter:_____ Telephone:_____

Affiliation of interpreter: ☐ Facility Interpreting Services
☐ Contracted Agency, specify:_____
☐ Family ☐ Friend ☐ Other, specify:_____

B. MANDATORY SUSPICIOUS INJURY REPORT (Pursuant to Pen. Code §11160)

1. Name of Person Making Mandated Telephone Report to Law Enforcement Agency | Date | Time

2. Name of Person Taking Telephone Report | Name of Law Enforcement Agency | ☐ OES 920 Written Report Submitted

C. RESPONDING OFFICER TO MEDICAL FACILITY ☐ Not Applicable

Law Enforcement Officer | Name of Law EnforcementAgency | ID Number

D. AUTHORIZATION FOR MEDICAL EVIDENTIARY EXAMINATION: Follow Local Policy ☐ Not Applicable

Law Enforcement Officer | Name of Law Enforcement Agency | ID Number

Telephone | Date | Time | Case Number

E. PATIENT INFORMATION

1. I understand that hospitals and health care professionals are required by Penal Code §§11160-11161 to report to law enforcement authorities cases in which medical care is sought when injuries have been inflicted upon any person in violation of any state penal law. The report must state the name of the injured person, current whereabouts, and the type and extent of injuries. ____(initial)
2. I have been informed that victims of crime are eligible to submit crime victim compensation claims to the California Victim Compensation Program (VCP) for out-of-pocket medical expenses, psychological counseling, loss of wages, and job retraining and rehabilitation. ____(initial)
3. I have been informed about domestic violence advocacy services or a social services professional who can provide me with counseling and support. ____(initial)

F. PATIENT CONSENT

1. I understand that a forensic medical examination for evidence of domestic violence can, with my consent, be conducted by a health care professional to discover and preserve evidence of the assault. If conducted, the report of the examination and any evidence obtained will be released to law enforcement authorities. I understand that the examination may include the collection of reference specimens at the time of the examination or at a later date. I understand that I may withdraw consent at any time for any portion of the examination. ____(initial)
2. I understand that collection of evidence may include audio/visual recordings and photographing injuries and that these photographs may include the genital area. ____(initial)
3. I hereby consent to a forensic medical examination for evidence of domestic violence. ____(initial)
4. I understand that data without patient identity from this report may be collected for health and forensic purposes, and provided to health authorities and other qualified persons with a valid educational or scientific interest. ____(initial)

☐ Patient ☐ Parent ☐ Guardian ☐ Surrogate

Print Name_____ Signature_____ Date_____

G. DISTRIBUTION OF OES 502 (check all that apply)

☐ Law Enforcement Officer - Original ☐ Crime Lab - Copy within evidence kit ☐ Medical or Agency Facility Records - Copy

H. CURRENT ASSAULT HISTORY

1. Examination audio and/or videotaped
☐ No ☐ Yes ☐ Audio ☐ Video

2. Name of person providing history | Relationship to Patient

3. Date(s) of Assault | Time/Time Frame of Assault

Patient Identification: **Date:**

4. Describe Physical Surroundings of Assault

5. Patient Description of Assault

☐ Additional attached pages

6. Assailant(s)

#1	Assailant's Name	DOB	Age	Gender	Ethnicity

Relationship to Patient: (check all that apply)
☐ Spouse ☐ Cohabitant/Domestic Partner ☐ Dating Relationship ☐ Child Together
☐ Former Spouse ☐ Former Cohabitant/Domestic Partner ☐ Former Dating Relationship ☐ Other
Current Whereabouts: ☐ Unknown ☐ In Custody ☐ Known Location

#2	Assailant's Name	DOB	Age	Gender	Ethnicity

Relationship to Patient: (check all that apply)
☐ Spouse ☐ Cohabitant/Domestic Partner ☐ Dating Relationship ☐ Child Together
☐ Former Spouse ☐ Former Cohabitant/Domestic Partner ☐ Former Dating Relationship ☐ Other
Current Whereabouts: ☐ Unknown ☐ In Custody ☐ Known Location:

7. Methods employed by assailant(s) and circumstances

	No	Yes	If yes:
Weapons	☐	☐	☐ Firearm ☐ Knife ☐ Blunt Object ☐ Other
Threatened?	☐	☐	Describe:
Displayed?	☐	☐	Describe:
Used?	☐	☐	Describe:
Injuries?	☐	☐	Describe:

Physical blows ☐ by hands ☐ by feet ☐ by head ☐ Other, describe:
☐ Grabbing ☐ Holding ☐ Pinching ☐ Slapping ☐ Punching ☐ Other, describe:
Hair pulling? ☐ No ☐ Yes ☐ If yes, describe:
Physical restraints ☐ No ☐ Yes ☐ If yes, describe:

Strangulation

One Hand	Two Hands	Forearm
Frontal Assault	Frontal Assault	Frontal Assault
Rear Assault	Rear Assault	Rear Assault

☐ Ligature, describe:

Bites ☐ No ☐ Yes, describe:
Burns ☐ Thermal ☐ Chemical ☐ Other
Threat(s) of harm ☐ No ☐ Yes If yes, target of threat: ☐ Patient ☐ Children ☐ Pet(s) ☐ Property ☐ Other, describe:
Describe what was said or done:

Sexual relations with assailant as part of this assault? ☐ No ☐ Unsure ☐ Yes If yes: ☐ Forced ☐ Coerced
Involuntary use of alcohol/drugs ☐ No ☐ Yes If yes: ☐ Forced ☐ Coerced ☐ Suspected
If yes: ☐ Alcohol ☐ Drugs Describe:

8. Injuries inflicted upon assailant(s) during assault ☐ No ☐ Unsure ☐ Yes, describe:

9. Post assault hygiene
☐ Bath / shower / wash ☐ Clothes change ☐ Other, describe:

I. CURRENT SYMPTOMS REPORTED BY PATIENT
(check all that apply)

Symptoms	From This Event	From Past Event(s)
Neurological		
Headache		
Dizziness		
Memory/Concentration Problems		
Lightheaded		
Visual Changes		
Hearing Changes		
Loss of Consciousness		
Numbness		
Weakness		
Other		
Psychological		
Acute Anxiety		
Depression		
Suicide Ideation		
Homicide Ideation		
Other		
Cardiorespiratory		
Voice Change		
Coughing		
Shortness of Breath		
Chest Pain		
Palpitations		
Other		
Gastrointestinal		
Sore Throat		
Difficulty Swallowing		
Nausea		
Vomiting		
Diarrhea		
Abdominal Pain		
Hematemesis		
Rectal Bleeding		
Rectal Pain		
Penis/Testicular Pain		
Other		
Urogenital		
Pelvic Pain		
Dysuria		
Vaginal Bleeding		
Vaginal Discharge		
Other		
Musculoskeletal		
Extremity Pain		
Neck Pain		
Back Pain		
Deformity		
Other		
Other		
Other		

Patient Identification: **Date:**

J. PATIENT HISTORY

1. **Disability** ☐ No ☐ Yes
   If yes: ☐ Cognitive ☐ Physical ☐ Blind ☐ Deaf/HOH ☐ Mental

2. **History of prior physical assault(s) with this assailant?**
   ☐ No ☐ Yes If yes, past injuries to patient? ☐ No ☐ Yes, describe: ____________

3. **Prior history of forced or coerced sexual relations with this assailant?** ☐ No ☐ Yes, describe:
   Approximate Date(s): ____________

4. **Has patient sought medical care for prior assault(s) by this assailant?** ☐ No ☐ Yes
   If yes, name of facility: ____________
   If yes, under what name(s)? ____________
   If yes, approximate date(s): ____________

5. **Obstetrical History** Pregnant? ☐ No ☐ Yes ☐ Unknown
   If yes, any possible problems related to current assault(s)?
   ☐ No ☐ Yes, describe: ____________
   Any possible problems in past pregnancies related to past assault(s) by this assailant?
   ☐ No ☐ Yes, describe: ____________

6. Name(s) of Children/Dependent Adults Living in Household	Present During Assault(s)			Gender	DOB or Age
	No	Yes	UNK		
				M F	
				M F	
				M F	
				M F	
				M F	

7. **Voluntary Use of Alcohol/Drugs** ☐ No ☐ Yes
   Any voluntary alcohol use within 12 hrs prior to assault? ☐ No ☐ Yes
   Any voluntary drug use within 96 hrs prior to assault? ☐ No ☐ Yes
   Any voluntary drug ☐ or alcohol ☐ use between time of assault and forensic exam? ☐ No ☐ Yes
   List drug(s) used: ____________

8. **Are there other ways the patient's life has been impacted by behaviors of this assailant?**

Note: For history of sexual assault (<72 hours), stop and consult with law enforcement prior to beginning physical exam to determine next steps.

K. GENERAL PHYSICAL EXAMINATION			
1. Blood Pressure	Pulse	Respiration	Temp
2. Describe general physical appearance			
3. Describe general demeanor			

Patient Identification: **Date:**

4. Describe condition of clothing upon arrival. Collect outer and under clothing if applicable. ☐ Not Applicable

5. Examine the face, head, ears, hair, scalp, neck, and mouth for injury. Document findings using photographs, diagrams, legend, and consecutive numbering system.

6. Collect dried and moist secretions, stains and foreign materials from the scalp, head and neck.

A

C

E

B

D

F

LEGEND: Types of Findings ☐ Findings ☐ No Findings ☐ Additional copies of this page attached

AB	Abrasion	**DS**	Dry Secretion	**IN**	Induration	**OI**	Other Injury (describe)	**TA**	Tooth Avulsed
BI	Bite	**EC**	Ecchymosis (bruise)	**IW**	Incised Wound	**PE**	Petechiae	**TD**	Tooth Decay
BU	Burn	**ER**	Erythema (redness)	**LA**	Laceration	**PS**	Potential Saliva	**TF**	Tooth Fractured
CS	Control Swab	**FB**	Foreign Body	**MS**	Moist Secretion	**SI**	Suction Injuries	**TM**	Tooth Missing
DE	Debris	**F/H**	Fiber/Hair	**OF**	Other Foreign Materials (describe)	**SW**	Swelling	**V/S**	Vegetation/Soil
DF	Deformity	**FT**	Frenulum Torn			**TE**	Tenderness		

Locator #	Type	Description	Locator #	Type	Description

K. GENERAL PHYSICAL EXAMINATION (continued)

7. Conduct a physical examination of body and extremities. Record findings using photographs, diagrams, legend, and a consecutive numbering system.
8. Collect dried and moist secretions, stains and foreign materials from body ☐ Findings ☐ No Findings
9. Collect fingernail scrapings/cuttings according to local policy ☐ Done ☐ Not Applicable

Patient Identification: **Date:**

G

H

LEGEND: Types of Findings ☐ Findings ☐ No Findings ☐ Additional copies of this page attached

AB	Abrasion	DS	Dry Secretion	IW	Incised Wound	PE	Petechiae
BI	Bite	EC	Ecchymosis (bruise)	LA	Laceration	PS	Potential Saliva
BU	Burn	ER	Erythema (redness)	MS	Moist Secretion	SI	Suction Injuries
CS	Control Swab	FB	Foreign Body	OF	Other Foreign Materials (describe)	SW	Swelling
DE	Debris	F/H	Fiber/Hair			TE	Tenderness
DF	Deformity	IN	Induration	OI	Other Injury (describe)	VS	Vegetation/Soil

Locator #	Type	Description	Locator #	Type	Description

K. GENERAL PHYSICAL EXAMINATION (continued)

10. Use diagrams I and J to record findings to lateral or medial aspect of trunk or extremities. Record findings.

11. If genital injuries sustained, use pages 6 and 7 from OES 923 Forensic Medical Report: Acute Adult/Adolescent Sexual Assault Examination form to document findings. Are OES 923 pages 6 & 7 attached? ☐ Yes ☐ No ☐ Not applicable

Patient Identification: **Date:**

I

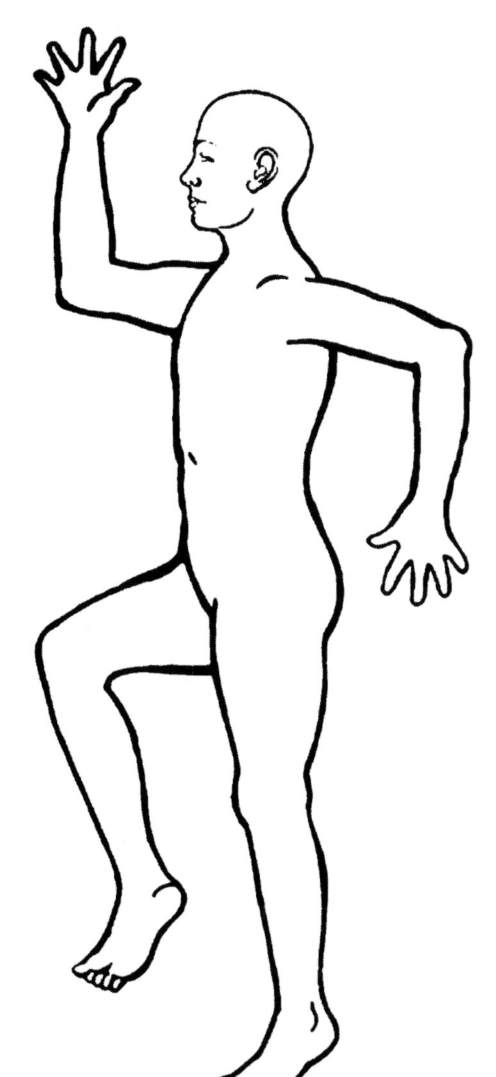

J

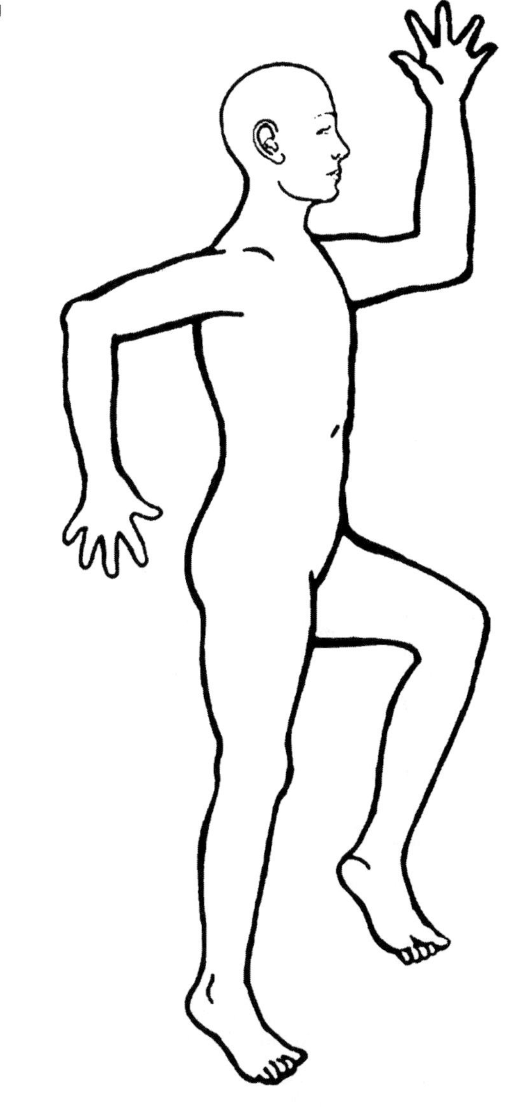

LEGEND: Types of Findings ☐ Findings ☐ No Findings ☐ Additional copies of this page attached

AB Abrasion
BI Bite
BU Burn
CS Control Swab
DE Debris
DF Deformity
DS Dry Secretion
EC Ecchymosis (bruise)
ER Erythema (redness)
FB Foreign Body
F/H Fiber/Hair
IN Induration
IW Incised Wound
LA Laceration
MS Moist Secretion
OF Other Foreign Materials (describe)
OI Other Injury (describe)
PE Petechiae
PS Potential Saliva
SI Suction Injuries
SW Swelling
TE Tenderness
VS Vegetation/Soil

Locator #	Type	Description	Locator #	Type	Description

L. EVIDENCE COLLECTED AND SUBMITTED TO CRIME LAB

1. Clothing Collected ☐ No ☐ Yes		Clothing Placed in Evidence Kit	Clothing Placed in Paper Bag
Bra	☐		
Dress/skirt	☐		
Jacket/sweater	☐		
Nylons	☐		
Pants/shorts	☐		
Shirt/top	☐		
Shoes (1 or 2)	☐		
Socks (1 or 2)	☐		
Underwear	☐		
Undershirt	☐		
Other	☐		

2. Foreign Materials Collected

	N/A	No	Yes	Collected by:
Swabs/suspected blood	☐	☐	☐	
Dried secretions	☐	☐	☐	
Fiber/loose hairs	☐	☐	☐	
Soil/debris/vegetation	☐	☐	☐	
Swabs/suspected saliva	☐	☐	☐	
Foreign body	☐	☐	☐	
Fingernail scrapings	☐	☐	☐	
Control swabs	☐	☐	☐	

Other, describe:__________

3. Laboratory Results Additional Page ☐ Yes ☐ No

Pregnancy ☐ Positive ☐ Negative

Additional Labs: ☐ No ☐ Yes, specify:__________

4. X-Ray/Imaging Results Additional Page ☐ Yes ☐ No

☐ No ☐ Yes, specify: __________

5. Toxicology Samples

	N/A	No	Yes	Time	Collected by:
Blood Alcohol / Toxicology	☐	☐	☐		
Urine Toxicology	☐	☐	☐		

6. Reference Samples ☐ Blood ☐ Saliva ☐ Buccal ☐ N/A

Collected by:__________

7. Photo Documentation

☐ No ☐ Yes **35mm** ☐ **Digital** ☐ **Instant** ☐ **Other** ☐______

Photography by:__________ # Rolls/images ______

Recommend follow-up photographs to be taken in 1-2 days

☐ No ☐ Yes ☐ Not applicable

8. Voice recording for strangulation injuries

☐ **No** ☐ **Yes** **If yes:** ☐ **Audio** ☐ **Audiovideo**

If yes, obtained by: ☐ Examiner ☐ Law Enforcement

M. SUMMARY OF KEY FINDINGS

Patient Identification: **Date:**

N. PERTINENT ISSUES AFFECTING EXAMINATION

O. PERSONNEL INVOLVED

Name (print clearly)			Phone
History taken by:			
Physical exam performed by:			
Specimens labeled and sealed by:			
Assisted by: ☐ N/A			
Additional narrative by: ☐ N/A			
Signature of Examiner	Date		License Number

P. DISTRIBUTION OF EVIDENCE

	Released To
Clothing (items not placed in evidence kit)	
Evidence Kit	
Reference samples	
Toxicology samples	
Recording(s) ☐ Audio ☐ Audiovideo	

Q. DISPOSITION AND FOLLOW UP

☐ Discharged ☐ Admitted ☐ Follow Up Exam Scheduled

☐ Cross Reporting to: ☐ CPS ☐ APS ☐ N/A

☐ Referral to domestic violence advocacy services

☐ Safety plan discussed with patient

☐ Referral to counseling, drug, and alcohol treatment services

☐ Referral to Victim Witness Assistance Program

☐ Referral for Protective Order **OR** EPO. ☐ PO or EPO Granted

R. SIGNATURE OF OFFICER

I have received the evidence indicated above:

Printed Name ID Number

Signature

Agency Telephone

State of California
Governor's Office of Emergency Services

FORENSIC MEDICAL REPORT: ELDER AND DEPENDENT ADULT ABUSE AND NEGLECT EXAMINATION

OES 602

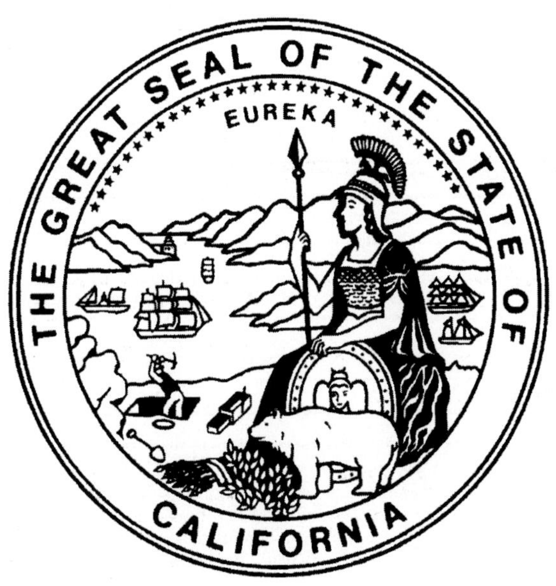

For more information or assistance in completing the OES 602, please contact University of California, Davis California Medical Training Center at: (888) 705-4141 or **www.calmtc.org**

This form is available on the following website:
http://www.oes.ca.gov
Criminal Justice Programs Division
Publications and Brochures

Forensic Medical Report: Elder and Dependent Adult Abuse & Neglect Examination State of California Governor's Office of Emergency Services OES 602 PART 1: INTERVIEW

Confidential Document: Restricted Release **Patient Identification:** **Date:**

A. GENERAL INFORMATION ☐ Elder Abuse Exam ☐ Dependent Adult Abuse Exam

1. Patient's Last Name First Name M.I.

2. Street Address	City	County	State	Zip Code	Telephone (Home) (Work)

3. Age	DOB	Gender	Ethnicity		
		☐ Female ☐ Male	☐ White ☐ Black / African American	☐ Hispanic / Latino ☐ Asian ☐ American Indian / Alaskan Native	☐ Native Hawaiian / Other Pacific Islander ☐ Other ________

4. Name and address of facility where exam performed	If patient transferred from another facility, name and address of facility

5. Patient Arrival		Patient Discharged		6. Exam Started		Exam Completed	
Date	Time	Date	Time	Date	Time	Date	Time

7. **Interpreter Used** ☐ No ☐ Yes Language Used: ________
Name of Interpreter: ________ Telephone: ________
Affiliation of interpreter: ☐ Facility Interpreting Services
☐ Contracted Agency, specify: ________
☐ Family ☐ Friend ☐ Other, specify: ________

B. MANDATORY REPORTING FOR ELDER AND DEPENDENT ADULT ABUSE

☐ Adult Protective Services ☐ Ombudsman ☐ Law Enforcement ☐ Other: ________ ☐ Telephone Report

Name of Person Taking Telephone Report Date Name of Agency ☐ Written Report Submitted

Name of Person Taking Telephone Report Date Name of Agency ☐ Written Report Submitted

C. RESPONDING PERSONNEL TO MEDICAL FACILITY ☐ Law Enforcement ☐ APS ☐ Ombudsman

Name	Agency	ID Number	Telephone

D. REQUEST AND AUTHORIZATION FOR MEDICAL EVIDENTIARY EXAM: Follow local policy ☐ Not Applicable

	Name	Agency	ID Number
☐ Law Enforcement Officer ☐ Adult Protective Services ☐ Ombudsman			

E. PATIENT INFORMATION

1. I understand that hospitals and health care professionals are required by Penal Code §11160-11161 to report to law enforcement authorities cases in which medical care is sought when injuries have been inflicted upon any person in violation of any state penal law. The report must state the name of the injured person, current whereabouts, and the type and extent of injuries. ____(initial)
2. I have been informed that victims of crime are eligible to submit crime victim compensation claims to the California Victim Compensation Program (VCP) for out-of-pocket medical expenses, psychological counseling, loss of wages, job retraining and rehabilitation. ____(initial)

F. PATIENT CONSENT

1. I understand that a medical evidentiary examination for evidence of abuse and/or neglect can, with my consent, be conducted by a health care professional to discover and preserve evidence. If conducted, the report of the examination and any evidence obtained will be released to investigative authorities. I understand that the examination may include the collection of reference specimens at the time of the examination or at a later date. I understand that I may withdraw consent at any time for any portion of the examination. ____(initial)
2. I understand that collection of evidence may include photographing injuries and that these photographs may include the genital area. ____(initial)
3. I hereby consent to a medical evidentiary examination for evidence of abuse and/or neglect. ____(initial)
4. I understand that data without patient identity from this report may be collected for health and forensic purposes, and provided to health authorities and other qualified persons with a valid educational or scientific interest for demographic and/or epidemiological studies. ____(initial)

☐ Patient ☐ Surrogate ☐ Conservator ☐ Other: ________

Print Name ________ Signature ________ Date ________

G. DISTRIBUTION OF OES 602 (check all that apply)

☐ Local Law Enforcement - Original ☐ Adult Protective Services - Copy ☐ Crime Lab - Copy ☐ Ombudsman - Copy ☐ Other Agency
☐ Medical Facility Records - Copy ☐ Bureau of Medi-Cal Fraud & Elder Abuse - Copy ☐ District Attorney - Copy Specify: ________

PART I: INTERVIEW
PATIENT HISTORY

H. SUSPECTED TYPES OF ABUSE BEING REPORTED

1. Interview audio and/or video taped ☐ No ☐ Yes

Patient Identification: **Date:**

2. Name(s) of person(s) providing history	**Relationship to patient**	**Telephone**

3. Form(s) of abuse and neglect described

	No	Yes	Unknown	Describe
Physical Abuse				
1. Physical blows and/or ☐ grabbing ☐ holding ☐ pinching ☐ pushing	☐	☐	☐	
2. Strangulation	☐	☐	☐	
3. Bites	☐	☐	☐	
4. Weapons ☐ Firearm ☐ Knife ☐ Blunt object ☐ Other	☐	☐	☐	
5. Burns ☐ Thermal ☐ Chemical	☐	☐	☐	
6. Physical restraints	☐	☐	☐	
7. Chemical restraints	☐	☐	☐	
8. Poisoning	☐	☐	☐	
9. Involuntary alcohol/drug use	☐	☐	☐	
Sexual Assault (Consult with law enforcement)	☐	☐	☐	
Financial				
1. Misappropriation of money	☐	☐	☐	
2. Property transfer	☐	☐	☐	
3. Other: ______	☐	☐	☐	
Abandonment				
1. Desertion	☐	☐	☐	
2. Patient left alone in unsafe circumstances	☐	☐	☐	
Isolation				
1. False imprisonment	☐	☐	☐	
2. Patient prevented from seeing family/social contacts	☐	☐	☐	
3. Patient prevented from receiving mail/phone calls	☐	☐	☐	
4. Patient prevented from keeping appointments with medical, legal, or other service providers	☐	☐	☐	
Abduction	☐	☐	☐	
Neglect				
1. Unsafe environment	☐	☐	☐	
2. Inadequate provision for heat or cooling	☐	☐	☐	
3. Malnutrition	☐	☐	☐	
4. Dehydration	☐	☐	☐	
5. Pressure ulcers	☐	☐	☐	
6. Medication not given as prescribed	☐	☐	☐	
7. Failure to provide patient with glasses, walker, wheel-chair, hearing aide, dentures, or assistive devices	☐	☐	☐	
8. Failure to seek physician services or follow physician orders	☐	☐	☐	
9. Care plan not followed	☐	☐	☐	
Self-Neglect				
1. Failure to live in a safe environment	☐	☐	☐	
2. Inability or failure to perform self-care tasks	☐	☐	☐	
Psychological Abuse				
1. Threats of harm/intimidation If yes, target of threat: ☐ patient ☐ family ☐ pet ☐ other	☐	☐	☐	
2. Harassment	☐	☐	☐	
3. Emotional abuse	☐	☐	☐	
Other:	☐	☐	☐	

I. ALLEGED PERPETRATOR(S)

Name(s)	Age/DOB	Gender	Ethnicity	Address	Telephone	Relationship to patient

J. LOCATION WHERE ABUSE AND NEGLECT OCCURRED

PART I: INTERVIEW
FUNCTIONAL, COGNITIVE, MENTAL HEALTH, AND SUBSTANCE ABUSE SCREENING

Patient Identification: **Date:**

K. FUNCTIONAL HISTORY: Indicate any limitations

	Independent	Needs Assistance	Totally Dependent	Unknown		Independent	Needs Assistance	Totally Dependent	Unknown
Bathing	☐	☐	☐	☐	Medication management	☐	☐	☐	☐
Dressing	☐	☐	☐	☐	Housekeeping	☐	☐	☐	☐
Going to toilet	☐	☐	☐	☐	Laundry	☐	☐	☐	☐
Transferring	☐	☐	☐	☐	Transportation management	☐	☐	☐	☐
Continence	☐	☐	☐	☐	Handling finances	☐	☐	☐	☐
Eating	☐	☐	☐	☐	Vision	☐	☐	☐	☐
Telephoning	☐	☐	☐	☐	Hearing	☐	☐	☐	☐
Shopping	☐	☐	☐	☐	Communication	☐	☐	☐	☐
Preparing meals	☐	☐	☐	☐	Judgement	☐	☐	☐	☐

L. DISABILITY? ☐ No ☐ Yes If yes, ☐ Cognitive ☐ Developmental ☐ Physical ☐ Blind ☐ Deaf/HOH ☐ Mental

M. COGNITIVE ASSESSMENT - MINI-MENTAL STATE EXAM (Score one point for each correct answer)

Max. Points	Patient Score	
		Orientation
5	( )	What is the (year) (season) (date) (day) (month)?
5	( )	Where are we (state) (county) (town/city) (building) (floor)?
		Registration
3	( )	Ask patient to name three common objects (e.g., "apple," "table," "penny") ____________ Take one second to say each. Then ask the patient to repeat all three after you have said them. Give one point for each correct answer. Then repeat them until he/she learns all three. Count trials and record. Trials: ( )
		Attention and Calculation
5	( )	Spell "world" backwards. The score is the number of letters in the correct order. (D__L__R__O__W__)
		Recall
3	( )	Ask for the three objects repeated above. Give one point for each correct answer. (Note: recall cannot be tested if all three objects were not remembered during registration.)
		Language
2	( )	Name a "pencil" and a "watch."
1	( )	Repeat the following: "no if's, and's, or but's."
3	( )	Follow a three-state command: "Take a paper in your right hand, fold it in half and put it on the floor."
1	( )	Read and obey the following: "Close your eyes"
1	( )	Write a sentence
1	( )	Copy this design
		Scoring **Number of years of education:** _______
30	( )	Total
	( )	Age/education corrected score (see instructions)

N. MENTAL HEALTH AND SUBSTANCE ABUSE SCREENING

Ask the patient:	No	Yes
1. Do you feel your life is empty?	☐	☐
2. Do you often feel sad?	☐	☐
3. Do you feel "pretty worthless" the way you are now?	☐	☐
4. Have you had recent thoughts of suicide?	☐	☐
5. Do you have a history of substance abuse?	☐	☐

O. INTERVIEWER FOR PART I

Signature

Printed Name ID No./License No.

Agency/Facility

Telephone Date

PART II: MEDICAL ASSESSMENT

P. ABUSE AND NEGLECT RELATED MEDICAL HISTORY | **Patient Identification:** | **Date:**

1. Date(s) of abuse and/or neglect | **Time/time frame of abuse and/or neglect**

2. Description of abuse and/or neglect: ______

3. Past history of abuse? ☐ No ☐ Yes ☐ Unknown When? ______
Reported? ☐ No ☐ Yes ☐ Unknown Where? ______

4. Any recent (60 days) surgeries, diagnostic procedures, psychiatric or medical treatment that may affect the interpretation of current physical or cognitive findings? ☐ No ☐ Yes ☐ Unknown If yes, describe ______

5. Any other pertinent medical condition(s) that may affect the interpretation of current physical findings?
☐ No ☐ Yes Unknown If yes, describe: ______

6. Any pre-existing physical injuries? ☐ No ☐ Yes ☐ Unknown If yes, describe: ______

7. Name(s) of current/prior health care providers	**Address**	**Telephone**

8. Current use of medication(s) ☐ **No** ☐ **Yes** ☐ **Unknown**	**Dose/frequency**	**Time of last dose**
Aspirin		
Nonsteroidal anti-inflammatory drugs		
Coumadin		

9. Abuse and/or neglect related cognitive change(s)?	No	Yes	Unknown	
Loss of memory?	☐	☐	☐	______
Change in level of consciousness?	☐	☐	☐	______
Recent consumption of alcohol?	☐	☐	☐	______
If yes, collection of toxicology samples is recommended according to local policy. ☐ Blood ☐ Urine				______
Other	☐	☐	☐	______

PART II: MEDICAL ASSESSMENT

Patient Identification: Date:

Q. GENERAL PHYSICAL EXAMINATION

1. Describe general physical appearance and hygiene.
2. Describe general demeanor/behavior during exam.
3. Describe condition of clothing. Collect, if indicated. ________________
4. Describe condition of glasses, dentures, hearing aides, wheelchairs, canes, walkers, etc. Collect, if indicated.

5. Status of nutrition

	No	Yes	Describe
Adequately nourished	☐	☐	
Cachexia	☐	☐	
Temporal wasting	☐	☐	
Status of hydration:			
Adequate hydration	☐	☐	
Dry mucous membranes	☐	☐	
Poor skin turgor	☐	☐	

6. Pain Scale

For verbal patients:
Patient's self-rated pain status:
1-10____________

Location(s) of pain:
____
____
____

For nonverbal patients:

0	1	2	3	4	5
NO HURT	HURTS LITTLE BIT	HURTS LITTLE MORE	HURTS EVEN MORE	HURTS WHOLE LOT	HURTS WORST

Observed evidence of pain:

7. Vital Signs

Blood pressure lying ____________ Sitting ____________ Standing ____________ Temperature____________

Pulse lying ____________ Sitting ____________ Respiration(s) ____________ Oxygen Saturation ____________

Height ____________ Weight ____________ Prior weight ____________ Date of prior weight ____________

8. Conduct a general physical exam and record findings.

	WNL	ABN	Not Examined	See Diagrams	Describe Abnormal Findings
Skin					
Head					
Eyes					
Ears					
Nose					
Mouth/pharynx					
Teeth					
Neck					
Thorax					
Back					
Breasts					
Cardiac					
Pulmonary					
Abdomen					
Rectal					
Genitalia					
Musculoskeletal					
Neurological Including gait					

PART II: MEDICAL ASSESSMENT
R. GENERAL PHYSICAL EXAMINATION

Examine the face, head, hair, scalp, neck and mouth for injury and foreign materials. Measure all findings. Record all findings using photographs, diagrams, legend, and a consecutive numbering system.

Patient Identification: **Date:**

A

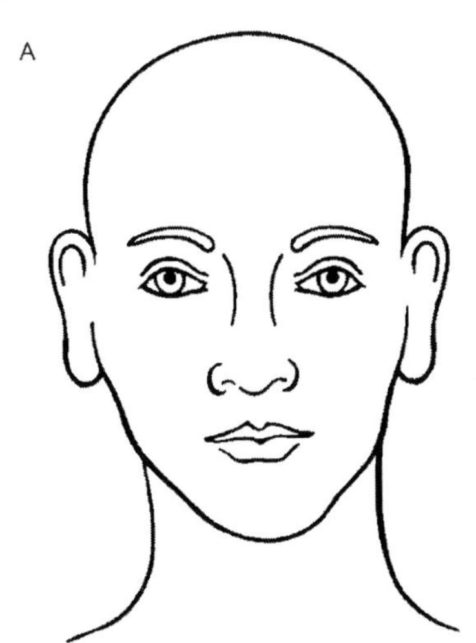

C

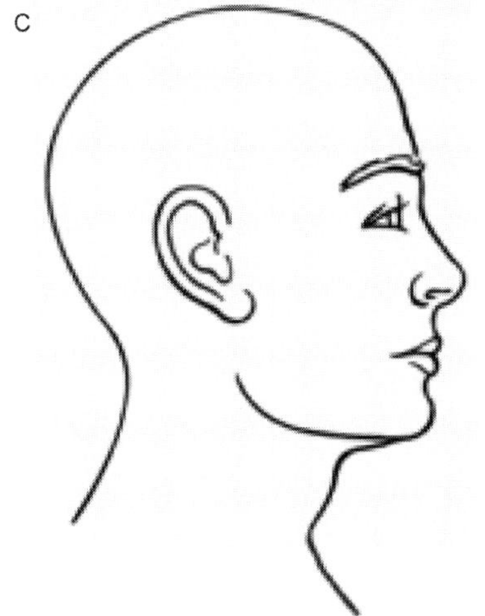

E

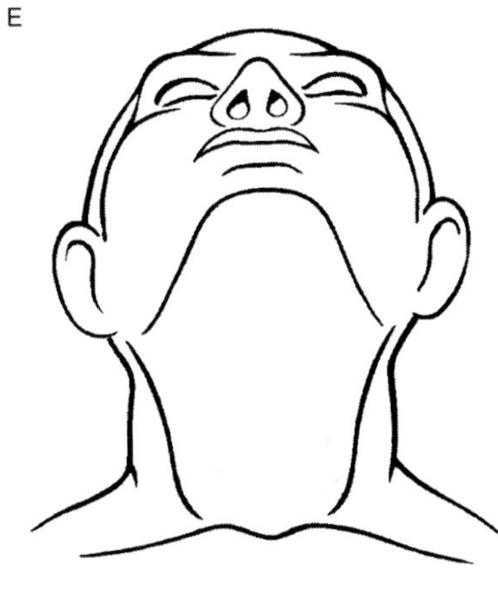

B

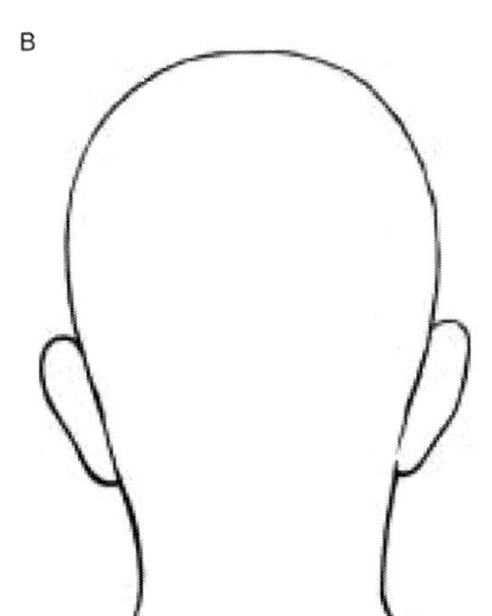

D

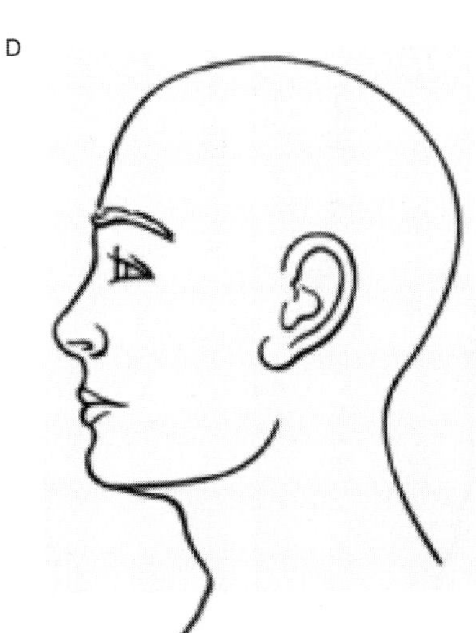

F

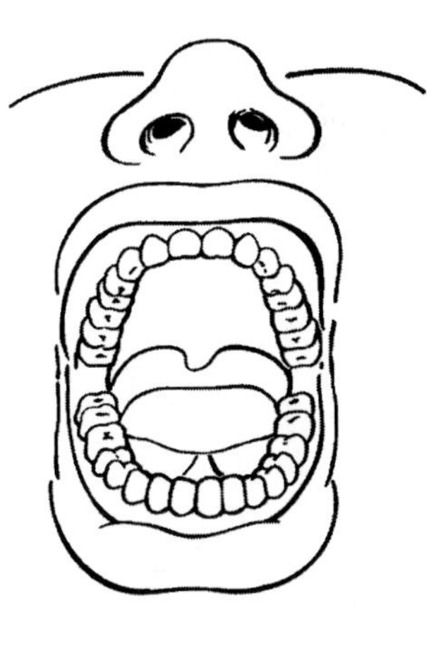

LEGEND: Types of Findings ☐ **Findings** ☐ **No Findings**

AB Abrasion
AL Alopecia
BI Bite
BU Burn
DE Debris
DEN Denture
DM Dry Mucous Membranes
DF Deformity
DS Dry Secretion
EC Ecchymosis (bruise) color
ED Edema
ER Erythema (redness)
FI Fecal Soiling
F/H Fiber/Hair
FB Foreign Body
FR Fracture
IN Induration
INF Infestation
IW Incised Wound
LA Laceration
OF Other Foreign Materials (describe)
OI Other Injury (describe)
PE Petechiae
PI Pattern Injury
PU Pressure Ulcer (indicate State I, II, III, IV)
SC Scratch
ST Skin Tears
TD Tooth Decay
UI Urinary Soiling

Locator #	Type	Description	Locator #	Type	Description

R. GENERAL PHYSICAL EXAMINATION (cont.)

Conduct physical examination of body and extremities. Record all findings using diagrams, legend and a consecutive numbering system. Measure all applicable findings.

Patient Identification: **Date:**

G

H

LEGEND: Types of Findings ☐ **Findings** ☐ **No Findings**

AB Abrasion
AL Alopecia
BI Bite
BU Burn
DE Debris
DM Dry Mucous Membranes
DF Deformity
DS Dry Secretion
EC Ecchymosis (bruise) color
ED Edema
ER Erythema (redness)
FI Fecal Soiling
F/H Fiber/Hair
FB Foreign Body
FR Fracture
IN Induration
INF Infestation
IW Incised Wound
LA Laceration
OF Other Foreign Materials (describe)
OI Other Injury (describe)
PE Petechiae
PI Pattern Injury
PU Pressure Ulcer (indicate State I, II, III, IV)
SC Scratch
ST Skin Tears
UI Urinary Soiling

Locator #	Type	Description	Locator #	Type	Description

R. GENERAL PHYSICAL EXAMINATION (cont.)

Use diagrams I and J to record findings to lateral or medial aspect of trunk and/or extremities. Record all findings using photographs, diagrams, legend and a consecutive numbering system. Measure all applicable findings.

Note: If genital injuries sustained, use pages 6 and 7 from OES 923 Forensic Medical Report: Acute Adult/Adolescent Sexual Assault Examination form to document findings.

Patient Identification: **Date:**

I

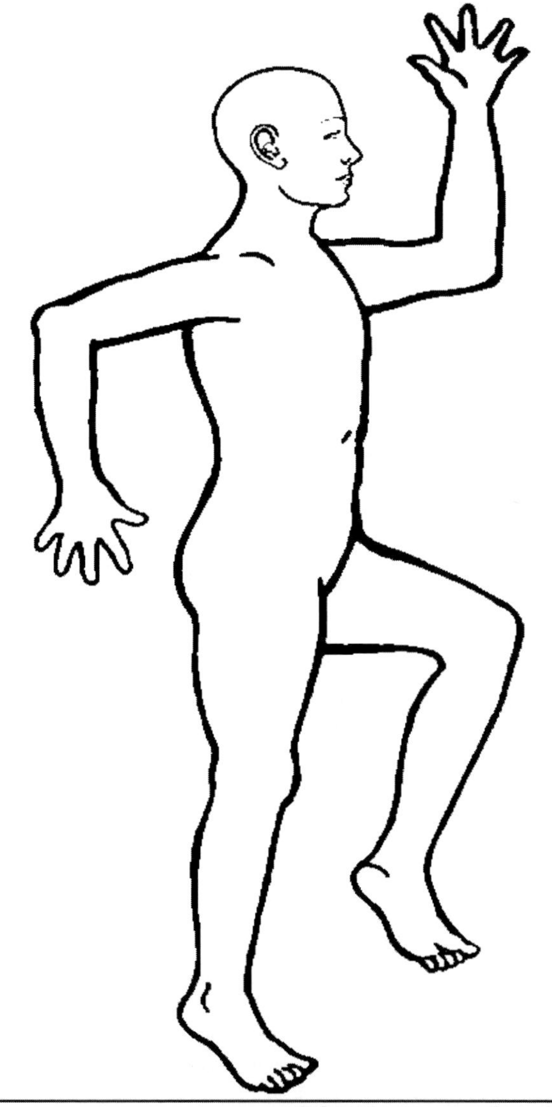

J

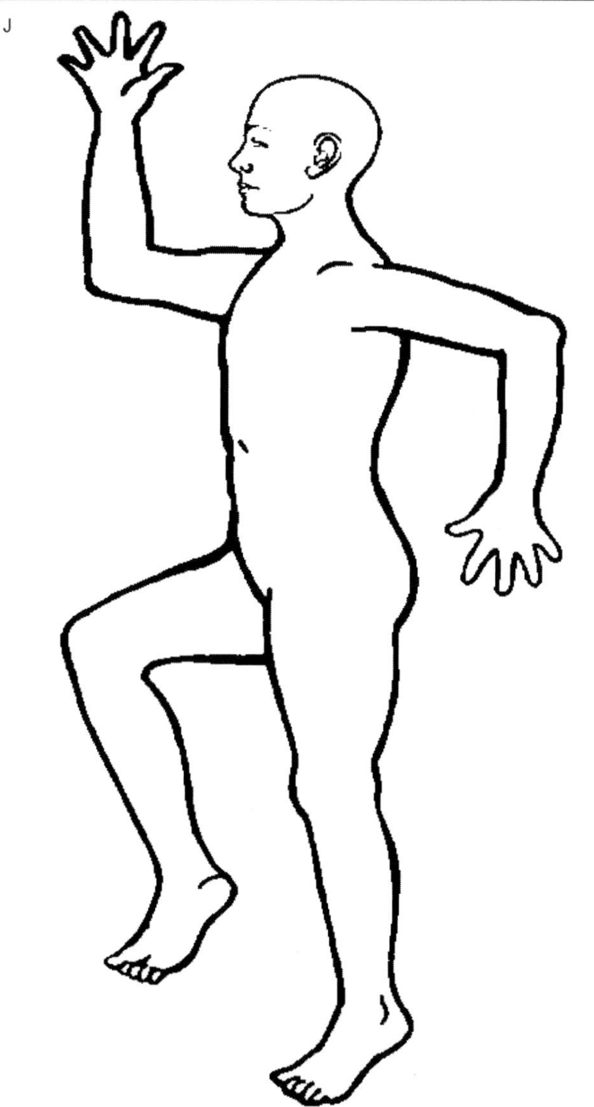

LEGEND: Types of Findings ☐ **Findings** ☐ **No Findings**

AB Abrasion
AL Alopecia
BI Bite
BU Burn
DE Debris
DM Dry Mucous Membranes
DF Deformity
DS Dry Secretion
EC Ecchymosis (bruise) color
ED Edema
ER Erythema (redness)
FI Fecal Soiling
F/H Fiber/Hair
FB Foreign Body
FR Fracture
IN Induration
INF Infestation
IW Incised Wound
LA Laceration
OF Other Foreign Materials (describe)
OI Other Injury (describe)
PE Petechiae
PI Pattern Injury
PU Pressure Ulcer (indicate State I, II, III, IV)
SC Scratch
ST Skin Tears
UI Urinary Soiling

Locator #	Type	Description	Locator #	Type	Description

PART II: MEDICAL ASSESSMENT
SUMMARY OF FINDINGS

Patient Identification: Date:

S. EVIDENCE COLLECTED AND SUBMITTED TO CRIME LAB

1. Clothing Collected	No ☐	Yes ☐	Placed in Evidence Kit	Placed in Paper Bag

2. Foreign Materials	N/A	No	Yes	Collected by:
Swabs/suspected blood	☐	☐	☐	
Dried secretions	☐	☐	☐	
Fibers/loose hairs	☐	☐	☐	
Soil/debris/vegetation	☐	☐	☐	
Swabs/suspected saliva	☐	☐	☐	
Foreign body	☐	☐	☐	
Fingernail scrapings	☐	☐	☐	
Control swabs	☐	☐	☐	
Other (specify)	☐	☐	☐	

T. CLINICALSTUDIES

	No	Yes	Pending	Additional Page
Laboratory Results:	☐	☐	☐	☐ No ☐ Yes
X-ray/Imaging Results:	☐	☐	☐	☐ No ☐ Yes

Toxicology Samples				Time	Collected by
Toxicology screen Results:	☐	☐	☐		
Blood alcohol/toxicology Results:	☐	☐	☐		
Urine toxicology Results:	☐	☐	☐		

Reference Samples

☐ No ☐ Yes ☐ Blood ☐ Saliva

U. PHOTO DOCUMENTATION

☐ No ☐ Yes ☐ 35 mm ☐ Digital ☐ Instant ☐ Other Optics

Photography by: ________ # Rolls/Images ________

☐ Retained ☐ Released to: ________

Recommend follow-up photographs to be taken in 1-2 days ☐ No ☐ Yes ☐ Not applicable

V. DISTRIBUTION OF EVIDENCE

V. DISTRIBUTION OF EVIDENCE	Released to:
Clothing (items not placed in evidence kit)	
Evidence Kit	
Reference Samples	
Toxicology Samples	
Recordings ☐ Audio ☐ Audiovideo	

W. VOICE RECORDING FOR STRANGULATION INJURIES

☐ No ☐ Yes If yes: ☐ Audio ☐ Audiovideo If yes, obtained by: ☐ Examiner ☐ Law Enforcement

X. SUMMARY AND INTERPRETATION OF FINDINGS: ________

If patient expires, contact medical examiner/coroner for an autopsy. ☐ **No, not applicable** ☐ **Yes**

Y. FOLLOW UP

Family/friend contact name	Telephone	Follow-up Exam Needed (specify reason):
Location/address of patient following examination	Telephone	

Z. EXAMINER for Part II	
Signature of Examiner	Printed name
Signature of Supervising Physician, if applicable	
Title	License Number
Medical Facility	Date
Address	Telephone

SIGNATURE OF LAW ENFORCEMENT OFFICER	
I have received the evidence indicated above	
Signature of Officer	Printed Name
ID Number	
Agency:	
Telephone	
Date:	

State of California

Governor's Office of Criminal Justice Planning

FORENSIC MEDICAL REPORT: SEXUAL ASSAULT SUSPECT EXAMINATION

OCJP 950

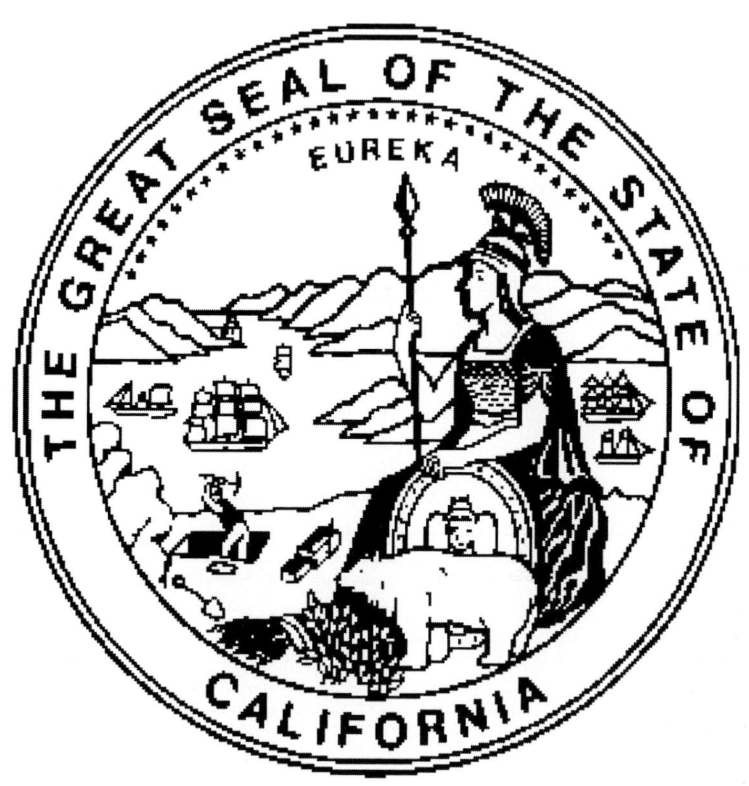

For more information or assistance in completing the OCJP 950 please contact University of California, Davis California Medical Training Center at: (916) 734-4141

This form is available on the following Web site: www.ocjp.ca.gov

FORENSIC MEDICAL REPORT:
SEXUAL ASSAULT SUSPECT EXAMINATION
STATE OF CALIFORNIA
OFFICE OF CRIMINAL JUSTICE PLANNING

OCJP 950

Confidential Document

Patient Identification

A. GENERAL INFORMATION (print or type) **Name of Medical Facility:**

1. Name of patient					Patient ID number			
2. Address			City		County		State	Telephone (W) (H)
3. Age	DOB	Gender M F	Ethnicity	Arrival Date	Arrival Time		Dishcarge Date	Discharge Time

B. AUTHORIZATION Jurisdiction (☐ city ☐ county ☐ other):

1. Name of Law Enforcement Officer	Agency	ID Number	Telephone

2. **I request a forensic medical examination for suspected sexual assault at public expense.**

Law enforcement officer signature　Date　Time　Case number

C. MEDICAL HISTORY

1. **Any recent (60 days) anal-genital injuries, surgeries, diagnostic procedures, or medical treatment that may affect the interpretation of current physical findings?** ☐ **No** ☐ **Yes**
   If yes, describe: ____
2. **Any other pertinent medical condition(s) that may affect the interpretation of current physical findings?** ☐ **No** ☐ **Yes**
   If yes, describe: ____
3. **Any pre-existing physical injuries?** ☐ **No** ☐ **Yes**
   If yes, describe: ____

D. RECENT HYGIENE INFORMATION ☐ Not applicable if over 72 hours

	No	Yes		No	Yes
Urinated	☐	☐	Bath/shower/wash	☐	☐
Defecated	☐	☐	Brushed teeth	☐	☐
Genital or body wipes	☐	☐	Ate or drank	☐	☐
If yes, describe: ____			Changed clothing	☐	☐
Oral gargle/rinse	☐	☐	If yes, describe: ____		

E. GENERAL PHYSICAL EXAMINATION

1. Blood Pressure	Pulse	Respiration	Temperature	2. Exam Started		Exam Completed	
				Date	Time	Date	Time
3. Height	Weight	Hair color	Eye color	☐ Right-handed ☐ Left-handed			

4. **Describe general physical appearance**

5. **Describe general demeanor**

6. **Describe condition of clothing upon arrival.**

7. **Collect outer and under clothing, if indicated.** ☐ **Not indicated**

DISTRIBUTION OF OCJP 950

☐ Original - Law Enforcement　☐ Copy within evidence kit - Crime Lab　☐ Copy - Medical Facility Records

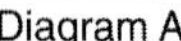

E. GENERAL PHYSICAL EXAMINATION

Record all findings using diagrams, legend, and a consecutive numbering system

8. **Conduct a physical examination. Record scars, tattoos, skin lesions, and distinguishing physical features.** ☐ Findings ☐ No Findings
9. **Collect dried and moist secretions, stains, and foreign materials from the body. Scan the entire body with a Wood's Lamp.** ☐ Findings ☐ No Findings
10. **Collect fingernail scrapings or cuttings according to local policy.**
11. **Collect chest hair reference samples according to local policy.**

Patient Identification

Diagram A

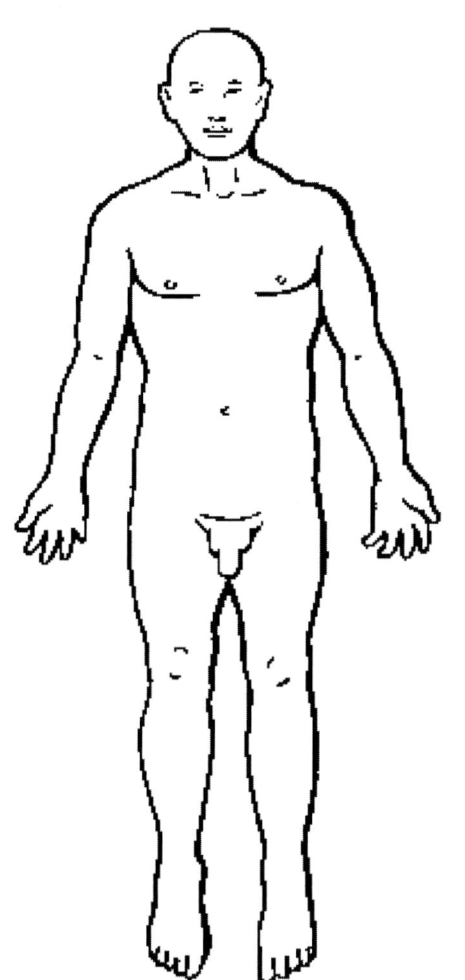

Diagram B

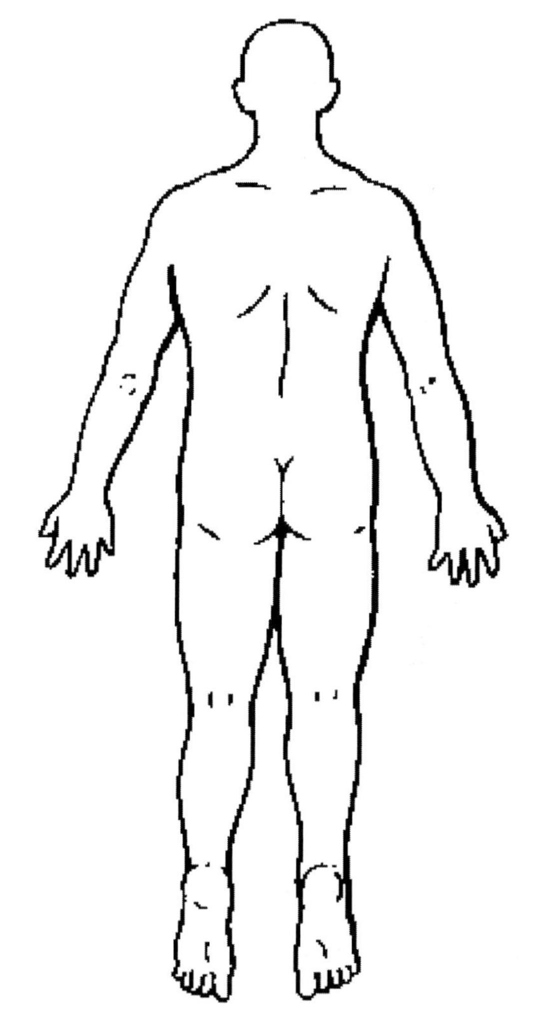

LEGEND: Types of Findings

AB	Abrasion	**DE**	Debris	**F/H**	Fiber/hair	**OF**	Other Foreign Materials (describe)	**SC**	Scars	**TA**	Tattoos
BI	Bite	**DF**	Deformity	**IN**	Induration			**SHX**	Sample Per History	**TB**	Toluidine Blue⊕
BP	Body Piercing	**DS**	Dry Secretion	**IW**	Incised Wound	**OI**	Other Injury (describe)			**TE**	Tenderness
BU	Burn	**EC**	Ecchymosis (bruise)	**LA**	Laceration	**PE**	Petechiae	**SI**	Suction Injury	**V/S**	Vegetation/Soil
CS	Control Swab	**ER**	Erythema (redness)	**MS**	Moist Secretion	**PS**	Potential Saliva	**SW**	Swelling	**WL**	Wood's Lamp⊕

Locator #	Type	Description	Locator #	Type	Description

RECORD ALL CLOTHING AND SPECIMENS COLLECTED ON PAGE 5

F. HEAD, NECK, AND ORAL EXAMINATION

Record all findings using diagrams, legend, and a consecutive numbering system.

1. **Examine the face, head, hair, scalp, and neck for injury and foreign materials.**
   ☐ Findings ☐ No Findings
2. **Collect dried and moist secretions, stains, and foreign materials from face, head, hair, scalp, and neck.**
   ☐ Findings ☐ No Findings
3. **Examine the oral cavity for injury and foreign materials (if indicated by assault history). Collect foreign materials.**
   Exam done: ☐ Not applicable ☐ Yes ☐ Findings ☐ No Findings
4. **Collect 2 swabs from the oral cavity up to 12 hours post assault and prepare one dry mount slide from one of the swabs.**
5. **Collect head and facial hair reference samples according to local policy.**

Patient Identification

Diagram C

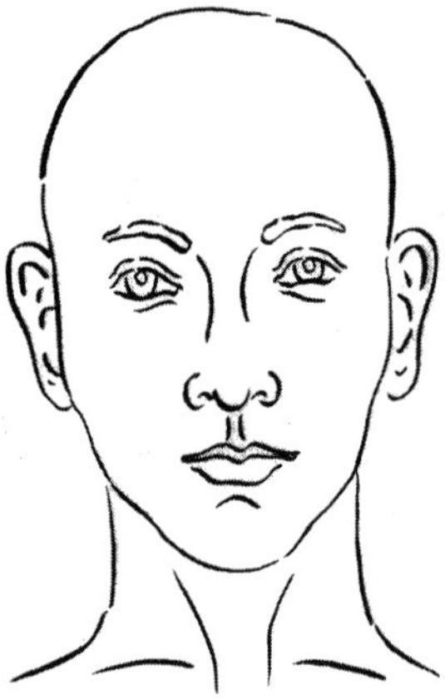

Diagram D

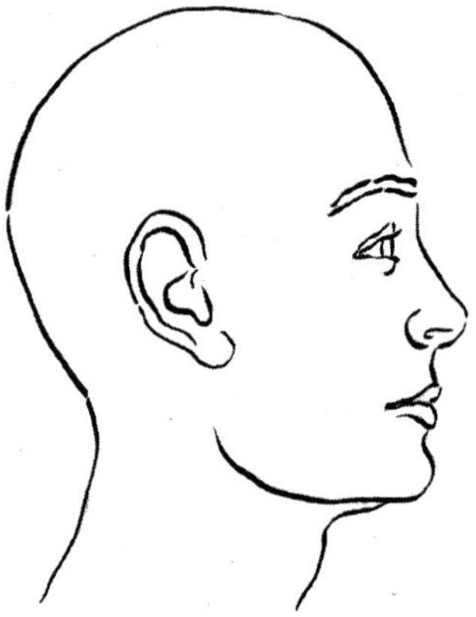

Diagram E

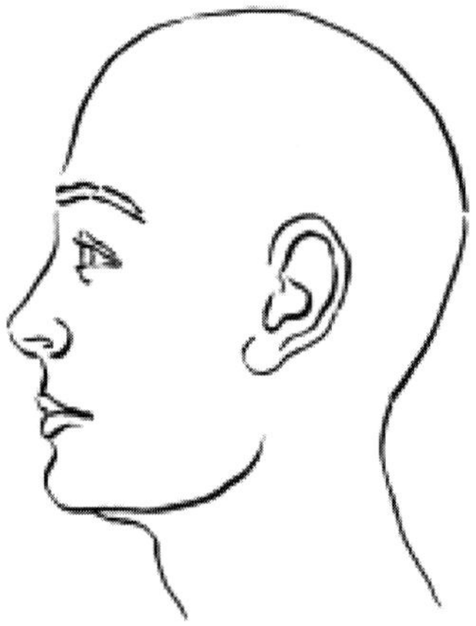

Diagram F

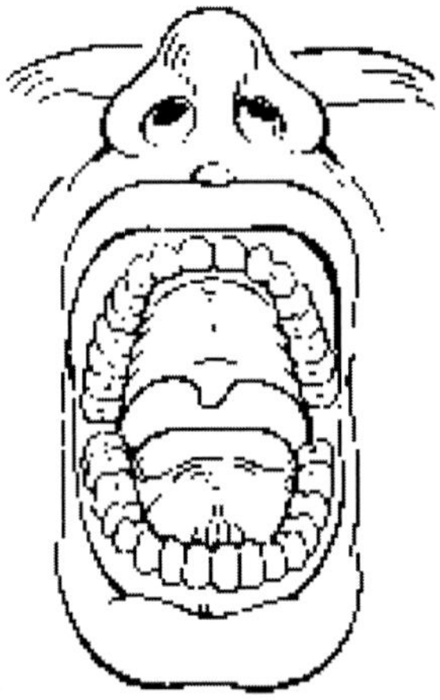

LEGEND: Types of Findings

AB	Abrasion	**DE**	Debris	**F/H**	Fiber/hair	**OF**	Other Foreign Materials (describe)	**SC**	Scars	**TA**	Tattoos
BI	Bite	**DF**	Deformity	**IN**	Induration			**SHX**	Sample Per History	**TB**	Toluidine Blue⊕
BP	Body Piercing	**DS**	Dry Secretion	**IW**	Incised Wound	**OI**	Other Injury (describe)			**TE**	Tenderness
BU	Burn	**EC**	Ecchymosis (bruise)	**LA**	Laceration	**PE**	Petechiae	**SI**	Suction Injury	**V/S**	Vegetation/Soil
CS	Control Swab	**ER**	Erythema (redness)	**MS**	Moist Secretion	**PS**	Potential Saliva	**SW**	Swelling	**WL**	Wood's Lamp⊕

Locator #	Type	Description	Locator #	Type	Description

RECORD ALL CLOTHING AND SPECIMENS COLLECTED ON PAGE 5

OCJP 950 (Rev 7/02) 3

G. GENITAL EXAMINATION

Record all findings using diagrams, legend, and a consecutive numbering system.

1. **Examine the inner thighs, external genitalia, and perineal area. Check the box(es) if there are assault related findings:**
   ☐ No Findings
   ☐ Inner thighs ☐ Glans penis ☐ Scrotum
   ☐ Perineum ☐ Penile shaft ☐ Testes
   ☐ Foreskin ☐ Urethral meatus
2. **Circumcised** ☐ **No** ☐ **Yes**
3. **Collect dried and moist secretions, stains, and foreign materials. Scan the area with a Wood's Lamp.** ☐ Findings ☐ No Findings
4. **Collect pubic hair combing or brushing.**
5. **Collect pubic hair reference samples according to local policy.**
6. **Collect 2 penile swabs, if indicated by assault history.** ☐ **N/A**
7. **Collect 2 scrotal swabs, if indicated by assault history.** ☐ **N/A**
8. **Record other findings per history.** ☐ **No** ☐ **Yes**
   If yes, describe:

Patient Identification

Diagram G

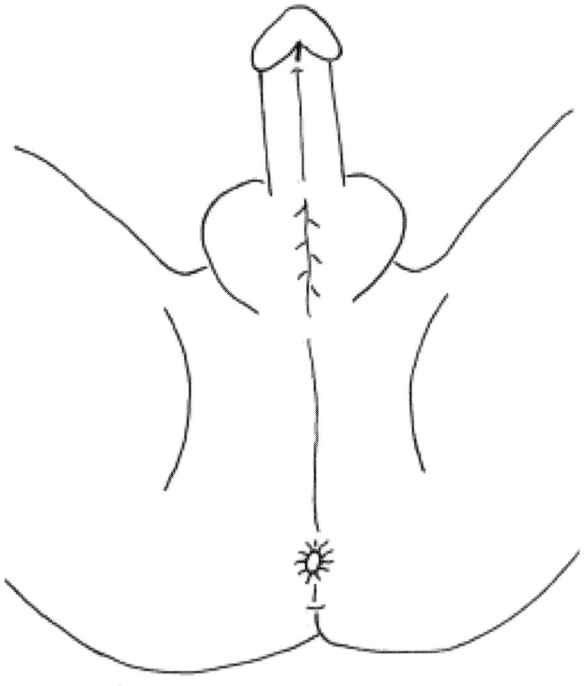

Diagram H

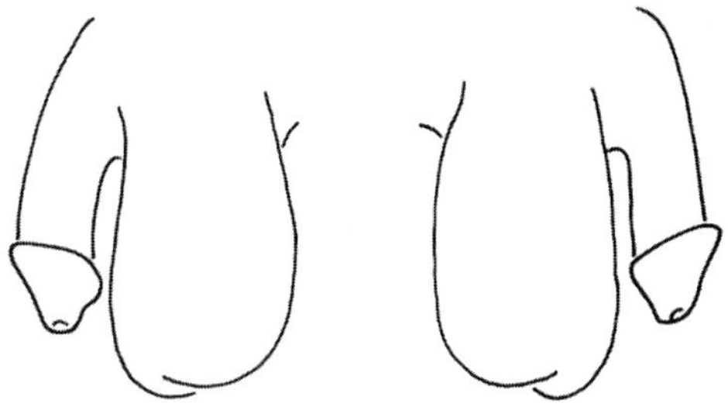

Diagram I

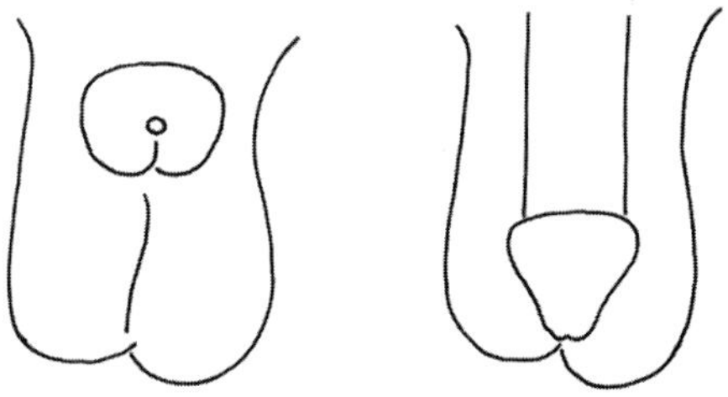

Diagram J

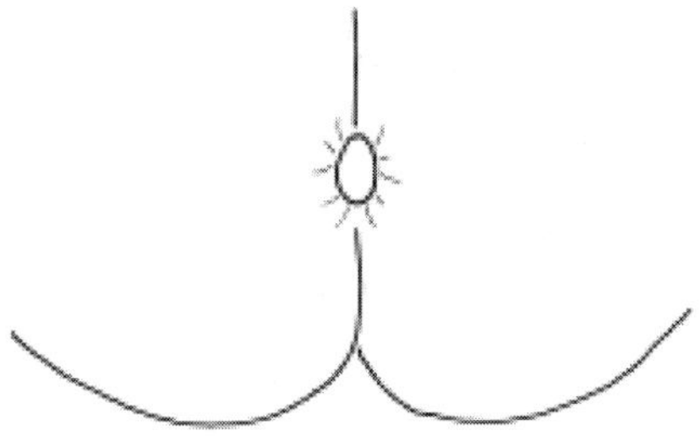

LEGEND: Types of Findings

AB	Abrasion	**ER**	Erythema (redness)	**PE**	Petechiae	**V/S**	Vegetation/Soil
BI	Bite	**F/H**	Fiber/hair	**PS**	Potential Saliva	**WL**	Wood's Lamp⊕
BP	Body Piercing	**IN**	Induration	**SC**	Scars		
BU	Burn	**IW**	Incised Wound	**SHX**	Sample Per History		
CS	Control Swab	**LA**	Laceration	**SI**	Suction Injury		
DE	Debris	**MS**	Moist Secretion	**SW**	Swelling		
DF	Deformity	**OF**	Other Foreign Materials(describe)	**TA**	Tattoos		
DS	Dry Secretion			**TB**	Toluidine Blue⊕		
EC	Ecchymosis (bruise)	**OI**	Other Injury (describe)	**TE**	Tenderness		

Locator #	Type	Description

RECORD ALL CLOTHING AND SPECIMENS COLLECTED ON PAGE 5

H. EVIDENCE COLLECTED AND SUBMITTED TO CRIME LAB

1. Clothing placed in evidence kit	Other clothing placed in bags

2. Foreign materials collected

	No	Yes	Collected by:
Swabs/suspected blood	☐	☐	
Dried Secretions	☐	☐	
Fiber/loose hairs	☐	☐	
Vegetation	☐	☐	
Soil/debris	☐	☐	
Swabs/suspected semen	☐	☐	
Swabs/suspected saliva	☐	☐	
Swabs/Wood's Lamp⊕ area(s)	☐	☐	
Control swabs	☐	☐	
Fingernail scrapings/cuttings	☐	☐	
Matted hair cuttings	☐	☐	
Pubic hair combings/brushings	☐	☐	
Other types	☐	☐	

If yes, describe:

3. Oral/genital samples

	# Swabs	# Slides	Time collected	Collected by:
Oral				
Penile		■		
Scrotal		■		

I. TOXICOLOGY SAMPLES

	No	Yes	Time	Collected by:
Blood alcohol/toxicology (gray top tube)				
Urine toxicology				

J. REFERENCE SAMPLES

	No	Yes	Collected by:
Blood (lavender top tube)			
Blood (yellow top tube)			
Blood Card (optional)			
Buccal swabs (optional)			
Saliva swabs			
Chest hair			
Facial hair			
Pubic hair			
Head hair			

K. PHOTO DOCUMENTATION METHODS

	No	Yes	Colposcope/35mm	Macrolens/35mm	Colposcope/ Videocamera	Other optics
Body	☐	☐	☐	☐	☐	☐ ______
Genitals	☐	☐	☐	☐	☐	☐ ______

Photographed by:

Patient Identification

L. RECORD EXAM METHODS

	No	Yes
Direct visualization only	☐	☐
Colposcopy	☐	☐
Other magnifier	☐	☐
Other	☐	☐

If yes, describe:

M. RECORD EXAM FINDINGS

☐ **Physical Findings** ☐ **No Physical Findings**

N. SUMMARIZE FINDINGS

O. PRINT NAMES OF PERSONNEL INVOLVED

History taken by:	Telephone
Exam performed by:	
Specimens labeled and sealed by:	
Assisted by: ☐ N/A	
Signature of examiner:	License No.

P. EVIDENCE DISTRIBUTION

	GIVEN TO:
Clothing (item(s) not placed in evidence kit)	
Evidence kit	
Reference blood samples	
Toxicology samples	

Q. SIGNATURE OF OFFICER RECEIVING EVIDENCE

Signature: ______

Print name and ID#: ______

Agency: ______

Date: ______ Phone: ______

OCJP 950 (Rev 7/02)

APPENDIX II Pediatric Forms

A. California Sexual Assault Pediatric Form—OCJP 930 264

B. Philadelphia Sexual Assault Pediatric Form 273

C. California Pediatric Abuse and Neglect Form—OES 900 279

State of California
Governor's Office of Criminal Justice Planning

FORENSIC MEDICAL REPORT: ACUTE (<72 HOURS) CHILD/ADOLESCENT SEXUAL ABUSE EXAMINATION

OCJP 930

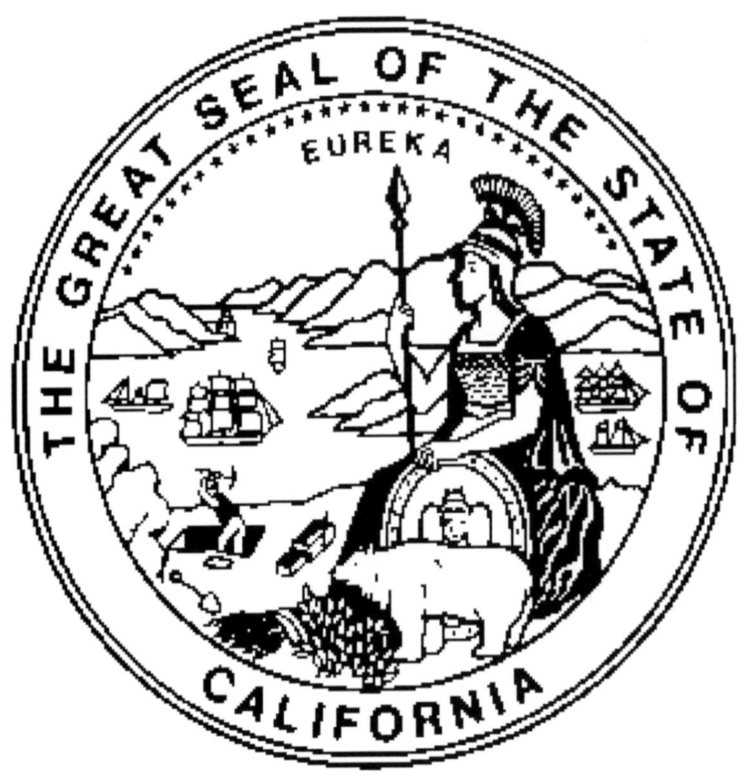

For more information or assistance in completing the OCJP 930 please contact University of California, Davis California Medical Training Center at:
(916) 734-4141

This form is available on the following Web site:
www.ocjp.ca.gov

FORENSIC MEDICAL REPORT: ACUTE (<72 HOURS)
CHILD/ADOLESCENT SEXUAL ABUSE EXAMINATION
STATE OF CALIFORNIA
OFFICE OF CRIMINAL JUSTICE PLANNING

OCJP 930

Confidential Document **Patient Identification**

A. GENERAL INFORMATION (print or type) Name of Medical Facility:

1. Name of patient — Patient ID number
2. Address — City — County — State — Telephone

3. Age	DOB	Gender M F	Ethnicity	Arrival Date	Arrival Time	Discharge Date	Discharge Time

4. Name of : ☐ Mother ☐ Stepmother ☐ Guardian — Address — City — County — State — Telephone W: H:
5. Name of : ☐ Father ☐ Stepfather ☐ Guardian — Address — City — County — State — Telephone W: H:

6. Name(s) of Siblings	Gender	Age	DOB	Name(s) of Siblings	Gender	Age	DOB
	M F				M F		
	M F				M F		

B. REPORTING AND AUTHORIZATION Jurisdiction (☐city ☐county ☐other):

1. **Telephone report made to** — Name — Agency — ID number — Telephone
   Law Enforcement ☐
   and/or
   Child Protective Services ☐
2. **Responding Personnel** (to medical facility) — Name — Agency — ID number — Telephone
   Law Enforcement ☐
   and/or
   Child Protective Services ☐
3. **Assigned Investigator (if known)** — Name — Agency — ID number — Telephone
   Law Enforcement ☐
   and/or
   Child Protective Services ☐
4. **Authorization for evidential exam requested by law enforcement or child protective services agency**
   I request a forensic medical examination for suspected sexual abuse at public expense.

Telephone Authorization
Agency:
Authorizing party:
ID number:
Date/time:

☐ **Law enforcement officer** — **ID number** — ☐ **Child Protective Services**

Telephone — **Date** — **Time** — **Case number**

C. CONSENT FOR EXAMINATION BY PATIENT/PARENT/GUARDIAN

Note: Parental consent is not required for a suspected child sexual abuse examination if the child is in protective custody. Family Code Section 6927 permits minors (12 to 17 years of age) to consent to medical examination, treatment, and evidence collection for sexual assault without parental consent. See instructions regarding parental notification requirements for minors.

- I hereby consent to a forensic medical examination for evidence of sexual abuse. I understand that collection of evidence may include photographing injuries and that these photographs may include the anal-genital area (private parts). I further understand that medical providers are required to notify child protective authorities of known or suspected child abuse; and, if child abuse is found or suspected, this form and any evidence obtained will be released to a child protective agency.
- I have been informed that victims of crime are eligible to submit crime victim compensation claims to the State Victims of Crime (VOC) Restitution Fund for out-of-pocket medical expenses, psychological counseling, loss of wages, and job retraining/rehabilitation.
- I understand that data without patient identity may be collected from this report for health and forensic purposes and provided to health authorities and other qualified persons with a valid educational or scientific interest for demographic and/or epidemiological studies.

Signature ______________________ ☐ Patient ☐ Parent ☐ Guardian

DISTRIBUTION OF OCJP 930

☐ Original – Law Enforcement ☐ Copy – Child Protective Services ☐ Copy within evidence kit – Crime Lab ☐ Copy – Medical Facility Records

D. PATIENT HISTORY

1. Record time or time frame of the incident(s)	Date(s)	Time or time frame
☐ Less than 72 hours		
☐ Multiple incidents over time		

2. Pertinent physical surroundings of abuse/assault:

Patient Identification

3. Record patient's name for:	4. Alleged perpetrator(s) name(s)	Age	Gender	Ethnicity	Relationship to Patient Known	Relationship to Patient Unknown
Female genitalia						
Male genitalia	#1.		M F			
Breasts	#2.		M F			
Anus	#3.		M F			

E. ACTS DESCRIBED BY HISTORIAN

Name of historian	Relationship to patient	History obtained by:	Telephone	Agency	☐ Not applicable

	No	Yes	Attempted	Unsure	N/A	Describe pain and/or bleeding and additional pertinent history:
Genital/vaginal contact/penetration by:						
Penis	☐	☐	☐	☐	☐	
Finger	☐	☐	☐	☐	☐	
Object (Describe)	☐	☐	☐	☐	☐	
Associated pain?	☐	☐		☐	☐	
Associated bleeding?	☐	☐		☐	☐	
Anal contact/penetration by:						
Penis	☐	☐	☐	☐	☐	
Finger	☐	☐	☐	☐	☐	
Object (Describe)	☐	☐	☐	☐	☐	
Associated pain?	☐	☐		☐	☐	
Associated bleeding?	☐	☐		☐	☐	
Oral copulation of genitals:						
Of patient by assailant	☐	☐	☐	☐	☐	
Of assailant by patient	☐	☐	☐	☐	☐	
Oral copulation of anus:						
Of patient by assailant	☐	☐	☐	☐	☐	
Of assailant by patient	☐	☐	☐	☐	☐	
Anal/genital fondling:						
Of patient by assailant	☐	☐	☐	☐	☐	
Of assailant by patient	☐	☐	☐	☐	☐	
Non-genital act(s)?	☐	☐				
If yes: ☐ Fondling ☐ Licking ☐ Kissing ☐ Suction Injury ☐ Biting						
Other acts? (Describe)	☐	☐	☐	☐	☐	
Did ejaculation occur?	☐	☐		☐	☐	

If yes, note location(s):
☐ Mouth ☐ Vagina ☐ Body surface ☐ On bedding
☐ Anus/Rectum ☐ On clothing ☐ Other

Contraceptive or lubricant products? ☐ No ☐ Yes ☐
If yes, note type/brand: ☐ Foam ☐ Jelly ☐ Lubricant ☐ Condom
Were force or threats used? ☐ No ☐ Yes ☐ Force ☐ Threats ☐
Were weapons used? ☐ No ☐ Yes ☐
If yes, describe: ______
Were pictures/videotapes taken ☐ or shown ☐? ☐ No ☐ Yes
If yes, note type(s): ☐ Pictures ☐ Videotapes
Were drugs ☐ or alcohol ☐ used? ☐ No ☐ Yes* ☐
Loss of memory? ☐ No ☐ Yes* ☐
Lapse of consciousness? ☐ No ☐ Yes* ☐
Vomited after act(s)? ☐ No ☐ Yes ☐
Behavioral changes in patient? ☐ No ☐ Yes ☐

***Collection of toxicology samples is recommended according to local policy.**

F. ACTS DESCRIBED BY PATIENT

1. Acts disclosed by patient to:
☐ Medical Examiner
☐ Social Worker
☐ Law Enforcement Officer
☐ Multi-disciplinary Interview Team
☐ Other:

	No	Yes	Attempted	Unsure	N/A
Genital/vaginal contact/penetration by:					
Penis	☐	☐	☐	☐	☐
Finger	☐	☐	☐	☐	☐
Object (Describe below)	☐	☐	☐	☐	☐
Associated pain?	☐	☐		☐	☐
Associated bleeding?	☐	☐		☐	☐
Anal contact/penetration by:					
Penis	☐	☐	☐	☐	☐
Finger	☐	☐	☐	☐	☐
Object (Describe below)	☐	☐	☐	☐	☐
Associated pain?	☐	☐		☐	☐
Associated bleeding?	☐	☐		☐	☐
Oral copulation of genitals:					
Of patient by assailant	☐	☐	☐	☐	☐
Of assailant by patient	☐	☐	☐	☐	☐
Oral copulation of anus:					
Of patient by assailant	☐	☐	☐	☐	☐
Of assailant by patient	☐	☐	☐	☐	☐
Anal/genital fondling:					
Of patient by assailant	☐	☐	☐	☐	☐
Of assailant by patient	☐	☐	☐	☐	☐
Non-genital act(s)?	☐	☐			☐

If yes: ☐ Fondling ☐ Licking ☐ Kissing ☐ Suction injury ☐ Biting

	No	Yes	Attempted	Unsure	N/A
Other acts? (Describe below)	☐	☐	☐	☐	☐
Did ejaculation occur?	☐	☐		☐	☐

If yes, note location(s):
☐ Mouth ☐ Vagina ☐ Body surface ☐ On bedding
☐ Anus/Rectum ☐ On clothing ☐ Other

Contraceptive or lubricant products? ☐ No ☐ Yes ☐
If yes, note type/brand: ☐ Foam ☐ Jelly ☐ Lubricant ☐ Condom
Were force or threats used? ☐ No ☐ Yes ☐ Force ☐ Threats
Were weapons used? ☐ No ☐ Yes ☐
If yes, describe: ____
Were pictures/videotapes ☐ taken or ☐ shown? ☐ No ☐ Yes ☐
If yes, note type(s): ☐ Pictures ☐ Videotapes
Were drugs ☐ or alcohol ☐ used? ☐ No ☐ Yes* ☐
Loss of memory? ☐ No ☐ Yes* ☐
Lapse of consciousness? ☐ No ☐ Yes* ☐
Vomited after act(s)? ☐ No ☐ Yes ☐
Behavioral changes? ☐ No ☐ Yes ☐

***Collection of toxicology samples is recommended according to local policy.**

2. Describe pain and/or bleeding (using patient's exact words) and additional pertinent history from above.

Patient Identification

G. MEDICAL HISTORY (to be completed by medical personnel)

1. Name of person providing history	Relationship to patient	Date	Time

	No	Yes
2. Any recent (60 days) anal-genital injuries, surgeries, diagnostic procedures, or medical treatment that may affect the interpretation of physical findings?	☐	☐
3. Any other pertinent medical conditions that may affect the interpretation of physical findings?	☐	☐
4. Any pre-existing physical injuries?	☐	☐
5. Any previous history of physical abuse and/or neglect?	☐	☐
6. Any previous history of sexual abuse?	☐	☐
7. Other intercourse? (For adolescents only)	☐	☐
If yes,		
anal (within past 5 days)? When ____	☐	☐
vaginal (within past 5 days)? When ____	☐	☐
oral (within past 24 hours)? When ____	☐	☐
If yes, did ejaculation occur?	☐	☐
If yes, where? ____		
If yes, was a condom used?	☐	☐
8. Menstrual periods? If yes, age of menarche: ____	☐	☐
Last menstrual period: ____	☐	☐

9. Other symptoms disclosed	by patient: No	by patient: Yes	by historian: No	by historian: Yes	by historian: Unk
Abdominal/pelvic pain	☐	☐	☐	☐	☐
Pain on urination	☐	☐	☐	☐	☐
Genital discomfort or pain	☐	☐	☐	☐	☐
Genital itching	☐	☐	☐	☐	☐
Genital discharge	☐	☐	☐	☐	☐
Genital bleeding	☐	☐	☐	☐	☐
Rectal discomfort or pain	☐	☐	☐	☐	☐
Rectal itching	☐	☐	☐	☐	☐
Rectal bleeding	☐	☐	☐	☐	☐
Constipation	☐	☐	☐	☐	☐
Other ____	☐	☐	☐	☐	☐

If yes, describe onset, duration, and intensity:

10. Post-assault hygiene activity
☐ Not applicable if over 72 hours

	by patient: No	by patient: Yes	by historian: No	by historian: Yes	by historian: Unk
Urinated	☐	☐	☐	☐	☐
Defecated	☐	☐	☐	☐	☐
Genital or body wipes	☐	☐	☐	☐	☐
If yes, describe: ____	☐	☐	☐	☐	☐
Douched					
If yes, with what? ____					
Removed/inserted ☐ tampon ☐ diaphragm	☐	☐	☐	☐	☐
Oral gargle/rinse	☐	☐	☐	☐	☐
Bath/shower/wash	☐	☐	☐	☐	☐
Brushed teeth	☐	☐	☐	☐	☐
Ate or drank	☐	☐	☐	☐	☐
Changed clothing	☐	☐	☐	☐	☐

If yes, describe:

H. GENERAL PHYSICAL EXAMINATION

Record all findings using diagrams, legend, and a consecutive numbering system.

1. BP	Pulse	Resp	Temp	Height	Weight	2. Exam Started		Exam Completed	
						Date	Time	Date	Time

3. Female Tanner Stage – Breast 1☐ 2☐ 3☐ 4☐ 5☐
4. Describe general physical appearance.
5. Describe general demeanor and relevant statements made during exam.
6. Describe condition of clothing upon arrival.
7. Collect outer and underclothing if indicated. ☐ Not indicated

Patient Identification

8. Conduct a physical examination. ☐ Findings ☐ No Findings
   General exam within normal limits: ☐ Yes ☐ No ☐ If no, describe:
9. Collect dried and moist secretions, stains, and foreign materials from the body. Scan the entire body with a Wood's Lamp.
   ☐ Findings ☐ No Findings
10. Collect fingernail scrapings or cuttings according to local policy.

Diagram A

Diagram B

LEGEND: Types of Findings

AB	Abrasion	CS	Control Swab	DS	Dry Secretion	HC	Hymenal Cleft	OI	Other Injury (describe)	PE	Petechiae	SW	Swelling
AHT	Absent Hymenal Tissue	CV	Congenital Variation	EC	Ecchymosis (bruise)	IN	Induration	OSC	Other Skin Condition	PGW	Possible Genital Wart	TB	Toluidine Blue⊕
AL	Anal Laxity	DE	Debris	ER	Erythema (redness)	IW	Incised Wound	OT	Other	PS	Potential Saliva	TE	Tenderness
BI	Bite	DF	Deformity	FB	Foreign Body	LA	Laceration	PW	Perianal Wart	SH	Submucosal Hemorrhage	V/S	Vegetation/Soil
BU	Burn	DI	Discharge	F/H	Fiber/Hair	MS	Moist Secretion			SHX	Sample Per History	VL	Vesicular Lesion
				GT	Granulation Tissue	OF	Other Foreign Materials (describe)			SI	Suction Injury	WL	Wood's Lamp⊕

Locator #	Type	Description	Locator #	Type	Description

RECORD ALL CLOTHING AND SPECIMENS COLLECTED ON PAGE 8

I. HEAD, NECK, AND ORAL EXAMINATION

Record all findings using diagrams, legend, and a consecutive numbering system.

1. **Examine the face, head, hair, scalp, and neck for injury and foreign materials.**
   ☐ Findings ☐ No Findings
2. **Exam method:**
   ☐ Direct visualization ☐ Colposcope ☐ Other magnification
3. **Collect dried and moist secretions, stains, and foreign materials from the face, head, hair, scalp, and neck.**
   ☐ Findings ☐ No Findings
4. **Examine the oral cavity for injury and foreign materials. Collect foreign materials.**
   ☐ Findings ☐ No Findings
5. **Collect 2 swabs from the oral cavity up to 12 hours post assault and prepare one dry mount slide from one of the swabs.**
6. **Collect head hair reference samples according to local policy.**

Patient Identification

Diagram C

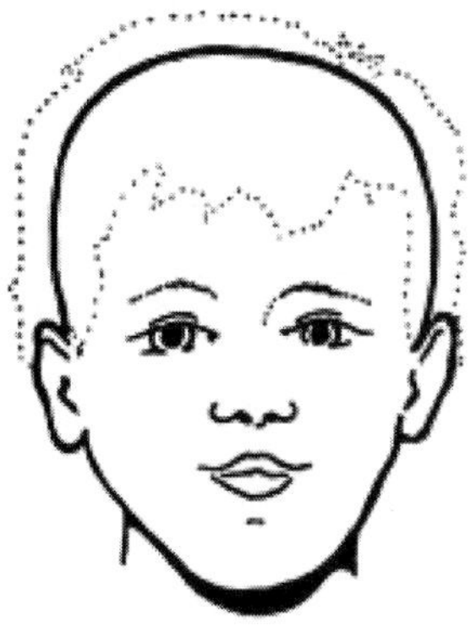

Diagram D

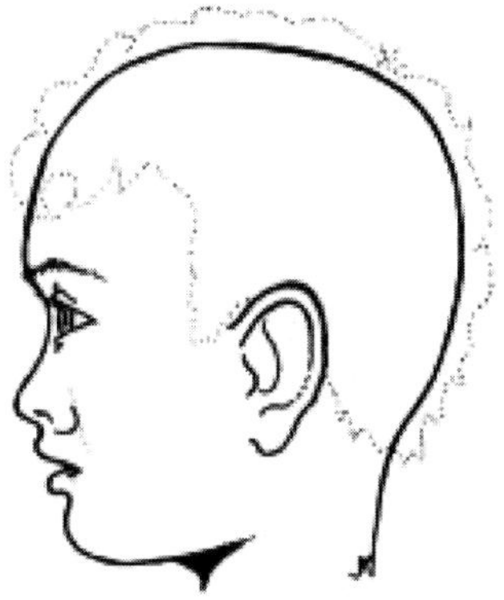

Diagram E

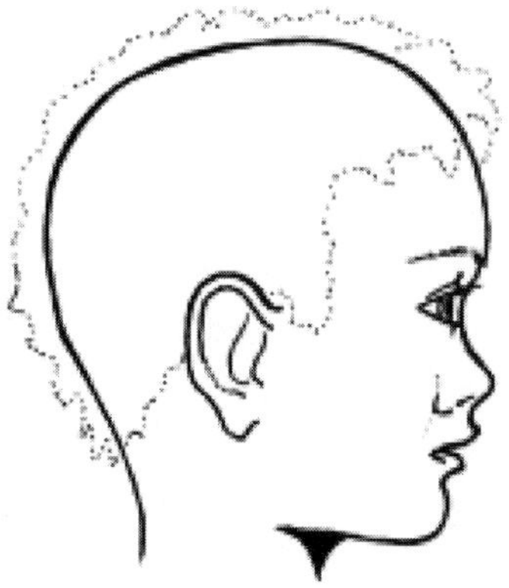

Diagram F

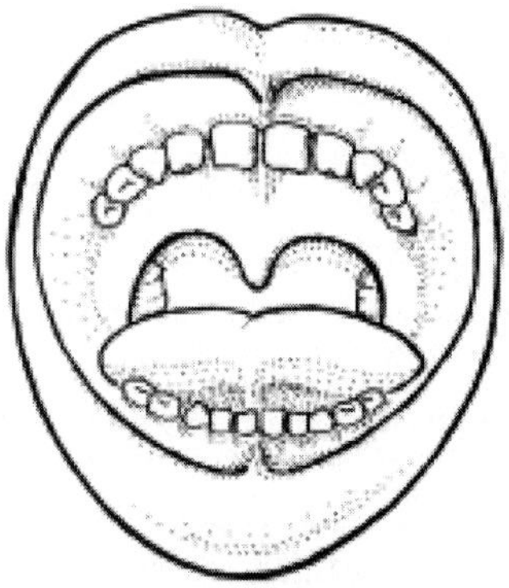

LEGEND: Types of Findings

AB	Abrasion	**CS**	Control Swab	**DS**	Dry Secretion	**HC**	Hymenal Cleft	**OI**	Other Injury (describe)	**PE**	Petechiae	**SW**	Swelling
AHT	Absent Hymenal Tissue	**CV**	Congenital Variation	**EC**	Ecchymosis (bruise)	**IN**	Induration	**OSC**	Other Skin Condition	**PGW**	Possible Genital Wart	**TB**	Toluidine Blue⊕
				ER	Erythema (redness)	**IW**	Incised Wound			**PS**	Potential Saliva	**TE**	Tenderness
AL	Anal Laxity	**DE**	Debris	**FB**	Foreign Body	**LA**	Laceration	**OT**	Other	**SH**	Submucosal Hemorrhage	**V/S**	Vegetation/Soil
BI	Bite	**DF**	Deformity	**F/H**	Fiber/Hair	**MS**	Moist Secretion	**PW**	Perianal Wart	**SHX**	Sample Per History	**VL**	Vesicular Lesion
BU	Burn	**DI**	Discharge	**GT**	Granulation Tissue	**OF**	Other Foreign Materials (describe)			**SI**	Suction Injury	**WL**	Wood's Lamp⊕

Locator #	Type	Description	Locator #	Type	Description

RECORD ALL CLOTHING AND SPECIMENS COLLECTED ON PAGE 8

J. GENITAL EXAMINATION - FEMALES

Record all findings using diagrams, legend, and a consecutive numbering system.

1. **Examine the inner thighs, external genitalia, and perineal area.**
2. **Exam method:** ☐ Direct visualization ☐ Colposcope ☐ Other magnification

Exam positions/methods:

	Separation	Traction	Knee Chest
Supine	☐	☐	☐
Prone	☐	☐	☐

☐ Saline/Water ☐ Moistened swab ☐ Toluidine Blue Dye
☐ Catheter ☐ Other:

3. **Genital Tanner Stage** 1☐ 2☐ 3☐ 4☐ 5☐
4. **Examine the genital structures. Check the ABN box(es) if there are abuse/assault related findings and describe.**

	WNL	ABN	Describe:
Inner thighs	☐	☐	
Inguinal adenopathy	☐	☐	
Labia majora	☐	☐	
Labia minora	☐	☐	
Clitoral hood	☐	☐	
Perineum	☐	☐	
Periurethral tissue/urethral meatus	☐	☐	
Perihymenal tissue (vestibule)	☐	☐	
Hymen ☐ Supine ☐ Prone	☐	☐	
Record morphology:			
☐ Annular			
☐ Crescentic			
☐ Imperforate			
☐ Septate			
Fossa navicularis	☐	☐	
Posterior fourchette	☐	☐	
Vagina (pubertal adolescents)	☐	☐	
Cervix (pubertal adolescents)	☐	☐	

Discharge ☐ No ☐ Yes
If yes, describe: ______
No Findings ☐

5. **Collect dried and moist secretions, stains, and foreign materials. Scan the area with a Wood's Lamp.** ☐ Findings ☐ No Findings
6. **Collect swabs and prepare slides.**
   - ☐ **Prepubertal female**
     - ☐ **Collect at least 2 vulvar and 2 vestibular swabs.**
   - ☐ **Pubertal female**
     - ☐ **Collect 4 swabs from the vaginal pool.**
     - ☐ **Prepare one wet mount and one dry mount slide.**
     - ☐ **Collect 2 cervical swabs (if over 48 hours post assault).**
7. **Collect pubic hair combing or brushing.** ☐ Not applicable
8. **Collect pubic hair reference samples according to local policy.** ☐ Not applicable

LEGEND: Types of Findings

AB	Abrasion	**DF**	Deformity	**LA**	Laceration	**SH**	Submucosal Hemorrhage
AHT	Absent Hymenal Tissue	**DI**	Discharge	**MS**	Moist Secretion	**SHX**	Sample Per History
AL	Anal Laxity	**DS**	Dry Secretion	**OF**	Other Foreign Materials (describe)	**SI**	Suction Injury
BI	Bite	**EC**	Ecchymosis (bruise)	**OI**	Other Injury (describe)	**SW**	Swelling
BU	Burn	**ER**	Erythema (redness)	**OSC**	Other Skin Condition	**TB**	Toluidine Blue⊕
CS	Control Swab	**FB**	Foreign Body	**OT**	Other	**TE**	Tenderness
CV	Congenital Variation	**F/H**	Fiber/hair	**PW**	Perianal Wart	**V/S**	Vegetation/Soil
DE	Debris	**GT**	Granulation Tissue	**PE**	Petechiae	**VL**	Vesicular Lesion
		HC	Hymenal Cleft	**PGW**	Possible Genital Wart	**WL**	Wood's Lamp⊕
		IN	Induration	**PS**	Potential Saliva		
		IW	Incised Wound				

Locator #	Type	Description

Patient Identification

Diagram the position that best illustrates your findings.

Diagram G Genitalia - Supine

Diagram H Genitalia - Knee-Chest

RECORD ALL CLOTHING AND SPECIMENS COLLECTED ON PAGE 8

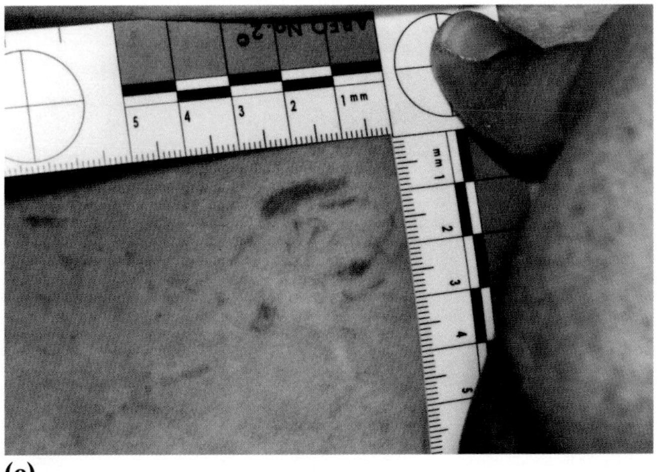

(c)

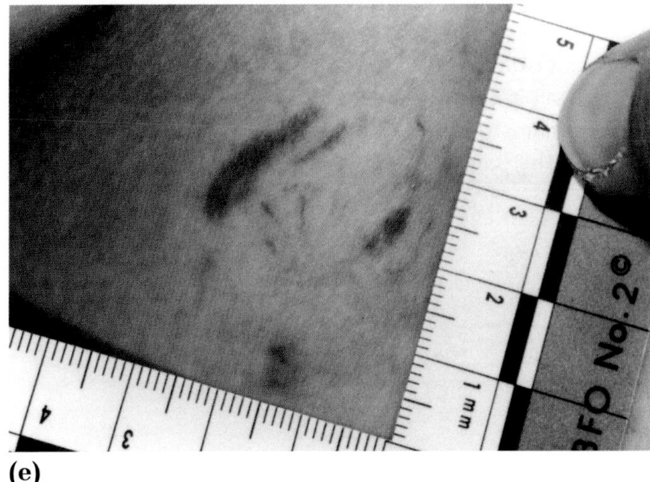

(e)

Color Plate 1: **45-year-old female who was sexually assaulted 40 hours prior to forensic examination. Injuries included multiple burns from a hot cigarette lighter pressed into the left upper quadrant of her abdomen several times. (c) Closer view showing scale for dimension. Note different positions of the scale reveal all findings. (e) Close-up view with scale showing best detail. (See Figure 7-5).**

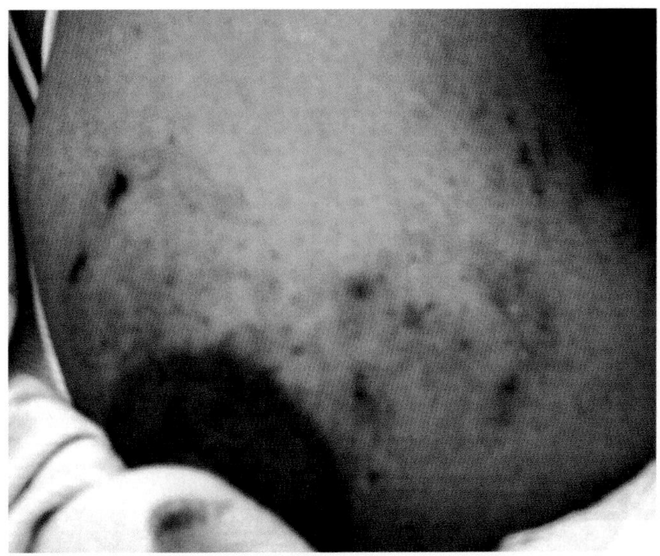

Color Plate 2: **Bite marks to a breast. (See Figure 8-1.)**

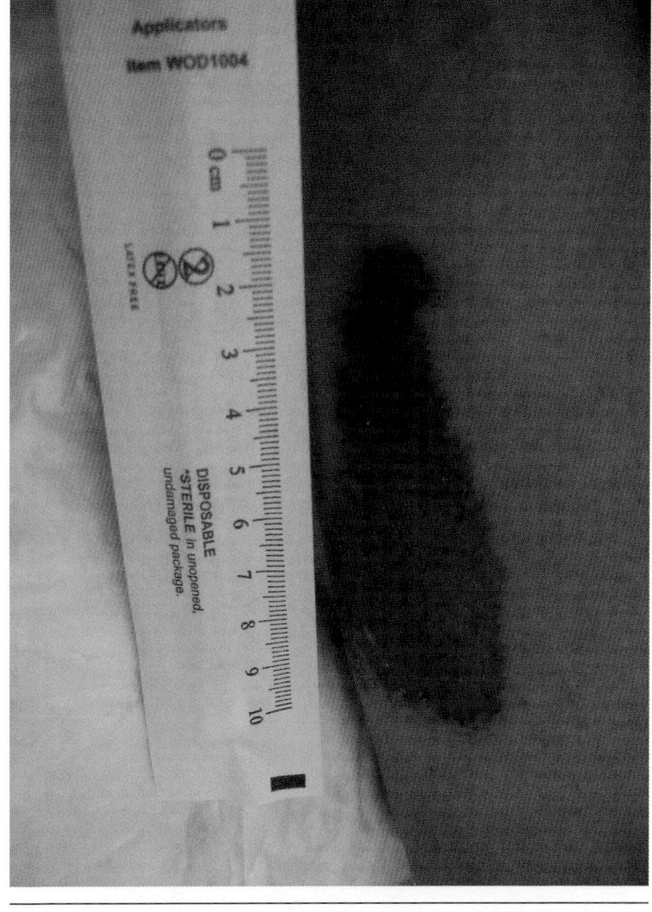

Color Plate 3: **Graze. This photo shows an example of a graze type wound, or brush burn abrasion. This injury, on the patient's forearm, occurred within hours after the patient fell off of his moped onto the pavement. (See Figure10-2.)**

Color Plate 4: ***(right)*** **Patterned abrasion. This photo shows an example of tire marks on the chest of the patient. The patient was struck and run over by a motorized vehicle. The strength of the impact left tire track impressions on the patient. (See Figure 10-4.)**

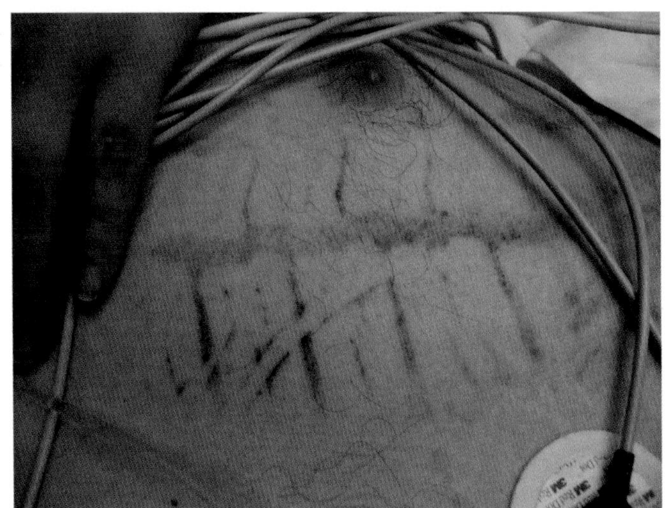

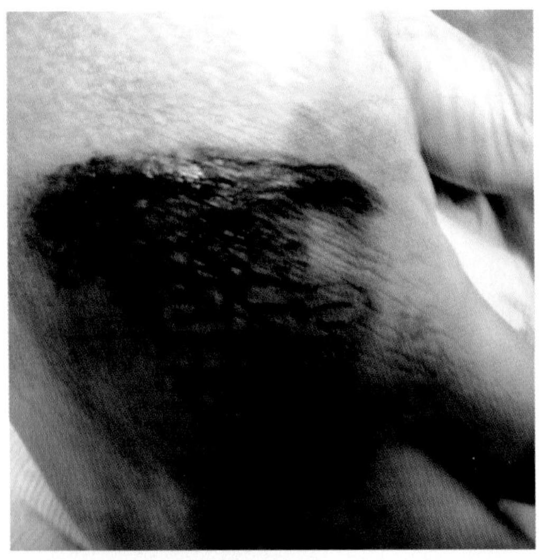

Color Plate 5: **Patterned abrasion-contusion. This photo shows the letters *SRS*, which stand for supplemental restraint system. The patient was the driver in a single-vehicle accident. The airbag deployed and struck her hand, leaving the imprint on the dorsum of her hand. (See Figure 10-5.)**

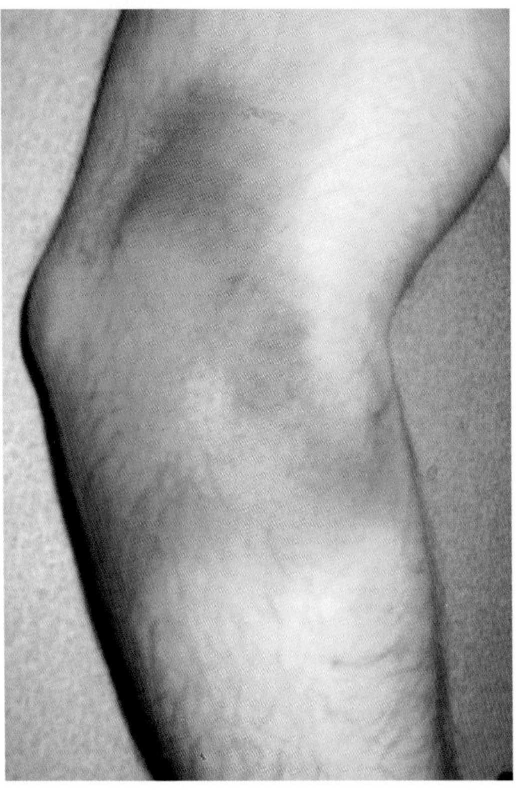

Color Plate 6: **Contusion. This photo shows a bruise in the second stage of healing. This wound to the elbow region was caused by another person's arm or foot—it was obtained during a Judo class. (See Figure 10-7.)**

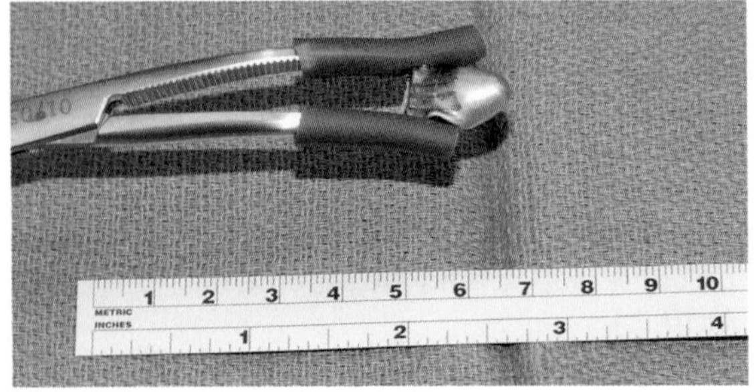

Color Plate 7: **Rubber-shodded hemostat used to extract a bullet from a patient. (See Figure 13-4.)**

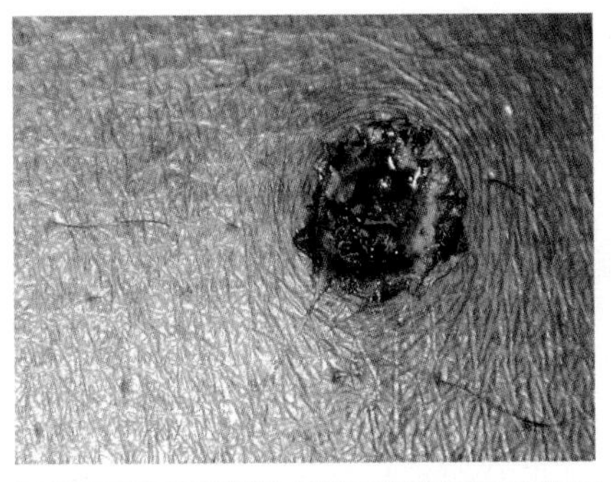

Color Plate 8: **Entrance gunshot wound with annular abrasion ring. (See Figure 13-8.)**

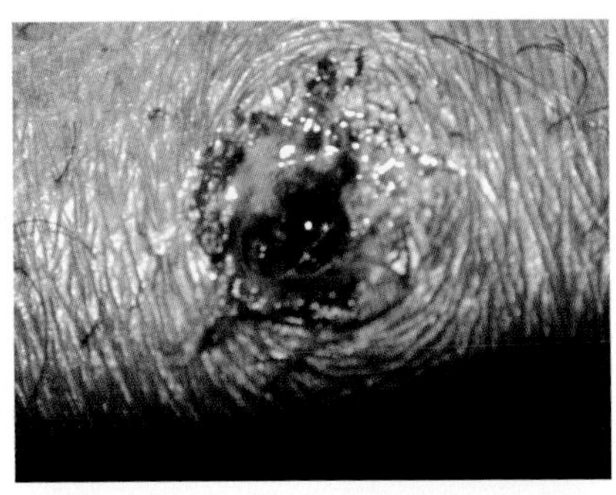

Color Plate 9: **Gunshot wound with jagged edges. (See Figure 13-9.)**

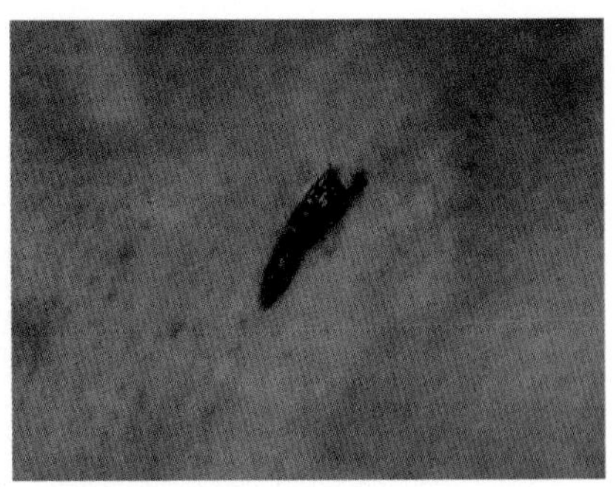

Color Plate 10: **Gunshot wound with slit-like exit. (See Figure 13-10.)**

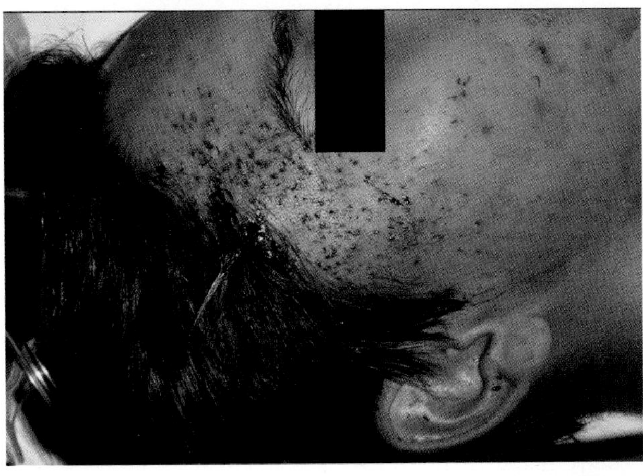

Color Plate 11: **Tattooing caused by close-range gunshot wound. (See Figure 13-12.)**

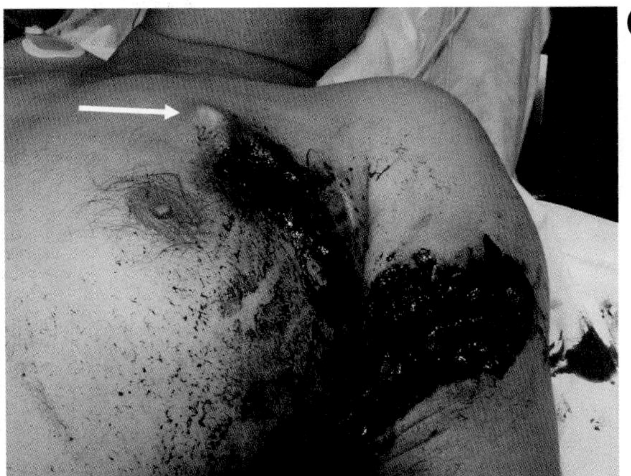

(b)

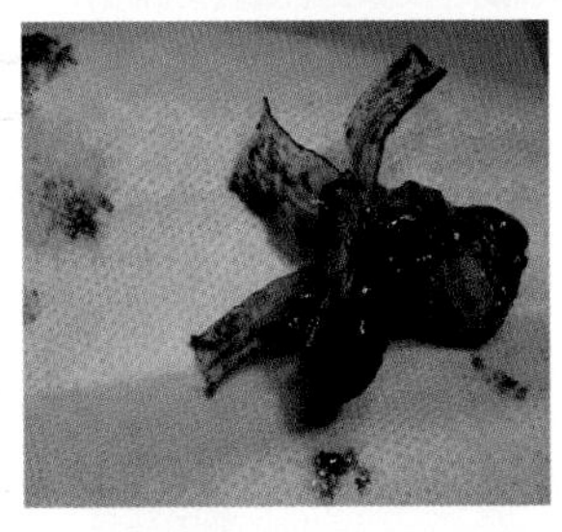

(c)

Color Plate 12: **Close-range shotgun wound: (b) tissue destruction obvious (arrow points to wadding embedded in wound); (c) wadding removed from patient. (See Figure 13-14 (b) and (c).)**

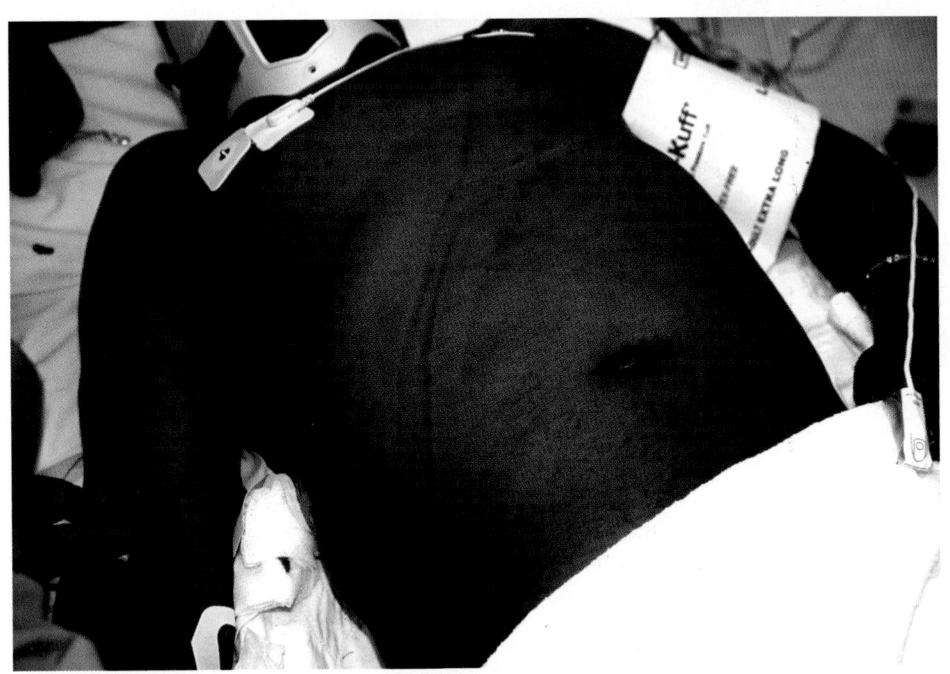

Color Plate 13: **Abdominal and chest linear ecchymosis from driver's side combined lap and shoulder belts. (See Figure 14-3.)**

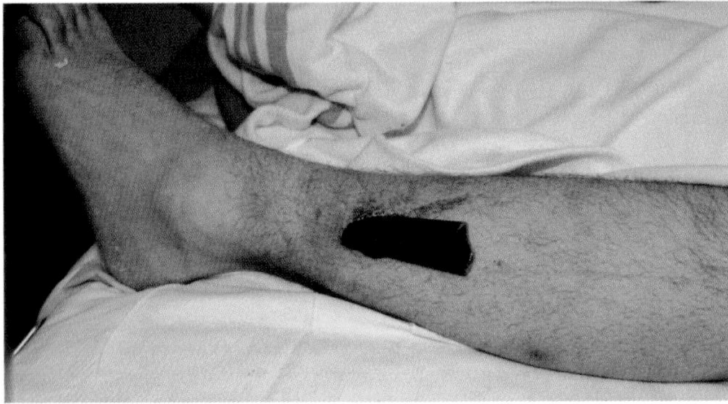

Color Plate 14: **Penetrating injury: (a) impaled brake pedal in lower leg. (See Figure 14-5 (a).)**

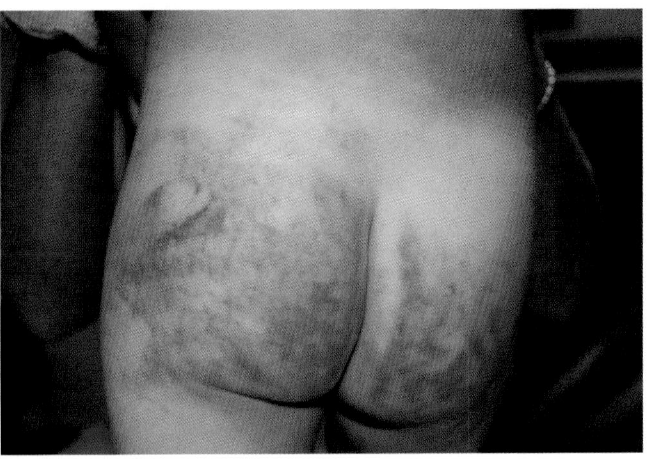

Color Plate 15: **Three-year-old male with ecchymosis to buttocks (medium-range photograph). Note patterned injury to left buttocks from "strap" used to discipline the child. (See Figure 19-1.)**

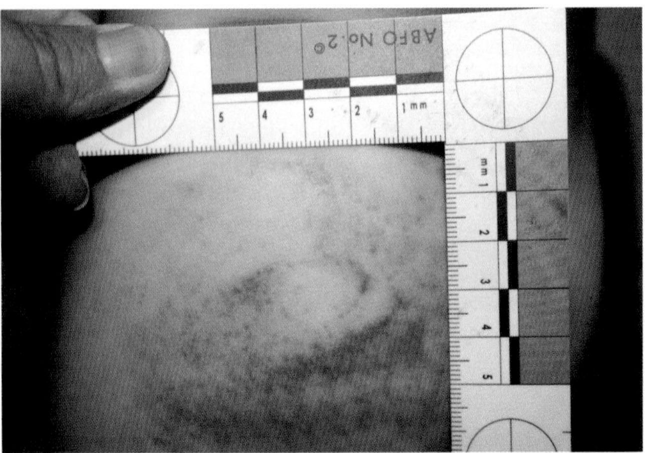

Color Plate 16: **Close-up photograph of patterned injury with a scale. (See Figure 19-2.)**

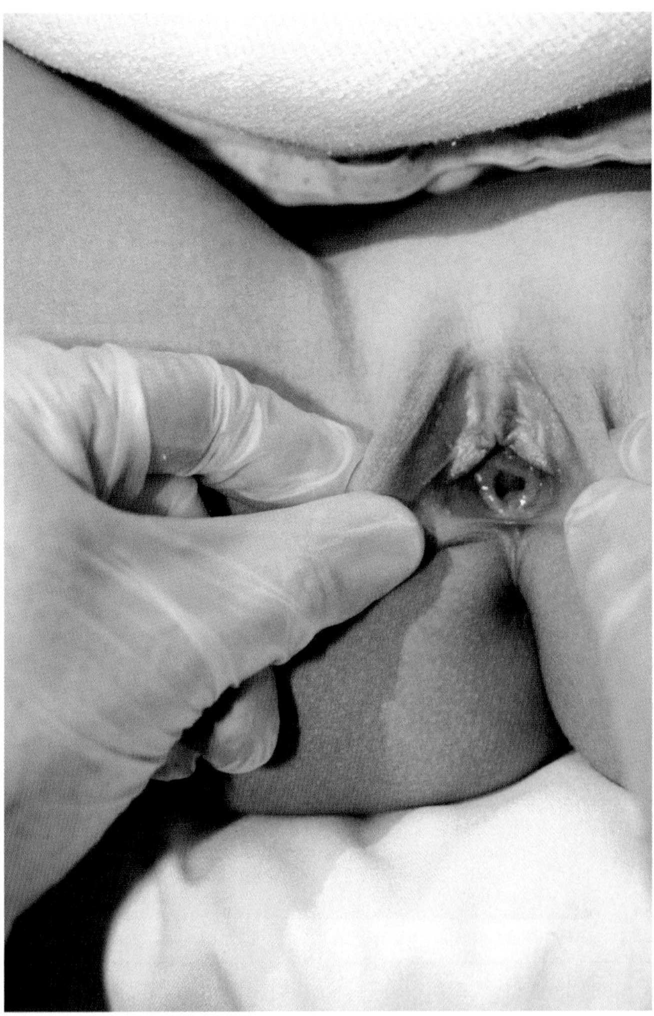

Color Plate 17: **Ten-year-old female examined using labial traction in the frog-leg position. A "bump" is noted at the 4 to 6 o'clock position. (See Figure 19-3.)**

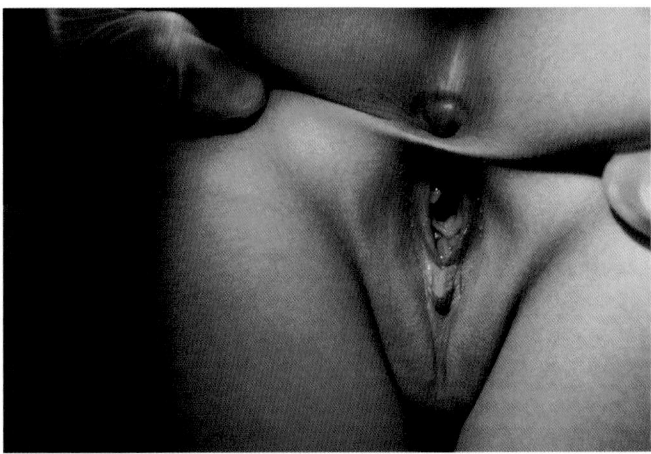

Color Plate 18: **Ten-year-old female examined using labial separation in the knee–chest position to confirm finding in the frog-leg position. (See Figure 19-4.)**

K. GENITAL EXAMINATION – MALES

Record all findings using diagrams, legend, and a consecutive numbering system.

1. **Examine the inner thighs, external genitalia, and perineal area.**
2. **Exam method:** ☐ Direct visualization ☐ Colposcope ☐ Other magnification
   Exam positions/methods:
   ☐ Supine ☐ Prone ☐ Moistened swab
   ☐ Toluidine Blue Dye ☐ Other:________
3. **Genital Tanner Stage** 1☐ 2☐ 3☐ 4☐ 5☐
4. **Circumcised:** ☐ No ☐ Yes
5. **Check the ABN box(es) if there are abuse/assault related findings and describe.**

	WNL	ABN	Describe:
Inner thighs	☐	☐	
Inguinal adenopathy	☐	☐	
Perineum	☐	☐	
Foreskin	☐	☐	
Glans Penis	☐	☐	
Penile shaft	☐	☐	
Urethral meatus	☐	☐	
Scrotum	☐	☐	
Testes	☐	☐	

Discharge ☐ No ☐ Yes If yes, describe: ________
No Findings ☐

6. **Collect dried and moist secretions, stains, and foreign materials. Scan the area with a Wood's Lamp.** ☐ Findings ☐ No Findings
7. **Collect pubic hair combing or brushing.** ☐ Not applicable
8. **Collect pubic hair reference samples according to local policy.** ☐ Not applicable
9. **Collect 2 penile swabs, if indicated by assault history.** ☐ Not applicable
10. **Collect 2 scrotal swabs, if indicated by assault history.** ☐ Not applicable

L. FEMALE/MALE ANAL AND RECTAL EXAMINATION

1. **Examine the buttocks, perianal skin, and anal folds for injury, foreign materials, and other findings.**
2. **Record exam positions, methods, observations:**
   ☐ Direct visualization ☐ Colposcope ☐ Other magnification

Exam positions	Observation	Observation with traction
Supine	☐	☐
Supine knee chest	☐	☐
Prone knee chest	☐	☐
Lateral recumbent	☐	☐

Exam methods: ☐ Moistened swab ☐ Toluidine blue dye ☐ Anoscopy ☐ Other:________

3. **Check the ABN box(es) if there are abuse/assault related findings and describe any abnormal or unusual findings.**

☐ No Findings	WNL	ABN	Describe:
Buttocks	☐	☐	
Perianal skin	☐	☐	
Anal verge/folds/rugae	☐	☐	
Rectum	☐	☐	

Anal dilation ☐ No ☐ Yes If yes: ☐ Immediate ☐ Delayed
Stool present in rectal ampulla ☐ No ☐ Yes ☐ Undetermined

4. Collect dried and moist secretions, stains, and foreign materials.
   ☐ Findings ☐ No Findings
5. **Collect 2 anal and/or rectal swabs and prepare one dry mount slide.**
6. **Rectal bleeding:** ☐ No ☐ Yes If yes, describe:

LEGEND: Types of Findings

AB	Abrasion	DF	Deformity	LA	Laceration	SH	Submcosal Hemorhage
AHT	Absent Hymenal Tissue	DI	Discharge	MS	Moist Secretion	SHX	Sample Per History
AL	Anal Laxity	DS	Dry Secretion	OF	Other Foreign Materials (describe)	SI	Suction Injury
BI	Bite	EC	Ecchymosis (bruise)	OI	Other Injury (describe)	SW	Swelling
BU	Burn	ER	Erythema (redness)	OSC	Other Skin Condition	TB	Toluidine Blue⊕
CS	Control Swab	FB	Foreign Body	OT	Other	TE	Tenderness
CV	Congenital Variation	F/H	Fiber/hair	PW	Perianal Wart	V/S	Vegetation/Soil
DE	Debris	GT	Granulation Tissue	PE	Petechiae	VL	Vesicular Lesion
		HC	Hymenal Cleft	PGW	Possible Genital Wart	WL	Wood's Lamp⊕
		IN	Induration	PS	Potential Saliva		
		IW	Incised Wound				

Locator #	Type	Description

Patient Identification

Diagram I - Penis

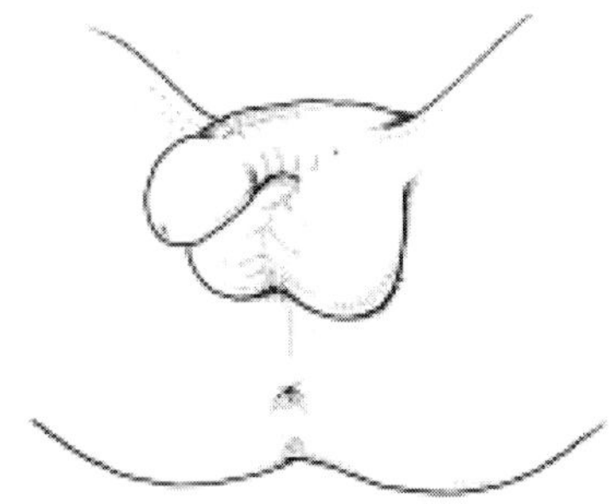

Diagram J - Penis

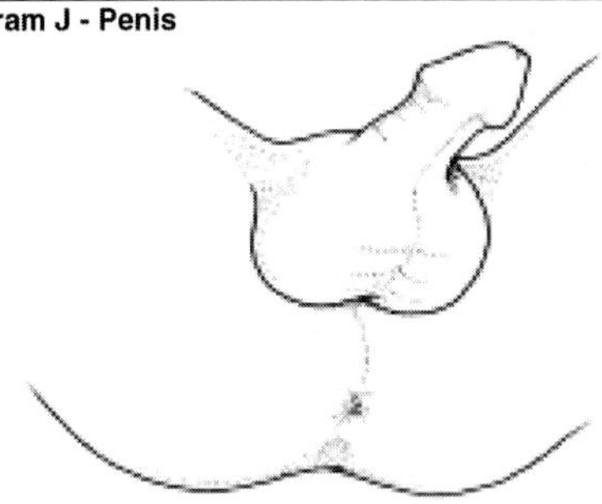

Diagram K - Anus Supine

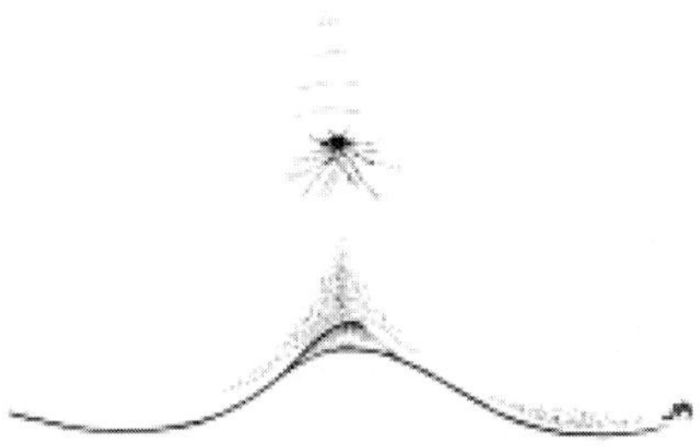

Diagram L - Anus Prone

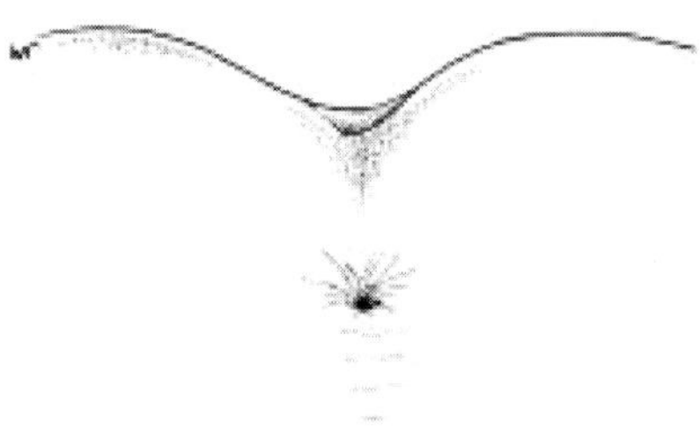

RECORD ALL CLOTHING AND SPECIMENS COLLECTED ON PAGE 8

M. EVIDENCE COLLECTED AND SUBMITTED TO CRIME LAB

1. Clothing placed in evidence kit	Other clothing placed in bags

2. Foreign materials collected

	No	Yes	Collected by:
Swabs/suspected blood	☐	☐	
Dried secretions	☐	☐	
Fiber/loose hairs	☐	☐	
Vegetation	☐	☐	
Soil/debris	☐	☐	
Swabs/suspected semen	☐	☐	
Swabs/suspected saliva	☐	☐	
Swabs/Wood's Lamp⊕ area(s)	☐	☐	
Control swabs	☐	☐	
Fingernail scrapings/cuttings	☐	☐	
Matted hair cuttings	☐	☐	
Pubic hair combings/brushings	☐	☐	
Intravaginal foreign body	☐	☐	
Describe:			
Other types	☐	☐	
If yes, describe:			

3. Oral/genital/anal/rectal samples

	# Swabs	# Slides	Time collected	Collected by:
Oral				
Vulvar		■		
Vestibular		■		
Vaginal				
Cervical		■		
Anal				
Rectal				
Penile		■		
Scrotal		■		
Aspirate/washings (optional) ☐ No ☐ Yes				

4. Vaginal wet mount slide

	No	Yes	Time	Examiner:
Slide prepared				
Motile sperm observed				
Non-motile sperm observed				

N. TOXICOLOGY SAMPLES

	No	Yes	Time	Collected by:
Blood alcohol/toxicology (gray top tube)				
Urine toxicology				

O. REFERENCE SAMPLES

	No	Yes	Collected by:
Blood (lavender top tube)			
Blood (yellow top tube)			
Blood Card (optional)			
Buccal swabs (optional)			
Saliva swabs			
Head hair			
Pubic Hair			

P. PHOTO DOCUMENTATION METHODS

	No	Yes	Colposcope/ 35mm	Macrolens/ 35mm	Colposcope/ Videocamera	Other Optics
Body	☐	☐	☐	☐	☐	☐
Genitals	☐	☐	☐	☐	☐	☐

Photographed by:

Patient Identification

Q. FINDINGS AND INTERPRETATION

1. **Anal-Genital Findings**
   - ☐ Normal anal-genital exam
   - ☐ Abnormal anal-genital exam
   - ☐ Indeterminate anal-genital exam
2. **Assessment of Anal-Genital Findings**
   - ☐ Consistent with history
   - ☐ Inconsistent with history
   - ☐ Limited/Insufficient history
3. **Interpretation of Anal-Genital Findings**
   - ☐ Normal exam: can neither confirm nor negate sexual abuse
   - ☐ Non specific: may be caused by sexual abuse or other mechanisms
   - ☐ Sexual abuse is highly suspected
   - ☐ Definite evidence of sexual abuse and/or sexual contact
4. ☐ **Need further consultation/investigation**
5. ☐ **Lab results or photo review pending (may alter assessment)**
6. **Additional comments regarding findings, interpretations, and recommendations:**

R. MEDICAL LAB TESTS PERFORMED

STD Cultures	GC	Chlamydia	Other	Describe:	Collected by:
Oral	☐	☐	☐		
Vestibular	☐	☐	☐		
Vaginal	☐	☐	☐		
Cervical	☐	☐	☐		
Rectal	☐	☐	☐		
Penile	☐	☐	☐		
Wet mount	☐	☐	☐		
Serology	Syphilis ☐	HIV ☐	Hepatitis ☐		
Pregnancy test	Blood ☐	Urine ☐			
Other test(s)					

S. PRINT NAMES OF PERSONNEL INVOLVED

History taken by:	Telephone
Exam performed by:	
Specimens labeled and sealed by:	
Assisted by: N/A	
Signature of examiner	License No.

T. EVIDENCE DISTRIBUTION

	GIVEN TO:
Clothing (item(s) not placed in evidence kit)	
Evidence Kit	
Reference blood samples	
Toxicology samples	

U. SIGNATURE OF OFFICER RECEIVING EVIDENCE

Signature:

Print name and ID#:

Agency:

Date: Telephone:

City of Philadelphia Department of Public Health

Suspected Sexual Maltreatment Form

Medical Record #:____________________

Patient Last Name: ________________ First Name: ________________________ Gender: ☐ Male ☐ Female

DOB: ________________________ Date of Visit: ____________ Time of Visit: ________________________

Race: ☐ Cauc. ☐ Black ☐ Asian ☐ Hispanic ☐ Other: ____________ Primary language spoken: __________________

Interpreter Name: ______________________________________ Interpreter relation to patient: ________________

Legal Guardian/ Primary caretaker: ____________________________ Relationship to Child: ____________________

Offender's Name: ______________________________________ Offender's age/DOB & gender: ________________

Offender's relationship to Child: _______________________ Race: ☐ Cauc. ☐ Black ☐ Asian ☐ Hispanic ☐ Other________

Place where offense occurred: ____

Date of Offense: _____________________________ Time of Offense: ___________________________________

Time elapse since offense: _______________________ Last known contact with offender: _________________________

History given by Adult: Relationship of Adult: ____

Continuation sheet attached? ☐Yes ☐No

History of Assault given by Child *(use exact words where possible)*: History obtained by *(name &title)*:__________________

Name and title of staff present:____

Continuation sheet attached? ☐Yes ☐No

Resident/Fellow/SAFE Name: ________________________ Attending Name: _____________________________________

Resident/Fellow/SAFE Signature: ______________________ Attending Signature: __________________________________

Page 1 of 6

City of Philadelphia Department of Public Health

Suspected Sexual Maltreatment Form

Child's current symptoms:

☐ headache	☐ eye pain	☐ ear pain	☐ sore throat
☐ difficulty breathing	☐ palpitations	☐ chest pain	
☐ abdominal pain	☐ vomiting	☐ diarrhea	☐ tenesmus
☐ dysuria	☐ urinary urgency	☐ urinary frequency	☐ vaginal / penile discharge
☐ neck pain	☐ back pain		
☐ extremity pain:	☐ RUE ☐ LUE	☐ RLE ☐ LLE	
☐ difficulty walking	☐ pain with walking		
☐ other symptoms:			

Past Medical History: ______ Immunizations UTD: ☐ Yes ☐ No
Past Surgical History: ______ Development Appropriate for Age: ☐ Yes ☐ No
Current Medications (incl. contraception): ______ Allergies: ______
Social history: ☐ Tobacco ☐ Alcohol ☐ Drugs: type ______
STD history (include treatment and doses): ______
Primary pediatrician Name: ______

GYN History: ☐ Premenarche Age at Menarche: ______ Gravida: ______ Para: ______
LMP: ______ ☐ Sexually active ☐ Condom used: ______
Last consensual sexual activity: ______ Area(s) of penetration: ______

Acts of Force: N = No Y = Yes U = Unsure NA = Not asked

Verbal	N	Y	U	NA
Choking	N	Y	U	NA
Hitting	N	Y	U	NA
Pushing	N	Y	U	NA
Gagging	N	Y	U	NA
Blindfold	N	Y	U	NA

Other: ______

Weapons:

Knife	N	Y	U	NA
Gun	N	Y	U	NA
Household object	N	Y	U	NA specify: ______

Other: ______

Drugs involved in assault: ☐ Yes ☐ No Type: ______
☐ unknown Describe: ______

Since assault, has patient:
Changed clothes? ☐ Yes ☐ No
Urinated / defecated? ☐ Yes ☐ No
Showered / wiped areas or fluid? ☐ Yes ☐ No
Eaten / brushed teeth / used dental floss? ☐ Yes ☐ No
Used tampon or pad? ☐ Yes ☐ No
Anything else? ______

Acts of sexual assault: N = No Y = Yes U = Unsure NA = Not asked

Kissing/Licking N Y U NA
Location(s): ______

Fondling Victim N Y U NA
Location(s): ______

Vaginal Penetration	N	Y	U	NA
Penis	N	Y	U	NA
Offender's fingers	N	Y	U	NA
Offender's tongue	N	Y	U	NA

Foreign Object ______
Other ______

Oral Penetration	N	Y	U	NA
Penis	N	Y	U	NA
Offender's fingers	N	Y	U	NA
Offender's tongue	N	Y	U	NA

Foreign Object ______
Other ______

Anal Penetration	N	Y	U	NA
Penis	N	Y	U	NA
Offender's fingers	N	Y	U	NA
Offender's tongue	N	Y	U	NA

Foreign Object ______
Other ______

Other oral acts

Victim mouth to Offender genitals	N	Y	U	NA
Victim mouth to Offender anus	N	Y	U	NA
Offender mouth to Victim genitals	N	Y	U	NA
Offender mouth to Victim anus	N	Y	U	NA

Did offender ejaculate?	N	Y	U	NA
Vagina	N	Y	U	NA
Anus	N	Y	U	NA
Mouth	N	Y	U	NA

Other ______

Resident/Fellow/SAFE Name: ______ Attending Name: ______

Resident/Fellow/SAFE Signature: ______ Attending Signature: ______

City of Philadelphia Department of Public Health

Suspected Sexual Maltreatment Form

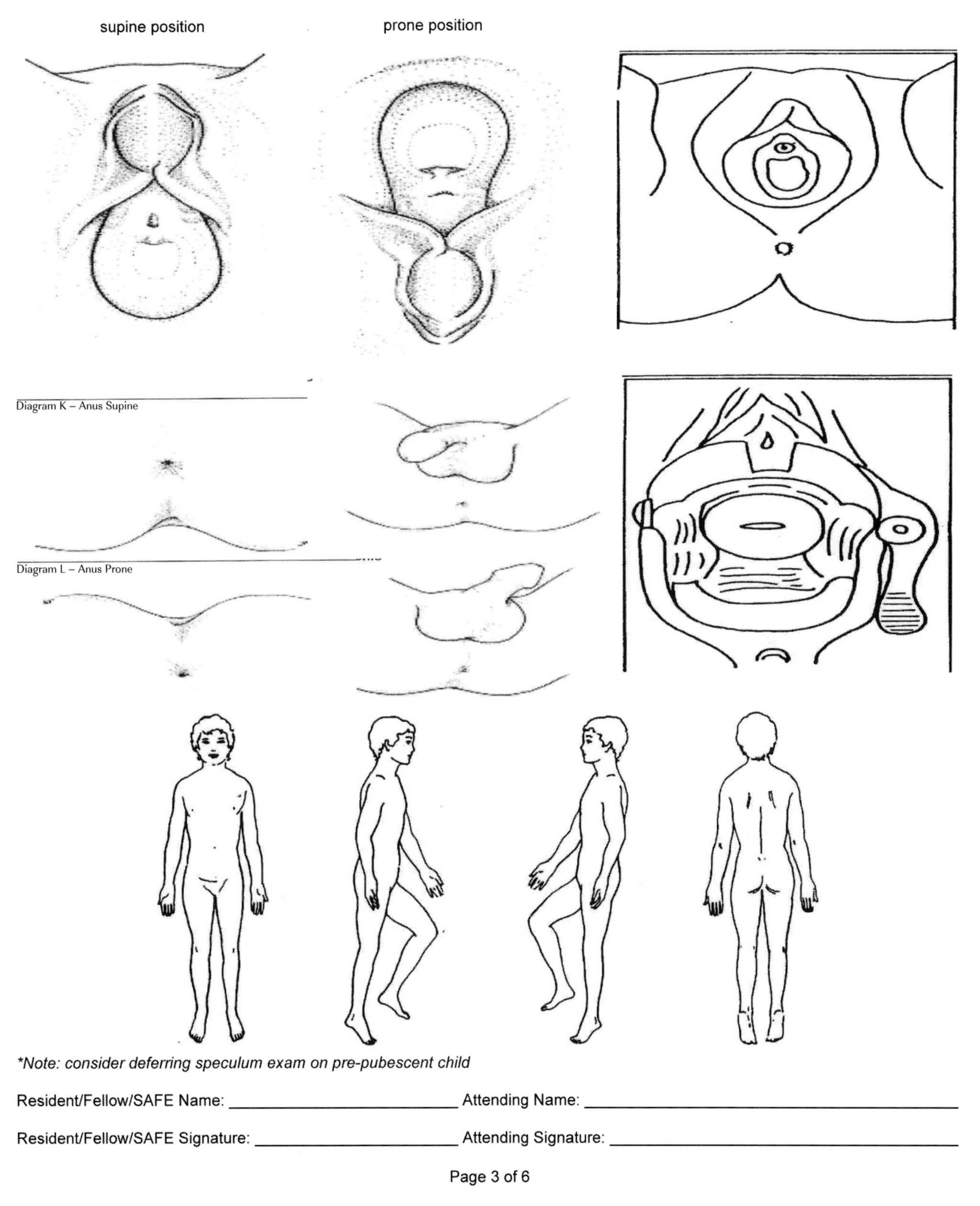

**Note: consider deferring speculum exam on pre-pubescent child*

Resident/Fellow/SAFE Name: ______________________ Attending Name: ______________________

Resident/Fellow/SAFE Signature: ______________________ Attending Signature: ______________________

City of Philadelphia Department of Public Health

Suspected Sexual Maltreatment Form

Physical Examination:

Vitals: Temp: ________ HR: ________ RR: ________ BP: ________ Weight: ________

General appearance: Describe ________

HEENT: ☐ Normal ☐ Abnormal ________

Chest: ☐ Normal ☐ Abnormal ________

Cardiovascular: ☐ Normal ☐ Abnormal ________

Abdomen: ☐ Normal ☐ Abnormal ________

Extremities: ☐ Normal ☐ Abnormal ________

Skin: Describe ________

Neuro: Level of consciousness: ________ DTR: ________

Cranial nerves: ________ Motor/Sensory: ________

Genitourinary Tanner Stage: ☐ I ☐ II ☐ III ☐ IV ☐ V

FEMALE *Please describe any abnormal findings--Refer to body diagrams on previous page*

Ext Genitalia ☐ Normal ☐ Abnormal ________

Labia Majora ☐ Normal ☐ Abnormal ________

Labia Minora ☐ Normal ☐ Abnormal ________

Fossa Navicularis ☐ Normal ☐ Abnormal ________

Posterior fourchette ☐ Normal ☐ Abnormal ________

Vagina ☐ Normal ☐ Abnormal ________

Cervix ☐ Normal ☐ Abnormal ________

Perineum ☐ Normal ☐ Abnormal ________

Bimanual Exam ☐ Normal ☐ Abnormal ________

Anus ☐ Normal ☐ Abnormal ________

Hymen ☐ Describe ________

MALE *Please describe any abnormal findings--Refer to body diagrams on previous page*

Penis: ☐ Normal ☐ Abnormal ________

Scrotum: ☐ Normal ☐ Abnormal ________

Testes: ☐ Normal ☐ Abnormal ________

Perineum: ☐ Normal ☐ Abnormal ________

Anus: ☐ Normal ☐ Abnormal ________

Resident/Fellow/SAFE Name: ________ Attending Name: ________

Resident/Fellow/SAFE Signature: ________ Attending Signature: ________

Page 4 of 6

City of Philadelphia Department of Public Health

Suspected Sexual Maltreatment Form

Laboratory

Urine:
☐ Urinalysis
☐ HCG: Pos Neg
☐ Urine toxicology
☐ PCR swab (GC and Chlamydia)

Blood:
☐ Blood Alcohol Level
☐ RPR
☐ Hepatitis B
☐ Hepatitis C
☐ HIV (with consent):

Cultures:
☐ Vaginal culture (routine): ☐ gram stain
☐ GC: ☐ oral ☐ urethral ☐ vaginal ☐ anal
☐ Chlamydia: ☐ urethral ☐ vaginal ☐ anal
☐ Herpes Simplex, location: ____________

Medications and Prophylaxis

☐ Pregnancy prophylaxis — Medication given: ____________
☐ Gonorrhea prophylaxis — Medication given: ____________
☐ Chlamydia prophylaxis — Medication given: ____________
☐ Trichomonas prophylaxis — Medication given: ____________
☐ HIV prophylaxis — Medication given: ____________
☐ Tetanus prophylaxis
☐ Hepatitis B prophylaxis
☐ Other Medications given: ____________

Agency Notification

☐ Social Work Notified — Social Worker's Name: ____________
☐ Child Line notified — Hot-line worker's name: ____________
Called by: ____________
CY - 47 completed by: ____________
☐ WOAR Notified
☐ Police notified — Police Officer's Name, District/Unit, and Badge #: ____________

Evidence collected

Clothing ☐ None
☐ panties / underpants/ describe: ____________
☐ shirt / blouse / describe: ____________
☐ pants / slacks / describe: ____________
☐ skirt / dress / describe: ____________
☐ bra / undershirt / describe: ____________
☐ jacket / coat / describe: ____________
☐ nightgown / PJs / describe: ____________
☐ other:

Rape Kit: ☐ None
☐ changing sheet
☐ oral swab ☐ bite mark-site: ____________
☐ vulva swab ☐ vaginal swab ☐ cervical swab
☐ rectal swab ☐ perineum swab
☐ debris: source: ________ description: ________
☐ secretions: source: ________ description: ________
☐ hair combings: source:
☐ blood / purple top

Photographs: Taken: ☐ Yes ☐ No
Number of photos: ____________
Type: ☐ camera ☐ colposcope
Photographer: ____________

Chain of Custody
☐ all checked items: labeled, sealed and secured:
Date: ________ Name/Title: ____________
☐ all checked items received from: ____________ Date: ____________
☐ all checked items given to: ____________ Badge number: ____________
Date: ________ Time: ________

Disposition

☐ Admitted ☐ Discharged To whom: ____________

Follow up services: ☐ Primary doctor ☐ Psychosocial counseling ☐ Immunology (with referral)
☐ SAFE/CARE Clinic ☐ Other: ____________

Resident/Fellow/SAFE Name: ____________ Attending Name: ____________

Resident/Fellow/SAFE Signature: ____________ Attending Signature: ____________

Page 5 of 6

City of Philadelphia Department of Public Health

Suspected Sexual Maltreatment Form

Consent: Authorization for Evaluation and Treatment of Possible Sexual Maltreatment

A. Conditions

1. I understand that the examination for medical treatment and sexual assault can, with my consent, be conducted by an examiner to discover and preserve evidence of the assault. I understand that I may refuse any portion of the examination.
2. Photographs and video prints may be taken as evidence. Like all evidence collected in this evaluation, these records are to be used for medical treatment and legal purposes.

B. Authorization

I give permission for ____________________ to evaluate me or ____________________

I certify that I have read, understand, and agree to the conditions described in section A.

____________________ ____________________ ____________________

Signature of legal guardian   Witness   Date / Time

I understand that the collection of evidence may include photographing injuries and in cases of sexual assault, may include the genital area. Knowing this, I consent to having photographs taken.

____________________ ____________________ ____________________

Signature of legal guardian   Witness   Date / Time

I understand that any photographs taken may be used for educational purposes and if used for such purposes, my identity will be kept confidential.

☐ I consent to the use of photography for educational purposes

☐ I refuse to consent to the use of photography for educational purposes

____________________ ____________________ ____________________

Signature of legal guardian   Witness   Date / Time

C. Release of information

I hereby authorize ____________________ to release medical information and reports regarding any examination and treatment for alleged assault to the Philadelphia Police and to the Philadelphia District Attorney's Office. Disclosure may include psychiatric, drug alcohol, and / or HIV related information.

Date/Time: ____________________   Patient signature: ____________________

Date/Time: ____________________   Parent / Guardian Signature: ____________________

Relationship to patient: ____________________

Witness: ____________________   Address: ____________________

____

____

Resident/Fellow/SAFE Name: ____________________ Attending Name: ____________________

Resident/Fellow/SAFE Signature: ____________________ Attending Signature: ____________________

Page 6 of 6

State of California
Governor's Office of Emergency Services

MEDICAL REPORT: SUSPECTED CHILD PHYSICAL ABUSE AND NEGLECT EXAMINATION

OES 900

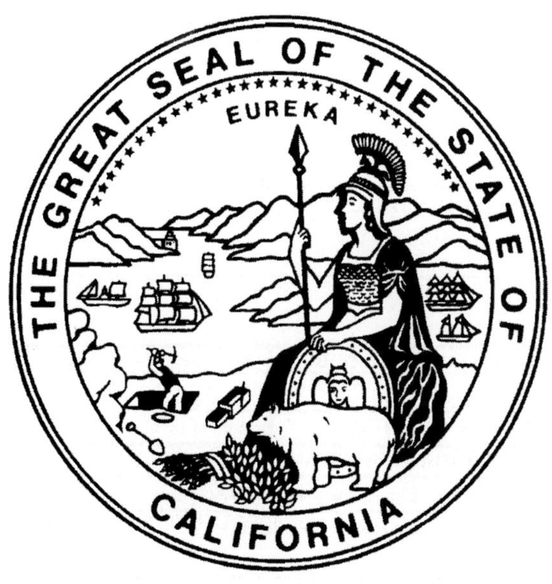

For more information or assistance in completing the OES 900, please contact University of California, Davis California Medical Training Center at: (888) 705-4141 or www.calmtc.org

Available at: **www.oes.ca.gov**
Criminal Justice Programs Division;
Publications and Brochures

MEDICAL REPORT: SUSPECTED CHILD PHYSICAL ABUSE AND NEGLECT EXAMINATION
State of California
Governor's Office of Emergency Services
OES 900

Confidential Document: Restricted Release | **Patient Identification:** **Date:**

A. GENERAL INFORMATION ☐ See Patient Label/Registration Face Sheet

1. Name of Medical Facility Where Exam Performed	Facility Address	2. Date of Exam	Time of Exam

3. Patient's Last Name	First Name	M.I.	Telephone	Cell Phone

4. Street Address	City	County	State	Zip Code

5. Age	Date of Birth	Gender ☐ Female ☐ Male	Ethnicity

6. Interpreter Used: ☐ No ☐ Yes Language Used: ______
Name of Interpreter: ______ Telephone: ______
Affiliation of interpreter: ☐ Facility Interpreting Services
☐ Contracted Agency, specify: ______
☐ Family ☐ Friend ☐ Other, specify: ______

7. Name of Child's Caregiver ☐ Parent ☐ Legal Guardian ☐ Other, specify: ______	Gender ☐ Female ☐ Male	Telephone (w) (h) (c)

Street Address	City	County	State	Zip Code

8. Name of Child's Caregiver ☐ Parent ☐ Legal Guardian ☐ Other, specify: ______	Gender ☐ Female ☐ Male	Telephone (w) (h) (c)

Street Address	City	County	State	Zip Code

9. Name(s) of Siblings	Gender	Age	DOB	Name(s) of Siblings	Gender	Age	DOB
	M F				M F		
	M F				M F		

B. MANDATORY REPORTING FOR SUSPECTED CHILD ABUSE AND NEGLECT

Mandatory Child Abuse/Neglect Report made to both Law Enforcement and CPS Agencies (Pursuant to Penal Code §11166):

	Name of Agency	Telephone	Date
☐ Law Enforcement ☐ Telephone Report ☐ Written Report Submitted Name of Person Taking Report:			
☐ Child Protective Services ☐ Telephone Report ☐ Written Report Submitted Name of Person Taking Report:			

C. RESPONDING PERSONNEL TO MEDICAL FACILITY

	Name	ID Number	Agency	☐ Unknown
Child Protective Services				
and/or				
Law Enforcement Officer				

D. PATIENT CONSENT AND AUTHORIZATION FOR EXAMINATION (See instructions)

☐ Law Enforcement Authorized ☐ CPS Authorized ☐ Placed in protective custody ☐ Physician authority pursuant to state law ☐ Parent/Guardian consent

E. DISTRIBUTION OF OES 900 (Check all that apply)

☐ Law Enforcement Agency (original) ☐ Hand Delivered ☐ Mailed ☐ Faxed	☐ Child Protective Services (copy) ☐ Hand Delivered ☐ Mailed ☐ Faxed
☐ Crime Laboratory (copy included with evidence)	☐ Medical Facility Records (copy)

F. PATIENT HISTORY

1. Name of Person(s) Providing History	Relationship to Patient

2. Child Accompanied to Facility By	Relationship to Patient

Patient Identification: **Date:**

3. History of Present Illness ☐ **See dictation for additional information.** ☐ **N/A**

If dictating, provide brief 2-3 sentence handwritten summary. Print or write legibly. Include date, time or timeframe, place of incident, and initial reporting party. Distinguish statements made by child in quotation marks from those statements made by other historians.

G. PAST MEDICAL HISTORY

	Yes	No	Unknown	Describe
Birth History (if applicable)	☐	☐	☐	
Physical Abuse History	☐	☐	☐	
Sexual Abuse History	☐	☐	☐	
Neglect History	☐	☐	☐	
Emotional Abuse History	☐	☐	☐	
Domestic Violence Exposure	☐	☐	☐	
Alcohol/Drug Exposure ☐ Prenatal ☐ Postnatal ☐ Alcohol ☐ Drug	☐	☐	☐	Specify types of drugs if known, and collect urine toxicology up to 96 hours after ingestion:
Hospitalization(s)	☐	☐	☐	
Surgery	☐	☐	☐	
Significant Illness/Injury	☐	☐	☐	
Any pertinent medical condition(s) that may affect the interpretation of findings?	☐	☐	☐	
Allergies	☐	☐	☐	
Medications	☐	☐	☐	
Immunizations Up To Date	☐	☐	☐	
Disabilities	☐	☐	☐	(Specify):
Growth & Development ☐ WNL ☐ ABN ☐ Unknown	☐	☐	☐	

H. REVIEW OF SYSTEMS ☐ Negative except as noted below

☐ See dictation for additional information ☐ N/A

I. NAME OF PERSON TAKING HISTORY (Print Name)	**Signature**	**Telephone**	**Date**

J. GENERAL PHYSICAL EXAMINATION

1. Temperature	Pulse	Respiration	Blood Pressure

2. Height (cm or in)	(%)	Weight (kg or lb)	(%)	Children under 2: (HC)	(%)

3. General physical appearance, demeanor, and level of physical discomfort/pain. Provide brief handwritten summary even if dictating. ☐ See dictation for additional information. ☐ N/A

Patient Identification: **Date:**

4. Record results of physical examination.

	WNL	ABN	Not Examined	See Body Diagram	Describe Abnormal Findings. ☐ N/A ☐ See dictation for additional information
Skin					
Head					
Eyes					
Ears					
Nose					
Mouth/Pharynx					
Teeth					
Neck					
Lungs					
Chest					
Heart					
Abdomen					
Back					
Buttocks					
Extremities					
Neurological					
Genitalia					

5. If genital injuries are sustained, use copies of page(s) 6 and 7 (if applicable) from OES 930 Forensic Medical Report: Acute (<72 hours) Child/Adolescent Sexual Abuse Examination Form or OES 925 Forensic Medical Report: NonAcute (>72 hours) Child/Adolescent Sexual Abuse Examination to document findings and attach to this form.

J. GENERAL PHYSICAL EXAMINATION (continued)

6. Conduct physical examination and record findings using the diagrams.

Patient Identification: **Date:**

A

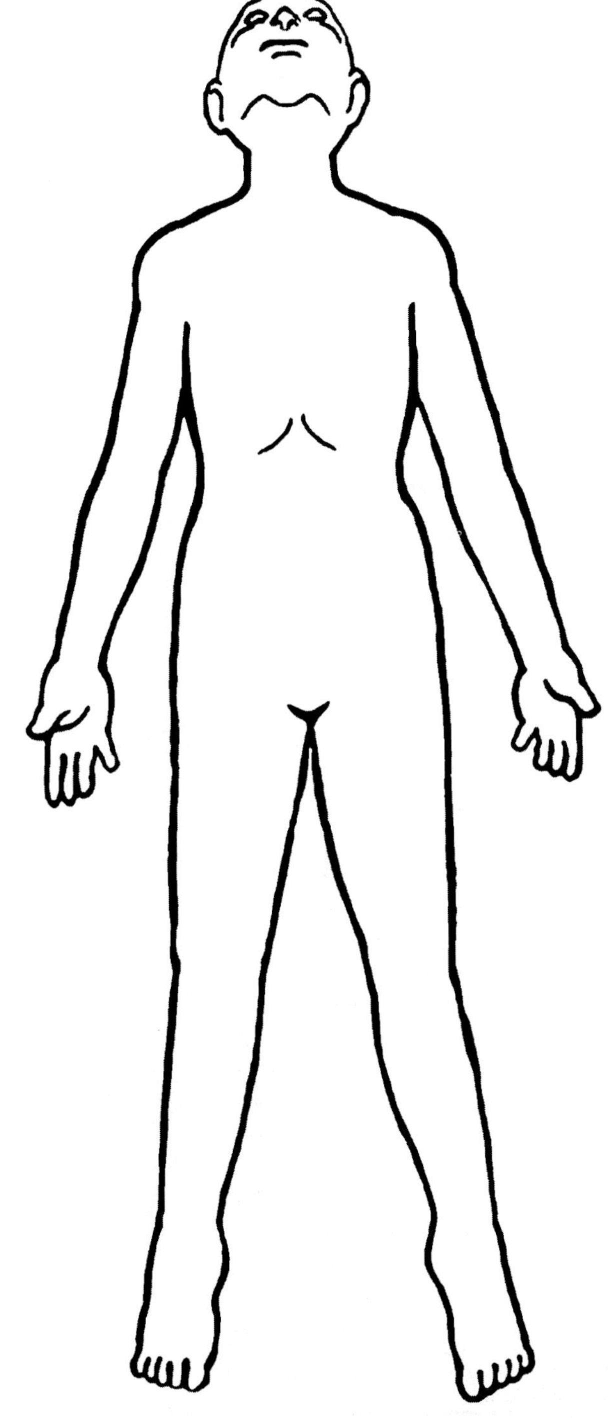

B

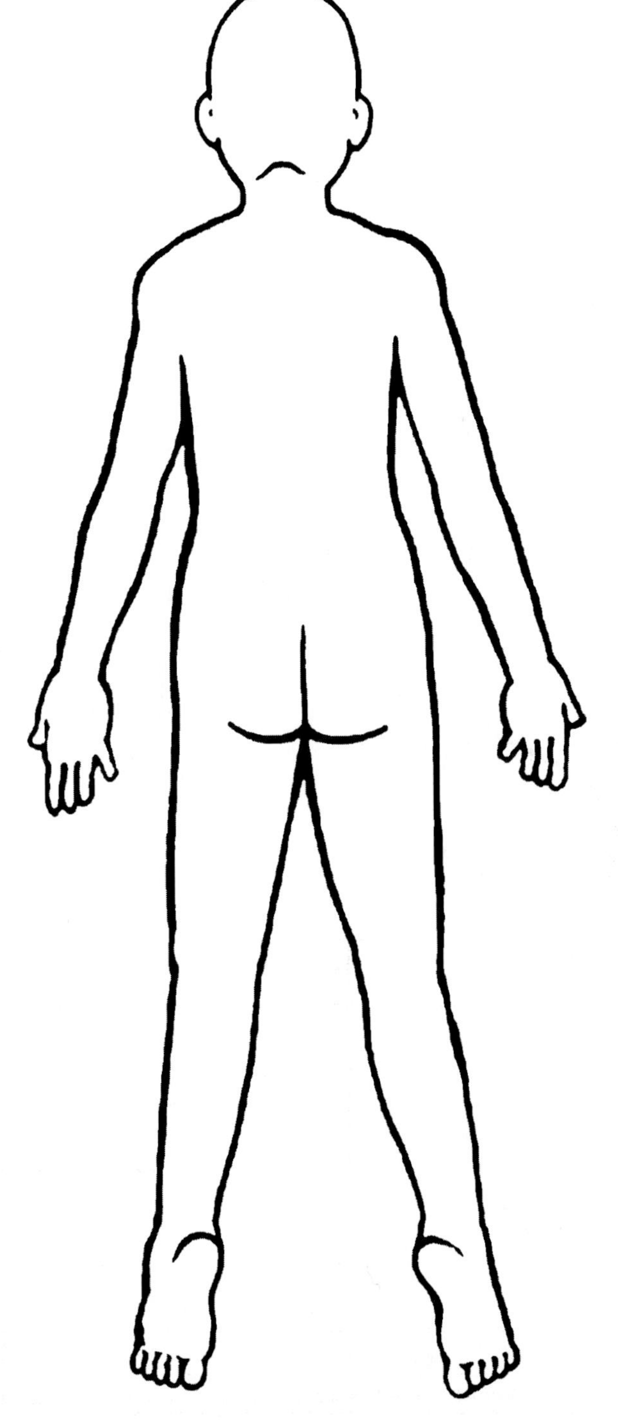

J. GENERAL PHYSICAL EXAMINATION (continued)

6. Conduct physical examination and record findings using the diagrams.

Patient Identification: **Date:**

C

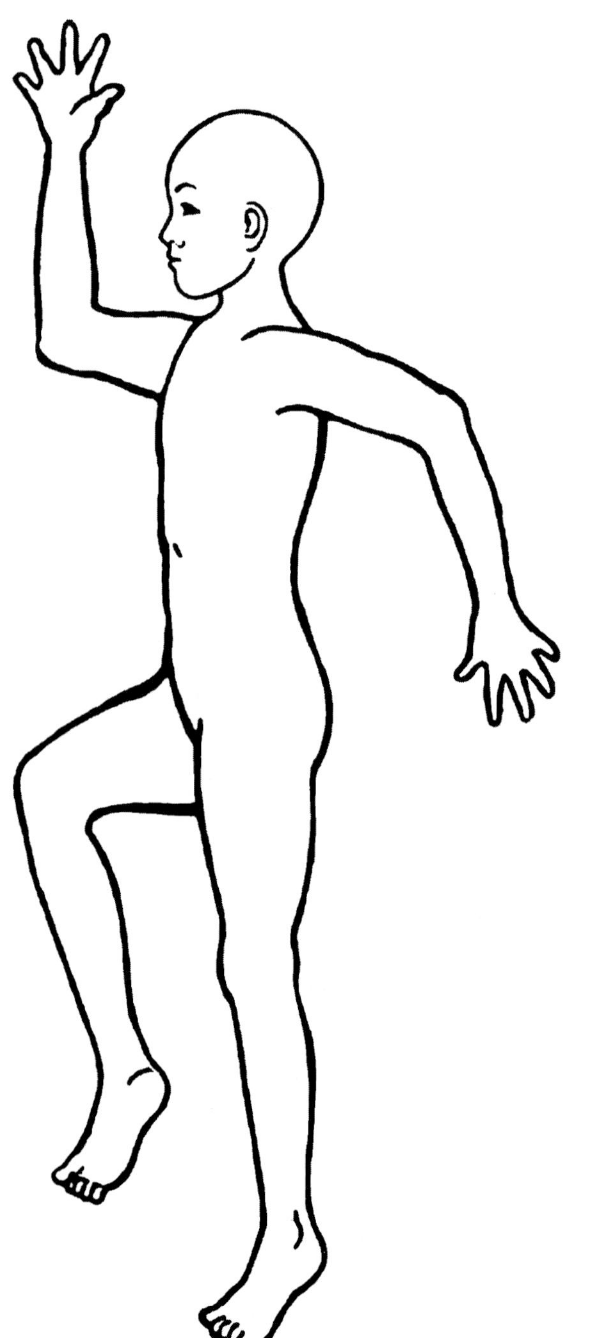

D

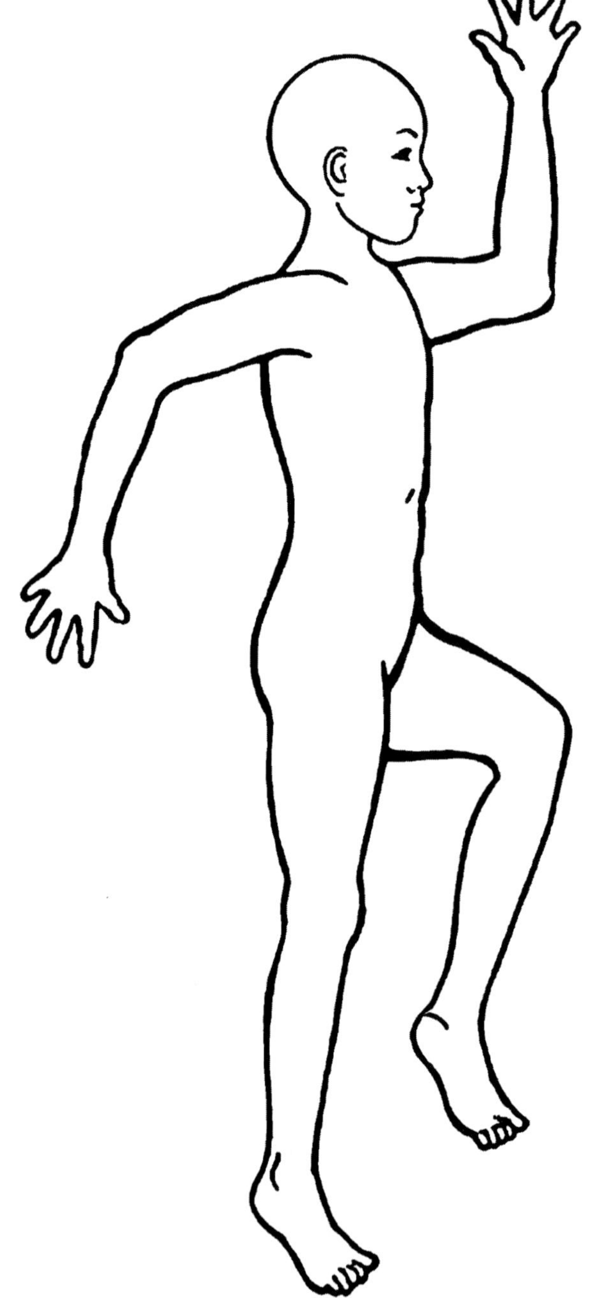

J. GENERAL PHYSICAL EXAMINATION (continued)

7. Examine the face, head, ears, hair, scalp, neck, and mouth for injury. Record findings using the diagrams.

Patient Identification: **Date:**

E

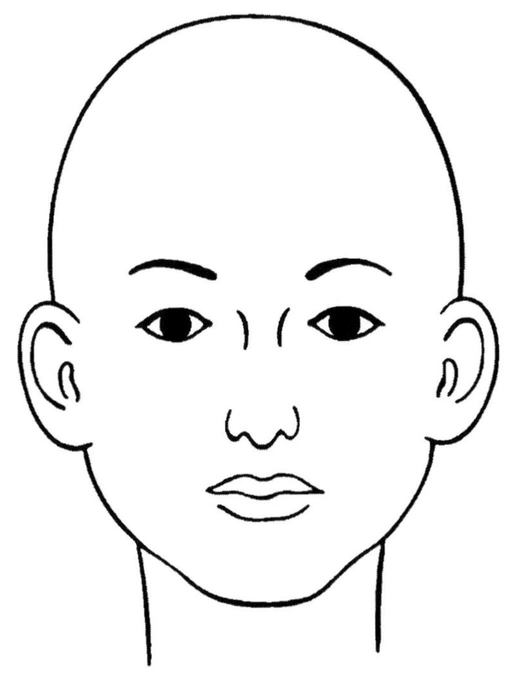

F

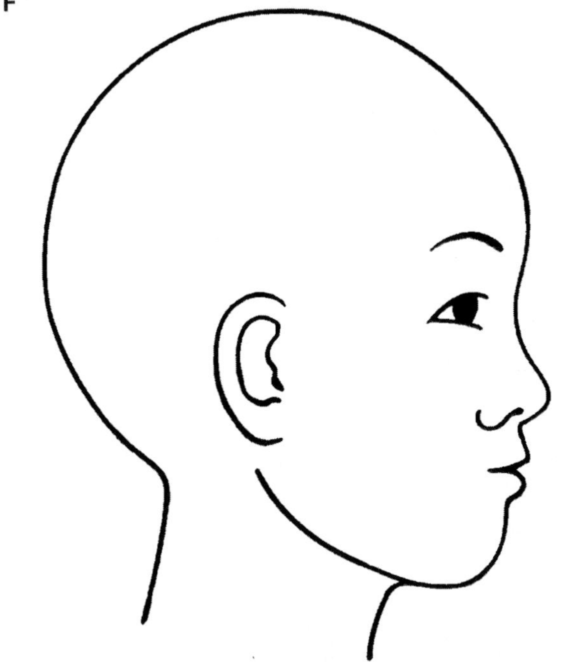

G

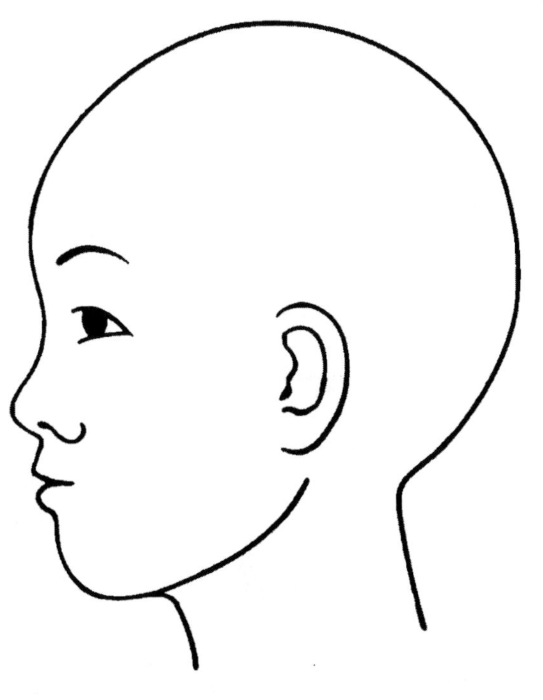

H

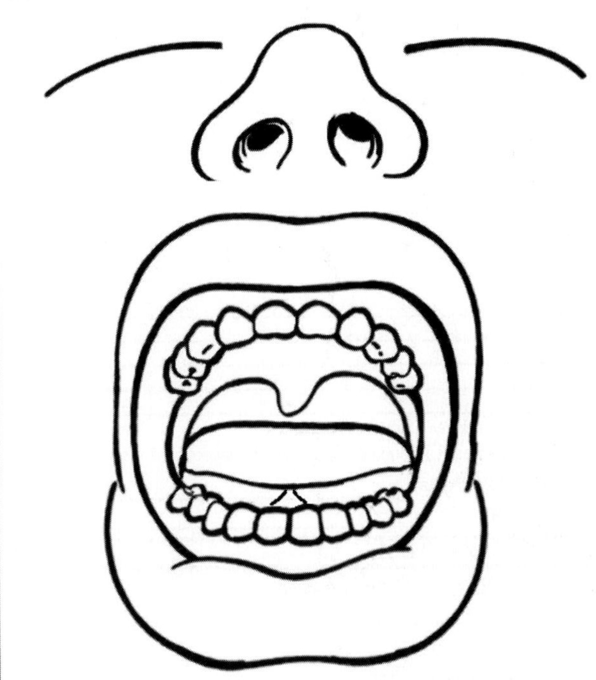

K. EVIDENCE COLLECTED AND SUBMITTED TO CRIME LAB

1. Clothing Collected ☐ No ☐ Yes ☐ N/A

Clothing Placed in Evidence Kit	Clothing Placed in Paper Bag

2. Foreign Materials Collected

	N/A	No	Yes	Collected by:
Swabs/suspected blood	☐	☐	☐	
Dried secretions	☐	☐	☐	
Fiber/loose hairs	☐	☐	☐	
Soil/debris/vegetation	☐	☐	☐	
Swabs/suspected saliva	☐	☐	☐	
Foreign body	☐	☐	☐	
Control swabs	☐	☐	☐	
Fingernail scrapings	☐	☐	☐	
Matted hair cuttings	☐	☐	☐	

Other types, describe:__________

L. TOXICOLOGY SAMPLES

	N/A	No	Yes	Time	Collected by:
Blood Alcohol / Toxicology	☐	☐	☐		
Urine Toxicology	☐	☐	☐		

M. REFERENCE SAMPLES

	N/A	No	Yes	Time	Collected by:
Blood (lavender top tube)	☐	☐	☐		
Blood card (optional)	☐	☐	☐		
Buccal swabs (optional)	☐	☐	☐		
Saliva swabs	☐	☐	☐		

N. DIAGNOSTIC STUDIES ☐ Refer to dictation

1. Laboratory:

	WNL	ABN	N/A	Pending	Results
☐ CBC	☐	☐	☐	☐	
☐ Platelets	☐	☐	☐	☐	
☐ INR, PTT, PT	☐	☐	☐	☐	
☐ SGOT, SGPT	☐	☐	☐	☐	
☐ Urinalysis	☐	☐	☐	☐	
☐ Toxicology Screen	☐	☐	☐	☐	
☐ Other	☐	☐	☐	☐	

2. Diagnostic Imaging

	WNL	ABN	N/A	Preliminary Reading	Final Report
☐ Skeletal Survey	☐	☐	☐	☐	☐
☐ CT Scan	☐	☐	☐	☐	☐
☐ M R I	☐	☐	☐	☐	☐
☐ Other	☐	☐	☐	☐	☐

Describe:

3. Exam Performed by Ophthalmologist:

☐ N/A ☐ No ☐ Yes ☐ Pending ☐ See Medical Record for Report

Name of Ophthalmologist:__________

Photographs Taken By:__________

O. PHOTO DOCUMENTATION

☐ No ☐ Yes ☐ N/A ☐ Film Retained

☐ Film Released to:__________

Photographs taken by:__________

35mm ☐ Digital ☐ Instant ☐ Other ☐ __________

Recommend follow-up photographs be taken in 1-2 days

☐ No ☐ Yes ☐ N/A

Patient Identification: **Date:**

P. REQUIRED SUMMARY AND INTERPRETATION OF HISTORY, EXAMINATION, AND DIAGNOSTIC STUDIES

Describe:

☐ Neglect

☐ Physical abuse

☐ Evaluation suspicious for physical abuse. Further information needed.

☐ Indeterminate cause

☐ Evaluation indicates non-abusive cause of medical findings.

☐ See Additional Dictation Dictation Reference Number:

Q. DISTRIBUTION OF EVIDENCE

	Released To
Clothing (items not placed in evidence kit) ☐ N/A	
Evidence Kit ☐ N/A	
Reference samples ☐ N/A	
Toxicology samples ☐ N/A	

R. PERSONNEL INVOLVED

Examination Performed By: (Print)		Signature of Examiner
License No.	Telephone	Date
Examination Assisted By: (Print)		Signature
License No.	Telephone	Date
Specimen labeled and sealed by:		Signature
License No.	Telephone	Date

S. PATIENT DISPOSITION

☐ Admitted ☐ Home ☐ Protective Custody

☐ Follow Up Exam Needed (specify reason):__________

Glossary

A

abrasion Removal of the outer layer of skin by either compression and/or sliding over a rough surface or object. Also known as scratches and grazes.

alternate light source A source of ultraviolet radiation emitting wavelengths of 320 to 400 nm used to help identify semen. Semen, urine, and other oily substances fluoresce a blue-green to orange color.

anal sodomy Contact of the penis to the anus.

anilingus Mouth to anus.

aperture The adjustable opening in a camera lens that controls the beam of light that enters. It is also known as f-stop and f-number.

avulsed bite A bite in which the bitten tissue is separated from the victim.

avulsion Injury where there is a tearing away of a structure or part. It is characterized by tissue loss.

B

biological evidence Evidence that originates from a body. This includes blood, semen, tissues and organs, bones, teeth, hair, nails, saliva, urine, and other biological fluids.

blunt force trauma Injury made by the crushing impact of or when a moving body strikes a blunt object. This includes abrasions, contusions, lacerations, and fractures.

bondage The use of physical restraints and devices that have sexual significance for the user.

bore The interior of a gun barrel in front of the chamber.

bullet wipe The discolored area on the immediate periphery of a bullet hole caused by bullet lubricant, lead, soot, bore debris, or possibly by jacket material.

C

caliber When used with firearms, the approximate diameter of the circle made by the tops of the lands of a rifled barrel. When used with ammunition, a numerical term (without the decimal point) included in a cartridge name to indicate the nominal bullet diameter.

cartridge A single unit of ammunition made up of the case, primer, and propellant.

cause of death The entity that initiated the sequence of events that ended in death, such as multiple injuries from a vehicle accident or a hemorrhage from a firearms injury.

cervical os Opening of the cervix (endocervix).

cervix Narrow lower or outer end of the uterus; neck of the uterus.

chain of custody Written documentation signifying the link formed between each person who handles evidence.

chamber The rear part of the barrel bore in a gun that has been formed to accept a specific cartridge.

child sexual abuse The use of power and control of a sexual nature where there is an age difference or caretaking responsibility between perpetrator and victim.

choking Blockage of an internal airway due to aspiration.

chop wounds Deep, gaping wounds often involving major structures and resulting from the use of relatively heavy, sharp objects such as meat cleavers, axes, and machetes. Chop wounds may display both sharp and blunt characteristics.

clinical forensic medicine The medical specialty that applies the principles and practice of clinical medicine to the elucidation of questions in judicial proceedings for the protection of the individual's legal rights prior to death.

clinical forensic nurse A nurse who evaluates and performs the root cause analyses of adverse patient events within a clinical setting and who has the ability to recognize forensic implications in any given patient care situation and to set in motion the appropriate chain of events.

clitoris Small erectile organ at the anterior or ventral part of the vulva; sole purpose is sexual stimulation; homologous to the penis.

close-up and macro lenses These camera lenses are necessary for detailed images. They allow the photographer to focus a few inches or centimeters from the subject.

club drugs Synthetic and designer drugs or illegally diverted and trafficked therapeutic drugs popularized at nightclubs and parties with the false perception that they do not cause serious, harmful effects.

CODIS (Combined DNA Index System) FBI program designed to type and catalog biological evidence for DNA typing, allowing scientists to identify or eliminate suspects in forensic settings; the national DNA data bank that enables states to compare their no-suspect profiles to a national DNA repository and solve additional crimes.

colposcope An instrument that provides illumination and magnification for the examination of the anogenital area. It is a stereoscopic or binocular microscope that can include magnification from 5× up to 30×, with a 150-watt halogen ring-light source for bright illumination, a 300-mm objective lens, and photographic capability.

colposcopy The examination of the vagina and cervix by use of an instrument with a magnifying lens system.

contusions or bruises Injuries resulting from the leakage of blood from vessels into soft tissues after sufficient force had been applied to distort soft tissue to tear vessels.

Convicted Offender Index CODIS data bank consisting of DNA typing of individuals convicted of felony sex crimes and other crimes, depending on state legislation.

coronal ridge The widest portion around the glans penis.

coroner An elected official who performs a legal role of death investigator within a given jurisdiction, but who does not necessarily possess medical or death investigation credentials.

cunnilingus Mouth to vulva contact.

cut A tissue wound resulting from a sharp object, under pressure, coming into contact with the skin.

D

defense wound A characteristic injury, either blunt or sharp, incurred in an attempt to ward off the blows or thrusts of a weapon wielded by an assailant.

depth of field A measurement of the zones in front of and beyond the subject of a photograph that are in acceptably sharp focus.

digital photography Electronically capturing an image through the use of a filmless camera.

dorsal vein Vein that runs along the dorsal surface of the penile shaft.

drug-facilitated sexual assault The use of chemical agents such as drugs and alcohol to assist in or procure sexual contact by impairing the victim.

E

elder abuse Abuse of the elderly by a caretaker, whether a relative, friend, or individual upon whom the elderly person is dependent. This can include sexual or physical abuse, financial abuse or exploitation, neglect, and emotional or psychological abuse.

epididymis A coiled tubing network folded against the back surface of each testis. Sperm cells spend several weeks in the epididymis while they mature. The epididymis then passes them to the vas deferens.

evidence Data presented to a court or jury to prove or disprove a claim; any item or information that may be submitted and accepted by a competent tribunal for the purpose of determining the truth of any matter it is investigating.

evidence recovery kit Supply kit that contains suitable containers to recover a variety of substances.

expert witness One who is qualified by the court, based on education, experience, employment, publications, or research, to render an opinion on certain facts where the knowledge is beyond that of a judge or jury; one who has special knowledge on the subject about which he or she is to testify.

F

fact witness A witness testifying to actual events or occurrences observed.

fellatio Any mouth to penis contact.

female circumcision Surgical removal of the labia minora.

female genital mutilation One of several procedures designed to alter the sexual responses of women by altering their reproductive structures.

financial abuse or exploitation The misuse of another individual's funds or assets without his or her knowledge or consent, for the perpetrator's benefit.

focal length The distance measured from the optical center of a camera lens to the film plane; it determines the reproduction ratio and thus the field that you see through the lens.

forensic Pertaining to courts of justice, it commonly refers to the application of science to the resolution of legal issues.

forensic anthropology The analysis and identification of human remains for criminal and legal investigation.

forensic archaeology Application of archaeological recovery techniques to death scene exhumations.

forensic botanist One who uses training in taxonomy, morphology, plant anatomy, and plant ecology to identify plant evidence for the purpose of placing a suspect at the crime scene or determining the time of death.

forensic entomologist One who analyzes insects and other invertebrates in determining manner of death, movement of a cadaver from one site to another, and length of the postmortem interval.

Forensic Index CODIS data bank consisting of DNA typing of individuals derived from lawfully collected specimens obtained during the course of a criminal investigation; contains DNA records from cases without a suspect.

forensic medicine Application of medical knowledge and skills to questions of law and/or patient treatment involving court-related issues.

forensic nurse A registered nurse qualified by education and experience in the evaluation and investigation of trauma, injury, or death involving individuals in need of medicolegal intervention and court-related evaluations.

forensic nurse death investigator A licensed nurse who carries out the duties of a death investigator in accordance with the performance standards and procedures established under the medical examiner's or coroner's system of death investigation and the jurisdictional standards of practice; one subspecialty of forensic nursing.

forensic nurse examiner The forensic nurse who provides a medicolegal examination whether physical, psychological, or sexual, for the documentation and recovery of trace and physical evidence, whether the patient is living or dead. Those who review and investigate or examine medical records and other documents of record and those who examine a crime scene.

forensic nursing The application of nursing to the law; the forensic aspects of health care combined with the bio/psycho/social/spiritual education of the RN in the scientific investigation and treatment of trauma or death of victims and perpetrators of violence.

forensic odontology The branch of dentistry that deals with the collection, evaluation, and proper handling of dental evidence to provide assistance to law enforcement and civil and criminal judicial proceedings; applying knowledge of development, structure, and function of the teeth to the identification or age of individuals.

forensic pathologist Pathologist who is specially trained to recognize, interpret, and document features of injury and disease in the human body.

forensic science The application of science to the just resolution of legal issues.

forensic toxicologist One who applies the science of the nature of poisons, their effects, and detection to legal causes.

forensic toxicology Investigation of drugs and poisons practiced within a legal domain for the purpose of upholding the law.

fossa navicularis Concave area immediately below the hymen, extending outward to the posterior fourchette.

fracture Discontinuity, break, or rupture of bone caused by blunt trauma; can be direct or indirect.

frottage Rubbing for the purpose of sexual gratification.

G

glans Head of the penis, which is an expansion of the corpus spongiosum, covered by a loose skin (foreskin or prepuce), which enables it to expand freely during exertion.

graze A wide area of abrasion.

H

hearsay rule A statement other than the one made by the declarant while testifying at the trial or hearing, offered in evidence to prove the truth of the matter asserted (Uniform Rules of Evidence, Rule 801). This means that a witness is not permitted to provide testimony about something that someone else has told him or her.

hematoma A localized mass of blood that is relatively or completely confined within an organ, tissue, space, or potential space, and which is usually or partly clotted.

hesitation marks/wounds Superficial, often parallel cuts made while attempting suicide, in an attempt to gain courage or attention, or arising from vacillation. Also referred to as trial, tentative, or decision cuts.

human bite The prototypical human bite is ovoid and circular and consists of two opposing U-shaped patterns separated at their bases by open space. Frequently there is a central area of ecchymosis or contusion between the opposing arches.

hymen Fine membranous tissue that partially or (rarely) completely covers the vaginal orifice. It separates the external genitalia from the vagina. Located at the junction of the vestibular floor and vaginal canal. All females have this structure; however, wide anatomic variations exist. During the forensic examination, hymenal configuration, symmetry, narrowing, and injuries are used. Terms such as "intact," "not intact," and "virginal" are *not* used.

hymenal findings

- ***bump*** Small rounded projection, which may indicate where a septate bridge once attached, an area of attachment of vaginal rugae, or a chronic inflammatory change.
- ***cleft*** V-shaped indentation, not extending to the base (junction of the hymen and vestibule). Also called notched.
- ***fimbriated*** Uneven edges with small projections.
- ***gaping*** Extra large hymenal diameter without stretching.
- ***rolled*** Tissue folded over on itself either inwardly or outwardly.
- ***scalloped*** Rounded series of half-circle tissue.
- ***smooth*** No breaks, bumps, or notches.
- ***thickened*** Fatter and less elastic.
- ***transected*** Torn, cut, or divided (usually used to describe a healed tear with edges that have not grown back together).

hymenal shapes

- ***annular*** Ring shaped; smooth, unfolded, 360 degrees.
- ***crescentic*** Half-moon; the anterior rim of tissue extending from 1 to 11 o'clock position may be absent.
- ***cribiform*** Multiple small openings.
- ***elongated*** Vertical diameter is longer than horizontal length.
- ***fimbriated*** Ruffled, redundant, uneven tissue.
- ***imperforate*** No opening. The vaginal orifice cannot be visualized.
- ***microperforate*** Small opening.
- ***septated*** Band of tissue crossing the vaginal orifice.
- ***sleevelike*** Ventrally displaced hymenal tissue with circular orifice; "kangaroo pouch."

I

incision A soft tissue wound created by a sharp object or instrument; characterized by a defect that is longer than it is deep and has clean-cut edges.

informed consent Permission given for a procedure after full disclosure of all aspects of the procedure, including risks, benefits, complications, consequences, and alternatives.

International Association of Forensic Nurses (IAFN) A professional organization of RNs working in the medicolegal nursing arena whose purpose is to develop, promote, and disseminate information about the science of forensic nursing.

J

JPEG format (Joint Photographic Experts Group) Digital files that are compressed to a fraction of their original size by a lossy compression method, resulting in lowered quality but faster uploading.

L

labia majora Outer skin folds of the vagina; covered with pubic hair after menarche.

labia minora Inner skin folds of the vagina.

laceration A defect in soft tissues resulting from blunt forces. Characterized by tissue bridging.

lividity Discoloration of tissue caused by settling or hypostasis of the blood after death. Blood is in the vessels.

Locard's principle A principle that states that when a person or object comes in contact with another person or object, there exists a possibility that an exchange of materials (a cross-transfer of evidence) will take place.

M

manner of death The fashion of circumstances in which the cause of death arose and whether it was natural, suicide, homicide, accidental, or undetermined.

median raphe Seamlike union extending from the scrotum to the rectum.

medical examiner A forensic pathologist who is appointed or hired to determine the cause and manner of death, and who possesses medical knowledge and skills associated with a medical degree and license to practice.

medicolegal or legal medicine Areas of common interest to medicine and law, where medical knowledge is applied to the administration of justice.

midline commissure Midline fusion external from the posterior fourchette; used in anatomic descriptions of children.

mitochondrial DNA typing A new forensic tool involving PCR amplification followed by direct sequencing of the DNA. The mitochondrial genome contains 16,569 base pairs of circular DNA. Mitochondrial DNA exists outside of the nucleus and is present in multiple copies per cell.

mons pubis Rounded eminence of fatty tissue on the pubic symphysis.

Munchausen by proxy Factitious disorder in which a parent or other caretaker fabricates or induces illness in a dependent, especially a child.

N

National DNA Index System (NDIS) The single central repository of DNA records submitted to the FBI by all participating states.

necropsy The evisceration and dissection of the dead; an examination of the dead; looking at the dead.

neglect The failure to fulfill a caretaking obligation to provide goods or services; typically involves acts of omission rather than commission and may or may not be intentional.

O

oral sodomy Mouth to vagina, anus, or penis.

orientation shots Initial photographs that include the person's face and the wound or wounds prior to taking close-up photos of individual injuries.

P

pectinate line Anal papilla and columns interdigitate with anal verge tissue (where squamous cells meet columnar cells).

penis External organ consisting of three parallel cylinders of erectile tissue that run the length of the penis; consists of the glans, prepuce, corona, shaft, and frenulum. Two of the tissue masses lie alongside each other and end behind the head of the penis. The third tissue mass lies beneath them and contains the urethra. The average length of a nonerect penis is 8.5–10.5 cm and the length of an erect penis averages 16 to 19 cm.

perineal body Mass of muscle and fascia that separates the lower end of the vagina from the rectum.

perineum, female Region bounded by the vulva in front, the buttocks behind, and laterally by the medial side of the thighs. A line drawn transversely across in front of the ischial tuberosities divides the space into two portions: the posterior (anal region) contains the termination of the anal canal, and the anterior (urogenital region) contains the external urogenital organs. The perineum is sometimes raised, rough, and/or pigmented. Its deep boundaries are the pubic arch and the arcuate ligament of the pubis in front, the tip of the coccyx behind, the inferior rami of the pubis and ischium on either side, and the sacrotuberous ligament.

perineum, male Region bounded by the scrotum in front, by the buttocks behind, and laterally by the medial side of the thighs.

periurethral tissue The immediate 360° area around the urethra not including the urethral meatus.

periurethral vestibular bands Bands lateral to the urethra, connected to the vestibule wall; support bands.

physical abuse The infliction of nonaccidental physical harm or injury through the use of excessive and inappropriate physical force. It can be hitting, slapping, punching, pinching, pushing, burning, or sexual abuse.

physical evidence Any matter, material, or condition that may be used to determine facts in a given situation.

physical violence Behavior that inflicts harm and includes threats and attempts to harm another individual.

point-and-shoot camera A camera system where the viewfinder is placed near the lens so that the photographer's view and camera's view are similar, but not exactly the same.

polymerase chain reaction DNA typing method whereby small segments of DNA are amplified (duplicated).

Population File CODIS data bank of DNA types and allele frequency data from anonymous persons intended to represent major population groups found in the United States. These are used to estimate statistical frequencies of DNA profiles.

posterior fourchette Area below the fossa navicularis; the point of fusion of the posterior labia minora.

prepuce or foreskin Fold of skin that covers the glans of the penis.

primer The ignition component of an ammunition cartridge.

profiler A forensic specialist who develops profiles of perpetrators based on evidence, situation reconstruction, and hypothetical constructs using experience and data collected from multiple cases.

prostate Located directly below the bladder and surrounding the urethra in males. Normally about the size of a chestnut; consists of muscular and glandular sections. The prostate produces about 30% of the seminal fluid; the rest is produced by the seminal vesicles.

psychiatric forensic nurse Professional RN who assesses perpetrators on issues of mental status, competency, legal sanity, and dangerousness.

psychological abuse Behaviors that are cruel, degrading, terrorizing, isolating, rejecting, demeaning, humiliating; intimidating verbal abuse.

R

rape An act of violence; nonconsensual sexual aggression involving the penetration of a body orifice; nonconsensual penile-vaginal or anal penetration.

rape kit A kit (box) that contains all the supplies (swabs, carriers, envelopes, paper sheet, blood tubes, envelopes) required to obtain and store biological evidence from a rape survivor. It can be customized to individual jurisdictions.

rape-trauma syndrome A two-stage syndrome of response to a sexual assault; a specific type of post-traumatic stress disorder pertaining to the consequences of trauma related to sexual assault or childhood sexual abuse.

rectum The terminal part of the intestine from the sigmoid flexure to the anus; not sensitive to pain.

Relatives of Missing Persons Index CODIS data bank of DNA typing from missing persons and their close relatives; used to identify individuals or body parts and relate them to a known group.

rigor mortis A postmortem change that presents as muscle rigidity; the stiffening of the body after death that is produced by chemical reactions in the muscle.

rimfire A flange-headed cartridge containing the priming mixture inside the rim cavity.

S

SANE-A Credentials used by a sexual nurse examiner who has passed the IAFN national certification examination for adults and adolescents.

scratch A superficial abrasion that is long and narrow.

scrotum This loose sac of skin under the penis containing the testicles.

self-harm A direct, deliberate, and often repetitive destruction or alteration of one's own body tissue without conscious suicidal intent; also known as self-mutilation, self-injury, and auto-aggression.

self-neglect The neglect of personal well-being and home environment.

seminal fluid The whitish sticky material that contains mature sperm from the body. Semen is discharged at male sexual climax. A single discharge, about 3.5 mL of semen, contains 120 million to 600 million spermatozoa. After vasectomy, sperm is no longer present in the ejaculate, but the volume of seminal fluid remains the same.

sexual assault Sexually explicit conduct used as an expression of interpersonal violence against another person; nonconsenting sexual acts achieved through the use of power and control.

sexual assault nurse examiner (SANE) An RN who has achieved education in forensic examination of sexual assault victims.

sexual assault response team (SART) A group of professionals who work together to facilitate the survivor's recovery and the investigation and prosecution of the assailant by providing information, support and crisis intervention, and evidence gathering and to facilitate the movement of the survivor through the legal system. SART members work to improve the response to victims within their own disciplines and to educate the community they serve.

shaft The cylindrical part of the penis located between the glans and body. The shaft contains vascular chambers that fill during arousal to produce an erection.

shaken baby syndrome Intracranial injuries produced by acceleration–deceleration forces associated with vigorous shaking; may or may not involve blunt head trauma; also called shaken impact syndrome.

short tandem repeats (STRs) Method of DNA typing whereby multiple short tandem repeats in a single reaction are studied by several fluorescent detection methods. Different STR types exhibit variation in the number of repeated core elements they contain and have tremendous discriminating power.

shutter speed The time that the shutter of a camera is open can vary from 1/8000th of a second or less to 30 seconds or more.

single-lens reflex camera A camera that allows the photographer to look through the viewfinder to see exactly what will be reproduced on the film.

smothering Asphyxia due to obstruction of external airways.

sodomy Legal term to describe anal intercourse.

spermatozoa Mature male sperm cells.

stab A soft tissue injury resulting from a relatively pointed and/or sharp object inward by a thrustlike force or by the forces created when a person falls onto something with enough force for the object to pass through the tissue, creating impalement. A stab wound is generally deeper than it is long.

stippling (tattooing) Small abrasions and minute hemorrhages created when particles of unburned or partially burned gunpowder strike the skin. These wounds are usually consistent with a range of fire of about 24 to 30 inches but can be as great as 4 feet. Can be interchanged with tattooing, but tattooing is the indriving of gunpowder particles when a weapon was relatively near; stippling is when the weapon was sufficiently far away that particles could not be driven into the skin.

strangulation Asphyxia due to hanging, ligature, or manual strangulation that obstructs the main airways and/or blood vessels supplying the brain, impairing oxygen delivery.

subpoena An official notification or court order to appear in court for the purpose of participating in a legal proceeding, usually to provide testimony.

suffocation Hypoxia or anoxia caused by the obstruction of the upper airways.

T

Tanner stage, pubic hair Development assessment used to stage gonadal maturation in terms of acquisition of secondary sexual characteristics. For females breast size and pubic hair distribution are assessed to categorize the stage of development. For males, scrotal, penile, and pubic hair distribution is used to stage development.
1. No hair or fine, vellus (peach fuzz) hair
2. Sparse, long pigmented hair
3. Increased density; dark, coarse, curly hair
4. Abundant hair, sparing the medial thigh
5. Abundant hair, spreading to the medial thigh

Tardieu spots Ecchymotic spots found in the dependent extremities due to vascular congestion and/or hypoxia.

telephoto lens A camera lens greater than the standard focal length for a particular size of camera. Behaves like a telescope.

three-dimensional bite A bite having all the components of a two-dimensional bite plus depth of penetration.

TIFF format Tagged image format file; a lossless compression method where data is compressed, not lost.

toluidine blue dye (TBD) An aqueous dye used as a nuclear stain, which adheres to abraded skin and microlacerations; used to mark denuded tissue.

traumagram Diagram used to annotate locations and types of injury on surfaces, anatomic parts, or within the human body cavities.

two-dimensional bite A bite having width and breadth but no penetration of the epidermis.

U

Unidentified Persons Index CODIS data bank of DNA typing of individuals with uncertain identities.

urethral meatus Orifice for the urethra.

V

vagina Tubular structure or canal extending from the hymen to the cervix.

vaginal introitus Located below the urethral meatus and situated behind the labia minora; the entrance to the vagina.

vaginal vestibule Space posterior to the clitoris between the labia minora into which the urethra and vagina open.

vas deferens The 16-in tube that connects the epididymis to the urethra. This tube is cut and sutured off during a vasectomy.

victim Legal term that describes a person against whom a crime has been committed.

Victims' Index CODIS data bank of DNA typing from victims, living or dead, from whom DNA may have been carried away by perpetrators.

violence The intentional use of physical force or power, threatened or real, against oneself, another person, or a group or community that results in or has a high likelihood of resulting in injury, death, psychological harm, maldevelopment, or deprivation.

VNTRs The most common type of genetic variation studied in forensic DNA analysis whereby length differences produced by variable number tandem repeats are studied.

vulva Region of the external genital organs of the female (includes the labia majora, labia minora, and mons pubis).

W

wide-angle lens A camera lens that is less than the standard size, allowing a wider than normal field of view.

witness Generally, a person who describes under oath what he or she has seen, heard, or otherwise observed, or, one who testifies to specific knowledge on issues relevant to the case.

Wood's lamp One type of an alternate light source.

Z

zoom lens A camera lens with variable focal lengths that can be used to adjust the framing of an image.

Photo and Illustration Credits

CHAPTER 3

page 12, Figure 3-1 Adapted from CDC/NCHS, National Vital Statistics System, Mortality

CHAPTER 7

page 47, Figure 7-1 Adapted from *Complete Digital Photography* 3rd Edition by Long. 2004. Reprinted with permission of Delmar Learning, a division of Thomson Learning: www.thomsonrights.com; Figure 7-2 Adapted from *Complete Digital Photography* 3rd Edition by Long. 2004. Reprinted with permission of Delmar Learning, a division of Thomson Learning: www.thomsonrights.com; **page 49,** Figure 7-3 Adapted from *Complete Digital Photography* 3rd Edition by Long. 2004. Reprinted with permission of Delmar Learning, a division of Thomson Learning: www.thomsonrights.com

CHAPTER 11

page 78, Figure 11-1 Photo courtesy of Johan A. Duflou, MMed, Department of Forensic Medicine, Central Sydney Laboratory Service, Sydney, Australia; Figure 11-2 Photo courtesy of Isidore Mihalakis, MD, Warren County Medical Examiner's Office, Phillipsburg, New Jersey; Figure 11-3 Photo courtesy of Johan A. Duflou, MMed, Department of Forensic Medicine, Central Sydney Laboratory Service, Sydney, Australia; **page 79,** Figure 11-4 Photos courtesy of Vincent Tranchida, MD, Office of the Chief Medical Examiner, New York, New York; **page 80,** Figure 11-5 Photos courtesy of Isidore Mihalakis, MD, Warren County Medical Examiner's Office, Phillipsburg, New Jersey (left) and Johan A. Duflou, MMed, Department of Forensic Medicine, Central Sydney Laboratory Service, Sydney, Australia (right); Figure 11-6 Photos courtesy of Isidore Mihalakis, MD, Warren County Medical Examiner's Office, Phillipsburg, New Jersey; Figure 11-7 Photo courtesy of Isidore Mihalakis, MD, Warren County Medical Examiner's Office, Phillipsburg, New Jersey; **page 81,** Figure 11-8 Photos courtesy of Vincent Tranchida, MD, Office of the Chief Medical Examiner, New York, New York; **page 82,** Figure 11-9 Photos courtesy of Vincent Tranchida, MD, Office of the Chief Medical Examiner, New York, New York (left) and Johan A. Duflou, MMed, Department of Forensic Medicine, Central Sydney Laboratory Service, Sydney, Australia (right); Figure 11-10 Photos courtesy of Isidore Mihalakis, MD, Warren County Medical Examiner's Office, Phillipsburg, New Jersey

CHAPTER 13

page 90, Figure 13-1 Courtesy of Anne Olson, Medical Illustrator; **page 91,** Figure 13-2 Courtesy of Anne Olson, Medical Illustrator; Figure 13-3 Photo courtesy of Roger Thompson; **page 95,** Figure 13-11 Courtesy of Anne Olson, Medical Illustrator; **page 96,** Figure 13-13 Courtesy of Anne Olson, Medical Illustrator

CHAPTER 14

page 101, Figure 14-4 Used with permission, Dickinson ET. *Fire Service Emergency Care.* Upper Saddle River, NJ: Brady-Prentice Hall; 1999; **page 102,** Figure 14-6 Used with permission, Dickinson ET. *Fire Service Emergency Care.* Upper Saddle River, NJ: Brady-Prentice Hall; 1999; Figure 14-7 Used with permission, Dickinson ET. *Fire Service Emergency Care.* Upper Saddle River, NJ: Brady-Prentice Hall; 1999; **page 103,** Figure 14-9 Used with permission, Dickinson ET. *Fire Service Emergency Care.* Upper Saddle River, NJ: Brady-Prentice Hall; 1999; **page 104,** Figure 14-13 Used with permission, Dickinson ET. *Fire Service Emergency Care.* Upper Saddle River, NJ: Brady-Prentice Hall; 1999; **page 105,** Figure 14-14 Used with permission, Dickinson ET. *Fire Service Emergency Care.* Upper Saddle River, NJ: Brady-Prentice Hall; 1999; **page 106,** Figure 14-16 Used with permission, Dickinson ET. *Fire Service Emergency Care.* Upper Saddle River, NJ: Brady-Prentice Hall; 1999

CHAPTER 18

page 143, Figure 18-2 (right) Photo courtesy of Stephen Selbst, MD, AI duPont Hospital for Children, Newark, DE; **page 145,** Figure 18-3 Photo courtesy of Christopher Haines, DO, St. Christopher's Hospital for Children, Philadelphia, PA; **page 146,** Figure 18-4 (top row) Photo courtesy of Christopher Haines, DO, St. Christopher's Hospital for Children, Philadelphia, PA; Figure 18-5 (middle row) Photo courtesy of Christopher Haines, DO, St. Christopher's Hospital for Children, Philadelphia, PA; Figure 18-6 (bottom left) Photo courtesy of Christopher Haines, DO, St. Christopher's Hospital for Children, Philadelphia, PA; **page 147,** Figure 18-7 Photo courtesy of Christopher Haines, DO, St. Christopher's Hospital for Children, Philadelphia, PA; **page 148,** Figure 18-8 Photo courtesy of Stephen Selbst, MD, AI duPont Hospital for Children, Newark, DE; Figure 18-9 Photo courtesy of Stephen Selbst, MD, AI duPont Hospital for Children, Newark, DE

CHAPTER 19

page 158, Figure 19-1 UVA ED & Forensic Nurse Examiner Program; Figure 19-2 UVA ED & Forensic Nurse Examiner Program; Figure 19-3 (left) UVA ED & Forensic Nurse Examiner Program; Figure 19-4 (bottom) UVA ED & Forensic Nurse Examiner Program

CHAPTER 21

page 177, Figure 21-1 Centers for Disease Control and Prevention. Guidelines for death scene investigation of sudden, unexplained infant deaths: recommendations of the Interagency Panel of Sudden Infant Death Syndrome. *MMWR.* 1996:45 (No. RR-10) [1-23]

CHAPTER 22

page 191, Figure-22-1 (a) and (b) Reprinted with permission from the Charlotte Gang Intelligence Unit; **page 192,** Figure 22-2 Reprinted with permission from the Charlotte Gang Intelligence Unit; **page 194,** Figure 22-3 Reprinted with permission from the Charlotte Gang Intelligence Unit; **page 195,** Figure 22-4 Reprinted with permission from the Charlotte Gang Intelligence Unit; Figure 22-5 Reprinted with permission from the Charlotte Gang Intelligence Unit; **page 196,** Figure 22-6 Reprinted with permission from the Security Threat Intelligence Unit; **page 197,** Figure 22-7 Reprinted with permission from Mitchell Goldman, DO; **page 199,** Figure 22-9 Courtesy of www.Chicagogangs.com; **page 201,** Figure 22-11 Reprinted with permission from the Charlotte Gang Intelligence Unit

Unless otherwise indicated, all photographs are under copyright of Jones and Bartlett Publishers, LLC, or have been provided by the authors.

Index

A

abandonment of elders, 167
abdominal injuries
  blunt force trauma, 69–71, 73–74
  child abuse suspicions, 135–138, 145
  firearm suicides, 13
  frontal impact crashes, 101
  intimate partner violence, 126
  seat belt syndrome, 99–100
  suspect evaluation/evidence collection, 208
ABFO (American Board of Forensic Odontology), 50, 56–57
ABO blood-typing, 31
abrasions
  bite mark, 71
  extremity, 75
  forensic importance of, 67, 69
  intimate partner strangulation, 126
  lacerations with, 71
  punching and kicking, 71
  sexual assault, 117
  stab wound, 78
  stages of healing, 67
  types of, 66–68
abuse
  child. *see* child abuse
  elder. *see* elder abuse and neglect
  institutional, 8
  intimate partner violence. *see* intimate partner violence
  male interpersonal violence, 128–132
  substance. *see* substance abuse
ACEP (American College of Emergency Physicians), 2–3, 124, 165
ACS (American College of Surgeons), 99
acute examination, pediatric sexual abuse, 157
adolescents
  autoerotic asphyxiation in, 17
  gang violence. *see* gang violence
  Russian roulette in, 15
  sexual assault genital injuries in, 118
adult protective services (APS), 167–169
adulteration, urine drug screens, 38
age, and sexual assault injury, 118
airbags
  injuries related to, 101
  reducing morbidity and mortality, 99
  side impact, 103
alcohol abuse
  driving accidents and, 40
  firearm-related suicide related to, 12
  forensic toxicology and, 40
  risk of suicide and, 11
  Russian roulette victims and, 15
  sexual assault and, 42, 111
  suicide by cop and, 14
alkaline phosphatase, 136
alopecia, 141
ALTEs (apparent life-threatening events), 135–136, 175–176
American Board of Forensic Odontology (ABFO), 50, 56–57
American College of Emergency Physicians (ACEP), 2–3, 124, 165
American College of Obstetricians and Gynecologists, 124
American College of Surgeons (ACS), 99
American Journal of Nursing, 2
American Medical Association, 124, 165
American Nurses Association (ANA), 5
ammunition
  cartridge parts, 86–87
  machine gun, 85
  shotgun, 87, 95
amnesia, in GHB toxicity, 42
amphetamines, detecting, 39
amputation, and rollover crashes, 105
angulation fractures, 71
animal bites, 55, 147
Annals of Emergency Medicine, 3
anogenital injuries
  male pediatric patients, 131
  pediatric sexual abuse, 157–159
  sexual assault, 117–118
anorectal examination, sexual assault
  conducting, 116
  determining consent to sexual activity, 119–120
  in male victims, 130
aortic injuries
  cocaine use, 41
  frontal impact crashes, 101
  lacerations, 70, 73
  rib fractures, 72
  side impact crashes, 103
aperture (f-stop), 46–49
apparent life-threatening events (ALTEs), 135–136, 175–176
APS (adult protective services), 167–169
argon ion laser light, 31
Aryan Brotherhood, 192–193
asphyxia suicides
  autoerotic asphyxiation, 17
  by gender, 11
  through strangulation, 15–17
  through suffocation, 15
assailant(s), sexual assaults, 112–113, 118
assault rifles, 85
auto loading rifles, 85
auto loading shotguns, 85
autoerotic asphyxiation, 17
automatics, firearm, 84–85
autopsies
  collecting toxicologic samples, 37
  in SIDS deaths, 173–175
  suicide death investigations, 12–15

B

Back to Sleep campaign, SIDS, 176
ballistics
  defined, 90
  external, 92–93
  internal, 90–92
  terminal, 93–94
barbiturates, 42
barrels, firearm, 84–86, 90–92
bathing suit pattern, 126
"Battered Child Syndrome" (Kempe), 133
batteries, digital camera, 48, 50
battering-ram effect, rear impacts, 103–104
behavior pathology
  intimate partner violence victims, 123–124
  male sexual assault victims, 131
benzodiazepines, 42
benzoylecgonine, 41
BESS (benign enlargement of the subarachnoid space), 139
biologic samples, specimen handling, 37
birdshot ammunition, 87, 95
bite marks, 54–58
  from blunt force trauma, 71
  collection of evidence, 56–57
  differential diagnosis, 55–56
  documenting, 57, 62–63
  identification of, 55
  intimate partner violence, 125
  location on body, 55
  overview of, 54
  references, 58
  from sexual assault, 117
  summary, 57–58
  suspicious of child abuse, 147
  treatment of, 57
BJS (Bureau of Justice Statistics), 40
bladder rupture, blunt force trauma, 74
blade, knife anatomy, 77–78
bleeding disorders, 142, 147
blood
  collecting as DNA evidence, 30
  on-site drug tests, 39
  postmortem specimen handling, 38
  serological screening of, 31
  as source of DNA evidence, 29–30
  specimen handling for living cases, 38
blood spatter, suicide vs. homicide, 14
Bloods (LA street gang), 189–190, 196–197
blunt force trauma
  abdominal and genitalia injuries, 73–74
  abrasions, 66–69
  bite marks, 71
  blunt trauma vs., 65
  cardiac injuries, 72–73
  child abuse, to abdomen, 145
  child abuse, to ears, 142
  contusions, 69–70
  diaphragmatic injuries, 73
  documentation of, 60–61, 66
  extremity injuries, 75
  fractures, 71
  frontal impact in motor vehicle crashes, 101–102
  head injuries, 75

intimate partner violence injuries, 125
lacerations, 70–71
orthopedic injuries, 74–75
pulmonary injuries, 73
punching and kicking injuries, 71
references, 75–76
rib and sternal fractures, 71–72
sexual assault injuries, 117
summary, 75
terminology, 65–66
blunt trauma, 65
body diagram maps
physical exam documentation, 60–63
suspect evaluation/evidence collection, 207
body language, gangs, 197
body surfaces exam, in sexual assault, 114–115
bolt action rifles, 85
bone
injuries from bullets striking, 94
mitochondrial DNA analysis of, 33
scintigraphy, child abuse, 137
serological screening of, 31
Border Brothers, 191
brain injury, child abuse, 138
branding, gang, 193–194
broken bottle injuries, 78
bruises. *see* contusions
brush abrasions, 66–67
brush burn abrasions, 66–67
buccal swabs, DNA evidence, 30
buckshot ammunition, 87, 95
built-in flash, forensic photography, 48
bullets
anatomy of, 86–87
autoloading pistols, 84
class characteristics of, 85
documenting, 62
evidence preservation guidelines, 21, 91–92
external ballistics, 92–93
firearm-related suicide vs. homicide, 14
forensic importance of, 86
internal ballistics, 90–91
measuring weapon caliber, 86
revolvers, 83–84
terminal ballistics, 93–94
Bureau of Justice Statistics (BJS), 40
burns
child abuse victims, 147–149
elder abuse victims, 167–168
intimate partner violence victims, 126
photographic documentation of, 51
sexual assault victims, 117
buttock injuries, intimate partner violence, 126

C

caliber, weapon, 85–86
canine teeth, identifying, 55
car accidents. *see* motor vehicle accidents
cardiac injuries. *see also* aortic injuries
blunt force trauma, 72–73
in-custody deaths from TASERS, 215–216
rib fractures and, 72
cardiopulmonary resuscitation, SIDS, 173
caregivers
evaluating for child abuse, 134–135
pediatric sexual abuse and, 157
carotid compression, 16
cartridges
assault rifles, 85
autoloading pistols, 84
firearm ammunition, 86–87
internal ballistics, 90
measuring weapon caliber, 86
case studies, 24–27
cases, cartridge, 86
cells, as DNA evidence, 30
center-weighted metering mode, 48
central nervous system (CNS), in suicide victims, 13
CEWs (conducted electrical weapons), 215–216
chain of custody (COC)
bullets, 91
developing, 24, 26
digital imaging and, 45
disadvantages of GC-MS testing, 39
form for, 92
gunshot victim case study, 27
hit-and-run victim case study, 26
in pediatric sexual abuse, 161
photographic documentation in, 7
during physical exam, 60
toxicologic specimen handling, 38
chain of evidence, 21
chambers, revolver, 83–84
Chance lumbar fracture, 99
chest injuries
blunt force trauma, 69–70
cardiac, 72–73
diaphragmatic, 73
firearm suicides and, 13
pulmonary, 73
rib and sternal fractures, 71–72
suspect evaluation/evidence collection, 208
Chicago-based gangs, 190–191
child abuse, 133–155. *see also* pediatric sexual abuse
abdominal injuries, 145
ALTEs and, 175–176
bite marks, 55–56
conclusion, 149–150
disposition and follow-up, 149
documentation of, 64
drownings/near drownings, 149
ears, 142
epidemiology, 134
evaluation: diagnostic testing, 136–138
evaluation: history, 134–136
evaluation: overall physical exam, 136
forensic nursing and, 8
injuries, 138–141
oral and dental aspects, 142–145
overview of, 134
references, 150–155
reporting, 149
retinal hemorrhages and ocular findings, 141–142
rotational fractures, 71
skin injuries, 145–149
skin injuries mimicking, 147
suspicious sudden infant deaths, 8, 173–174
children. *see also* adolescents
airbag-related injuries, 101
car vs. pedestrian impacts in, 106
pediatric sexual abuse. *see* pediatric sexual abuse
sexual abuse of male, 131
skin conditions mimicking bite marks, 56
chokes, shotgun, 97
chop injuries, 79–80
classic metaphyseal lesions (CMLs), 144
classification
bullets, 85
of death as suicide, 11–12
of gunshot wounds, 87–88
tooth types, 55
clinical forensic medicine, 1–2
clinical toxicology, 36
close-ups, forensic composition, 50–51
clothing, evidence preservation
as DNA evidence, 30
in firearm injuries, 27, 62
in gang violence, 193–194
guidelines for, 20–21, 95
in gunshot wounds, 95
hit-and-run victim case study, 24
patient as crime scene, 24
in sexual assault, 111–112, 114, 116
in sharp force injuries, 79–81
in stabbing suicides vs. homicides, 18–19
suspect evaluation/evidence collection, 207
in victims of violent crime, 6–7
CMLs (classic metaphyseal lesions), 144
CNS (central nervous system), in suicides, 13
coagulation studies, trauma in children, 136
COC. *see* chain of custody (COC)
cocaine, forensics, 41
coding, gang, 189, 197
CODIS (Combined DNA Index System), 29–30, 32–34
color balance, digital cameras, 46
colors, gang, 193
colposcope magnification instrument, 115–116
Combined DNA Index System (CODIS), 29–30, 32–34
commotio cordis, 72–73
community factors, and youth gangs, 188
compact digital cameras, 48–49
Complete Digital Photography, 3rd Edition (Long, 2004), 47
composition, forensic photography, 50–52
compound rib fractures, 72
computed tomography (CT) scans
blunt force injuries to abdomen, 74
child abuse, 137–138
seatbelt injuries, 99–100
computer support, digital imaging, 48, 50
conducted electrical weapons (CEWs), 215–216
confirmatory toxicologic analysis (GC-MS), 39
congenital dermatologic manifestations, 147
consent, in sexual assault, 108–109, 119–120
contact wounds
from bullets, 87–88, 95
from burns, 148–149
children's head trauma, 139
in firearm-related suicide, 12–13
contusio cordis, 72
contusions
age dating in sexual assault, 117
bite mark, 71
blunt force trauma, 69–70
cardiac, 72
cerebral, 75
documentation errors in, 60–61
elder abuse, 166
extremities, 75
intimate partner violence victims, 125
lacerations with, 71

myocardial, 72
punching and kicking injuries, 71
from sexual assault, 117
stab wound, 78
Convicted Offender Index, CODIS, 33
co-oximetry, 38
copper deficiency, in children, 144
coroners, 1, 11–12, 20
correctional nurses, forensic, 6
crime scene
forensics for EMS, 210–213
photography. *see* forensic photography
processing patient as, 23–24
criminal cases, and DNA analysis, 31
criminal justice system, sexual assault, 108
Crips (LA street gang), 189–190, 196–197
crush fractures, 71
CT scans. *see* computed tomography (CT) scans
cuts
lacerations vs., 70
sharp objects causing, 60
by young women, 18
cycle of violence, 123
cylinders, revolver, 83–84

D

D1S80, DNA analysis, 32
Daguerreotype arrest photographs, 45
data banks, DNA, 33–34
date, of sexual assault, 112
date rape drugs, 42
DAWN (Drug Abuse Warning Network), 40
death
in ED, 8, 24
investigating scene of SIDS, 174–175
in police custody, 214–218
defensive wounds
extremity injuries from blunt force, 75
intimate partner violence victims, 126
from sharp force, 60, 81–82
demographics
intimate partner violence victims, 123–124
sudden infant death syndrome, 172
suicide, 11
suicides vs. homicides, 13
dental impressions, bite mark evidence, 55–56, 71
dermalogic conditions, mimicking bite marks, 55
diagnostic peritoneal lavage (DPL), 74
diagnostic testing
suspect evaluation/evidence collection, 206–209
suspected child abuse, 136–138, 150
diagrammatic documentation
blunt force trauma wounds, 66, 73
collected DNA evidence, 31
of physical exam, 60
sexual assault injuries, 114
using body diagram maps, 60–63
working with, 20
dicing injuries, 63
diffuse injuries, head trauma, 139
digital cameras, 45–50
digital zoom, digital cameras, 46
direct rib fractures, 72
displaced rib fractures, 72
distant gunshot wounds, 87–88
disuse osteoporosis, in children, 144
DNA evidence, 29–35
analysis, 31–34
bite marks and, 56, 71
challenges of, 34
collection of, 30
references, 34–35
serological screening and, 31
sexual assault and, 111, 113, 130
sources of, 29–30
summary, 34
documentaries, gang, 187
documentation
of bite marks, 57, 62–63
of blunt force trauma wounds, 60–61, 66
of bullets, 86
causes of failure in, 59
chain of custody. *see* chain of custody (COC)
of declarations by dying or injured at crime scene, 211
diagrammatic. *see* diagrammatic documentation
of DNA evidence. *see* DNA evidence
drug-facilitated sexual assaults, 42
firearm injuries, 61–62
forcible entry tools at crime scene, 212
forensic patient and case management, 7–8
of gunshot injuries, 27, 88, 89–90
of history, 60
of interpersonal violence victims, 64
of intimate partner violence injuries, 126
of motor vehicle injuries, 24, 63–64
photo. *see* photographic documentation
physical exam, 60
references, 64
of sexual assault, 109–113
sharp force injuries, 60–61
of sharp force injuries, 81
of SIDS cases, 174
suggested readings, 64
of suicides, 10
summary, 64
suspect evaluation/evidence collection, 207
of suspected elder abuse, 169
of suspicious deaths, 20
written. *see* narrative documentation
domestic violence
intimate partner. *see* intimate partner violence
male sexual assault and, 129–130
double-action revolvers, 83
double-edged knives, 77–78
down and under pathway, frontal impacts, 101–102
DPL (diagnostic peritoneal lavage), 74
DQA1 test, DNA analysis, 32
dragging abrasions, 66
drive-by shootings, 187
driving while intoxicated (DWI), and toxicology, 37
drowning, 19, 149
drug abuse. *see* substance abuse
Drug Abuse Warning Network (DAWN), 40
drug reactions, bite marks mimicking, 55
drug trade, and gangs, 190, 192
DWI (driving while intoxicated), and toxicology, 37

E

ear injuries, and child abuse, 142
economic impact, of gang violence, 187
ecstasy (drug), forensics, 41
ED (emergency department)
common forensic mistakes in, 1
emergency medicine and forensics, 2–3
evidence collection in. *see* evidence collection/preservation in ED
forensic nursing in. *see* forensic nursing in ED
forensic photography in, 45
gang-related violence in, 198–210
in-custody death and, 217–218
managing SIDS in, 173
suicide and, 19–21
trends in drug use and abuse, 40
egress route, 206
EKGs, 176
elder abuse and neglect
contusions from blunt trauma, 69
defining, 166–167
documentation of, 64
forensic nursing and, 7–8
in institutional setting, 8
legal aspect, 167–168
overview of, 165–166
prevention and intervention, 168–169
references, 169–170
signs of, 167
elderly, motor vehicle accidents and, 103, 106
EM (emergency medicine), curriculum topics, 3
e-mailing, digital forensic photos, 45
emergency medical services (EMS), forensics
on arrival, 211
conclusion, 213
crime scene, 211
forcible entry, 211–212
Haz-Mat, 211
observation, 212–213
overview of, 210
subject vs. vehicle scenario, 212
suggested reading, 213
emergency medicine (EM), curriculum topics, 3
emotions
provoked by suicide, 10
signs of elder abuse, 166
EMS. *see* emergency medical services (EMS), forensics
energy, motor vehicle crashes and, 98
environmental toxicology, 36
epidemiology, child abuse, 134
epidural hematomas, in blunt force trauma, 75
epidural hemorrhages, in child abuse, 139
epithelial regeneration stage, abrasions, 67
equipment, forensic photography, 48–50
errors, forensic photography, 51–52
erythema multiforme, 56
esophageal injuries, in child abuse, 142
euphoria
in cocaine toxicity, 41
in ecstasy and methamphetamine use, 41
in heroin use, 41
in marijuana toxicity, 41
evidence collection form, 24–25
evidence collection/preservation in ED, 22–28. *see also* trace evidence
bite marks, 56–58
case studies, 24–27
chain of custody for. *see* chain of custody (COC)
collection of, 205

DNA. *see* DNA evidence
emergency medicine and, 2
forensic photography. *see* photographic documentation
forensics for EMS, 210–213
intimate partner violence, 125–126
overview of, 22, 205
Patient's Bill of Rights and, 205–206
pediatric sexual abuse, 161–162
during physical exam, 60
processing patient as crime scene, 23–24
references, 27
sexual assault, 111, 113, 116
by sexual assault nurse examiners, 6
sharp force injuries, 81
suggested reading, 27–28
summary, 24
suspicious deaths and, 20–21
tools for processing patient, 23
value of, 205
violence victims, 23
Exchangeable Image File Format (EXIF), 52
excited delirium, 216
EXIF (Exchangeable Image File Format), 52
exposure mode, forensic photography, 46–50, 52
external ballistics, 92–93
extragenital injuries, sexual assault, 117
extremities
blunt force trauma injuries, 75
suspect evaluation/evidence collection, 208

F

facial injuries, and child abuse, 145
fading, gang fashion, 195–196
falls, child abuse evaluation, 135
fame, and suicide, 10
family factors, youth gangs, 188
fashions, gang, 193–194
FAST (Focused Assessment Sonography in Trauma), 73
FCCs (fired cartridge cases), 86
feet, sharp force defensive injuries on, 81
female gangs, 188, 193
femur fractures, and child abuse, 144
fight bites, 55
file formats, digital images, 46, 50
film cameras, 45–46
financial exploitation of elders, 166
fingernail scratches, 125
fingerprinting, DNA. *see* DNA evidence
firearm-related suicides
by cop, 14–15
as most common suicide, 11
overview of, 12–14
risk factors for, 11
Russian roulette victims, 15
firearms, 83–88. *see also* gunshot injuries
ammunition, 86–87
forensic guidelines for, 88
gang-related homicides using, 187
handguns, 83–85
machine guns, 85
rifles, 85
rifling, 85
shotguns, 85
submachine guns/machine pistols, 85
suggested reading, 88
weapon caliber and, 85–86
fired cartridge cases (FCCs), 86
firing pins, revolvers, 83–84
flail chest, 72
flash, digital settings, 50
flunitrazepam (Rohypnol), 42
FMJ (full metal jacket) bullets, 93–94
focal fractures, 71
focal injuries, children's head trauma, 139
focus, digital cameras, 48, 52
Focused Assessment Sonography in Trauma (FAST), 73–74
Folk Nation (Chicago-based gang), 190, 196
forcible entry, forensics, 211–212
forensic correctional nurses, 6
forensic documentation. *see* documentation
forensic drug testing, 36
forensic emergency medicine, 1–3
Forensic Index, CODIS, 33
Forensic Medicine Section, ACEP, 3
forensic nurse examiners, 6
forensic nurse investigators, 6
forensic nursing in ED, 4–9
education of, 5
history of, 2, 5
International Association of Forensic Nurses, 5
overview of, 4–5
patient and case management, 6–7
references, 9
resources, 9
roles of, 6
success of, 2
suggested reading, 9
summary, 9
team environment, 5
vicarious trauma in ED, 7–8
forensic photography. *see* photographic documentation
forensic psychiatric nurses, 6
forensic record, sexual assault, 109–111
forensic toxicology, 36–43
alcohol, 40–41
barbiturates, 42
benzodiazepines, 42
cocaine, 41
defined, 36
detecting marijuana toxicity using, 41
drug-facilitated sexual assault, 42
ecstasy and methamphetamine, 41
gamma-hydroxybutyrate (GHB), 42
heroin, 41
interpreting analysis, 39–40
investigation, 37–38
marijuana, 41
overview of, 36–37
phencyclidine (PHP), 41–42
references, 43
summary, 43
toxicologic analysis, 38–39
trends in drug use and abuse, 40
in utero and newborn drug exposure, 43
forensics, defined, 4
forms, standard documentation, 60
fractures
blunt force trauma, 71
diagnosing elder abuse, 166
extremity injuries, 75
in intimate partner violence victims, 126
in punching and kicking injuries, 71
rib and sternal, 71–72
skull, 75
spinal, 74–75
suspicious of child abuse, 137, 142–145
frangible bullets, 93
frontal impact crash mechanisms, 101–104
f-stop (aperture), 46–49
full metal jacket (FMJ) bullets, 93–94
fully automatic rifles, 85

G

gamma-hydroxybutyrate (GHB), 42
gang violence, 186–203
Chicago-based gangs, 190–191
drive-by shootings, 187
economic impact, 187
female gangs, 193
firearm morbidity and mortality, 187
gang symbols and coding, 196–200
hate gangs, 192–193
healthcare prevention strategies, 197–201
hybrid gangs, 193–196
initiation and recruitment, 188–189
LA-based gangs, 189–190
Latin gangs, 191–192
motorcycle gangs, 192
overview of, 186–187
prison gangs, 192
references, 202
risk factors for involvement in, 188
street gangs, 189
gaping stab wounds, 78
gashes. *see* lacerations
gauge, shotgun, 86, 95
gays, and intimate partner assaults, 130
gender
autoerotic asphyxiation and, 17
bite marks and, 54, 55
drowning suicides and, 19
firearm-related suicide and, 12
intimate partner assaults and, 123–124
stabbing suicide and, 18
suicide causes by, 11
genital examination
pediatric sexual abuse, 158–159
sexual assault, 115–116
genital injuries
age and sexual experience affecting, 118
from blunt force trauma, 73–74
detection, characterization and documentation of, 117–118
determining consent to sexual activity, 119–120
intimate partner violence victims and, 126
other factors related to, 118–119
visualizing, 118
GHB (gamma-hydroxybutyrate), 42
glutaric aciduria type I, 139
gothic gangs, 193, 196–197
Grand Theft Auto: San Andreas, 187
granuloma annulare, 55
grazes, classifying, 66–67
grips, knife, 77–78
guard, knife, 77–78
gunpowder residue, 90
documenting firearm injuries, 62
internal ballistics, 90
suspect evaluation/evidence collection, 207
testing suicide victim for, 13–14
gunshot injuries, 89–97. *see also* firearms

acknowledgments, 97
classifying, 87–88
external ballistics, 92–93
forensic documentation of, 61–62
in-custody death from, 215
internal ballistics, 90–92
morphology of, 94–95
overview of, 89
references, 97
shotgun wounds, 96–97
terminal ballistics, 93–94
testing suicide victim for residue, 13–14
victim case study, 27

H

hair
postmortem specimen handling, 39
as source of DNA evidence, 30
youth gang styles, 195–196
hallucinations
in cocaine toxicity, 41
in ecstasy and methamphetamine use, 41
in heroin use, 41
in marijuana toxicity, 41
hammers, revolver, 83–84
hand signs, gangs, 189–190, 197–198
handguns
automatics or pistols, 84–85
revolvers, 83–84
rifling of, 85
weapon caliber of, 85–86
hands, sharp force defensive injuries on, 81
hanging
asphyxia suicide from, 16
in autoerotic asphyxiation, 17
in intimate partner violence victims, 125–126
hate gangs, 192–193
hazing process, gangs, 189
Haz-Mat (Hazardous Materials), EMS assessment of, 211
head injuries
in blunt force trauma, 75
diagnosing child abuse, 135
in intimate partner violence victims, 126
suspect evaluation/evidence collection, 208
head-on collisions, 101–102
headstamps, cartridge cases, 86
hematuria, child abuse evaluation, 136
hemopneumothorax, 72
hemorrhagic disease of newborn, misdiagnosing, 139–140
hemothorax, 72
Henoch-Schonlein purpura (HSP), 56
hereditary multiple exostoses (HMEs), 144–145
Hermanos de la Frontera, 191
heroin, forensics, 41
hesitation marks, 18, 60, 79
high velocity weapons, 92–93
hinge fracture, skull, 75
Hispanic gangs, 189, 191–192, 195–197
history
child abuse evaluation, 134–136
forensic documentation, 60
male sexual assault, 130
sexual assault examination, 110–111, 120
SIDS deaths, 172, 173–174
suspect evaluation/evidence collection, 207
hit-and-run victim case study, 24–26
HIV postexposure prophylaxis, 130
HLA histocompatibility antigens, 31
HLAs (human leukocyte antigens), 31
HMEs (hereditary multiple exostoses), 144–145
hollow point bullets, 93
homeopathic remedies, mimicking child abuse, 147
homicide
asphyxia suicide vs., 15–17
bite mark locations in, 55
drowning suicide vs., 19
firearm-related suicide vs., 13
gang-related, 187
of infants. *see* infanticide
intimate partner violence and, 123–124
stabbing suicide vs., 18–19
suicide vs., 11
Hoover, Larry, 192
HSP (Henoch-Schonlein purpura), 56
HSR (human sexual response), determining consent, 119
human leukocyte antigens (HLAs), 31
human performance, forensics, 36
human sexual response (HSR), determining consent, 119
hybrid gangs, 193–196
hymenal injuries
pediatric sexual abuse, 159
sexual assault, 118

I

IFAN (International Association of Forensic Nursing), 2, 4–5, 9
image enhancement, 45
immunoassays, 39–41
impact abrasions, 67
in utero drug exposure, 43
incarceration
examination of patient under, 206–209
suicidal hangings during, 16
incised wounds
defined, 70
lacerations vs., 70, 71
from sharp force, 79
incision wounds, 18, 60
in-custody death, 214–218
conducted electrical weapons causing, 215–216
excited delirium causing, 216
gunshot wounds and suicide by cop causing, 215
implications for emergency physician, 217–218
oleoresin capsicum causing, 216
overview of, 214–215
references, 218
sudden, 216–217
Indexes, CODIS DNA data bank, 33
indirect rib fractures, 72
infanticide
diagnosed as SIDS, 136
percentage of SIDS deaths as, 173–174
statistics, 134
infection
causing retinal hemorrhages, 141–142
in SIDS deaths, 173
skin findings mimicking child abuse, 147
infrared (IV), photodocumentation, 56–57
initiations, gang, 188–189
injuries, wounds vs., 65
institutional abuse or neglect, 8
instruments, weapons vs., 65
intermediate gunshot wounds, 87–88
intermediate wound patterns, 13
internal ballistics, 90–92
International Association of Forensic Nursing (IFAN), 2, 4–5, 9
interpersonal violence, intimate partner. *see* intimate partner violence
interpersonal violence, male, 128–132
intimate partner violence, 122–127
behavior pathology, 123
care, intervention and reporting, 124–125
documenting victims of, 64
forensic nurses for, 7
gathering forensic evidence, 125–126
impact on society, 123
male interpersonal violence, 128–132
morbidity and mortality, 123
overview of, 122
in pregnancy, 123
prevalence of, 123
references, 127
screening for, 124
suggested reading, 127
summary, 126–127
victim demographics, 122–124
intoxicants, SICDS and, 217
intracerebral hemorrhages, 75
intracranial hemorrhages, 75, 137
intracranial injuries, 139–140
investigators, forensic nurse, 6
ISO rating, digital cameras, 46, 49–50

J

jacketed ammunition, 86
JCAHO (Joint Commission on Accreditation of Healthcare Organizations), 2, 124
Joint Commission on Accreditation of Healthcare Organizations (JCAHO), 2, 124
Joint Photographic Experts Group (JPEG), 46, 50
JPEG (Joint Photographic Experts Group), 46, 50
Juggalos, 195
jugular compression, in strangulation, 16

K

KE (kinetic energy), ballistics, 92–94
kicking injuries, 71
knives, 77–79
Koop, Everett, MD, 5

L

LA-based gangs, 189–190
labial fusion, in pediatric sexual abuse, 159
laboratory studies, 136, 161
lacerations
bite mark, 71
blunt force trauma causing, 60, 70–71, 73–74
cardiac, 72–73
diaphragmatic, 73
extremity, 75
incised wounds vs., 78
myocardial, 72
punching and kicking, 71
lactate, 136
landmarks, blunt force trauma wounds, 66

lands, of gun barrel, 91
lateral compression pelvic fractures, 74–75
Latin gangs, 191–192
Latin Kings, 191–192
law enforcement
 controlling crime scene safety, 211
 forensic nurse investigators as, 6
 forensic patient and case management, 6–7
 on increase in gang membership, 196–200
 motorcycle gangs interacting with, 192
 sexual assault cases and, 108
 suspect evaluation/evidence collection using, 206
LCD screen, digital cameras, 46
lead bullets, 86
lead shot, shotguns, 87
legal issues
 elder abuse and neglect, 167–168
 evidence. *see* evidence collection/preservation in ED
 forensic photography, 52–53
 legal nurse consultants, 6
 nurse attorneys, 6
 sexual assault, 108–109
legal nurse consultants, 6
lenses, digital cameras, 46
lesbians, and intimate partner assaults, 130
less-lethal weapons, and in-custody death, 215–216
lever action rifles, 85
lever action shotguns, 85
ligature strangulation, 16–17, 125–126
lighting, digital photography, 48
linear abrasions, 66–67
lines of Langer, 78
lip injuries, and child abuse, 142
liver injuries
 blunt force trauma, 73
 and child abuse, 145
liver/pancreatic enzymes, 136
location on body
 documenting bite marks, 62
 documenting firearm injuries, 62
 sexual assault, 112
 using landmarks to reference wounds, 60
logos. *see* symbols, gang
Long-Term Care Ombudsman Program (LTCOP), 167–168
lossless images, 46
lossy images, 46
love bites, 55
lower incisors, 55
LTCOP (Long-Term Care Ombudsman Program), 167–168

M

machine guns, 85
machine pistols, 85
magazines, 84
magnetic resonance imaging (MRI), 138
male interpersonal violence
 domestic violence, 129–130
 overview of, 128–129
 pediatric male patients, 131
 references, 131–132
 role of healthcare provider, 130–131
 sequelae of male sexual assault, 131
 summary, 131
 unique patient populations, 131
manual focus, digital cameras, 48
manual strangulation, 17, 125
Mara Salvatrucha (MS-13s), 191
marijuana abuse, 41–42
masochism, autoerotic asphyxiation and, 17
ME. *see* medical examiner (ME)
mechanisms of injury (MOI), as triage tool, 99
medical examiner (ME)
 approach to sexual assault patient, 109–116
 classifying death as suicide, 11–12
 investigating deaths in ED, 8
 investigating suspicious deaths, 1
 reporting suicidal death to, 20
medical records, sexual assault, 109–111, 130–131
medical screening exam (MSE), sexual assault patients, 110, 113, 130
memory, and sexual assault, 111
memory cards
 downloading images onto computer, 52
 file formats for storage on, 46
 having extra, 48, 50
 storing digital data on, 45
mental health disorder, and suicide, 11
mental impairment, alcohol toxicity, 40
mesenteric injuries, blunt force, 74
metabolic abnormalities, in ALTE and SIDS, 176
metacarpophalangial joint, fight bites, 55
metal jacketed bullets, 86
metering mode, forensic imaging, 48, 50
methamphetamine, 41
Mexican street gangs, 191
microwave oven burns, 149
midrange views, forensics, 51
military, male sexual assault in, 131
mini crime scene scope, 31
mitochondrial DNA (MtDNA) analysis, 31, 33
MOI (mechanisms of injury), as triage tool, 99
Mongolian spots, 56, 147
motor vehicle accidents
 documentation of, 64
 drug/alcohol use and, 40
 forcible entry tools at scene of, 212
 suicide by, 19
motor vehicle crashes, mechanisms of injury, 98–106
 airbag-related, 101
 car vs. pedestrian impacts, 105–106
 essential principles of physics, 98–99
 frontal impacts, 101–103
 rear impacts, 103
 references, 106
 rollovers, 105
 side impacts, 103–104
 summary, 106
 as triage tool, 99–100
 vehicle restraint and safety systems as, 99–100
motorcycle gangs, 192, 196
mouth injuries, and child abuse, 142
MRI (magnetic resonance imaging), 138
MS-13s (Mara Salvatrucha), 191
MSE (medical screening exam), sexual assault, 110, 113, 130
MtDNA (mitochondrial DNA) analysis, 31, 33
MVCs. *see* motor vehicle crashes, mechanisms of injury
myocardial contusions/lacerations, blunt force, 72

N

nails, postmortem specimen handling, 39
narrative documentation
 blunt force trauma, 66
 sexual assault, 114
 working with, 20
National DNA Database (NDNAD), 33
National Institutes of Child Health and Human Development (NICHD), 172
Native American gangs, 197
near-contact gunshot wounds, 12–13, 87–88
neck injuries
 intimate partner violence, 126
 suspect evaluation/evidence collection, 208
neurotransmitters, SIDS deaths, 173
newborn drug exposure, 43
Newton's first law of physics, 99
NICHD (National Institutes of Child Health and Human Development), 172
No. 2 Angled Rule, forensic photography, 50
nonacute examination, pediatric sexual abuse, 157
nonconsent, and sexual assault, 119–120
nurse attorneys, 6
nursing homes, institutional abuse, 8

O

observation, forensics for EMS, 212–213
occult or gothic gangs, 193, 196–197
occupational-related toxicologic investigations, 38
offensive wounds, 75
Office on Violence Against Women, 124
OI (osteogenesis imperfecta), diagnosing, 144
oleoresin capsicum (OC), death from, 216
on-site drug tests, 39
open-book pelvic fractures, blunt force, 74
opiates, detecting, 39
optical zoom, digital cameras, 46
oral cavity examination
 sexual assault, 115
 suspect evaluation/evidence collection, 208
 suspected child abuse, 142
oral contact, sexual assault exam, 112–113
orienting shots, forensic composition, 50–51
orthopedic injuries, blunt force, 74–75
osteogenesis imperfecta (OI), diagnosing, 144
osteopenia, 144

P

Paint Data Query (PDQ), 24
pancreatic injuries, 74, 145
paternity testing, DNA analysis, 31
pathologists, 36
Patient's Bill of Rights, 205–206
patterned injury
 abrasions, 67–68
 assessing wounds, 60
 contusions, 69
 documenting blunt force, 66
 extragenital injuries in sexual assault, 117
 intimate partner violence, 125–126
 scald burns in children, 148
 sexual assault forensic examination, 112
 skin injuries to children, 146
PCR. *see* polymerase chain reaction (PCR)
pedestrians, vs. car collisions, 105–106
pediatric sexual abuse, 156–164

conclusion, 163
conditions mimicking, 162
evidence collection, 161–162
lab investigations, 161
overview of, 156
patient interview, 157
physical exam, 157–159
references, 163–164
symptoms and signs, 160
team approach to, 162–163
pelvic injuries
fractures in blunt force trauma, 74–75
suspect evaluation/evidence collection, 208
penetrating fractures, 71
penetrating gunshot wounds, 87–88
penetrating injury, frontal impacts, 101–102
penis, male sexual assault, 130
People Nation (Chicago-based gang), 190–191, 196
pepper spray, and in-custody death, 216
perforating gunshot wounds, 87–88
phencyclidine (PHP), 41–42
photographic documentation
basics of, 46–48
bite mark evidence, 56–57, 62, 147
blunt trauma contusions, 70
bruises, 61
collected DNA evidence, 31
common errors, 51–52
digital imaging, 45–46
in ED, 45
equipment and setup, 48–50
forensic patient and case management, 7–8
forensics for EMS, 212
gunshot victims, 27
history of, 45
hit-and-run victims, 26
legal issues, 52–53
overview of, 44–45
physical exam, 60, 136
sexual assault, 114–116
summary, 53
techniques and composition, 50–51
workflow, 52
working with, 20
PHP (phencyclidine), 41–42
physical abuse, elder, 166–167
physical evidence, value of, 205
physical examination
child abuse evaluation, 136
forensic documentation using, 60
intimate partner violence, 125
male sexual assault, 130
pediatric sexual abuse, 157–159
sexual assault, 113
SIDS cases, 174
physicians, forensic training of, 2–3
physics, motor vehicle crash injuries, 98–99, 101
pistols, 84–86
pityriasis rosea, 55
pixels, 45–46
PM (polymarker) test, DNA analysis, 32
pneumonia, 72
pneumothorax, 72
point-and-shoot cameras, 48
point-of-care tests, 39
poisoning, suicide by, 11
police crime laboratory, 6
police-assisted suicide, 14–15
polymarker (PM) test, DNA analysis, 32
polymerase chain reaction (PCR)
CODIS storage and research of, 33
collecting bite mark evidence, 56
DNA analysis using, 31–32
STR technology using, 32–33
Population File Index, CODIS, 33
pornography, autoerotic asphyxiation, 17
positional asphyxia, restraint and, 216–217
positive physical findings, SAFE, 120
postassault hygiene activities, 111
postmenopausal women, sexual assault genital injuries, 118
postmortem
bruising, 70
collecting toxicologic samples, 37
forensic toxicology in, 36
specimen handling, 38
post-traumatic stress disorder, 8
powder tattooing, 13
PowerPoint presentations, digital forensic photos, 45
preassault sexual activity, 111
pregnancy
intimate partner violence during, 123
testing after pediatric sexual abuse, 161
prenatal care, and SIDS, 174
primary injury, 139
primer, ammunition, 86–87
prison gangs, 191–192, 196–197
prisons, male sexual assault in, 131
propellant, firearm ammunition, 86
psychiatric nurses, forensic, 6
psychological impact, of sexual assault, 109, 131
pubic hair samples, sexual assault, 115
pulmonary injuries, blunt force trauma, 73
pump action shotguns, 85
punching injuries, blunt force trauma, 71

R

radiographic studies
of gunshot wounds, 95
identifying child abuse, 136–138
suspect evaluation/evidence collection, 208–209
rape. *see also* sexual assault
crisis resources for, 109
defined, 108
evidence kit for, 113, 130
male sexual assault, 128–132
trauma syndrome, 109
rat-holed wounds, 13
RAW (uncompressed) format, 46
razor blades, suicide using, 79
RBC (red blood cell) antigen systems, 31
rear impact crash mechanisms, 103
recruitment, gang, 188–189
rectal examination, 208
red blood cell (RBC) antigen systems, 31
regression stage, abrasions, 67
Relatives of Missing Persons Index, CODIS, 33
religion
Chicago-based gangs, 190
view on suicide, 10
reporting
child maltreatment, 149–150
elder abuse, 168
of EMS on abuse and assault, 213
intimate partner violence, 124
male interpersonal violence and, 129–130
resolution, digital imaging, 46, 50
respiratory depression, 40–41
restraint systems, motor vehicle crashes, 99–100
restriction fragment length polymorphism (RFLP), 31–33
retinal hemorrhages, child abuse, 139, 141–142
revolvers, 83–84
RFLP (restriction fragment length polymorphism), 31–33
Rh blood typing system, 31
rib fractures, 71–73, 143–144
ricasso, knife anatomy, 77–78
rickets, diagnosing in children, 144
rifles, 85–86
rifling, 85, 91
risk factors
for elder abuse, 167
for suicide, 11
youth gang involvement, 188
risk taking practices, Russian roulette, 15
Rohypnol (flunitrazepam), 42
rollover motor vehicle crashes, 105
rope burns, 125
rotational force, stab wounds, 78
rotational fractures, 71
Russian roulette, 15

S

SAFE. *see* sexual assault forensic examination (SAFE)
safety systems, motor vehicle crashes, 99–100
saliva
collecting bite mark evidence, 56
laboratory finding of sexual abuse, 161
serological screening of, 31
as source of DNA evidence, 30
SANE (sexual assault nurse examiner), 6–7, 30
SBS (shaken baby syndrome), 138–140
scab formation stage, abrasions, 67
scald burns, 148
scaling images, 50, 51
school factors, youth gang involvement, 188
scintigraphy, 137
scissor injuries, 78, 80
The Scope and Standards of Forensic Nursing Practice, ANA, 5
scrape abrasions, 66
scratches, classifying, 66–69
screwdriver injuries, 79, 80
scurvy, diagnosing in children, 144
SDH (subdural hemorrhages), 138–139
seat failures, rear impact collisions, 103
seatbelt syndrome, 99
seatbelts, 99–100
secondary injury, children's head trauma, 139
security protocols, for hospitals, 200
self-inflicted injuries, sharp force, 79–82
self-neglect, in elders, 167
seminal fluid
autoerotic asphyxiation, 17
laboratory finding of sexual abuse, 161
serological screening of, 31
as source of DNA evidence, 29–30
seminal fluid, sexual assault evidence
body surfaces exam, 114–115
examining genitals, 116
physical exam collecting, 113
physical surrounding of assault, 112

postassault hygiene activities, 111
sexual acts of assailant(s), 112–113
victim's clothing, 114
sensitivity (speed or ISO rating), digital cameras, 46
serological screening, 31
serrated-edge knives, 77–78
serum protein markers, 31
sexual abuse
of elders, 166–167
pediatric. *see* pediatric sexual abuse
as suicide risk factor, 11
sexual assault
age, sexual experience and, 118
anogenital injuries, 117–118
body surfaces exam, 114–115
clothing, 114
collecting DNA evidence, 30
consent vs. nonconsent, 119–120
debriefing, 116–117
defined, 7
drug-facilitated, 42
extragenital injuries, 117
factors related to genital injury, 118–119
general description of patient, 114
genital exam, 115–116
legal issues, 108–109
male victims, 128–132
managing victims, 7, 107–108
medical screening exam and vital signs, 113
oral cavity exam, 115
physical exam and evidence collection, 113
psychological impact of, 109
references, 120–121
summary and accountability, 116
suspect evaluation/evidence collection, 208
systematic forensic approach to patient, 113–116
time frames, 113
toxicologic specimen handling, 38
visualizing injuries, 118
sexual assault forensic examination (SAFE)
assailant(s), 112–113
assault-related signs and symptoms, 111–112
forensic and medical records in, 109–110
overview of, 109
sexual assault history, 110–111
sexual assault nurse examiner (SANE), 6–7, 30
sexual experience, and age, 118
sexually transmitted infection (STIs), pediatric sexual abuse, 157, 161
shaken baby syndrome (SBS), 138–140
Shakur, Tupac, 187
sharp force injuries, 77–82
anatomy of knife, 77
chop injuries, 79–80
defensive injuries, 81–82
evidence handling and documentation, 81
forensic documentation of, 60–61
incised wounds, 79
other wounds, 79–80
overview of, 77
references, 82
self-inflicted injuries, 79–82
during sexual assault, 117
stab wounds, 78–79
summary, 81–82
short tandem repeats (STRs)
collecting bite mark evidence, 56
DNA analysis using, 32–33
Y-chromosome, 34
shot pattern, shotguns, 96
shotguns, 85–87, 96–97
shutter speed, digital cameras, 46–49
SICDS (sudden in-custody death syndrome), 216–217
side impact crash mechanisms, 103–104
SIDS. *see* sudden infant death syndrome (SIDS)
SIDS Act of 1974, 172
simple rib fractures, 72
single shot rifles, 85
single shot shotguns, 85
single-action revolvers, 83
single-edged knives, 77–78
single-lens reflex (SLR) cameras, 48
single-vehicle accidents, as suicide, 19
skeletal survey
identifying fractures from child abuse, 137
mitochondrial DNA analysis, 33
SIDS cases, 174
suspicious fractures of child abuse, 142–143
skin injuries
suspect evaluation/evidence collection, 207
suspicious of child abuse, 145–149
skinheads, 193, 197
Skinheads Against Racial Prejudice (SHARP), 193
skull fractures
from blunt force trauma, 75
child abuse evaluation, 135, 137, 142–143
sliding abrasions, 66, 69
SLR (single-lens reflex) cameras, 48
slugs, shotgun, 87
Smock, William, 2
smothering, asphyxia by, 15
SOPs (standard operating procedures), forensic photography, 52–53
specimen handling, for living cases, 37–38, 208
spectrochemical tests, 38
spinal fractures, blunt force trauma, 74–75
spine, knife anatomy, 77–78
splenic injuries, blunt force trauma, 73
sports utility vehicle (SUV) rollover crashes, 105
spot focus, digital cameras, 48
spot metering, 48
sprains, 126
stab wounds, 78–79
stabbing suicides, 17–19
standard operating procedures (SOPs), forensic photography, 52–53
stellate wounds, 95
sternal fractures, 71–72
STIs (sexually transmitted infection), pediatric sexual abuse, 157, 161
stomach laceration, blunt force trauma, 74
storage
of collected DNA evidence, 31
digital imaging, 46, 48, 50
strangulation
defined, 15
hangings, 16
intimate partner violence, 125–126
ligature, 16–17
manual, 17
street gangs, 189, 197
STRs. *see* short tandem repeats (STRs)
subacute cutaneous lupus erythema, 55
subarachnoid hemorrhages, blunt force, 75
subdural hematomas, blunt force, 75
subdural hemorrhages (SDH), 138–139
subepidermal regeneration stage, abrasions, 67
submachine guns, 85
substance abuse. *see also* forensic toxicology
facilitating sexual assault, 112
forensic nursing and, 7, 8
Russian roulette victims and, 15
sexual assault and, 111
suicide by cop victims and, 14
as suicide risk factor, 11
suicides vs. homicides and, 19
trends in, 40
sudden in-custody death syndrome (SICDS), 216–217
sudden infant death syndrome (SIDS), 171–185
apparent life-threatening events, 175–176
child abuse evaluation, 136
clinical history, 173–174
death scene investigation, 174
demographics, 172
diagnosing, 175
history of, 172
investigating deaths in ED, 8
managing in ED, 173
mortality rates, 172
overview of, 171–172
physical exam, 174
postmortem imaging and pathology, 174–175
presentation of, 172–173
prevention of, 176
references, 185
reporting form, 177–184
Sudden Unexplained Infant Death Investigation Report Form (SUIDIRF), 174
suffocation, 15. *see also* asphyxia suicides
suicide, 10–21
by asphyxia, 15–19
classification, 11–12
by cop, 14–15, 215
by drowning, 19
emergency department and, 19–21
epidemiology of, 11
by firearm, 12–15
overview of, 10–11
references, 21
risk factors, 11
by sharp force injury, 79–82
by single-vehicle accidents, 19
by stabbing, 17–18
summary, 21
Surgeon General's Workshop on Violence and Public Health, 5
suspect evaluation/evidence collection, 204–209
evidence, 205
examination of patient, 206–209
incarcerated patients, 206
overview of, 204–205
Patient's Bill of Rights, 205–206
references, 209
value of evidence, 205
SUV (sports utility vehicle) rollover crashes, 105
symbols, gang, 189–191, 193–200

T

Tagged Image File Format (TIFF) files, 46
Takayama microcrystal test, 31
TASERS, 215–216

tattoos
close-range gunshot wound, 95
gang, 191–192, 196–197, 199
teams
forensic nursing, 5
pediatric sexual abuse, 162–163
tears. *see* lacerations
teeth
bite marks. *see* bite marks
diagnosing child abuse, 142
terminal ballistics, 93–94
THC (tetrahydrocannibinol), marijuana toxicity, 41
therapeutic rib fractures, 71–72
thermal injuries, intimate partner violence, 126
time of sexual assault, 112–113
tin ear syndrome, 142
tinea corporis, 55
tissue bridges, lacerations, 70
toluidine blue dye, 115–116, 118, 130
tongue, and child abuse, 142
toxicology, branches of, 36
toxicology, forensic. *see* forensic toxicology
trace evidence
gunshot victim case study, 27
hit-and-run victim case study, 24
in lacerations, 71
recovered bullets, 86–87
trap-door lacerations, 70
trauma in ED
mechanisms of injury as triage tool, 99
vicarious, 8
triage tool, motor vehicle crashes, 99–100
triggers, firearm, 83–84
tripods, forensic photography, 48, 52

U

ultrasounds, 138
Unidentified Persons Index, CODIS, 33
up and over pathway, frontal impacts, 101–102
urinalysis, trauma in children, 136
urine
postmortem specimen handling, 38
specimen handling for living cases, 38
urine drug screens
adulteration of, 37, 39–40
detecting cocaine toxicity, 41
in drug-facilitated sexual assault, 42
drugs typically detected, 39
ecstasy and methamphetamine, 41
GHB toxicity, 42
heroin, 41
immunoassays, 39
on-site drug tests, 39
UV light, photodocumentation, 56

V

vaginal delivery, and retinal hemorrhages, 141
Valsalva maneuvers, 142
variable number tandem repeats (VNTRs), 31
vasculitis, and retinal hemorrhages, 142
vehicle accidents. *see* motor vehicle accidents
vertebral column fractures, 74–75
vertical compression fractures, 71
vertical shear pelvic fractures, 75
vicarious traumatization, in ED, 8–9
victim-precipitated homicide, 14
Victims Index, CODIS, 33
violence
bite marks. *see* bite marks
blunt force trauma. *see* blunt force trauma
collecting DNA evidence, 30
domestic. *see* intimate partner violence
evidence collection. *see* evidence collection/preservation in ED
firearms. *see* firearms
forensic patient and case management, 6–7
gang. *see* gang violence
homicide. *see* homicide
interpersonal. *see* intimate partner violence
male interpersonal, 128–132
recognizing ED patient as victim of, 23
sexual assault. *see* sexual assault
sharp force injuries. *see* sharp force injuries
trends in drug use and abuse, 40
Violence Against Women Act, 1994, 124
Vitamin D deficiency, 144
VNTRs (variable number tandem repeats), 31
vomitus, sexual assault, 111

W

wadcutter bullets, 93
wadding, shotgun, 95
WB (white balance), 46, 50
weapon caliber
on cartridge case headstamps, 86
overview of, 85–86
weapons
asphyxia suicides, 15–17
firearm-related suicides, 12–15
firearms. *see* firearms
gang-related violence in ED, 198–201
instruments vs., 66
knives. *see* knives
LA street gangs, 190
processing patient as crime scene, 24
single-vehicle accidents, 19
stabbing suicides, 17–19
white balance (WB), 46, 50
white supremacists, 192–193, 196–197
Wilson, Mary Ellen, 133
Wood's lamp, 161
workflow, forensic photography, 52
wounds
abrasions, 66–69
bite marks. *see* bite marks
blunt force trauma. *see* blunt force trauma
contusions, 69–70
diagrammatic documentation of suspicious deaths, 20
documenting, 60
documenting elder or child abuse, 64
documenting firearm injuries, 62
documenting motor vehicle injuries, 63
fractures, 71
injuries vs., 65
lacerations, 70–71
sharp force. *see* sharp force injuries

X

X-rays, 95, 137

Y

yawed bullets, 93
Y-chromosome STRs, 34
youth. *see* adolescents

Z

zoom, digital camera, 46, 50